Protocols in
Neonatal Nursing

Protocols in Neonatal Nursing

Carole Kenner, D.N.S., R.N.C., F.A.A.N.
Professor and Department Head
Parent Child Health Nursing
College of Nursing and Health
University of Cincinnati
Cincinnati, Ohio

Stephanie Rockwern Amlung, R.N.C., Ph.D.
Research Associate, Institute for Nursing Research
College of Nursing and Health
University of Cincinnati
Cincinnati, Ohio

Ann Applewhite Flandermeyer, R.N.C., Ph.D.
Assistant Director, Clinical Services
Kendle Research
Cincinnati, Ohio

W.B. SAUNDERS COMPANY

A Division of Harcourt Brace & Company

Philadelphia   London   Toronto   Montreal   Sydney   Tokyo

W.B. SAUNDERS COMPANY
A Division of Harcourt Brace & Company

The Curtis Center
Independence Square West
Philadelphia, Pennsylvania 19106

Library of Congress Cataloging-in-Publication Data

Kenner, Carole.

Protocols in neonatal nursing / Carole Kenner, Stephanie Rockwern Amlung,
Ann Applewhite Flandermeyer.

p.   cm.

ISBN 0–7216–6117–3

1. Infants (Newborn)—Diseases—Nursing.   I. Amlung, Stephanie
  Rockwern.   II. Flandermeyer, Ann Applewhite.   III. Title.
  [DNLM: 1. Neonatal Nursing—methods.   WY 157.3 K34p 1998]

RJ253.K464 1998   610.73′62—dc21

DNLM/DLC   97–48248

PROTOCOLS IN NEONATAL NURSING   ISBN 0–7216–6117–3

Printed in the United States of America.

Last digit is the print number: 9   8   7   6   5   4   3   2   1

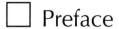 Preface

Neonatal nurses need to have reference materials that are quick and easy to use to meet the diverse needs of their client population. This text is derived from *Comprehensive Neonatal Nursing: A Physiologic Perspective, Second Edition,* edited by Carole Kenner, Judy Wright Lott, and Ann Applewhite Flandermeyer, and presents material in a quick protocol format. This format provides easy access to key information for staff nurses in levels II and III nurseries, transport nurses, and graduate students. It presents pathophysiology, signs and symptoms, assessment, necessary diagnostic tests, pertinent laboratory values, and patient outcomes. The format reflects JCAHO guidelines for documentation and accreditation. Tables and figures support the protocols that are aimed at neonatal management, safe early discharge, and necessary follow-up.

For more detailed information, the reader is referred to the comprehensive text for a complete discussion of physiology and rationales for care. We hope that you find this pocket guide to be a useful edition to your clinical handbooks.

Carole Kenner, D.N.S., R.N.C., F.A.A.N.
Stephanie Rockwern Amlung, R.N.C., Ph.D.
Ann Applewhite Flandermeyer, R.N.C., Ph.D.

DRUG NOTICE

☐ Acknowledgments

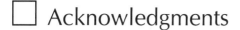

We would like to thank Carol Phipps for her efforts in typing and preparing the manuscript. We wish to acknowledge the work of the contributors from *Comprehensive Neonatal Nursing: A Physiologic Perspective, Second Edition,* whose contributions in that work formed the basis for the rationales in this text.

Cynthia Margaret Acree, R.N., M.S.N., N.N.P.
Neonatal Nurse Practitioner, Children's Hospital Medical Center, Cincinnati, Ohio

Helen Archer-Dusté, M.S.N., R.N.
Kaiser Foundation Health Plan, San Francisco, California

Vicky L. Armstrong, M.S.N., R.N.C.
Clinical Nurse Specialist, Perinatal Outreach Program, Children's Hospital, Columbus, Ohio

Gail A. Bagwell, M.S.N., R.N.
Clinical Nurse Specialist/Case Manager, Children's Hospital, Columbus, Ohio

Kathy Bergman, M.S.N., R.N.C., C.C.E.
Faculty, Department of Nursing, Xavier University, Cincinnati, Ohio

Susan M. Berns, M.S.N., R.N.C., N.N.P.
Volunteer Clinical Faculty, University of Cincinnati; Neonatal Nurse Practitioner, Good Samaritan Hospital, Cincinnati, Ohio

Kim Bivens, M.S.N., R.N., C.N.S.
Trauma Clinical Nurse Specialist, Children's Hospital Medical Center, Cincinnati, Ohio

Susan Tucker Blackburn, Ph.D., R.N.C., F.A.A.N.
Professor, Department of Family and Child Nursing, University of Washington, Seattle, Washington

Susan M. Broughton, R.G.N., R.M., G.D.M.S., B.H.Sc.(Hons), P.G.Dip.Ed.
Midwifery Lecturer, Division of Midwifery, School of Human and Health Sciences, The University of Huddersfield, West Yorkshire, England

Lois A. Brown, M.S.N., R.N.C., N.N.P.
Neonatal Nurse Practitioner, Riverside Methodist Hospitals, Columbus, Ohio, Good Samaritan Hospital, Cincinnati, Ohio

Kimberly S. Burton, R.N.C., B.S.N.
Clinical Nurse III, Regional Center for Newborn Intensive Care, Children's Hospital Medical Center, Cincinnati, Ohio

Joyce Butler, M.S.N., R.N.C., N.N.P.
Neonatal Nurse Practitioner Coordinator, The University of Mississippi Medical Center, Jackson, Mississippi

Waldemar A. Carlo, M.D.
Professor of Pediatrics and Director, Division of Neonatology, School of Medicine, University of Alabama at Birmingham; Director, Newborn Nurseries, University of Alabama Medical Center and the Children's Hospital of Alabama, Birmingham, Alabama

Javier Cifuentes, M.D.
Instructor in Pediatrics, University Hospital, Pontificia Universidad Catolica de Chile, Santiago, Chile

Marguerite Degenhardt, M.S., R.N., N.D.
Lisle, Illinois

Sergio DeMarini, M.D.
Attending Physician, Division of Neonatology, Ospedale Civile, Udine, Italy

Edward F. Donovan, M.D.
Professor of Pediatrics, University of Cincinnati Medical Center; Attending Staff, University of Cincinnati Hospital, Children's Hospital Medical Center, Cincinnati, Ohio

Donna A. Dowling, Ph.D., M.N., R.N.
Assistant Professor of Nursing, Frances Payne Bolton School of Nursing, Case Western Reserve University, Cleveland, Ohio

Kathleen M. Driscoll, J.D., M.S., B.S.N., R.N.
Associate Professor, College of Nursing and Health, University of Cincinnati, Cincinnati, Ohio

Jody Farrell, B.S.N., R.N.
Coordinator, Fetal/Neonatal Care, Pediatric Surgery, University of California, San Francisco, San Francisco, California

Dianne M. Felblinger, M.S.N., Ed.D., R.N.
Associate Professor, College of Nursing and Health, University of Cincinnati, Cincinnati, Ohio

Linda Sturla Franck, Ph.D., R.N.
Assistant Professor, School of Nursing, University of California, San Francisco; Nursing Research Coordinator, Pediatric Clinical Research Center, University of California, San Francisco, San Francisco, California

Vivian Gamblian, M.S.N., R.N.
President, Gamblian Enterprises, Inc. (Healthy Homecomings), Plano, Texas

Lynda Hutt Hall, M.N., R.N.C., N.N.P., P.N.P.
Nursing Faculty Consultant, University of Phoenix, Phoenix, Arizona

Jeanne Harjo, R.N.
Staff Nurse, Clinical Nurse III, Children's Hospital, Cincinnati, Ohio

Judith S. Harmon, M.S., R.N., C.F.N.P.
Adjunct Faculty, College of Nursing, Grand Canyon University, Phoenix, Arizona; Women and Infants' Health and Certified Family Nurse Practitioner, Samaritan Family Health Center, Payson, Arizona

Rosanne C. Harrigan, Ed.D., C.P.N.P., F.A.A.N.
Dean and Professor, University of Hawaii at Manoa, Honolulu, Hawaii

Kathleen Haubrich, R.N.C., Ph.D.
Assistant Professor, Department of Nursing, Miami University, Hamilton, Ohio; Clinical Nurse, Obstetrical Special Care Unit, University of Cincinnati Medical Center, Cincinnati, Ohio

James L. Haywood, M.D.
Associate Professor of Pediatrics, School of Medicine, University of Alabama at Birmingham; Medical Director, Newborn Intensive Care Unit, Children's Hospital of Alabama, Birmingham, Alabama

Carol Hetteberg, M.S.N., R.N.
Assistant Professor of Clinical Nursing, College of Nursing and Health, University of Cincinnati, Cincinnati, Ohio

Marcia A. Hilse, M.S.N., R.N.
In Vitro Fertilization Coordinator, Center for Human Reproduction, Glenview, Illinois

Diana Holditch-Davis, Ph.D., R.N., F.A.A.N.
Associate Professor, School of Nursing, University of North Carolina at Chapel Hill, Chapel Hill, North Carolina

Lori J. Howell, M.S., R.N.
Clinical Associate, University of Pennsylvania School of Nursing; Program Manager, Surgery Advanced Practice Nurse Program, The Center for Fetal Diagnosis and Treatment, Philadelphia, Pennsylvania

Maribeth Inturrisi, M.S.N.
Associate Professor, Department of Family Health Care Nursing, School of Nursing, University of California, San Francisco; Clinical Nurse Specialist (Obstetrics), UCSF Medical Center, San Francisco, California

Nia Johnson-Crowley, M.N., R.N., Ph.D.(C)
Doctoral Candidate, Educational Psychology, Department of Education, University of Washington, Seattle, Washington

Karen Katz, R.N.C., N.N.P., M.S.N.(C)
MSN-CNS Student, Beth-El College of Nursing, Colorado Springs, Colorado; RNC, NNP Level II Nursery, Columbia North Suburban Medical Center, Thornton, Colorado; RNC, NNP–Locum Tenens, Innovative Health Care, Inc., Denver, Colorado

Charlotte A. Kenreigh, Pharm.D.
Manager, Clinical Education and Training, Merck-Medco Managed Care, L.C.C., Columbus, Ohio

Caroline Hoell Kistler, M.S.N., R.N.C., N.N.P.
Adjunct Clinical Instructor, Neonatal Nurse Practitioner Program, College of Nursing Health, University of Cincinnati; Neonatal Nurse Practitioner, Family Birthing Center, Jewish Hospital Kenwood, Cincinnati, Ohio

Tracey A. Kleeman, M.S.N., R.N.C., N.N.P.
Envision Group, Inc., Cincinnati, Ohio

Joanne McManus Kuller, M.S.N., R.N.
Assistant Clinical Professor, School of Nursing, University of California, San Francisco, San Francisco, California; Education Resource Specialist, Children's Hospital Oakland, Oakland, California

Rita Maria Kunk, M.S.N., R.N.C., N.N.P.
Neonatal Nurse Practitioner, Winchester Medical Center, Winchester, Virginia

Linda Lefrak, M.S., R.N., N.N.P.
Assistant Clinical Professor, University of California, San Francisco, San Francisco, California; Assistant Clinical Professor, School of Nursing, University of Illinois, Chicago, Illinois; Neonatal Clinical Nurse Specialist, Children's Hospital, Oakland, California

Judy Wright Lott, D.N.S., R.N.C., N.N.P.
Associate Professor, University of Cincinnati College of Nursing and Health, Cincinnati, Ohio

Denise Lucas, M.S.N., R.N.C.
Staff Nurse, Labor and Delivery, Bethesda Hospital, Cincinnati, Ohio

Carolyn Houska Lund, M.S.N., R.N., F.A.A.N.
Assistant Clinical Professor, School of Nursing, University of California, San Francisco, San Francisco, California; Assistant Clinical Professor, School of Nursing, University of Illinois, Chicago, Illinois; Neonatal Clinical Nurse Specialist and ECMO Coordinator, Intensive Care Nursery, Children's Hospital, Oakland, California

Linda L. McCollum, Ph.D., R.N.C., C.N.N.P.
Regional Education Coordinator, Emory Regional Perinatal Center, Emory University School of Medicine; Adjunct Clinical Faculty, Nell Hodgson Woodruff School of Nursing, Emory University, Atlanta, Georgia

Lisa M. Moles, M.S.N., R.N., C.P.N.P.
Pediatric Nurse Practitioner, Division of Cardiothoracic Surgery, Children's Hospital Medical Center, Cincinnati, Ohio

Jane A. Nichols, M.Ed.
Coordinator of Bereavement Services, Children's Hospital Medical Center of Akron, Akron, Ohio

Elaine Nishioka, M.S.N., R.N., C.P.N.P.
Pediatric Nurse Practitioner, Healthy Steps Specialist, Eastover Pediatrics, Presbyterian Healthcare System, Charlotte, North Carolina

Susan H. Pedersen-Ryckman, M.S.N., R.N., P.N.P.
Visiting Assistant Professor, Miami University, Oxford, Ohio; Pediatric Nurse Practitioner, Cardiac Care Center, Children's Hospital Medical Center, Cincinnati, Ohio

Dennis Perez, Ph.D.
Staff Psychologist, University of Illinois at Chicago, Chicago, Illinois

Cynthia Prows, M.S.N., R.N.
Adjunct Instructor of Clinical Nursing, College of Nursing and Health, University of Cincinnati; Clinical Nurse Specialist, Human Genetics Department, Children's Hospital Medical Center, Cincinnati, Ohio

Linda L. Rath, M.S.N.
Assistant Professor, University of Texas Medical Branch, Galveston, Texas; Adjunct Clinical Instructor, University of Texas Health Science Center–Houston, Houston, Texas

Madeline Ross, M.S.N., C.R.N.P., C.N.S.
Manager, Clinical Specialist Group, Ohmeda, Inc.; Consultant for NICU, Brookwood Medical Center; Neonatal Nurse Practitioner, NNP Services of Alabama, Birmingham, Alabama

Frederick C. Ryckman, M.D.
Associate Professor of Surgery, University of Cincinnati; Director, Pediatric Transportation, Children's Hospital Medical Center, Cincinnati, Ohio

Jonathan E. Schwartz, M.D.
Neonatal Fellow, Children's Hospital Medical Center, Cincinnati, Ohio; Staff Neonatologist, Neonatal Associates of Jacksonville, Jacksonville, Florida

Nancy Shaw, M.S.N., R.N., N.N.P.
Auxiliary Faculty, University of Utah; Neonatal Nurse Practitioner, Primary Children's Medical Center, Salt Lake City, Utah

Sheila M. Southwell, M.S.N., M.B.A.
Director of Patient Care Services, Pediatrics, Sinai Hospital of Baltimore, Baltimore, Maryland

Frances Strodtbeck, D.N.S., R.N.C., N.N.P.
Coordinator, Neonatal Nurse Practitioner Program, Rush University College of Nursing; Neonatal Nurse Practitioner, Rush-Presbyterian-St. Luke's Medical Center, Chicago, Illinois

Catherine Jursich Theorell, M.S.N., R.N.C., N.N.P.
Instructor, Rush University College of Nursing; Director, Neonatal Nurse Practitioner Services, University of Chicago Children's Hospital, Chicago, Illinois

Janet L. Thigpen, M.N., R.N.C., C.N.N.P.
Clinical Associate, Nell Hodgson Woodruff School of Nursing, Emory University; Neonatal Nurse Practitioner, Division of Neonatal Medicine, Department of Pediatrics, Emory University School of Medicine, Atlanta, Georgia

Reginald C. Tsang, M.B.B.S.
Professor of Pediatrics, University of Cincinnati; Associate Chairman,
Pediatrics, Executive Director, Children's Center for Bone Research and
Health, University of Cincinnati/Children's Hospital Medical Center,
Cincinnati, Ohio

Kathleen A. VandenBerg, M.A.
Director, Infant Development Program NICU, Director, Stanford NIDCAP
Training Center, Division of Neonatal and Developmental Medicine,
Department of Pediatrics, Stanford University School of Medicine, Palo
Alto, California

Linda Timm Wagner, Pharm.D.
Senior Manager, Clinical Practice and Education, Merck-Medco Managed
Care, L.L.C., Columbus, Ohio

Elizabeth Elder Weiner, Ph.D., R.N.
Professor, College of Nursing and Health, Director, Center for Academic
Technologies, University of Cincinnati, Cincinnati, Ohio

Tina Leigh Weitkamp, M.S.N., R.N.
Associate Professor of Clinical Nursing, College of Nursing and Health,
University of Cincinnati; Staff Nurse, Mercy Hospital–Anderson,
Cincinnati, Ohio

Contents

Neonatal Nursing Care: A Collaborative Practice Arena

. . . .

CHAPTER 1

Neonatal Nursing and Its Role in Comprehensive Care

Neonatal nursing practice consists of (1) implementing nursing therapy, (2) collaborating with other health care providers, and (3) assisting with medical care. The interrelationship of these three components centers on improving or maintaining neonatal and family health. Nursing therapy consists of assessment, planning, intervention, and evaluation of newborns and their families to provide developmentally appropriate environments, physical care, feeding, and parent care. Neonatal nursing care is protective, generative, and nurturant and focuses on the needs of neonates as embodied persons rather than as biologic systems.

Protective nursing services include early identification and evaluation of risk factors and anticipatory guidance and teaching. *Generative nursing activities* include developing new behaviors and modifying environments and roles for the neonate and family. *Nurturant nursing* behaviors provide surveillance of physiologic variables, comfort for the infant, and family teaching about infant's health and illness.

ROLE OF THE NEONATAL NURSE

The skills required of neonatal nurses have continued to evolve over the past 20 years, with orientation costs exceeding $8000 (Swanson, S., personal

1

communication, 1991). Generic-level nursing programs (associate, diploma, and baccalaureate levels) currently contain very little preparation in the knowledge and skills necessary for practice in neonatal intensive care units (NICUs).

Changes in medical education have resulted in residents spending progressively less NICU time and thus less time in becoming proficient in procedures. Funds for nursing continuing education at all levels of career development are diminishing (Aiken, Gwyther, & Whelan, 1996). The impact of managed care on neonatal nursing roles has not been clearly delineated in the literature. However, neonates are being discharged earlier and there is an emerging need for home care nurses who possess and maintain neonatal management competencies. There is even a need for the provision of high-tech care in the home where nurses do not have the personnel or equipment back-up found in hospital settings.

DEVELOPMENTAL ASPECTS OF NEONATAL NURSING PRACTICE

Beginning Practitioners

The beginning neonatal nurse must learn to perform critical elements of the role under *direct supervision*. In other words, a new nurse must begin by helping a more seasoned nurse preceptor with an assignment (Perez, 1981). The beginning nurse's role might include the following:

- Routine work assignments
- Activities focused on helping, learning, and following directions
- Rationale for decision-making discussed with preceptors

After orientation, the novice should be assigned a resource nurse for help and questions. Assignments should then become progressively more challenging.

Technical Competency of the Novice

The second developmental stage is *independence*. Transition is accomplished by establishing a reputation as a technically competent professional who can work independently to produce designated patient outcomes. This nurse has primary responsibility for a small number of patients and no longer requires close supervision. Technical skills have evolved to a high level. The nurse may establish an area of subspecialization in which expertise is recognized by peers (Perez, 1981). Examples of skills at this level of competence are given below:

- Begins to place importance on peer relationships
- Begins to develop personal views on specific situations
- Begins to develop individual performance standards
- Develops an awareness of a professional value system
- Develops competence and judgment

Often a supervisory position is taken during this stage. Lack of technologic expertise undermines the manager's self-confidence as well as the staff's confidence. Successful achievement of developmental tasks is extremely important in the process of long-term career development. Many nurses remain in this stage throughout their careers, making a substantial professional contribution to patient care.

Communicators and Translators of Care Practices

During this stage the nurse begins to take responsibility for influencing, guiding, directing, and developing others. The nurse is also ready to become a full member of the collaborative practice team. The nurse's interest broadens to professional activities at regional and national levels. Many nurses at this level return to school. Examples of characteristics of this stage are as follows:

- Acts as an informal mentor
- Is expected to perform more work because of evolving capabilities
- Becomes innovative
- Influences others
- Begins to be sensitive to the needs of other nurses
- Assumes responsibility for interdisciplinary collaboration
- Learns to cope with "being in the middle"
- Assists others in developing confidence by providing guidance and freedom
- Learns to experience success through others' accomplishments
- Must be psychologically willing to take responsibility for the output of another
- Technical skills must be maintained, or stagnation and inability to keep up with younger competitors occurs

Shapers and Generators of Care Delivery Systems

Some nurses move on to another developmental stage. These nurses become "shapers." They interface and negotiate with key segments of the NICU organization, developing new ideas, procedures, or services that lead to new areas of activity for the staff or directing the resources of the organization toward specific goals. They formulate policy and initiate and approve new programs.

Summary

Career stages assist nurses in planning what needs to occur and how much time will be needed if they want to move on to another stage, and they assist the NICU staff in developing a structure that promotes career development (Harrigan, 1995). Career stages also provide a viable structure for the development of a career ladder.

ADVANCED-PRACTICE NEONATAL NURSES: EXTENDED AND EXPANDED NEONATAL NURSING ROLES

The development of effective NICUs has increased the demand for experienced personnel available on a 24-hour basis to manage emergency neonatal problems. To help meet this demand, the American Academy of Pediatrics (AAP), in 1977, recommended the use of neonatal nurse practitioners in the NICU (Harper, Little, & Sia, 1982). The AAP believed that nurses with extended roles could adequately meet the demands for a portion of the personnel requirements. However, recent concern about the need for cost containment has slowed the emergence of this role (Hickey, 1996). In a number of settings neonatologists have become concerned about the impact of advanced-practice neonatal nurses on their job security.

The employment of neonatal nurse practitioners who would be responsible for the medical management of patients required a redefinition of the traditional bounds of nursing practice. The scope of nursing practice extends into the realm of medical practice and increases the need for collaborative planning.

Practice lines are blurring. There is an intense professional interest in and a recognized social need for the leadership of enterprising nurses and the availability of financial resources to support expanded and extended nursing practice (Hickey, 1996).

Three activities of advanced practitioners have contributed to the improvement of neonatal care:

- Innovation and refinement of practice
- Acceptance of control of neonatal nursing practice
- Development of a research basis for practice

Nursing has been unwilling to determine what level of education is needed to deliver competent neonatal nursing care. The American Nurses' Association suggests that specialist and practitioner roles will be merged (American Nurses' Association, 1991).

Advanced-practice nurses have a responsibility to the profession and to society to know the field of neonatal nursing extremely well. In addition, advanced-practice neonatal nurses have a responsibility to know a great deal about neonatal medicine. Mastery over this domain will yield public confidence in neonatal nurses.

Managed care and the implementation of care paths and care maps demand that neonatal nurses move away from a process focus and develop an outcome-oriented practice focused on improving the care outcomes (Harrigan, 1995). Common ground between the health professions is emerging and serves as the foundation of neonatal health care.

PRACTICE AND CREDENTIALING OF NEONATAL NURSES

There should be a relationship between the certification standards, requirements and options, and titles and content of curricula used to prepare advanced practitioners of nursing. Legislation to control the development of advanced practice should not be sought. This control is a responsibility of the professional organization, and it has been accepted by the National Association of Neonatal Nurses (NANN) (1994).

The public also has a right to reasonable expectations about the competencies of nurse providers. The credibility and trustworthiness of all neonatal nurses are compromised when any nurse or specialist decides to use the title of advanced-practice nurse without having the credentials or knowledge deemed appropriate by the profession.

Expert neonatal nurses must (1) be able to use appropriate knowledge, (2) have sufficient expertise to evaluate knowledge for its appropriateness in improving quality of life, and (3) contribute to the development of a body of knowledge relevant to neonatal health care (Sherwen, 1990). This is not possible unless the neonatal nurse is competent in both a technical and a theoretical sense. Thus, the nurse's education should occur in a graduate realm.

Standardization of education on the master's level also provides a service to the profession by gaining educational parity with other health care professions (e.g., social work, pharmacy). Policy makers are very aware of formal educational credentials. When the advanced-practice nurse possesses a "universal degree," such as a master's degree in science, it adds credibility to negotiating issues surrounding scope of practice, such as prescriptive authority and third-party payment.

REFERENCES

Aiken, L. H., Gwyther, M. E., & Whelan, E-M. (1996). Federal support of graduate nursing education: Rationale and policy options. *Nursing Outlook, 44*(1), 11–17.

American Nurses' Association. (1991). *The American nurse.* Kansas City, MO: Author.

Harper, R. G., Little, G. A., & Sia, C. G. (1982). The scope of nursing practice in level III neonatal intensive care units. *Pediatrics, 70*(6), 875–878.

Harrigan, R. C. (1995). Health care reform: Impact of managed care on perinatal and neonatal care delivery and education. *Journal of Perinatal Neonatal Nursing, 8*(4), 47–58.

Hickey, J. V. (1996). Advanced practice nursing: Moving into the 21st century in practice, education, and research. In J. V. Hickey, R. M. Ouimette, & S. L. Venegoni (Eds.), *Advanced practice nursing: Changing roles and clinical application.* (pp. 349–360). Philadelphia: J. B. Lippincott.

National Association of Neonatal Nurses (1994). *Position statement on advanced practice nursing.* Petaluma, CA: Author.

Perez, R. (1981). *Protocols for perinatal nursing practice.* St. Louis: C. V. Mosby.

Sherwen, L. (1990). Interdisciplinary collaboration in perinatal/neonatal health care: A worthwhile challenge. *Journal of Perinatology, 10*(1), 1–2.

• •

CHAPTER 2

Legal Aspects of Perinatal Care

LAW AS A DISPUTE RESOLUTION MECHANISM

Elements of Negligence

In law, a negligence suit may be brought when the careless, as opposed to the intentional, acts of an individual bring harm to a person to whom one has a duty of care. The following are the four legal elements necessary to prove negligence:

- Duty
- Breach of duty
- Injury
- Causation

Litigation results when the presence of these elements is disputed. The process of litigation is an attempt by plaintiff and defendant to get a disinterested third party—a judge or a jury—to believe a particular version of the facts. The plaintiff seeks monetary damages. The defendant seeks exoneration.

If parents sue the nurse in neonatal practice, they must show that the nurse owed the neonate a duty of care. Demonstration of institutional employment, assignment to the neonatal intensive care unit (NICU), and provision of direct or supervisory care to a particular infant establishes the nurse's duty of care. The plaintiff must then show breach of that duty of care. Evidence of deviation from the expected standard of care through an action or omission establishes breach of duty.

Violation of the standard of care must then be causally tied or connected to the actual injury. Injury must always occur for negligence to be proved.

Malpractice Versus Negligence

Malpractice describes negligence of individuals who violate a standard of care that can be known only by virtue of education in a field. *Negligence* that is not malpractice violates a standard of care a lay person would know.

Because NICU nursing is a specialized area of practice, it would be rare for a nurse to deviate from the standard of care in such a way that a lay jury could understand the deviation without some explanation. Expert witnesses may be used for this explanation. Conversely, commonly understood acts of negligence, such as leaving the crib's side rail down, would not need an expert's explanation.

Statutes of Limitations

Statutes of limitations are laws that set time frames during which certain legal actions must be brought. Their purpose is to prevent claims that have lost their credibility because information bases and persons knowledgeable about events are long removed from the event precipitating the suit. The time frames set in the statute are intended to provide sufficient time for plaintiffs to discover injuries and bring suit, while assuring potential defendants that they are not at risk forever.

Actions against neonatal nurses can be brought even beyond the ordinary statutory time limitation because the law has recognized that an injustice may occur if parents do not bring an action on behalf of their child during the usual statutory time frame. The remedy for this potential injustice is to permit individuals to bring actions on their own behalf within the ordinary statutory time frame after they reach the age of majority. For example, a child injured as a result of breach of the standard of care in an NICU has until age 18 plus the usual statutory time frame for bringing an action. A 1-year statute of limitations for physician suits would leave liability open through the child's reaching age 19. A 3-year statute of limitations for hospitals would leave liability open through the child's reaching age 21. Statutes of limitations vary from state to state.

Professional Liability Insurance

There are two types of professional liability coverage: *claims-made* and *occurrence* coverage.

Claims-made coverage pays damages only for claims brought during the period in which the policy is in force. Thus, any claim in negligence brought during the policy period, even if the event occurred many years ago, is covered. *Occurrence coverage* provides for claims brought many years after the precipitating event has occurred, even though the nurse no longer carries professional liability insurance.

Claims-made policies are advantageous to the insurer because the insurer receives premiums in an amount judged sufficient to cover claims during a certain period of time. Occurrence policies are advantageous to the nurse because it is not necessary to continue insurance coverage after ceasing to work or on retirement.

Nurses are often informed by health care facility employers that they do not need to carry personal professional liability insurance coverage. The reason given is that facilities purchase insurance to cover the negligent acts or omissions of their employees. Although health care facilities are generally well-meaning in proffering this advice (in terms of saving nurses' money), they ignore the probably minor but real risk that the nurse may independently practice outside the facility setting. Personal professional liability insurance serves as insulation for the nurse from loss of personal possessions through negligence or malpractice. Professional liability insurance does not insulate assets from intentional acts. A nurse who defames a parent, threatens a parent, or deliberately harms an infant will not be protected. This lack of protection is the case even if criminal charges have not been upheld before a civil suit is brought.

Standards of Care

Standards are general guidelines to practice. Accountable professionals practice prudently and reasonably based on their education and experience.

Knowing and practicing nursing according to current standards helps ensure that a legal challenge to one's practice can be successfully defended.

Professional accountability is defined as carrying out the nursing process. *Legal accountability* is defined by giving a positive orientation to the legal elements of negligence. Documentation provides evidence of both professional and legal accountability.

Specialty professional associations may provide specific guidelines to practitioners in the neonatal area. These are updated by professional consensus mechanisms based on changing knowledge in the field. The National Association for Neonatal Nurses (NANN), for example, has Neonatal Nursing Transport Standards and Guidelines (NANN, 1994) and Standards of Care for Neonatal Nursing Practice (NANN, 1993).

The development and widespread distribution of guidelines in neonatal care set by professional associations such as the American Academy of Pediatrics (AAP) and the American College of Obstetricians and Gynecologists (ACOG) (AAP/ACOG, 1997) are among the influences that have led states to recognize standards of care as being national rather than local in origin. Other influences have included ready accessibility of information about care in professional journals as well as the need for adherence to national standards to receive accreditation through the Joint Commission on Accreditation of Healthcare Organizations (JCAHO). Attendance at continuing education programs in the specialty area, referring to recognized texts when questions about care arise, and keeping abreast of state licensing standards also keep the nurse current in practice.

Health care facilities have a corporate duty of care. Thus, they have a responsibility to ensure conditions of employment that permit meeting the expected standard of care in areas like NICUs. Plaintiffs will look at the hospital's responsibility to meet JCAHO accreditation standards by examining hospital policy and procedure. Policy and procedure manuals should reflect these current standards of care.

CHANGING NURSING CARE DELIVERY STANDARDS OF CARE

The redesign of nursing care delivery systems to include use of unlicensed assistive personnel (UAPs) to perform nursing care most recently reserved to licensed staff is cause for concern about patient safety. While skill, experience, and numbers are, no doubt, critical components of quality and certainly safety in care, finding a proper staffing mix in the face of changing interventions, changing reimbursements, and changing delivery sites is not so certain (Huston, 1996).

Before delegating care to UAPs the nurse must be aware of their education and experience. Facilities have the responsibility for developing policies to ensure transmission of this vital information to staff nurses. Records of UAP education, both content and competency, must be retained (Ohio Board of Nursing, 1995).

The nurse must keep in mind that he or she cannot delegate patient assessment and, therefore, the judgment calls changing nursing care plans and collaborating with other providers. Because redesign increases the number of patients for whom the nurse is responsible, some reliance on UAPs for information about patient status is inevitable. Consistency in patient care teams is one risk management approach to ensure necessary information is transmitted from UAP to nurse.

At the national level the American Nurses' Association (ANA) has called for nurses to act as advocates in alerting the public to unsafe staffing conditions (American Nurses' Association, 1995a). Concurrently, the ANA has called for an increasing focus on quality of care research (ANA, 1995b). At the state level, nursing boards are moving to regulate UAPs under their nursing standards authority. Ohio is an example (Ohio Board of Nursing, August 1995 Hearing Notice).

Steps in the Litigation Process

The steps in the litigation process are as follows:

- A parent or previous NICU patient who has reached the age of majority who is unhappy with the result of neonatal care has the right to sue.
- Legal advice will be sought from an attorney and an expert in the field to determine sufficient cause to initiate a suit.
- Medical records are critical to the conduct of a lawsuit and are admissible as evidence—a true record of events. Evidence that records have been tampered with immediately decreases credibility of the defendant institution and nurse.
- If negligence is ascertained from a reading of the records, a complaint will be filed in the appropriate court. Simultaneously, the defendant will be served with a copy of the complaint.
- The defendant hospital will notify its insurance carrier.
- The carrier will notify its defense law firm.
- Response must occur within a specified period of time. Statutory rules of civil procedure govern the time period for receiving this answer. An answer offers the opportunity to state a defense to the action.
- The plaintiff may then have an opportunity to reply.

Settlement of a lawsuit can occur any time before a trial or even while a trial is in session.

MANAGEMENT OF RISK

Individual Nursing Practice and Management of Risk

A nurse must promptly record deviations and appropriate actions. When following protocols it is important to take into consideration infant responses that are not covered by the protocol. "Cookbook" responses, to the extent that they are knee-jerk rather than thoughtful reactions, are not good practice.

Today's monitoring equipment reduces the risk of providing too much fluid, but the possibility of human error remains in the initial rate-setting process. Guidelines to reduce risks associated with fluid administration are similar to those for administering pharmacologic agents: the right time, right dose, right route, right medication, and right person should be checked and rechecked. The infant patient, not just the equipment, requires constant assessment for reaction to fluid administration.

The nurse must have sufficient working knowledge of the operation of equipment to recognize equipment malfunction. Risk management requires that the nurse leave repair of malfunctions to trained persons.

Resuscitation events require careful documentation of both the sequence of events that precipitated resuscitation efforts and the sequence of interventions occurring during those resuscitation efforts. Assigning an individual to document the sequence of resuscitation efforts is critical to establishing the standard of care that was followed should questions later arise. Similarly, oxygen support for infants requires meticulous documentation to demonstrate that oxygen levels were commensurate with need and fine-tuned to the infant's developmental stage.

As care patterns move infants home quickly, nurses become more vulnerable to suits rooted in communication failure. Parents who have not sufficiently understood and practiced complicated technologic care—and even the seemingly low technology of breastfeeding—will bring suit if their child suffers harm because of their lack of understanding or ability to provide care. Clear documentation of teaching that includes evidence of both parent understanding and practice opportunities will serve in the nurse's defense. Written instructions and follow-up home visits are additional risk management measures for these situations.

Communication and Documentation

Communication and documentation are the linchpins of professional practice. Timely and clear *communication* among nurse, physician, and family acknowledges and values the roles of each in the care of the infant. Communication with family serves the added purpose of warding off misunderstandings that could lead to later lawsuits.

As the business record of the health care facility, the medical record is the enduring evidence of the activities of assessment, planning, implementation, and evaluation of the neonate's care. Interventions that reflect new professional thought or a more conservative standard of care than usual deserve a notation indicating their rationale.

Documentation is the legal evidence of professional accountability. Assessments, interventions, evaluations and reevaluations, and communications not documented are presumed not to have occurred. Without documentation the nurse who asserts at deposition or trial that an activity occurred can expect a deserved assault on his or her credibility.

Incident Reports

Incident or variance reports detail occurrences that pose a risk of monetary loss for a health care facility. A lawsuit need not occur for this financial loss to be realized. Incident reports need to be filed not only when actual injury has occurred but also when the potential for injury exists.

Incident reports should contain *facts* surrounding the event. Conclusory or blaming statements should be absent from the report. The report should reflect the steps taken to assess for and alleviate any actual injury that might have occurred.

SOCIAL AND PUBLIC POLICY CONCERNS IN PERINATAL CARE

Decision-Making in Infant Care

Infants in particular have no experience with life, nor for that matter can they speak for themselves in relation to choice of treatments. As the natural guardians of children, parents are presumed to act in the child's best interests in making choices about treatment. By providing information, health care providers should assist parents in the decision-making process. Unfortunately, health care providers may be at ethical or clinical odds with parental choices, resulting in legal action in the form of case law, statutory law, and regulatory law.

INFORMED CONSENT

A nurse's legal role in obtaining consent is generally limited to witnessing the consent form signed by the parents or legal guardian of the infant. By law, the responsibility for obtaining informed consent for treatments belongs to the physician.

THE LEGAL LEGACY OF BABY DOE

When withholding or withdrawing care from a handicapped newborn becomes a question, social policy introduces a further constraint on the decision maker. A 1982 case precipitated public outcry against the parents' nontreatment decision for a newborn with Down syndrome and esophageal fistula (*Indiana* ex rel. *Infant Doe* v. *Monroe Circuit Court*, 1982). With nutrition and treatment withheld the child died.

Issues about use of life-sustaining measures with infants continue. Fairfax Hospital in Virginia requested a declaratory judgment that withholding a ventilator from an anencephalic infant when the infant suffered respiratory distress would not violate state or federal law. Both District and Circuit courts found withholding the ventilator support would violate the Emergency Medical Treatment and Active Labor Act (1986) (In the Matter of Baby K, 1993, 1994; Capron, 1994). The Supreme Court declined to hear the case. With ventilator support when needed, the child lived to be 2½ years old.

Research on Infants and Children

Federal law establishes criteria for conduct of research on children according to varying degrees of risk (45 Code of Federal Regulations S 46.404–46.407, 1983). Familiarity with the provision of regulations guiding research is critical to the nurse who assumes an advocacy role for the child.

There are four categories of risk:

1. Research not involving greater than minimal risk
2. Research with greater than minimal risk but representing the prospect of direct benefit to the individual subjects
3. Research involving greater than minimal risk and no prospect of direct benefit to individual subjects
4. Research not otherwise approvable that presents an opportunity to understand, prevent, or alleviate a serious problem affecting the health or welfare of children

The regulations in all four categories call for assent of children capable of participating in the decision-making process, with consent coming from parents or guardians. Clearly, assent does not apply to neonates. The second category, greater than minimal risk with possible benefit to subjects, requires that the risk be justified by the anticipated benefit and that the anticipated benefit be at least as favorable to the subjects as available alternatives. The third category, greater than minimal risk with no prospect of direct benefit, is approvable if (1) the risk is only a minor increase over minimal risk; (2) the intervention presents experiences commensurate with what the subjects might experience in their actual or expected medical, dental, psychological, social, or educational situations; and (3) the intervention is likely to yield generalizable knowledge of vital importance for the understanding or amelioration of the subject's disorder or condition. Before approval of the fourth category of research, the Secretary of the Department of Health and Human Services must consult with a panel of experts and afford opportunity for public review. Following this review procedure, the research must satisfy either the conditions for the first three categories of risk or (1) be determined to present a reasonable opportunity of further understanding, prevention, or alleviation of a serious problem affecting the health or welfare of children (the category purpose); (2) be conducted in accordance with sound ethical principles; and (3) fulfill the necessary consent requirements.

Only federally funded research falls under the law. However, many institutional review boards (IRBs) apply federal regulations to all research projects conducted within the institution. The IRBs review research proposals to ensure protection for human subjects under the regulations.

Perinatal Maternal Substance Abuse

Nurses should be aware of the policy issues raised by suggestions that the definition of child abuse be extended to include fetal abuse or that the mother be viewed as a criminal guilty of delivering drugs to a minor. Until recently, however, the law has been satisfied to find women who abuse drugs during pregnancy in violation only of child protective laws. The policy goal is reunification of families. The law directs that parental skills be taught and successful completion of drug rehabilitation programs be documented.

Recently, prosecutors have begun to bring criminal charges against drug-abusing pregnant women. The women have been charged under a number of criminal statutes: delivering cocaine to a newborn child through the umbilical cord, involuntary manslaughter, and criminal neglect (Curriden, 1990).

REFERENCES

American Academy of Pediatrics/American College of Obstetricians and Gynecologists. (1997). *Guidelines for perinatal care* (4th ed.). Elk Grove Village, IL: Author.

American Nurses' Association. (1995a). *Nursing report card for acute care settings: A tool for protecting our patients, February 2, 1995*. Washington, DC: Author.

American Nurses' Association. (1995b). *Summary of the Lewin-VHI, Inc. Report: Nursing report card for acute care settings, February 2, 1995*. Washington, DC: Author.

Capron, A. M. (1994). At law—medical futility: Strike two. *Hastings Center Report, 24*(5), 42–43.

Curriden, M. (1990). Holding mom accountable. *American Bar Association Journal, 76*(3), 50–53.

Emergency Medical Treatment and Active Labor Treatment Act of 1986, 42 U.S.C. S 1395 dd.

Huston, C. L. (1996). Unlicensed assistive personnel: A solution to dwindling health care resources or the precursor to the apocalypse of registered nursing? *Nursing Outlook, 44*(2), 67–73.

In the matter of Baby K, 832 F.Supp. 1022 (E.D. Va 1993).

In the matter of Baby K, 16 F.3d590 (4th Cir. 1994), cert. Denied, 115 U.S.91 (1994).

National Association of Neonatal Nurses. (1993). *Standards of care for neonatal nursing practice*. Petaluma, CA: Author.

National Association of Neonatal Nurses. (1994). *Neonatal nursing transport standards and guidelines*. Petaluma, CA: Author.

Ohio Board of Nursing. (1995, August). Notice of hearing to establish parameters for the delegation of certain nursing tasks by registered nurses to licensed practical nurses and by licensed nurses to trained unlicensed persons in all settings, including dialysis centers (rules 4723-13-01 through 4723-13-10).

The Prenatal Environment: Maternal-Fetal Interactions

CHAPTER 3

Fetal Development: Environmental Influences and Critical Periods

EARLY FETAL DEVELOPMENT

Mitotic cell division occurs after fertilization as the zygote passes down the uterine tube, resulting in the formation of two blastomeres. *Cleavage* describes the mitotic cell division of the zygote. When the number of cells reach approximately 16 (usually on the third day), the zygote is called a *morula*, because of its resemblance to a mulberry. This is the time it enters the uterus.

About the fourth day after fertilization, the fluid-filled spaces fuse, forming a large cavity known as the blastocyst cavity. The morula is now called the *blastocyst*.

Implantation

Two layers of trophoblasts develop. The inner layer is made up of cytotrophoblasts, and the outer layer is composed of syncytiotrophoblasts. A syncytiotrophoblast has finger-like projections that produce enzymes capable of further eroding the endometrial tissues. By the end of the seventh day, the blastocyst is superficially implanted. The primary chorionic villi form at about the same time. These finger-like projections of the chorion develop into the chorionic villi of the placenta.

The inner cell mass differentiates into two layers: the hypoblast (endoderm), a layer of small cuboidal cells, and the epiblast (ectoderm), a layer of high columnar cells. The two layers form a flattened, circular *bilaminar embryonic disk*.

During the development of the amniotic cavity, other trophoblastic cells form a thin extracoelomic membrane, which encloses the primitive yolk sac. The yolk sac produces fetal red blood cells.

By the end of the second week, there is a slightly thickened area near the cephalic region of the hypoblastic disk, known as the prochordal plate, that marks the location of the mouth.

Formation of the Trilaminar Embryonic Disk

The third week of development is marked by rapid growth, the formation of the *primitive streak,* and the differentiation of the three germ layers, from which all fetal tissues and organs are derived.

Gastrulation is the process by which the bilaminar disk is expanded to a trilaminar embryonic disk. It is the most important event that occurs during early fetal formation.

On days 14 to 15, a groove and thickening of the ectoderm (epiblast), called the *primitive streak,* appear caudad in the center of the dorsum of the embryonic disk. The primitive groove develops in the primitive streak.

Cells from the primitive knot migrate craniad and form the midline cellular notochordal process. The *notochordal process* grows craniad between the ectoderm and endoderm until it reaches the prochordal plate, which is attached to the overlying ectoderm, thus forming the oropharyngeal membrane. The cloacal membrane, caudal to the primitive streak, develops into the anus.

The *notochord* is the structure around which the vertebral column is formed. *Neurulation* is the process by which the neural plate, neural folds, and neural tube are formed. The neural crest cells give rise to the spinal ganglia, the ganglia of the autonomic nervous system, and a portion of the cranial nerves. Neural crest cells also form the meningeal covering of the brain and spinal cord and the sheaves that protect nerves. The neural crest cells contribute to the formation of pigment-producing cells, the adrenal medulla, and skeletal and muscular development in the head.

During formation of the neural tube, the intraembryonic mesoderm on each side thickens, forming longitudinal columns of paraxial mesoderm. At about 20 days, the paraxial mesoderm begins to divide into paired cuboidal bodies known as *somites.* The somites give rise to most of the skeleton and associated musculature and much of the dermis of the skin. The somites develop in a craniocaudal sequence. In all, 42 to 44 somites develop, although only 38 develop during the "somite" period. These somite pairs can be counted and give an estimate as to fetal age before a crown–rump measurement is possible.

The intraembryonic cavity first appears as a number of small spaces within the lateral mesoderm and the cardiogenic mesoderm. It divides the lateral mesoderm into the parietal (somatic) and visceral (splanchnic) layers. The intraembryonic cavity gives rise to the pericardial cavity, the pleural cavity, and the peritoneal cavity.

PLACENTAL DEVELOPMENT AND FUNCTION

The rudimentary maternal-fetal circulation is intact by the fourth week. The placenta is mature and completely functional by 16 weeks of development. If the corpus luteum begins to regress before this 16th week and fails to produce enough progesterone (the hormone responsible for readying the uterine cavity for the pregnancy), the pregnancy will be aborted.

Placental-Fetal Circulation

By 28 days, unidirectional circulation is established. Deoxygenated fetal blood leaves the fetus by means of the umbilical arteries and enters the capillaries in the chorionic villi, where gaseous and nutrient exchange takes place. Oxygenated blood returns to the fetus through the umbilical veins. Initially there are two arteries and two veins, but eventually only two arteries and one vein remain, because one of the veins degenerates. If only one artery is present, a congenital anomaly, especially a renal one, should be suspected.

Placental Function

The function of the placenta is determined by the following:

- Synthesis of glycogen, cholesterol, and fatty acids, which provide nutrients and energy for early fetal development.
- Production and transport of hormones that maintain the pregnancy and promote growth and development of the fetus. Chorionic gonadotropin, a protein hormone produced by the syncytiotrophoblast, is excreted in maternal serum and urine and is used as a test for pregnancy. Human placental lactogen (hPL), a protein hormone produced by the placenta, acts as a fetal growth-promoting hormone by giving the fetus priority for maternal glucose.
- Production of progesterone throughout pregnancy, which is responsible for the maintenance of the pregnancy.
- Estrogen production, which depends on stimulation by the fetal adrenal cortex and liver.
- Placental transport to fetus of maternal antibodies, providing fetus with passive immunity to certain viruses. IgG antibodies are actively transported across the placental barrier, providing humoral immunity to the fetus. IgA and IgM antibodies do not cross the placental barrier, placing the neonate at risk for neonatal sepsis. However, failure of IgM antibodies to cross the placental membrane explains the lower incidence of a severe hemolytic process in ABO blood type incompatibilities as compared with Rh incompatibilities.
- Selective transfer of substances across the placenta. This selectivity does not screen out viral, bacterial, and protozoal organisms or toxic substances such as drugs and alcohol.

EMBRYONIC PERIOD: WEEKS 4 THROUGH 8

The embryonic period lasts from the beginning of week 4 through the end of week 8. All major organ systems are structurally formed during this period (Baraitser & Winter, 1996).

Folding of the Embryo

In the trilaminar embryonic disk, the growth rate of the central region exceeds that of the periphery, so that the slower growing areas fold under the faster growing areas, forming body folds. The head fold appears first, as a result of craniocaudal elongation of the notochord and growth of the brain, which projects into the amniotic cavity. The folding downward of the cranial end of the embryo forces the septum transversum (primitive heart), the pericardial cavity, and the oropharyngeal membrane to turn under onto the ventral surface. After the embryo has folded, the mass of mesoderm cranial to the pericardial cavity, called the septum transversum, lies caudad to the heart. The septum transversum later develops into a portion of the diaphragm. The foregut ends blindly at the oropharyngeal membrane, which separates the foregut from the primitive mouth cavity (stomodeum).

The tail fold occurs after the head fold as a result of craniocaudal progression of growth. Growth of the embryo causes the caudal area to project over the cloacal membrane. After completion of the head and tail folding, the connecting stalk is attached to the ventral surface of the embryo, forming the umbilical cord.

Folding also occurs laterally, producing right and left lateral folds. The lateral body wall on each side folds toward the median plane, causing the embryo to assume a cylindrical shape.

Organogenesis: Germ Cell Derivatives

The three germ cell layers (ectoderm, mesoderm, and endoderm) give rise to all tissues and organs of the embryo. The germ cells follow specific patterns during the process of organogenesis. The development of each major organ system is discussed separately. The embryonic period is the most critical period of development because of the formation of the internal and external structures.

FETAL PERIOD: WEEK 9 THROUGH BIRTH

The fetal period begins at the ninth week and extends through the duration of the pregnancy. It is characterized by further fetal growth and development. Vernix caseosa, lanugo, and scalp hair appear. The eyelids open at 24 to 26 weeks. The fetus has the potential for survival at 23 to 24 weeks, but there are many physiologic difficulties that impact on survival. The last part of the fetal period provides preparation for transition to the extrauterine environment.

DEVELOPMENT OF SPECIFIC ORGANS AND STRUCTURES

Nervous System

The origin of the nervous system is the neural plate. The cranial end of the neural tube forms the three divisions of the brain: the forebrain, the midbrain, and the hindbrain. The cerebral hemispheres and diencephalon arise from the forebrain; the pons, cerebellum, and medulla oblongata arise from the hindbrain. The midbrain makes up the adult midbrain.

The cavity of the neural tube develops into the ventricles of the brain and the central canal of the spinal column. The neuroepithelial cells lining the neural tube give rise to nerves and glial cells of the central nervous system.

The peripheral nervous system consists of the cranial, spinal, and visceral nerves and the ganglia. The somatic and visceral sensory cells of the peripheral nervous system arise from neural crest cells as do Schwann cells responsible for the myelin sheaths.

Cardiovascular System

The fetal cardiac system, the first functional system, appears at 18 to 19 days, and circulation is present by about 21 days of gestation. The heart and blood develop from the middle layer (mesoderm) of the trilaminar embryonic disk. Tissue from the lateral mesoderm migrates up the sides of the embryonic disk, forming a horseshoe-shaped structure that arches and meets above the oropharyngeal membrane. With further development, paired heart tubes form, which then fuse into a single heart tube. The vessels that make up the vascular system throughout the body develop from mesodermal cells that connect to each other, with the developing heart tube and the placenta. Thus, by the end of the third week there is a functional cardiovascular system.

As the heart tube grows, the folding of the embryonic disk results in the movement of the heart tube into the chest cavity. The heart tube differentiates into three layers: the endocardial layer, which becomes the endothelium; the cardiac jelly, which is a loose tissue layer; and the myoepicardial mantle, which becomes the myocardium and pericardium.

The single heart tube is attached at its cephalic end by the aortic arches and at the caudal end by the septum transversum. The attachments limit the length of the heart tube. Continued growth results in dilated areas and bulges, which become specific components of the heart. First, the atrium, ventricle, and bulbus cordis can be identified. The sinus venosus and truncus arteriosus follow. To accommodate continued growth, two separate bends in the heart occur. It first bends to the right to form a U-shape, and the next bend results in an S-shaped heart. The bending of the heart is responsible for the typical location of cardiac structures.

Initially, the heart is a single chamber. Partitioning of the heart into four chambers occurs from the fourth to the sixth weeks. The changes that cause the partitioning of the heart occur simultaneously. The atrium is separated from the ventricle by endocardial cushions. Endocardial cushions are thickened areas of endothelium that develop on the dorsal and ventral walls of

the open area between the atrium and ventricle. The endocardial cushions fuse with each other to divide the atrioventricular canals into right and left atrioventricular canals.

Partitioning of the atrium occurs through invagination of tissue toward the endocardial cushions, forming the septum primum. As the septum primum grows toward the endocardial cushions, it stretches very thin and perforates. The perforation becomes the foramen ovale. The septum primum does not completely fuse with the endocardial cushions; it has a lower portion that lies beside the endocardial cushions. Overlapping of the septum primum and the septum secundum forms a wall if the pressures in both atria are equal. In utero, the pressure on the right side is increased, allowing blood to flow across the foramen ovale from the right side of the heart to the left side.

The ventricle is also partitioned by a septum, which is membranous and muscular. The muscular portion of the septum develops from the fold of the floor of the ventricle. With blood flowing through the atrioventricular canal, ventricular dilation occurs on either side of the fold or ridge, causing it to become a septum. The membranous septum comes from ridges inside the bulbus cordis. These ridges, continuous into the bulbus cordis, form the wall that divides the bulbus cordis into the pulmonary artery and the aorta. The bulbar ridges fuse with the endocardial cushions to form the membranous septum. The membranous and muscular septa fuse to close the intraventricular foramen, resulting in two parallel circuits for blood flow. The pulmonary artery is continuous with the right ventricle, and the aorta is continuous with the left ventricle.

The blood flowing through the bulbus cordis and truncus arteriosus in a spiral causes the formation of ridges. The ridges fuse to form two separate vessels that twist around each other once. Thus, the pulmonary artery exits the right side of the heart and is in the left upper chest; the aorta exits the left side of the heart and is located close to the sternum.

The pulmonary veins grow from the lungs to a cardinal vein plexus. Concurrently, a vessel develops from the smooth wall of the left atrium. As the atrium grows, the pulmonary vein is incorporated into the atrial wall. The atrium and its branches give rise to four pulmonary veins that enter the left atrium. These pulmonary vessels, connected to the plexus of the cardinal vein, provide a continuous circulation from lung to heart.

The pulmonary and aortic valves (semilunar valves) develop from dilations within the pulmonary artery and aorta. The tricuspid and mitral valves develop from tissue around the atrioventricular canals that thicken and then thin out on the ventricular sides, forming the valves.

Respiratory System

The development of the respiratory system is linked to the development of the face and the digestive system. The respiratory system is composed of the nasal cavities, nasopharynx, oropharynx, larynx, trachea, bronchi, and lungs.

Development of the lungs occurs in four overlapping stages, which extend from the fifth week of gestation until about 8 years of life. For adequate functioning of the respiratory system, there must be a sufficient number of

alveoli, adequate capillary blood flow, and an adequate amount of surfactant produced by the secretory epithelial cells or the type II pneumatocytes.

Muscular System

The muscular system develops from mesodermal cells called myoblasts. Striated skeletal muscles are derived from myotomal mesoderm (myotomes) of the somites. The majority of striated skeletal muscle fibers develop in utero. Almost all striated skeletal muscles are formed by 1 year of age. Growth is achieved by an increase in the diameter of the muscle fibers, rather than the growth of new muscle tissue. Smooth muscle fibers arise from the splanchnic mesenchyme surrounding the endoderm of the primitive gut. Smooth muscles lining vessel walls of blood and lymphatic systems arise from somatic mesoderm.

As smooth muscle cells differentiate, contractile filaments develop in the cytoplasm, and the external surface is covered by an external lamina. As the smooth muscle fibers develop into sheets or bundles, the muscle cells synthesize and release collagenous, elastic, or reticular fibers.

Cardiac muscle develops from splanchnic mesenchyme from the outside of the endocardial heart tube. Cells from the myoepicardial mantle differentiate into the myocardium. Cardiac muscle fibers develop from differentiation and growth of single cells rather than from fusion of cells. Cardiac muscle growth occurs through the formation of new filaments. The Purkinje fibers develop late in the embryonic period. These fibers are larger and have fewer myofibrils than other cardiac muscle cells. The Purkinje fibers function in the electrical conduction system of the heart.

Skeletal System

The skeletal system develops from mesenchymal cells. In the long bones, condensed mesenchyme forms hyaline cartilage models of bones. By the end of the embryonic period, ossification centers appear, and these bones ossify by endochondral ossification. Other bones, such as the skull bones, are ossified by membranous ossification in which the mesenchyme cells become osteoblasts.

The vertebral column and the ribs arise from the sclerotome compartments of the somites. The spinal column is formed by the fusion of a condensation of the cranial half of one pair of sclerotomes with the caudal half of the next pair of sclerotomes.

The skull can be divided into the neurocranium and the viscerocranium. The neurocranium forms the protective covering around the brain. The viscerocranium forms the skeleton of the face. The neurocranium is made up of the flat bones that surround the brain and the cartilaginous structure, or chondrocranium, which forms the bones of the base of the skull. The neurocranium (chondrocranium) is made up of a number of separate cartilages, which fuse and ossify by endochondral ossification to form the base of the skull.

Gastrointestinal System

The gastrointestinal system is primarily derived from the lining of the roof of the yolk sac. The primitive gut, consisting of the foregut, midgut, and hindgut, is formed during week 4.

The structures that arise from the foregut include the pharynx, esophagus, stomach, liver, pancreas, gallbladder, and part of the duodenum. The esophagus and trachea have a common origin, the laryngotracheal diverticulum. A septum, formed by the growing tracheoesophageal folds, divides the cranial part of the foregut into the laryngotracheal tube and the esophagus. Smooth muscle develops from the splanchnic mesenchyme that surrounds the esophagus. The epithelial lining of the esophagus, derived from the endoderm, proliferates, partially obliterating the esophageal lumen. The esophagus undergoes recanalization by the end of the embryonic period.

The stomach originates as a dilation of the caudal portion of the foregut. The characteristic greater curvature of the stomach results because the dorsal border grows faster than the ventral border. As the stomach develops further, it rotates in a clockwise direction around the longitudinal axis.

The duodenum is derived from the caudal part of the foregut and the cranial portions of the foregut and the midgut. The junction of the foregut and midgut portions of the duodenum is normally distal to the common bile duct.

The liver, gallbladder, and biliary ducts originate as a bud from the caudal end of the foregut. The liver is formed by growth of the hepatic diverticulum, which grows between the layers of the ventral mesentery, forming two parts. The liver forms from the largest, cranial portion. Hepatic cells originate from the hepatic diverticulum. Hematopoietic tissue and Kupffer cells are derived from the splanchnic mesenchyme of the septum transversum. The liver begins its hematopoietic function by week 6.

The smaller portion of the hepatic diverticulum forms the gallbladder. The common bile duct is formed from the stalk connecting the hepatic and cystic ducts to the duodenum. The pancreas is derived from the pancreatic buds that arise from the caudal part of the foregut.

The structures that are derived from the midgut include the remainder of the duodenum, the cecum, the appendix, the ascending colon, and the majority of the transverse colon.

The intestines must undergo extensive growth during the first weeks of development. The liver and kidneys occupy the abdominal cavity, restricting the space available for intestinal growth. The phenomenal growth of the intestines is accommodated through a migration out of the abdominal cavity by the umbilical cord. A series of rotations occurs before the intestines return to the abdomen. The first rotation is counterclockwise, around the axis of the superior mesenteric artery. At about the 10th week, the intestines return to the abdomen, undergoing further rotation. When the colon returns to the abdomen, the cecal end rotates to the right side, entering the lower right quadrant of the abdomen.

The cecum and appendix arise from the cecal diverticulum, a pouch that appears in the fifth week on the caudal limb of the midgut loop.

The hindgut is the portion of the intestines from the midgut to the cloacal membrane. The cloacal membrane consists of the endoderm of the cloaca and ectoderm of the anal pit. The cloaca is divided by the urorectal septum. As the septum grows toward the cloacal membrane, folds from the lateral walls of the cloaca grow together, dividing the cloaca into the rectum and upper anal canal dorsally and the urogenital sinus ventrally.

By the end of the sixth week, the urorectal septum fuses with the cloacal membrane, forming a dorsal anal membrane and a larger ventral urogenital membrane. At about the end of week 7, these two membranes rupture, forming the anal canal.

Urogenital System

The development of the urinary and genital systems is closely related. The urogenital system develops from the intermediate mesoderm, which extends along the dorsal body wall of the embryo. During embryonic folding in the horizontal plane, the intermediate mesoderm is moved forward and is no longer connected to the somites. This mesoderm forms the urogenital ridge on each side of the primitive aorta. Both the urinary and genital systems arise from this urogenital ridge. The area from which the urinary system is derived is called the nephrogenic cord. The genital ridge is the area from which the reproductive system is derived.

There are three stages of development of the kidney: the pronephros, the mesonephros, and the metanephros. The *pronephros*, a nonfunctional organ, appears in the first month and then degenerates, contributing only a duct system for the next developmental stage. The *mesonephros* utilizes the duct of the pronephros and develops caudad to the pronephros. The mesonephros may function in urine formation during the development of the metanephros. The mesonephros degenerates by the end of the embryonic period. Remnants of the mesonephros persist as genital ducts in males or vestigial structures in females. The *metanephros* appears in the fifth week of gestation and becomes the permanent kidney. The metanephros begins to produce urine by about the 11th week of gestation.

The urinary bladder and the urethra arise from the urogenital sinus and the splanchnic mesenchyme. The caudal portion of the mesonephric ducts is incorporated into the bladder, giving rise to the ureters.

Although the genetic sex of the embryo is determined at conception, the early development of the genital system is indistinguishable until the seventh week, when the gonads begin to be differentiated. The ovaries and the testes are derived from the coelomic epithelium, the mesenchyme, and the primordial germ cells.

Development of female sexual organs occurs in the absence of hormonal stimulation precipitated by the H-Y antigen gene carried on the Y chromosome. If the Y chromosome is present, testes develop; otherwise, ovaries develop.

CONGENITAL DEFECTS

Congenital defects or anomalies are structural or anatomic abnormalities present at birth. Most congenital defects result from an interaction between genetic and environmental factors. This type of transmission of defects is categorized as multifactorial inheritance.

Incidence

The incidence of all defects (including both minor and major defects) is approximately 14 percent. Almost 20 percent of all perinatal deaths are caused by congenital defects.

Critical Periods of Human Development

Environmental influences during the first 2 weeks after conception may prevent successful implantation of the blastocyst and cause abortion of the embryo. The most sensitive period for the embryo is the period of organogenesis, especially from days 15 to 60. Each organ has a critical period during which its development is most likely to be adversely affected by the presence of teratogenic agents. Critical periods for each major organ system are shown in Figure 3–1.

Teratogens

Teratogens are agents that may adversely affect embryonic development. About 7 percent of all congenital defects are caused by exposure to teratogenic agents. Known teratogenic agents include drugs or other chemicals,

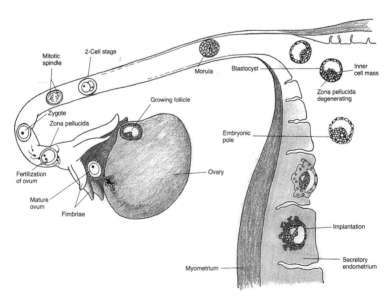

FIGURE 3–1. Fantastic voyage: from fertilization to implantation. The journey through the fallopian tubes takes approximately 4 days. During this time, mitotic cell division occurs. Implantation occurs on about day 9 through day 12.

TABLE 3–1. Drugs and Their Adverse Fetal/Neonatal Effects

Drug	Adverse Effect
Alcohol	Fetal alcohol syndrome
	Craniofacial abnormalities, limb deformities, and cardiovascular effects; growth deficiency and mental retardation
Lysergic acid diethylamide (LSD)	Limb abnormalities and central nervous system abnormalities
Phencyclidine, marijuana	Congenital anomalies
Crack cocaine	Anomalies secondary to vasoconstriction to developing fetal tissue (e.g., gastroschisis if cocaine taken during critical period of gut formation); also fetal stroke, arrhythmias from abrupt increase in blood pressure
Antibiotics	
Tetracycline	Brown discoloration of teeth and diminished long bone growth
Streptomycin and dihydrostreptomycin	Hearing defects and damage to cranial nerve VIII
Sulfonamides	Kernicterus
Anticonvulsants	
Diphenylhydantoin (Phenytoin)	Craniofacial defects, nail and digital hypoplasia, intrauterine growth retardation, microcephaly and mental retardation
Trimethadione (Tridione)	Facial dysmorphia, cardiac defects, cleft palate, and intrauterine growth retardation
Paramethadione (Paradione)	Same as trimethadione
Warfarin	Craniofacial abnormalities, optic atrophy, microcephaly, mental retardation
Antineoplastic agents	
Aminopterin and methotrexate	Major congenital malformations, especially of central nervous system; potentially harmful to individuals receiving and administering these agents
Antipsychotic and antianxiety agents	
Phenothiazine and lithium	Congenital defects
Diazepam	Cleft lip with or without cleft palate
Meprobamate and chlordiazepoxide	Congenital defects
Hormones	
Androgenic agents (progestins)	Masculinization of female fetuses
Diethylstilbestrol (DES)	Vaginal and cervical cancer in female children, abnormalities of reproductive system causing reproductive dysfunction
Propylthiouracil and potassium iodide	Neonatal goiter and mental retardation
Amphetamines	Oral clefts and heart defects
Salicylates (aspirin)	In utero closure of patent ductus arteriosus
Retinoic acid (vitamin A)	Teratogenic

Table continued on following page

TABLE 3–1. Drugs and Their Adverse Fetal/Neonatal Effects *Continued*

Drug	Adverse Effect
Isotretinoin (acne treatment)	Craniofacial abnormalities, cleft palate, thymic aplasia defects, and neural tube defects
Environmental chemicals, pollutants, fungicides, food additives, and defoliants	Congenital defects
Mercury	Neurologic manifestations
Radiation	Microcephaly, skull defects, spina bifida, blindness, and cleft palate
Infectious agents	
Rubella during first trimester	Heart defects, deafness, and cataracts
Cytomegalovirus (CMV)	In first trimester: miscarriage
	In second or third trimester: microcephaly and microphthalmia
Herpes simplex	Infection before delivery: microcephaly, microphthalmia, retinal dysplasia, and mental retardation
Toxoplasma gondii (protozoal parasite)	Hydrocephalus, cerebral calcification, microphthalmia, and ocular defects
Treponema pallidum (syphilis)	Serious fetal infection, congenital deafness, and mental retardation
Hyperthermia	Congenital defects

radiation, and infectious organisms. Some agents have been identified as teratogenic after exposure to the agent resulted in an increased incidence of defects (Kenner, 1991). The limited knowledge about safety of all substances makes it prudent for women to avoid all potential teratogens before conception and during pregnancy.

Drugs and Chemicals

Drugs and chemicals account for 2 to 3 percent of congenital defects. Drugs of various classifications have been identified as being teratogenic (Kuller, 1990). Table 3–1 includes a listing of teratogenic drugs and their possible adverse effects.

REFERENCES

Baraitser, M., & Winter, R. M. (1996). *Color atlas of congenital malformation syndromes.* St. Louis: C. V. Mosby.

Kenner, C. (1991). Genetic risks and other hazards for the NICU nurse. *Neonatal Network, 10*(1), 37–40, 49–51.

Kuller, J. M. (1990). Effects on the fetus and newborn of medications commonly used during pregnancy. *Journal of Perinatal and Neonatal Nursing, 3*(4), 73–87.

CHAPTER 4

High-Risk Pregnancy

MATERNAL-FETAL UNIT

Placenta

A healthy placenta is integral to producing a well-nourished, healthy infant. The four main organ or system functions of the placenta include the following:

- Fetal lung or respiratory function for exchange of oxygen and carbon dioxide
- Fetal kidney for the metabolic side of acid–base balance, regulating the excretion of wastes and electrolyte balance
- Fetal gastrointestinal tract for storage and release of nutrients
- Fetal skin for temperature control

Circulation of essential components to and from the fetus depends on the following:

- Placental surface area and integration of villi
- Blood flow in the intervillous spaces where nutrient and waste exchange occurs
- Umbilical cord: two arteries and one vein
- Maternal cardiovascular system

Under healthy circumstances, all blood flow to the uterus and through the placenta occurs through a low-pressure system with widely dilated vessels.

Amniotic Fluid

Most of the fluid contained within the amniotic sac is initially derived from maternal blood. Later, the fetus contributes to this quantity by excreting urine into the amniotic fluid. Amniotic fluid is also normally swallowed by the fetus and absorbed into the gastrointestinal tract.

Fetal renal malfunctions may lead to less amniotic fluid, whereas gastrointestinal anomalies may cause greater amniotic fluid. Nutritional deficiencies are often associated with a smaller placenta and lower amniotic fluid volume. The most common occurrence of decreased amniotic fluid is with postterm pregnancy, in which both fetal and maternal contribution to the volume is reduced.

Amniotic fluid has a number of functions:

- Permits symmetrical growth and development
- Prevents adherence of the amnion to the embryo
- Cushions the fetus against jolts
- Helps to control fetal body temperature
- Enables fetal movement, aiding musculoskeletal development

- Protects the umbilical cord
- Provides antimicrobial protection

These functions may be impaired in the presence of oligohydramnios or polyhydramnios (Creasy & Resnik, 1994).

Maternal Nutrition

A 25 percent deficit in needed calories and protein can interfere with the synthesis of DNA. As a result, during the first 2 to 3 months of pregnancy a deficit in nutrients can have teratogenic effects or lead to spontaneous fetal loss. After 2 to 3 months, a maternal nutritional deficit can impede fetal growth, resulting in an infant who may be small for gestational age or have small brain growth.

Protein, 75 to 100 g/day, is important in supporting embryonic and fetal cell growth, in promoting necessary increased maternal blood volume, and possibly in facilitating prevention of pregnancy-induced hypertension (PIH). To prevent maternal anemia, which affects oxygenation and neonatal red blood cell mass, an adequate maternal intake of iron, folic acid, and vitamins B_6 and B_{12} is needed. Supplemental iron of at least 300 mg in maternal stores is necessary for the fetus to draw upon.

During pregnancy, the diet should contain 30 to 50 mg/day of zinc. Zinc is found in such foods as nuts, meats, whole grains, legumes, and dairy products. A deficiency of zinc during pregnancy increases the risk of premature rupture of membranes and preterm labor.

Restricted sodium intake of less than 2.5 g/24 hr can impede adequate maternal blood volume increase, which, in turn, can activate the renin-angiotensin-aldosterone cycle and lead to vasoconstriction. Excess sodium intake can also cause vasoconstriction through an increased sensitivity of the blood vessel wall to angiotensin.

To meet the growing needs of the fetus for maternal storage of fat and protein, there should be an increase of 300 to 500 calories per day above normal caloric requirements. The formation and storage of fat and lean body tissue act as a reserve for the fetus during the last part of pregnancy, as well as provide an energy source for labor, delivery, and lactation. Social habits such as alcohol intake, smoking, and drug abuse interfere with adequate absorption of nutrients in the fetus and the mother.

MATERNAL HEALTH AND EFFECTS ON THE FETUS

Postterm Pregnancy

INCIDENCE

Postmaturity in the fetus is the second leading cause of intrapartum asphyxia. Approximately 10 percent of all pregnancies continue 14 or more days beyond term. Of these, 20 to 40 percent result in postmature neonates with a perinatal mortality rate three times that of term newborns. Mortality rates show that 35 percent of the deaths occur antepartum, 47 percent intrapartum, and 18 percent in the neonatal period (Creasy & Resnik, 1994).

ETIOLOGY

The postmature neonate is affected because of some degree of placental insufficiency. The actual onset of labor appears to be explained by alterations in estrogen:progesterone ratios, which ultimately release prostaglandins from the uterine muscle through contractions. Prostaglandins, in turn, pave the way for oxytocin to increase the intensity of the contractions. Maternal oxytocin is released because of stimulation from increased mature fetal adrenocortical activity (Gilbert & Harmon, 1997).

PATHOPHYSIOLOGY

After 36 weeks' gestation, the placenta begins to age by laying down fibrinoid material on the surface of the villi. By 42 weeks, the available surface area of the placenta for oxygen and carbon dioxide exchange diminishes. In addition, a decreased quantity of amniotic fluid is formed by diminished maternal blood flow. Thus, the fetus is at risk for both uteroplacental insufficiency and cord entrapment (Gilbert & Harmon, 1997).

SIGNS AND SYMPTOMS

Signs and symptoms of postterm pregnancy include the following:

- Maternal weight loss of greater than 2 lb/wk
- Oligohydramnios of less than 300 ml
- Meconium-stained amniotic fluid
- Advanced bony maturation of fetal head
- Prolonged labor (Gilbert & Harmon, 1997)

FETAL AND NEONATAL EFFECTS

A postterm pregnancy may affect the fetus or neonate in several ways:

- Failure of growth
- Dehydration
- Dry, cracked, wrinkled, parchment-like skin
- Long, thin arms and legs
- Advanced hardness of the skull
- Absence of vernix and lanugo
- Skin maceration, especially in folds
- Brownish green skin discoloration
- Increased appearance of alertness

ANTEPARTUM COMPLICATIONS

When antepartum complications are noted, they may include any of the following:

- Failure of growth
- Cord accident
- Hypoxia manifested by decreased fetal movement, late deceleration

with contraction stress testing, or absent long- and short-term variability on fetal heart rate (FHR) monitoring strips

INTRAPARTUM COMPLICATIONS

Intrapartum complications may also occur:

- Increased cesarean birth rate due to lack of cephalic molding and high arrest of fetal head or to fetal response to labor stressors
- Intrauterine fetal hypoxia due to placental insufficiency or cord compression
- Traumatic vaginal birth

TREATMENT

At between 40 and 42 completed weeks of gestation, decisions regarding intervention in the pregnancy should be made. If the physician or midwife and the pregnant woman elect to continue the pregnancy and await the onset of labor, antepartum FHR monitoring is ordered. FHR monitoring may be done with biweekly nonstress tests, contraction stress tests, amniotic fluid volume indices, biophysical profiles, or some combination of these tests.

The medical management also includes decisions regarding delivery time and route. With careful antepartum FHR monitoring and a fetus who is continuing to show well-being in utero, the pregnancy can continue uninterrupted until 42 weeks. At that time, a trial induction is usually opted for so that advanced rapid placental aging is less likely to affect the outcome adversely. Induction of labor is usually either preceded by prostaglandin gel ripening of the cervix or done immediately with an oxytocin drip. Careful FHR and maternal monitoring during the intrapartum period improves the outcome, but a cesarean birth is more likely if the fetus does not tolerate labor or if the mother does not progress in labor (Creasy & Resnik, 1994).

NURSING MANAGEMENT

Assessment

The nurse should perform the following:

- Note first day of last menstrual period.
- Ask if conception was preceded by normal menses.
- Review ultrasonogram dated before 20 weeks' gestation.
- Ask if first fetal movement was felt between 18 and 20 weeks' gestation.
- Perform Doptone FHR monitoring at 12 to 13 weeks and fetoscope FHR monitoring at 18 to 19 weeks.
- Note that fundal height growth rates at 22 weeks do not vary by 3 cm or more from the number of weeks of gestation.

Signs and symptoms of increased risk are listed below:

- Previous postterm delivery
- Previous cesarean birth for failure to progress
- Previous unexplained stillbirth before estimated date of confinement. The nurse should begin this reassessment before 40 weeks' gestation

- Decreased fetal movement in patient doing daily counts
- Maternal weight loss greater than 2 to 3 lb in 1 week without identified cause
- Hard, bony fetal head palpated at symphysis with no early cervical changes

The nurse should evaluate and educate the pregnant woman according to needs for fetal movement daily counts. Usually four kicks per hour is adequate. FHR monitoring needs to be explained. The purpose of challenging fetal well-being should be understood, as well as interpretation of good, bad, and equivocal results. The patient should be prepared for the potential of a cesarean birth.

Intrapartum care should include the following:

- Review of all dating information and general health history
- Knowledge about any FHR monitoring results
- Fundal height evaluation with position and engagement and Leopold's maneuver to estimate fetal size, presentation, and position
- Careful electronic FHR monitoring or intermittent auscultation to rule out FHR patterns of cord compression or insufficient uteroplacental transfer of oxygen
- If nonreassuring patterns are identified, prompt independent treatment is expected by the nurse and should include the following:
  - Turning patient to left side or side to side
  - Improving maternal circulating volume with intravenous fluid challenge (usually with lactated Ringer's solution)
  - Discontinuing labor stimulation, if used
  - Administering oxygen at 8 to 10 L by face mask
  - Notifying physician or nurse-midwife
  - Preparing for expeditious delivery if not improved within 30 minutes
  - Having suction equipment available if meconium is present

Preterm Delivery

INCIDENCE

Preterm delivery occurs in 8 to 10 percent of all live births in the United States. Despite current therapies for halting preterm labor, this incidence has remained unchanged for the past 25 years. Preterm delivery accounts for 75 to 80 percent of all neonatal morbidity and mortality (Gilbert & Harmon, 1997).

ETIOLOGY

The exact cause is unknown. Risk factors fall into four main categories:

- Past medical and pregnancy history, including the following factors:
  - Maternal diabetes, hypertension, renal disease, heart disease, systemic lupus erythematosus
  - More than two spontaneous or elective abortions
  - Previous preterm labor or delivery or both (increases the likelihood of repetitive preterm labor or delivery or both by 40 percent)

- Diethylstilbestrol exposure
- Uterine anomalies
- Current pregnancy:
  - Abruptio placentae
  - Placenta previa
  - Preeclampsia or PIH
  - Multiple gestation
  - Urinary tract infection
  - Febrile illness
  - Abdominal or cervical surgery
  - Small stature or weight (<5 feet or <100 lb)
- Socioeconomic factors:
  - Employment outside the home
  - Less than 12th grade education
  - Single mother
  - Younger than 17 or older than 39 years
  - Late prenatal care
  - Poor nutritional resources
  - Two or more toddlers in the home
- Daily habits and lifestyle (Gilbert & Harmon, 1997):
  - Smoking more than a half of a pack of cigarettes per day
  - Substance use and abuse (e.g., nicotine, alcohol, cocaine, heroin)
  - Long commute to health care or work
  - Inadequate rest during the day
  - Poor nutritional habits

PATHOPHYSIOLOGY

Preterm events that may trigger preterm labor are listed below:

- Increased estrogen in relation to progesterone
- Increased stretch of uterine muscle, leading to release of arachidonic acid
- Fetal stress, leading to increased fetal cortisol
- Increased amounts of prostaglandins
- Increased maternal oxytocin (Gilbert & Harmon, 1997)

SIGNS AND SYMPTOMS

The definition of preterm labor consists of the following occurrences between 20 and 37 weeks of gestation:

- Painless or uncomfortable contractions
- More than four contractions per hour
- Contractions greater than 30 seconds in duration
- Contractions leading to cervical changes

The signs and symptoms may include the following:

- Low abdominal cramping or pressure
- Rhythmic "tightening" and relaxation of the abdomen
- Low backache

- Tingling down the thighs
- Increase in or "watery" vaginal discharge
- Brownish or pink vaginal discharge
- Diarrhea with or without abdominal cramping
- "Feeling bad" (Gilbert & Harmon, 1997)

TREATMENT

Preterm labor requires immediate attention to avert preterm delivery, especially before 32 weeks' gestation, because prematurity is responsible for significant neonatal morbidity and mortality. The following therapeutic modalities are included in the treatment of preterm labor.

Drugs used as labor suppressants include magnesium sulfate ($MgSO_4$); beta-sympathomimetics (terbutaline, ritodrine); prostaglandin inhibitors (indomethacin, ibuprofen); and calcium channel blockers. The first two agents are accepted methods of halting labor; the last two are experimental. All appear to be effective if signs and symptoms are detected, reported, and responded to in early stages of preterm labor.

Adjunct treatment includes cervical cerclage and early bed rest or restricted activities. Home uterine contraction monitors or terbutaline pumps for subcutaneous infusion therapy are also effective if augmented with professional nursing care and education of the client (*Obstetrics & Gynecology* Supplement, 1990)

Cortisol has also been administered as an adjunct when successful halting of labor is doubtful. It is theorized that at between 28 and 32 weeks' gestation, cortisol stimulates a cascade of events that stabilizes lecithin, stimulating production of fetal surfactant and therefore promoting lung function. Cortisol has been widely researched, with diverse opinions about its efficacy (Creasy & Resnik, 1994; *Obstetrics & Gynecology* Supplement, 1990).

Patient education is central to early detection and halting the preterm labor. Nurses should do the following:

- Implement creative programs that meet the needs of the population being served for both accessibility and acceptability.
- Systematically screen all pregnant women for the previously discussed risk factors.
- Educate all pregnant women about the physical signs of preterm contractions and how to use their hands to self-detect rhythmic abdominal tightening.
- Instruct and encourage women's self-advocacy when reporting self-detected signs and symptoms of preterm labor (Gilbert & Harmon, 1997; *Obstetrics & Gynecology* Supplement, 1990).

Third-Trimester Bleeding

The two major sources of third-trimester bleeding are placental adherence and an implantation problem. These may result in placental abruption or placenta previa.

ETIOLOGY

The actual cause of placental abruption is unknown. Conditions associated with abruption are listed here:

- PIH or chronic hypertension, present in 4 percent
- Maternal age older than 35 years
- Multiparity greater than five pregnancies
- Previous abruption: 10 percent increased risk after one abruption, and 25 percent increased risk after two abruptions
- Trauma from a direct blow to the abdomen or needle puncture during an amniocentesis
- Short umbilical cord
- Folic acid deficiency
- Cigarette smoking, cocaine use, and polysubstance abuse, causing vasoconstriction of spiral arterioles and leading to decidual necrosis

The cause of placenta previa is also unknown. Predisposing factors include the following:

- Abortion
- Cesarean birth
- Increased parity
- Prior previa
- Uterine infection
- Closely spaced pregnancies
- Uterine tumors
- Multiple pregnancy
- Maternal age older than 35 years

PATHOPHYSIOLOGY

Theoretically, abruption of the placenta is believed to occur when the spiral arterioles, which nourish the decidua (endometrium) and the placenta, begin the process of degeneration. As necrosis takes place, the blood vessels rupture and bleed into the site, leading to separation of the placenta as pressure of the bleeding increases. Abruption may occur at the marginal edges of the placenta, outward to the edges. An abruption is classified, by the quantity of the surface involved, as mild (less than 15 percent), moderate (15 to 60 percent), or severe (greater than 60 percent) (Creasy & Resnik, 1994; Gilbert & Harmon, 1997).

SIGNS AND SYMPTOMS

Signs and symptoms of placental abruption include the following:

- Uterine tenderness or rigidity and low back pain
- Dark-red vaginal bleeding
- Fetal symptoms of stress
- Maternal signs of shock and disseminated intravascular coagulation (DIC)

Signs and symptoms of previa rarely occur before the early third trimester. The initial onset of symptoms is usually mild, and their recurrence is unpredictable. The signs and symptoms of placenta previa are listed below:

- Painless bleeding, usually bright red and initially slight in amount
- High presenting fetal part
- Subsequent recurrences of bleeding in increasingly significant amounts and associated signs of fetal stress (Gilbert & Harmon, 1997)

FETAL AND NEONATAL EFFECTS

The major effects of third-trimester bleeding on the fetus are related to inadequate oxygen–carbon dioxide exchange by means of the placenta, the potential maternal imperative for premature delivery, or a combination of factors (Gilbert & Harmon, 1997).

TREATMENT

Treatment of abruptio placentae or placenta previa depends on three major factors: severity of blood loss, fetal maturity, and fetal well-being. When bleeding is mild and ceases readily and the fetus is immature without evidence of being distressed, expectant management is chosen. This care plan includes the following (Creasy & Resnik, 1994):

- Hospitalization; bed rest for at least 72 hours
- Close observation for bleeding
- Continuous FHR monitoring
- Maternal red blood cell replacement as necessary
- No maternal vaginal examinations
  - Preparation for cesarean birth; vaginal birth is not safe for mother or infant in the presence of continual abruption or partial or complete previa
  - Discharge to home, undelivered, only if bleeding subsides and ceases, or, if previa is present, it is incomplete; instructions given for bed rest with restricted activity and preterm labor prevention

Fetal maturity needs to be assessed to determine the risk:benefit ratio of prolonging the pregnancy with a compromised uteroplacental unit. If fetal well-being is compromised by maternal bleeding, emergency cesarean section is indicated.

NURSING MANAGEMENT

Assessment

- Provide risk screening in early prenatal care.
- Monitor FHR for presence, absence, or compromise of fetal well-being in the presence of maternal bleeding.
- Visually inspect and quantify maternal blood loss.
- Be aware that any rapid change in fundal height or maternal vital signs or both is associated with abdominal or back pain.

Intervention

- If bleeding is life-threatening to mother or distressing to fetus or both, prepare for emergent delivery, usually by cesarean birth.
- If management is expectant, educate mother for prevention of preterm labor.
- Prepare parents for potential preterm delivery.

Hypertensive Disorders of Pregnancy

The Committee on Terminology of the American College of Obstetricians and Gynecologists has developed a classification of the various hypertensive states in pregnancy:

- PIH
- Gestational hypertension: development of hypertension after 20 weeks' gestation without proteinuria; blood pressure normotensive within 10 postpartum days
- Preeclampsia: development of hypertension with or without edema after 20 weeks' gestation or early post partum
- Eclampsia: development of convulsions or coma in a preeclamptic patient
- Superimposed preeclampsia or eclampsia in a patient with chronic hypertension
- Concurrent hypertension and pregnancy: chronic hypertension—hypertension that develops before pregnancy or before 20 weeks' gestation and is not pregnancy associated
- HELLP syndrome—a complex of symptoms described as a severe forerunner of PIH that has a sudden onset and is diagnosed from signs and symptoms of *h*emolysis, *e*levated *l*iver enzymes, and *l*ow *p*latelets

RISK FACTORS

Risk factors for a hypertensive disorder include the following (Gilbert & Harmon, 1997):

- First pregnancy
- Lower socioeconomic group
- Family history
- Diabetes
- Multiple gestation
- Polyhydramnios
- Persistent hypertension
- Hydatidiform mole
- RH incompatibility

ETIOLOGY

The etiology is largely unknown. Four theories are widely accepted as associated with PIH: nutritional deficiency, immunologic deficiency, genetics, and uterine ischemia.

PATHOPHYSIOLOGY

In PIH disorders there is an increased vascular sensitivity to angiotensin II. This increased sensitivity occurs before the onset of hypertension. When the normal pregnancy resistance to angiotensin II is lost, blood vessel spasms occur, causing vasoconstriction and a rise in blood pressure.

Blood flow to most organs is decreased, especially to the uterus, placenta, kidneys, liver, and brain, impairing their function by 40 to 60 percent. Impaired blood flow results in pathophysiologic changes (Creasy & Resnik, 1994):

- Decreased uterine and placental blood flow, resulting in premature, exaggerated degeneration of the placenta. Uterine activity is increased.
- Decreased blood supply to the kidney and reduced glomerular filtration rate, causing degenerative changes in the glomerulus, which result in the following:
  - Sodium and water retention
  - Decreased serum albumin and decreased plasma colloid osmotic pressure
  - Fluid shifts and generalized edema
- Decreased blood supply to the liver, impairing liver function
- Decreased blood supply to the eyes, with retinal arteriolar spasms and blurred vision
- Loss of fluid from blood vessels in the brain, leading to cerebral edema and hemorrhages
- Damage to blood vessel wall, occurring with progression of the disease. Platelets, fibrinogen, immunoglobulin, and components of complement are deposited at the damaged sites, and DIC occurs.

SIGNS AND SYMPTOMS

Two cardinal signs of PIH are (1) proteinuria and blood pressure of 140/90 mm Hg or greater on two occasions within 6 hours and (2) an increase of 50 mm Hg systolic or 15 mm Hg diastolic or both over the baseline blood pressure (Gilbert & Harmon, 1997).

FETAL AND NEONATAL EFFECTS

Perinatal mortality related to PIH ranges from 1 to 8 percent and, if allowed to progress to eclampsia or HELLP syndrome, to as high as 35 percent. The majority of perinatal losses are directly related to placental insufficiency, resulting in intrauterine fetal demise or early neonatal death in an already compromised premature infant.

Placental insufficiency in PIH usually leads to some degree of nutritional intrauterine growth retardation. The fetus is asymmetrically affected, in that head size is close to normal for gestation but general body size and fat deposition are decreased. This nutritional deprivation causes the fetus to be more vulnerable to the effects of labor contractions and other stressors. During antepartum or intrapartum monitoring, the fetus is more likely to show signs of fetal stress when oxygen and carbon dioxide exchange is mildly compromised over a shorter period of time.

The growth-retarded fetus is more often associated with decreased amounts of amniotic fluid as well. Any repetitive occlusion of the umbilical cord during contractions, or with fetal movement, may cause stress. Signs of fetal stress evident on FHR monitoring may include the following (Gilbert & Harmon, 1997):

- Tachycardia: rate above 160 beats per minute, or more than 20 beats per minute rise from previous baseline value
- Absence of long- or short-term variability
- Late decelerations with or without cord compression (variable decelerations), tachycardia, or absent long- or short-term variability

TREATMENT

The only cure for PIH is delivery. The risk of deteriorating maternal status must be weighed against the risk of prematurity.

Antepartum treatment is directed at improving maternal status to gain gestational time for the fetus. Treatment consists of the following (Creasy & Resnik, 1994):

- Pharmacologic treatment of maternal hypertension with drugs such as hydralazine, alpha-methyldopa, clonidine, or sodium nitroprusside
- Intermittent evaluation of fetal well-being through contraction stress or nonstress tests or biophysical profiles
- Ultrasound evaluation for growth of fetus every 2 to 3 weeks
- High-protein maternal diet (more than 100 g/day)
- Monitoring of maternal laboratory studies (i.e., uric acid, platelets, liver enzymes) and clinical signs for worsening disease

Diuretics and severe sodium restriction have no place in the treatment of PIH and, in fact, may worsen the disease. Likewise, long-term expectant management is not likely to result in improved maternal or fetal status and is therefore not practiced in most centers (Creasy & Resnik, 1994).

Intrapartum treatment is aimed at obtaining and maintaining immediate stabilization of the mother and then delivering the premature or mature fetus. Stabilization consists of the following (Creasy & Resnik, 1994):

- Pharmacologic therapy for prevention of central nervous system irritability with intravenous magnesium sulfate and treatment of maternal hypertension above 160/100 mm Hg with hydralazine or other fast-acting antihypertensive agents
- Plasma volume expanders, which may be used as a temporary therapy
- A delivery route based on whether labor can be induced (cervical ripening), gestation of the fetus, and fetal tolerance to stress of labor. A surgical delivery may not be safe for a woman with signs of DIC or HELLP syndrome because of the potential for hemorrhage. On the other hand, continuing the pregnancy through labor may not be tolerated by the fetus or may progress to eclampsia in the mother with HELLP syndrome because of diminished clotting factors; epidural anesthesia may be contraindicated because of increased potential epidural space bleeding. Therefore, a surgical delivery with general anesthesia is the best choice.

NURSING MANAGEMENT

Assessment

- Fetal: monitor for signs of fetal stress intermittently antepartum with contraction stress tests or nonstress tests or continuously during intrapartum period.
- Maternal: monitor blood pressure and laboratory studies.

Intervention

- Treat signs of fetal stress with maternal bed rest in left lateral position. Provide oxygen therapy and prevent volume depletion.
- Administer antihypertensive agents intravenously only in conjunction with continuous FHR monitoring.
- Educate pregnant women identified at risk for developing PIH to recognize and report early signs and symptoms.

Diabetes in Pregnancy

White's classification system is used primarily to make decisions for timing fetal surveillance and to evaluate for maternal complications:

Class A_1: gestational onset, normal fasting blood sugar; requires diet control.

Class A_2: gestational onset, abnormal fasting blood sugar; requires insulin therapy.

Class B: onset after age 20; requires insulin therapy.

Class C: onset after age 10, less than 10 years' duration, no vascular complications; requires insulin therapy.

Class D: onset before age 10 or greater than 10 years' duration or early vascular complications; requires insulin therapy.

Class F: renal changes; requires insulin therapy.

Class R: renal and retinal changes; requires insulin therapy.

Class H: heart complications, often older than age 35 with early-age onset of diabetes, 50 percent obstetrical maternal mortality; requires insulin therapy.

Class T: postrenal transplant; requires insulin therapy.

INCIDENCE

Diabetes exists in 1 to 2 percent of all pregnancies. Women can readily be screened for gestational onset with a 50-g glucola load and a blood glucose study done 1 hour later. Levels above 120 to 140 mg/dl are then evaluated for the requirement of insulin with a 3-hour glucose tolerance test that has two or more abnormal results or when fasting blood glucose levels rise above 110 mg/dl while treated by altering the diet.

ETIOLOGY

Diabetes exists when insufficient amounts of effective insulin are produced by the beta cells in the islets of Langerhans in the pancreas. Pregnancy has been likened to a diabetogenic state because of increases in metabolism of protein, fat, and carbohydrate, requiring additional insulin. The increased production of estrogen, progesterone, human placental lactogen, and cortisol produces an antagonistic effect on insulin that is produced or taken exogenously. Women at risk for developing gestational-onset diabetes have the following characteristics (Gilbert & Harmon, 1997):

- Age older than 35 years
- Chronic hypertension
- Obesity
- Multiparity with a previous unexplained stillbirth; more than two or three spontaneous miscarriages; a previous macrosomic infant, especially if larger than 9 lb, at term
- Women with strong, positive family history of diabetes or history of frequent vaginal candidal infections or current history of glucosuria

FETAL AND NEONATAL EFFECTS

The following fetal effects are possible:

- Interference with DNA-RNA transfer as a result of maternal high blood glucose level before and at the time of conception.
- Increased, rapid fetal body growth
- Decreased fetal brain growth
- Decreased fetal body growth

The following neonatal effects occur (Creasy & Resnik, 1994; Gilbert & Harmon, 1997):

- Hypoglycemia in the transitional period because of high insulin production and loss of maternal glucose supply
- Hyperbilirubinemia from increased "sugar"-coated fetal hemoglobin and breakdown of this in the early neonatal period
- Hypercalcemia, hypokalemia, and other abnormalities in electrolytes
- Increased incidence of cesarean birth
- Increased incidence of traumatic vaginal birth, usually from shoulder dystocias
- Neonatal respiratory distress syndrome even after 36 weeks. High maternal blood glucose level, high placental glucose storage, high placental production of cortisol, low fetal production of cortisol, and low surfactant production leading to decreased lung maturity at expected gestation

TREATMENT

Treatment of a pregnancy complicated by diabetes includes the following:

- Maintenance of euglycemia before conception and throughout the entire pregnancy through diet, insulin administration, and regular activity
- Careful evaluation of maternal estimated date of delivery
- Early maternal evaluation for diabetic vascular complications in insulin-requiring diabetes may include glycosylated hemoglobin, 24-hour urine

evaluation for protein and creatinine, recent eye examination, and electrocardiogram

Antepartum fetal surveillance includes the following:

- Maternal serum alpha-fetoprotein to screen for neural tube defects
- Ultrasonic evaluation between 15 and 20 weeks' gestation for congenital developmental problems
- Ultrasonic evaluation for growth rate, usually between 26 and 30 weeks' gestation and near to expected delivery (37 to 38 weeks)
- Amniocentesis for fetal lung maturity at the time of the last ultrasonic evaluation
- Fetal movement counts daily, biweekly nonstress tests, weekly contraction stress tests, weekly ultrasound biophysical profile evaluation, or some combination of testing weekly. These may begin anytime before 38 weeks and after 25 weeks, depending on fetal risk and maternal complications.

Intrapartum management includes the following:

- Insulin drip for an insulin-requiring labor patient
- Continuous FHR monitoring to detect onset of signs of fetal stress

NURSING MANAGEMENT

Antepartum Assessment

- Provide patient education.
- Assess fetus with evaluation of fetal movement counts, nonstress tests, or contraction stress tests.
- Check for maternal complications of polyhydramnios, PIH, urinary tract infections, or preterm labor, or abnormal persistent blood glucose levels.

Antepartum Intervention

- Educate the pregnant woman and her support system for the following:
  - Dietary management
  - Blood glucose determination four to six times daily
  - Insulin injections and changes in dose
  - Activity schedule and modification
  - Effects of diabetes and pregnancy on self and fetus
- Explain reason for testing for maternal and fetal complications.
- Provide support and assistance with time management and financial stressors from increased testing.

Cardiac Disease and Pregnancy

Cardiac disease has four classifications:

Class I: asymptomatic
Class II: symptomatic with increased exercise
Class III: symptomatic with normal exercise
Class IV: symptomatic at rest

Although the classification does not increase with pregnancy, the increased workload on the heart may increase symptoms by one or two classifications (Gilbert & Harmon, 1997).

INCIDENCE

The incidence of cardiac disease in pregnancy varies from 0.5 to 2.0 percent. Rheumatic fever is responsible for about 50 percent, and congenital heart disease in the mother is responsible for the other half.

ETIOLOGY

Cardiac disease in pregnancy may take one of several forms: rheumatic fever, valve deformities, congenital heart disease, congestive cardiomyopathies, or cardiac dysrhythmias. Several conditions may predispose a pregnant women to a greater than 50 percent maternal mortality rate: Marfan's syndrome with aortic arch dissection, primary pulmonary hypertension or Eisenmenger's syndrome, and diabetes complicated by heart disease.

During pregnancy, the heart of a pregnant woman complicated by heart disease may be unable to respond efficiently to the increased circulating volume. As blood is shunted to essential organs for the mother, it may bypass the growing uterus, placenta, intervillous space, and, thus, the fetus to some extent.

FETAL AND NEONATAL EFFECTS

Antenatal effects of decreased maternal placental blood flow include the following:

- Diminished fetal body growth
- Diminished brain growth
- Higher incidence of fetal wastage and pregnancy loss

During the intrapartum period the following may occur:

- Signs of fetal stress during labor may include deceleration patterns such as late decelerations because of insufficient uteroplacental blood flow or variable decelerations because of insufficient amniotic fluid to protect the umbilical cord from compression.

The following effects may be noted in the neonate:

- An increased rate of prematurity occurs if the neonate was delivered early for maternal reasons.
- If maternal congenital heart disease is present, there is also an increased risk of fetal congenital heart abnormalities.

FETAL ASSESSMENT

Antepartum Assessment

- Perform ultrasonography for growth rate.
- Perform nonstress or contraction stress tests, biophysical profiles, or

some combination of these on a weekly or biweekly basis after 26 weeks' gestation.

- Prevent development of associated maternal complications, such as anemia or severe preeclampsia, that might further compromise fetal well-being.

Intrapartum Assessment

- Carefully monitor labor for problems with maternal cardiac preload or afterload, often with central-line hemodynamic invasive monitoring.
- Provide continuous FHR monitoring, often with the pregnant woman on her left side with oxygen therapy.
- Shorten and assist with second stage of labor, usually with epidural anesthesia or analgesia to reduce pain and cardiac workload as well as preload (Hodnet, 1996; Lowe, 1996).

Urinary Tract Disease in Pregnancy

INCIDENCE

Urinary tract infections (UTIs) occur in 4 to 7.5 percent of childbearing women. Approximately 30 percent of pregnant women with untreated asymptomatic bacteriuria develop pyelonephritis during pregnancy.

PATHOPHYSIOLOGY

Escherichia coli, staphylococci, and streptococci are the common causative agents of UTIs. The inflammation occurring in bladder or renal tissue may result in fever and increased prostaglandin production. Increase in prostaglandin production predisposes a pregnant woman to preterm labor and thus the fetus to preterm delivery. If maternal sepsis occurs, fetal fever and potential infection from amnionitis often occur.

UTIs and fever must be treated with appropriate antibiotics therapeutically, prophylactically, or both. Renal disease is rare. Treatment of renal disease, which may temporarily worsen in pregnancy in response to increased renal blood flow and work, is usually aimed at clearing maternal blood of ureal wastes.

NURSING MANAGEMENT

Management is aimed at prevention of infection, of reinfection, and of preterm labor. This is best accomplished through prenatal education regarding the need for the following:

- Increased oral fluids to 6 to 8 oz per waking hour
- Perineal hygiene, cleaning front to back and urinating after intercourse
- Recognition of early signs of preterm labor
- Reporting of early signs of infection and preterm labor

REFERENCES

Creasy, R., & Resnik, M. (1994). *Maternal-fetal medicine: Principles and practice* (3rd ed.). Philadelphia: W. B. Saunders.

Gilbert, E., & Harmon, J. (1997). *Manual of high risk pregnancy and delivery* (2nd ed.). St. Louis: C. V. Mosby.

Hodnet, E. (1996). Nursing support of the laboring woman. *JOGNN, Journal of Obstretric, Gynecologic, and Neonatal Nursing, 25*(3), 257–264.

Lowe, N. K. (1996). The pain and discomfort of labor and birth. *JOGNN, Journal of Obstetric, Gynecologic, and Neonatal Nursing 25*(1), 82–92.

Obstetrics and Gynecology Supplement. (1990). 76(1).

The Intrapartal Environment: Maternal-Child Interactions

• •

CHAPTER 5

Resuscitation and Stabilization of the Neonate

ASPHYXIA

Asphyxia occurs when the organ of gas exchange fails or is prevented from carrying out its function. For the fetus, that organ is the placenta; for the neonate, it is the lungs. When the fetus or neonate becomes asphyxiated, the immediate consequence is progressive hypoxia and hypercarbia with mixed (metabolic + respiratory) acidosis.

The well-defined sequence of events is depicted in Figure 5–1.

Shortly after the onset of asphyxia, these physiologic changes occur:

- Rapid gasping begins. If the gasping does not relieve the asphyxia within about a minute, all respiratory activity ceases (primary apnea).
- Thrashing of the extremities occurs.
- The heart rate is briefly elevated.
- The heart rate begins to fall.
- The episode lasts about 60 seconds and is followed by a series of spontaneous deep gasps.

If the asphyxia persists, then the following occur (Banagale & Donn, 1986):

- The gasping respirations become progressively weaker.
- Respirations stop completely after 4 to 5 minutes.

45

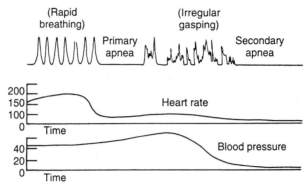

FIGURE 5–1. Effect of asphyxia on breathing, heart rate, and blood pressure. (From Bloom, R. S., & Cropley, C. [1994]. *Textbook of neonatal resuscitation*. Elk Grove Village, IL: American Academy of Pediatrics and American Heart Association. Reprinted with permission.)

- Secondary apnea (or terminal apnea) follows the last gasp and begins about 8 minutes after the anoxic event began.
- Heart rate continues to fall.
- Hypotension develops.
- If the asphyxia is not reversed within several minutes, extensive organ damage and, ultimately, death occur.

The passage of meconium in utero is estimated to occur in 10 to 15 percent of all fetuses and is considered a marker of antepartum or intrapartum asphyxia. It can lead to meconium-stained amniotic fluid and meconium aspiration.

Preventive Measures

Measures to prevent asphyxia include the following:

- Ongoing monitoring of the fetal status (by heart rate monitoring, scalp pH, or the observation of meconium)
- Expeditious delivery, once asphyxia has been identified
- Treatment for secondary apnea of all who are apneic or demonstrate evidence of cardiorespiratory depression (because it is difficult to distinguish between primary and secondary apnea) and urgent provision of resuscitative care
- Stimulation and supplemental oxygen

If the asphyxia is truly secondary apnea, the event has been long enough to result in central nervous system involvement. The patient is hyporeflexive and hypotonic and is unresponsive to stimulation alone and may require ventilation and aggressive therapy to maintain or improve cardiorespiratory function.

Urgency of intervention cannot be overstressed. Consequently, any event that causes delayed onset of respiration can potentially lead to hypoxia, hypercarbia, and acidosis. Under these circumstances, the pulmonary vasculature will remain constricted and the pulmonary vascular resistance will remain high, which, in turn, may cause a return to right-to-left shunting across the foramen ovale and ductus arteriosus.

CARDIORESPIRATORY DEPRESSION IN THE NEWBORN

The causes of cardiorespiratory depression in the newborn are listed in Table 5–1. Some arise during the intrapartum period (e.g., cord prolapse), but most occur during gestation (e.g., placenta previa) or even before conception (e.g., maternal diabetes). Each can become manifest as neonatal cardiorespiratory depression.

TABLE 5–1. Conditions Associated With Asphyxiation of Newborns

Site or Source of Problem	Conditions
Maternal	Amnionitis
	Anemia
	Diabetes
	Pregnancy-induced hypertension
	Heart disease
	Hypotension
	Respiratory disease
	Maternal genetic
	Drugs
	Infection
	Maternal deformities
Uterine	Preterm labor
	Prolonged labor
	Multiple pregnancies
	Abnormal fetal presentations
Placental	Placenta previa
	Abruptio placentae
	Placental insufficiency
	Postterm pregnancy
Umbilical	Cord prolapse
	Cord entanglement
	Compression
Fetal	Cephalopelvic disproportion
	Congenital abnormalities
	Erythroblastosis fetalis
	Iatrogenic:
	Mechanical
	Difficult forceps delivery
	Drugs
	Intrauterine infection

The mnemonic TAMMSS can be used as a simple but effective way of remembering these etiologic groups:

T—Trauma
A—Asphyxia (intrauterine)
M—Medication
M—Malformation
S—Sepsis
S—Shock (hypovolemia)

Trauma

Traumatic injury to the central or peripheral nervous system can result in either immediate or delayed respiratory depression.

Asphyxia (Intrauterine)

Of all the categories, the most common cause of cardiorespiratory depression at birth is fetal hypoxia and asphyxia. Any condition that reduces oxygen delivery to the fetus may be at fault. These factors are listed below:

- Maternal hypoxia (e.g., due to hypoventilation or hyperventilation, respiratory or heart disease, anemia, postural hypotension)
- Maternal vascular disease causing placental insufficiency (e.g., pre-existing or pregnancy-induced diabetes, primary or pregnancy-induced hypertension)
- Accidents involving the umbilical cord (compression, entanglement, or prolapse)
- Postterm pregnancies due to placental aging and progressive placental insufficiency

Medication

Pharmacologic agents given to the mother during the intrapartum period may affect the fetus both directly and indirectly. Indirectly, these agents may cause maternal hypoventilation, hypotension, and/or adversely effect placental perfusion. Some effects include those listed here:

- Hypnotic, analgesic, or anesthetic drugs may depress maternal respirations, resulting in reduced oxygen intake and delivery to the tissues and organs, including the uterus and placenta.
- Anesthetic agents, because of their effect on the sympathetic nervous system, may also cause peripheral vasodilation, decreased cardiac output, and hypotension with decreased placental perfusion.
- Pitocin may cause uterine hyperstimulation and reduced placental perfusion time.
- Narcotic analgesics rapidly cross the placenta and may directly depress neonatal respiratory drive.

Malformations

Malformations that may cause cardiorespiratory depression include the following:

- Congenital anomalies causing most concern during the first few minutes of life are those with associated facial or upper airway deformities and conditions leading to pulmonary hypoplasia. Suspicion should be raised if oligohydramnios or polyhydramnios is reported.
- Oligohydramnios is seen with prolonged rupture or leaking of membranes and in infants with renal agenesis or dysplasia or urethral obstruction. If fluid is lost or diminished, fetal structures may be compressed, leading to micrognathia or pulmonary hypoplasia.
- Polyhydramnios is associated with impaired swallowing ability (e.g., anencephaly and neuromuscular disorders); with real or functional obstruction high in the gastrointestinal trachea (e.g., esophageal atresia); with the leakage of large amounts of cerebrospinal fluid, which contributes to the volume of amniotic fluid (neural tube defects); with diaphragmatic hernia; and with hydrops fetalis.

Sepsis

The fetus may acquire bacterial or viral agents from infected amniotic fluid, from maternal blood crossing the placenta, or by direct contact on passage through the birth canal. Premature infants (who are relatively immunocompromised) and those with premature rupture of membranes or maternal history of infection or chorioamnionitis are especially prone to sepsis. If infection is acquired in utero, the lungs tend to be heavily involved and the alveoli may be filled with exudate. The infant may be apneic at birth or slow to establish a spontaneous and regular breathing pattern or may exhibit frank signs of respiratory distress.

Shock (Hypovolemia)

Most of the blood lost during delivery is from the maternal side of the placenta and of no consequence to the newborn. Blood lost from the fetal side of the placenta due to abruptio placentae or placenta previa can lead to acute hypovolemia and cardiovascular collapse. Whereas the normal umbilical cord is unusually strong, ruptures are possible if cord tension is suddenly increased (e.g., precipitous delivery) or if the vessels are superficially implanted into the placenta (velamentous insertions). Rarely, acute hypovolemia may occur without frank hemorrhage. With severe cord compression, for instance, the umbilical cord is compressed and blood flow to the fetus is impeded. The umbilical arteries, however, are much more resistant to compression and continue to pump blood back to the placenta. The effects of hypovolemia and asphyxia may be superimposed. Infants with chronic blood loss (e.g., fetal-to-maternal hemorrhage, twin-to-twin transfusions) are generally asymptomatic immediately after delivery.

PREPARATION FOR DELIVERY

Success of resuscitation depends on three factors: (1) anticipation, (2) trained and available personnel, and (3) the necessary equipment and supplies.

Anticipation

The maternal history must be reviewed to identify those at risk for being delivered of an infant in cardiorespiratory depression. A fetus who clinically is depressed demonstrates the effects of asphyxia—nonreassuring fetal heart rate pattern (particularly bradycardia and loss of beat-to-beat variability), acidosis demonstrated by fetal scalp blood sampling, and/or meconium-stained amniotic fluid—and is especially worrisome.

Personnel

At least one person competent in neonatal resuscitation should be present at every delivery (American Heart Association, 1992; Bloom & Cropley, 1994). When a team is required, the role each member is to play in the resuscitation should be predetermined. The "head" of the team is generally the person to establish and maintain the airway, the one responsible for ventilation and intubation. The second person is responsible for monitoring the heart rate and initiating chest compressions, if necessary. If intravenous medications are required, two additional persons will be needed—one to catheterize the umbilical cord and administer the drugs and the other to pass equipment and prepare the medications. This fourth individual may also be responsible for documenting the resuscitation process, but a fifth person is preferable because minute-to-minute notations must be made. The individual delivering the infant is not considered to be a part of the team.

Equipment and Supplies

The newborn is predisposed to heat loss (particularly evaporative and radiant losses) and if unprotected can quickly become *cold stressed*. The consequences of such stress include hypoxemia, metabolic acidosis, and rapid depletion of glycogen stores. All are conditions that may exacerbate asphyxia and, in turn, may make resuscitation more difficult.

Measures to Prevent Hypothermia

The nurse should implement the following measures to avoid hypothermia (American Heart Association, 1992):

- Keep delivery room warm.
- Preheat radiant warmer.
- Prewarm linens, towels, and head coverings.
- Wear gloves, gowns, masks, and protective eye wear during procedures that are likely to generate droplets or splashes of blood or other bodily fluids.

The additional equipment and supplies needed to carry out a full resuscitation are listed in Table 5–2. As the delivery nears, the team should check daily all supplies and make sure the equipment is in working order. Hospital infection control policies will dictate how far in advance packaged supplies can be opened, connected to tubing, and otherwise prepared. A back-up or duplicate set of materials should be maintained in case of equipment failure,

---

TABLE 5–2. Equipment and Supplies for Neonatal Resuscitation

Suction Equipment
Bulb syringe
Mechanical suction
Suction catheters, 5 French or 6 French, 8 French, 10 French
8 French feeding tube and 20-ml syringe
Meconium aspirator

Bag-and-Mask Equipment
Neonatal resuscitation bag with a pressure-release valve or pressure gauge—the bag
   must be capable of delivering 90% to 100% oxygen
Face masks, newborn and premature sizes (cushioned rim masks preferred)
Oral airways, newborn and premature sizes
Oxygen with flowmeter and tubing

Intubation Equipment
Laryngoscope with straight blades, No. 0 (preterm) and No. 1 (term)
Extra bulbs and batteries for laryngoscope
Endotracheal tubes, 2.5, 3.0, 3.5, 4.0 mm
Stylet
Scissors
Gloves

Medications
Epinephrine 1:10,000—3-ml or 10-ml ampules
Naloxone hydrochloride 0.4 mg/ml—1-ml ampules, or 1.0 mg/ml—2-ml ampules
Volume expander, one or more of these:
   5% Albumin-saline solution
   Normal saline
   Ringer's lactate
Sodium bicarbonate 4.2% (5 mEq/10 ml)—10-ml ampules
Dextrose 10%, 250 ml
Sterile water, 30 ml
Normal saline, 30 ml

Miscellaneous
Radiant warmer
Stethoscope
Cardiotachometer with electrocardiograph (oscilloscope desirable)
Adhesive tape, ½ or ¾ inch
Syringes, 1, 3, 5, 10, 20, 50 ml
Needles, 25, 21, 18 gauge
Alcohol sponges
Umbilical artery catheterization tray
Umbilical tape
Umbilical catheters, 3.5 French, 5 French
Three-way stopcocks
Feeding tube, 5 French

....

From Bloom, R. S., & Cropley, C. (1994). *Textbook of neonatal resuscitation.* Elk Grove Village, IL: American
Academy of Pediatrics and American Heart Association. Reprinted with permission.

contamination, or multiple births. Obviously, all items used should be promptly restocked after a resuscitation (Cropley, 1995; Elliott, 1994).

GENERAL CONSIDERATIONS
Resuscitation Goals

Resuscitation goals include the following:

- Removal or amelioration of the underlying cause of asphyxia
- Reversal or correction of the associated chain of events (hypoxia, hypercarbia, acidosis, bradycardia, and hypotension)

To achieve these ends, resuscitation management should be centered on attempts to expand, ventilate, and oxygenate the lungs with cardiac assistance provided as necessary.

The Apgar score provides a shorthand description of the infant's condition at specific intervals after birth. It is often poorly correlated with other indicators of well-being, such as cord pH (Fields, Entman, & Boehm, 1983). Its usefulness is suspect with extremely preterm infants who may have poor respiratory drive and be relatively hyporeflexive and hypotonic due to immaturity rather than distress (Catlin et al., 1986). Finally, waiting until the first Apgar score is assigned at 1 minute of age causes unnecessary delay in care. For these reasons, the Apgar score should not be used to determine the need or course of resuscitation (American Heart Association, 1992; Bloom & Cropley, 1994).

Need for resuscitation is based on three signs: (1) respiratory effort, (2) heart rate, and (3) color. As soon as the infant is positioned under a radiant warmer, thoroughly dried, and suctioned, these signs are assessed at 30-second intervals with subsequent actions carried out accordingly. Figure 5–2 provides an overview describing the step-by-step approach currently recommended by the American Heart Association and the American Academy of Pediatrics.

Airway Control
POSITIONING

For airway control the patient must be positioned in the following manner:

- Place infant in a flat supine position. Placing the infant in a slight head-down tilt (Trendelenburg position) has been abandoned.
- Place neck in a neutral or slightly extended "sniffing" position. This slight extension moves the tongue and epiglottis away from the posterior pharyngeal wall and opens up the airway
- Avoid full extension, which narrows the airway
- Use a safe extension posture—no more than 15 to 30 degrees from neutral.
- If the tongue is unusually large, place an oral airway.
- Use shoulder roll (up to 1 inch thick) to raise the chest and align the cervical vertebrae.
- If these procedures fail, intubation is indicated (American Heart Association, 1992; Bloom & Cropley, 1994; Todres, 1993).

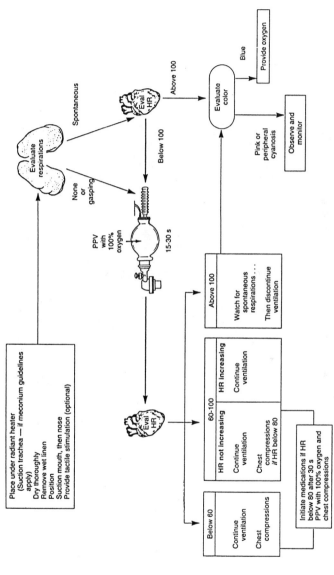

FIGURE 5–2. Overview of resuscitation in the delivery room. (From Bloom, R. S., & Cropley, C. [1994]. *Textbook of neonatal resuscitation.* Elk Grove Village, IL: American Academy of Pediatrics and American Heart Association. Reprinted with permission.)

SUCTIONING

If time permits, the mouth, nose, and posterior pharynx should be suctioned while the head is on the perineum before the thorax has been delivered. After delivery, the infant is placed on the bed and quickly dried and positioned and the airway is more thoroughly cleared using a bulb syringe. Because the very process of suctioning may provide inadvertent stimulation and gasping, the mouth should always be suctioned before the nose. Mechanical suction is often mentioned as an alternative to the bulb syringe, but its use should generally be avoided immediately after delivery because of vagal stimulation and potential unnecessary trauma. If mechanical suction is required (i.e., meconium removal), it should be applied for no more than 5 seconds at a time using an 8 or 10 French suction catheter and the equipment set to produce no more than 100 mm Hg (136 cm H_2O) negative pressure (American Heart Association, 1992; Bloom & Cropley, 1994).

If meconium is present in the amnionic fluid, endotracheal suctioning may be needed to achieve the most thorough clearing of the airway. This suction is performed *before* the infant is dried or otherwise stimulated and is conducted under laryngoscopy with suction directly applied to the trachea, using the endotracheal tube as a suction catheter. Although there is some controversy regarding the benefit of endotracheal suctioning if the infant is vigorous and the meconium is thin, it is generally recommended that suctioning be performed if the infant is depressed or the meconium is thick or particulate (Wiswell & Bent, 1993; Wiswell, Tuggle, & Turner, 1990). The suction is applied as the endotracheal tube is slowly withdrawn and the procedure is repeated as needed until the meconium has been cleared. Techniques involving mouth suction should not be used, owing to the risk of exposing personnel to blood and other body fluids. Also, passing a suction catheter through the endotracheal tube and directly intubating the trachea with a suction catheter are both inadequate as substitutions for the endotracheal tube. These catheters with their small bore are easily clogged with the thick, tenacious meconium (American Heart Association, 1992; Bloom & Cropley, 1994).

Tactile Stimulation

Drying and suctioning generally produces enough stimulation to induce effective respirations in the mildly depressed infant. If the respiratory rate and depth are nevertheless diminished, the newborn's spine should be rubbed or the soles of the feet should be flicked. Ten to 15 seconds of stimulation should be sufficient to elicit a response. Longer and more vigorous methods of stimulation should be avoided (American Heart Association, 1992; Bloom & Cropley, 1994).

OXYGENATION AND VENTILATION

Oxygenation and ventilation are the sine qua non of neonatal resuscitation. Early administration of 100 percent oxygen is critical and may be delivered by multiple means. The potential risks associated with oxygen excess should not be a concern during the brief period of time required for resuscitation.

Free-Flow Administration

An infant who is breathing spontaneously but fails to become pink in room air needs supplemental oxygen. Oxygen is provided directly from the end of the oxygen tube held in a cupped hand or by a funnel or face mask attached to the tubing or an anesthesia-type ventilation bag. The flow should be set to deliver at least 5 L/min, and the tubing, funnel, or mask should be held close to the face to maximize the inhaled concentration (Bloom & Cropley, 1994).

Ventilation

If the infant still fails to become pink with free-flow oxygen or demonstrates other signs of cardiorespiratory decompensation (apnea or gasping respirations or heart rate less than 100 beats per minute), positive-pressure ventilation should be instituted. Ventilation should provide the following:

- Initial breaths at pressures of 30 to 40 cm H_2O should be given to inflate the lungs.
- Succeeding breath pressures vary according to individual needs.
- The ventilation rate should be 40 to 60 breaths per minute.

VENTILATION BAGS

Two types of ventilation bags are available for neonatal use—the self-inflating bag and the anesthesia bag. Self-inflating bags do not require gas flow for use but do require a reservoir to deliver high concentrations of oxygen. There is a "pop-off" valve preset at 30 to 40 cm H_2O pressure. Anesthesia bags are closed systems and need a compressed gas source. They provide more reliable oxygen concentrations (particularly at low flow rates), better control of inspiratory times, and greater range of peak inspiratory pressures and can be used to provide free-flow oxygen.

METHODS OF VENTILATION

In mask ventilation, a face mask is used to provide an oxygen-enriched "microenvironment." The mask should cover the tip of the chin, the mouth, and the nose but not the eyes. Its disadvantages include the following:

- Difficulty achieving and maintaining a good seal between the mask and the infant's face
- Air leaks resulting in underventilation
- Considerable amount of dead space, which should not exceed 5 ml. Sufficient tidal volume must be delivered to prevent accumulation and rebreathing of carbon dioxide.
- Gastric distention, which can be avoided by insertion of an 8 French orogastric tube

If mask ventilation is ineffective (as evidenced by poor chest rise or continuing bradycardia) or if prolonged ventilation is anticipated, an endotracheal tube should be inserted. Premature infants (certainly those weighing < 1000 g) who have diminished lung compliance, immature respiratory musculature, and decreased respiratory drive may also benefit from early intubation (American Heart Association, 1992; Bloom & Cropley, 1994). Infants with suspected diaphragmatic hernia, hydrops fetalis, or certain airway or gastrointestinal abnormalities also benefit from immediate intubation. Uncuffed tubes with a uniform internal diameter are to be used. The proper tube size (Table 5–3) and depth of insertion are determined by the infant's weight.

Most neonatal endotracheal tubes have a black line (vocal cord guide) near the tip of the tube that serves as a guide for insertion. When this guide is placed at the level of the vocal cords, the tube should be properly placed with its tip in the midtrachea. As an alternative, the distance from the midtrachea (tube tip) to the infant's upper lip appropriate centimeter marking on the side of the endotracheal tube may be calculated using the simple "tip to lip" formula:

$$\text{Weight (in kg)} + 6 = \text{"tip to lip" distance}$$

When properly situated, the centimeter marking on the side of the tube at the level of the upper lip should be at or near the "tip to lip" distance. That is, infants weighing 1 kg are intubated to a depth of 7 cm ($1 + 6 = 7$), those weighing 2 kg, to a depth of 8 cm ($2 + 6 = 8$), and so on. Tubes with metallic markers or fiberoptic illumination at the tip may make it possible to transdermally determine the depth of the tube (by observing a circle of light on the skin or hearing an audible signal from a transcutaneous locator instrument), but these modifications do not allow one to differentiate between endotracheal and esophageal intubation and therefore offer no advantage in the emergency situation (Heller & Heller, 1994). Similarly, use of capnometers during resuscitation to measure end tidal carbon dioxide and thus confirm tube placement in the trachea may be very inaccurate when pulmonary blood flow is poor or absent (Bhende & Thompson, 1995).

TABLE 5–3. Endotracheal Tube Size and Placement

Weight (kg)	Tube Size (mm)	Insertion Depth (cm)
<1	2.5	<7
1–2	3.0	7–8
2–3	3.5	8–9
>3	3.5–4.0	<9

Data from American Heart Association, Emergency Cardiac Care Committee and Subcommittees. (1992). Guidelines for cardiopulmonary resuscitation and emergency cardiac care (part VII): Neonatal resuscitation. *Journal of the American Medical Association, 268,*2276–2281; and Bloom, R. S., & Cropley, C. (1994). *Textbook of neonatal resuscitation.* Elk Grove Village, IL: American Academy of Pediatrics and American Heart Association. Reprinted with permission.

Correct placement is best demonstrated by the "tried but true" methods—improved clinical signs (heart rate, color, and activity), symmetrical chest rise, bilateral and equal breath sounds (as auscultated in the axillae), and fogging of the tube on exhalation. Air should not be heard entering the stomach, and there should be no abdominal distention. If there are any doubts, tube placement can be checked by repeat laryngoscopy; the tube should be clearly seen passing through the glottic opening (American Heart Association, 1992; Bloom & Cropley, 1994).

Endotracheal intubation is the definitive technique for airway management and ventilation. The laryngeal mask airway (LMA), approved by the Food and Drug Administration in 1991, offers most of the advantages of intubation but does not require laryngoscopy for placement. The LMA device is a relatively long tube with a bag connector and inflation port at one end and an inflatable soft cuff at the other that is blindly passed into the hypopharynx so that the tip of the cuff lodges in the esophageal opening. Inflated, the cuff provides a seal around the larynx. The tube is then connected to a bag that delivers oxygen by ventilation through the central aperture of the laryngeal mask. Because of its size, current use is largely restricted to term infants, although successful use in very small infants (1.0 to 1.5 kg) has been anecdotally reported. The LMA does not provide access to the lower airway and is therefore not suitable for meconium removal or drug administration, nor does it preserve the airway during laryngospasm.

CHEST COMPRESSIONS

Chest compressions are rarely required for delivery room resuscitation. Chest compressions are begun if the heart rate is less than 60 beats per minute or between 60 and 80 beats per minute but not improving (American Heart Association, 1992; Bloom & Cropley, 1994).

Either of two techniques may be used to perform chest compressions. The first is the *thumb method.* Both hands encircle the chest, the fingers support the back, and the thumbs (pointing cephalad either side-by-side or one on top of the other, depending on the size of the infant) are used to press the sternum downward. The second is the *two-finger method.* One hand supports the back from below while two fingers of the free hand are held perpendicular to the chest and the fingertips are used to apply downward pressure on the sternum.

For both methods, the pressure is applied to the lower third of the sternum (just below the nipple line but above the xiphoid process) where the right ventricle lies closest to the sternum (Finholt et al., 1986). Just enough force is used to depress the sternum ½ to ¾ inch (American Heart Association, 1992; Bloom & Cropley, 1994). One must remember the following:

- Positive-pressure ventilation with 100 percent oxygen must be continued while chest compressions are performed.
- Chest compressions must be interposed with ventilations at a 3:1 ratio.
- Every fourth compression is dropped to allow delivery of a single, effective breath.

Over the course of a full minute, 90 compressions and 30 ventilations are given (American Heart Association, 1992; Bloom & Cropley, 1994). Faster rates only increase the chance of administering simultaneous compressions and ventilations (Trautman, 1995).

MEDICATIONS

Epinephrine

Epinephrine is a direct-acting catecholamine with both alpha- and beta-adrenergic effects. These lead to peripheral vasoconstriction, acceleration of the heart rate, and an increase in the forcefulness of cardiac contractions. The net effect is a sharp rise in blood pressure (pressor effect) and increased cardiac output. Also, the marked pressor effect in combination with the increased aortic diastolic pressure in turn increases cerebral and myocardial perfusion pressure, thereby maintaining blood flow to these critical organs during resuscitation (Berkowitz et al., 1991).

Epinephrine is the drug of choice in a newborn with asystole or persistent bradycardia (heart rate < 80 bpm) despite adequate ventilation with 100 percent oxygen and chest compressions. For newborns, the recommended dose is 0.1 to 0.3 ml/kg of 1:10,000 solution (0.01 to 0.03 mg/kg) (American Heart Association, 1992; Bloom & Cropley, 1994). The dose may be repeated every 3 to 5 minutes as indicated.

Administration is by endotracheal or intravenous or umbilical venous catheter (IV or UVC) routes. Because IV or UVC placement may be difficult and time consuming during resuscitation, initial doses tend to be given by endotracheal tube. In the rare situation when line placement is unattainable and the infant has failed to respond to standard doses given by endotracheal tube, higher doses of 1 to 2 ml/kg (0.1 to 0.2 mg/kg) may be considered (American Heart Association, 1992; Bloom & Cropley, 1994).

Routine use of high dose IV or UVC epinephrine is not recommended in the newborn. Only the standard dose of epinephrine (0.1 to 0.3 ml/kg) should be given by IV or UVC route.

Volume Expanders

Use of volume expanders is indicated when there is evidence or suspicion of acute blood loss with signs of hypovolemia:

- Pallor in spite of oxygen therapy
- Hypotension with weak pulses despite a normal heart rate
- Failure to respond to resuscitation
- Low hematocrit and hemoglobin, which are diagnostic of blood loss but may be within normal range even with acute blood loss

The basic requirement for any replacement solution is that its electrolyte and protein composition be roughly equivalent to that which was lost (Wayne & Fosburg, 1993). Otherwise, an osmotic pressure gradient will be created and fluids will be driven out of the capillaries into the interstitial tissue. The expansion of circulatory volume will be only transient and the infant will be placed at risk for secondary problems, particularly pulmonary edema. Correction of the blood loss should be as follows:

- Whole blood is the fluid of choice.
- Use fresh, O-negative blood crossmatched against the mother.
- When blood is not available, 5 percent albumin-saline (or other plasma substitute) or isotonic fluids (normal saline or Ringer's lactate) may also be used.
- Glucose-containing fluids, such as 5 percent dextrose in water (D_5W) or 10 percent dextrose in water ($D_{10}W$), should *not* be given by bolus, owing to the risk of profound hyperglycemia (Zaritsky, 1993).
- For emergency treatment of hypovolemia, 10 ml/kg of volume expander is given slowly over 5 to 10 minutes by IV or UVC route (AHA, 1992; Bloom & Cropley, 1994).
- Rapid infusion must be avoided because abrupt changes in vascular pressure in the vulnerable matrix capillaries place the infant at risk for an intracranial bleed.
- If hypovolemia continues, a second volume replacement may be given.
- Persistent failure beyond this point probably indicates some degree of "pump failure," and further improvement will not likely occur until cardiac function is improved.

Use of sodium bicarbonate (to correct metabolic acidosis) or an inotropic agent (such as dopamine) should be considered (Bloom & Cropley, 1994).

Dopamine

When vascular volume has been restored but hypotension still exists due to myocardial decompensation ("pump failure"), dopamine may be used to increase cardiac output, increase blood pressure, and increase peripheral and organ perfusion. Dopamine, a precursor of norepinephrine, is a naturally occurring catecholamine. If the duration of the hypotension is greater than or equal to 10 minutes, dopamine must be given by continuous intravenous infusion. After prolonged resuscitation, an initial dose of 5 μg/kg/min is given and titrated (increments of 3 to 5 μg/kg/min up to 20 μg/kg/min maximum) until blood pressure and perfusion improve. Heart rate and rhythm and blood pressure must be continuously monitored. Dopamine, like all catecholamines, is inactivated by alkaline solutions and should therefore *not be mixed with sodium bicarbonate* (Young & Mangum, 1997).

Sodium Bicarbonate

If the resuscitation is prolonged, alkali therapy may be helpful (American Heart Association, 1992; Bloom & Cropley, 1994). The administration of sodium bicarbonate is discouraged for brief resuscitation or episodes of bradycardia (American Heart Association, 1992). The recommended dose is 4 ml/kg of 4.2 percent solution (2 mEq/kg) by IV or UVC route. This is a hypertonic solution containing 0.5 mEq/ml. It should be given slowly over at least 2 minutes (1 mEq/kg/min) (Bloom & Cropley, 1994). A blood sample should be drawn for analysis from whatever site is available to confirm metabolic acidosis.

Naloxone

Maternal narcotic analgesics rapidly cross the placenta and can therefore cause neonatal respiratory depression. Peak fetal narcotic levels occur 30 minutes to 2 hours after maternal administration. Affected infants present with decreased respiratory effort and muscle tone but typically have adequate heart rate and perfusion. If these signs are demonstrated and the mother has received a narcotic within 4 hours of delivery, a narcotic antagonist should be given (American Heart Association, 1992; Bloom & Cropley, 1994; Wimmer, 1994).

Naloxone hydrochloride is a synthetic narcotic antagonist designed to reverse narcotic-induced respiratory depression. The American Academy of Pediatrics Committee on Drugs recommends use of either the 0.4 mg/ml or the 1.0 mg/ml preparations. Neonatal naloxone (0.02 mg/ml) *should not* be used, owing to the fluid volume that would be given.

The dose is 0.1 mg/kg, and this may be repeated every 2 to 3 minutes as needed. Administration by IV or UVC or endotracheal routes is preferred, but naloxone can also be given intramuscularly or subcutaneously. Rapid onset of action is obtained by IV or UVC route (generally apparent within 2 minutes), but intramuscular injection produces a more prolonged effect. Adequate ventilatory assistance must be provided until reversal is complete. Close monitoring should continue 4 to 6 hours after administration. If signs reappear, additional doses of naloxone should be given. Naloxone is contraindicated in infants born to narcotic-dependent mothers; it may precipitate seizures (withdrawal reaction). Ventilation should be assisted until the respiratory drive is adequate.

TERMINATION OF RESUSCITATION

The law and its underlying ethical principles mandate that treatment be provided and continued as long as it is judged to be effective in ameliorating or correcting underlying pathophysiology. There is evidence that neonates with birth weights of less than 750 g who require cardiac compressions in the delivery room do not survive to discharge (Davis, 1993). Survival is also unlikely at any birth weight if the Apgar score remains 0 after 10 minutes of aggressive resuscitation (Jain et al., 1991).

POST-RESUSCITATION STABILIZATION

The goal after resuscitation is to reverse the causes of cell death and tissue injury (hypoxia, ischemia, acidosis) and avoid any exacerbating conditions (hypothermia, hypoglycemia). The mnemonic STABLE can be used as a helpful aid to remembering the basic components of the stabilization process (Karlsen, 1994):

S—Sugar
T—Temperature
A—Artificial breathing
B—Blood pressure
L—Laboratory studies
E—Emotional support for the family

Sugar

Serial screening of the blood glucose level must be instituted with the first test done as soon as possible after emergency measures have been de-escalated. Hypoglycemia can be effectively managed and perhaps prevented by supplying a continuous dextrose infusion (4 to 6 mg/kg/min). Bolus administration is not advised because it may precipitate rebound hypoglycemia and transient hyperosmolarity, which may injure cerebral circulation (Jacobs & Phibbs, 1989).

Temperature

Temperature should be monitored and the radiant warmer or isolette regulated by servocontrol by means of a skin probe to maintain the infant's temperature between 35.5°C and 36.5°C (Boyd & Lenhart, 1996). If additional heat sources are required, they must be judiciously applied to avoid skin damage.

Blood Pressure

If the infant has survived severe asphyxia, postasphyxial myocardiopathy may occur secondary to ischemic injury. The heart becomes enlarged, myocardial contractility is diminished, and pulmonary edema may develop. True myocardiopathy is vigorously treated, usually with assisted ventilation, correction of any residual acidosis, and, if necessary, the administration of dopamine (Jacobs & Phibbs, 1989).

Continuous cardiorespiratory monitoring is recommended. Normal blood pressure is proportional to birth weight. The electrocardiogram should be checked for wave changes (Jacobs & Phibbs, 1989).

Laboratory Studies

Renal injury with oliguria (< 1 ml/kg/hr of urine), azotemia (elevated blood urea nitrogen level), and elevated serum creatinine levels frequently occur, probably as a consequence of the redistribution of blood flow during asphyxia (Perlman, 1989). Sodium levels may be either decreased or increased. Hyponatremia is most frequently the result of inappropriate secretion of antidiuretic hormone whereas hypernatremia is usually iatrogenic in infants who received large quantities of sodium bicarbonate during resuscitation. Hypocalcemia may occur due to anoxic stimulation of calcitonin. This thyroid hormone lowers blood calcium levels by inhibiting calcium resorption from the bone and increasing calcium excretion by the kidneys. Hypomagnesemia, in association with hypocalcemia, may also be noted (Banagale & Donn, 1986). Finally, release of potassium by lysed cells, transcellular shifts of potassium, and decreased renal excretion of potassium can lead to hyperkalemia. The following laboratory studies are ordered:

- Urine output
- Specific gravity
- Serum and urine electrolytes and osmolality

Hydration is evaluated by skin turgor and weight changes. Infants are kept NPO, and IV fluids are initially infused at a rate to provide 60 to 80 ml/kg/day, depending on the infant's gestational age. If renal damage becomes apparent, fluids may be restricted to 40 to 60 ml/kg/day to avoid overload.

DOCUMENTATION

No resuscitative event can go unrecorded. Descriptive charting is most appropriate to this situation. The record should include pertinent perinatal factors, physical findings, the activities performed, and the infant's response to them; but definitive diagnoses should not be offered. Factual data such as vital signs and blood gases should be recorded without adding an interpretation. Ventilation, chest compressions, and the administration of medications are essential items for documentation, but the basics should not be dismissed. It is just as important to note that attempts were made to keep the infant dry and warm (Holzman, 1993, 1994).

Accurate timing of notes can be critical because actions will be judged by the minute-to-minute changes noted in the chart. Using a preprinted recording tool will not only be helpful in this regard but can also provide a structure for evaluation and decision-making. It is recommended that any form used be printed in triplicate. One copy (the original) is retained for the medical record, the second is sent to the pharmacy so medications can be quickly restocked, and the third is used for quality assessment purposes (McCulloch & Vidyasagar, 1993; Thigpen, 1995).

REFERENCES

American Heart Association, Emergency Cardiac Care Committee and Subcommittees. (1992). Guidelines for cardiopulmonary resuscitation and emergency cardiac care (part VII): Neonatal resuscitation. *Journal of the American Medical Association, 268*(16), 2276–2281.

Banagale, R. C., & Donn, S. M. (1986). Asphyxia neonatorum. *Journal of Family Practice, 22*(6), 539–545.

Berkowitz, I. D., Gervais, H., Schleien, C. L., et al. (1991). Epinephrine dosage effects on cerebral and myocardial blood flow in an infant swine model of cardiopulmonary resuscitation. *Anesthesiology, 75*(6), 1041–1050.

Bhende, M. S., & Thompson, A. E. (1995). Evaluation of an end-tidal CO_2 detector during pediatric cardiopulmonary resuscitation. *Pediatrics, 95*(3), 395–399.

Bloom, R. S., & Cropley, C. (1994). *Textbook of neonatal resuscitation.* Elk Grove Village, IL: American Academy of Pediatrics and American Heart Association.

Boyd, H., & Lenhart, P. (1996). Temperature control: Servo versus nonservo—which is best? *Neonatal Network, 15*(2), 75–76.

Catlin, E. A., Carpenter, M. W., Brann, B. S., et al. (1986). The Apgar score revisited: Influences of gestational age. *Journal of Pediatrics, 109*(5), 865–868.

Cropley, C. (1995). How to make sure you can find what you are looking for when you need it. *NRP News Intermountain West, 2*(4), 1.

Davis, D. J. (1993). How aggressive should delivery room cardiopulmonary resuscitation be for extremely low birth weight neonates? *Pediatrics, 92*(3), 447–450.

Elliott, R. D. (1994). Neonatal resuscitation: The NRP guidelines. *Canadian Journal of Anaesthesia, 41*(8), 742–753.

Fields, L. M., Entman, S. S., & Boehm, F. H. (1983). Correlation of the one-minute

Apgar score and the pH value of umbilical arterial blood. *Southern Medical Journal, 76*(12), 1477–1479.

Finholt, D. A., Kettrick, R. G., Wagner, H. R., & Swedlow, D. B. (1986). The heart is under the lower third of the sternum. *American Journal of Diseases of Children, 140*(7), 646–649.

Heller, R. M., & Heller, T. W. (1994). Experience with the illuminated endotracheal tube in the prevention of unsafe intubations in the premature and full-term newborn. *Pediatrics, 93*(3), 389–391.

Holzman, I. (1993). Delivery room scenario may prompt legal tangles. *AAP News, 9*(8), 3, 13.

Holzman, I. (1994). Legal defense requires precise medical records. *AAP News, 10*(9), 4.

Jacobs, M. M., & Phibbs, R. H. (1989). Prevention, recognition, and treatment of perinatal asphyxia. *Clinics in Perinatology, 16*(4), 785–807.

Jain, L., Ferre, C., Vidyasagar, E., Nath, S., & Sheftel, D. (1991). Cardiopulmonary resuscitation of apparently stillborn infants: Survival and long-term outcome. *Journal of Pediatrics, 118,* 778–782.

Karlsen, K. A. (1994, September). *A mnemonic approach to neonatal stabilization: "Transporting newborns the S.T.A.B.L.E. way." Development of an outreach educational program.* Abstract presented at the 6th National Outreach Conference, Telluride, CO.

McCulloch, K. M., & Vidyasagar, D. (1993). Assessing adherence to standards for neonatal resuscitation taught throughout the perinatal referral area. *Pediatric Clinics of North America, 40*(2), 431–438.

Perlman, J. M. (1989). Systemic abnormalities in term infants following perinatal asphyxia: Relevance to long-term neurologic outcome. *Clinics in Perinatology, 16*(2), 475–484.

Thigpen, J. (1995). Neonatal resuscitation record. *Neonatal Network, 14*(1), 57–58.

Todres, I. D. (1993). Pediatric airway control and ventilation. *Annals of Emergency Medicine, 22*(2 part 2), 440–444.

Trautman, M. S. (1995). Neonatal resuscitation: Be prepared. *Contemporary Pediatrics, 12*(3), 101–110, 113.

Wayne, A. S., & Fosburg, M. T. (1993). Therapeutic plasma exchange and cytapheresis. In D. G. Nathan & F. A. Oski (Eds.), *Hematology of infancy and childhood* (Vol. 2, pp. 1819–1831). Philadelphia: W. B. Saunders.

Wimmer, J. E. (1994). Neonatal resuscitation. *Pediatrics in Review, 15*(7), 255–265.

Wiswell, T. E., & Bent, R. C. (1993). Meconium staining and the meconium aspiration syndrome: Unresolved issues. *Pediatric Clinics of North America, 40*(5), 955–981.

Wiswell, T. E., Tuggle, J. M., & Turner, B. S. (1990). Meconium aspiration syndrome: Have we made a difference? *Pediatrics, 85*(5), 715–721.

Young, T. E., & Mangum, O. B. (1997). *Neofax '97: A manual of drugs used in neonatal care* (8th ed.). Columbus, OH: Ross Products Division, Abbott Laboratories.

Zaritsky, A. (1993). Pediatric resuscitation pharmacology. *Annals of Emergency Medicine, 22*(2 part 2), 445–455.

CHAPTER 6

Neonatal Thermoregulation

INFANT ASSESSMENT

The first step in thermoregulation is a thorough assessment to identify normal and extraordinary thermal needs. The following assessment guide may be used (Tappero & Honeyfield, 1993):

I. Gestational age
   A. Comparison to size (appropriate, small, or large for gestational age)
   B. Degree of prematurity (influencing skin's permeability and ability to flex or extend)
II. Neurologic status
   A. Presence of central nervous system (CNS) defects
      1. Absent hypothalamus or anencephaly
      2. Myelomeningocele or encephalocele
   B. Neurologic insult
      1. Intracranial hemorrhage
      2. Prolonged hypoxia or asphyxia
III. Use of drugs that inhibit thermoregulatory response
   A. Maternal use during late pregnancy or labor
      1. Diazepam
      2. Meperidine
      3. Reserpine
      4. CNS depressants
   B. Infant drug intake
      1. CNS depressants
      2. Prostaglandins E_1 and E_2 (can cause increase in temperature)
      3. Atropine (may increase infant temperature)
IV. Cardiorespiratory response
   A. Cardiac insufficiency
      1. Cardiac failure
      2. Congenital heart disease
   B. Respiratory insufficiency
      1. Respiratory distress syndrome
      2. Persistent pulmonary hypertension
      3. Artificial ventilation
   C. Hypoxemia
   D. Exchange transfusion
V. Endocrine response
   A. Maternal use of thiourea compounds, leading to transient infant hypothyroidism
   B. Infant hypothyroidism
VI. Nutritional response
   A. Sufficient intake of calories

    B. Use of oral feedings (may improve heat production)

    C. Excess energy in the ingestion of nutrients

    D. Balance of electrolytes, especially sodium and potassium

VII. Infection

Temperature measurement instruments range from single-use paper thermometers to glass and mercury thermometers to a variety of electronic thermometers. Each method is satisfactory for accurate temperature measurement when used correctly.

Rectal temperature historically has been considered the most accurate measurement of core body temperature. The core temperature does not decline until the infant has lost the ability to produce heat (Dodman, 1987).

Axillary or skin surface temperatures may be lower than rectal temperature by as much as 1°C, but there is generally a difference of less than 0.4°C (Haddock, Vincent, & Merrow, 1986). Skin temperature readings taken over the site of large brown fat stores may yield a falsely high reading, because these skin areas tend to remain warmer (Dawes, 1968). High evaporative losses may produce falsely high readings in abdominal skin temperature measurements (Hey, 1994). Inguinal site temperature measurement may be more closely aligned to rectal temperature and provide a less traumatic site for core temperature measurement (Bliss-Holtz, 1989).

Infrared tympanic thermometers are used because the ear canal is a highly vascular region whose blood perfusion is the same as that which perfuses the hypothalamic region, the area responsible for temperature control. Temperature readings are obtained by placing a small probe into the ear canal, which should approximate the core temperature. When the tympanic thermometer is used correctly, there is only about a 0.3°C to 0.5°C difference compared with an axillary temperature, which is lower.

Physiologic Response

A change in measured temperature may not occur until the infant has lost the ability to generate heat. The infant may display subtle signs of distress:

- Tachycardia
- Tachypnea
- Short-term response: changes in behavior and response
- Long-term responses: poor growth patterns and behavioral changes

In cold stress, tachypnea results from an increased need for oxygen as the result of an increase in metabolism. In heat stress, the infant becomes tachypneic to increase expiratory heat losses.

Temperature Stability

Following temperature fluctuations over a period of time using the same method of assessment is *more* important in evaluating thermoregulation than the actual temperature value at one point in time. Assessing the infant for other factors, such as growth, oxygen needs, and feeding tolerance, also contributes to the determination of appropriate thermal control. Review of growth charts, of F_{IO_2} needs, and of feedings and emesis provides ready access to these data.

Growth

Changes in normal growth patterns are frequently overlooked as indicators of temperature instability. Energy demands for temperature control take precedence over the demands for growth. The infant who is experiencing slow weight gain or erratic growth patterns may be experiencing poor thermal control.

Oxygen Requirements

Using energy to produce heat also requires an increase in oxygen consumption. The infant who has increased demands for oxygen or has decreased ability to maintain basic oxygen needs through normal respiration is also at risk for impaired heat generation. As tissue oxygen levels decline, anaerobic metabolism of glucose yields relatively few heat energy molecules. The hypoxic tissues continue to metabolize greater stores of glucose and glycogen to meet energy demands, depleting limited supplies. The anaerobic glucose response in the cold-stressed infant is amplified (Maniscaleo & Warshaw, 1978).

The infant responds to thermal stress and energy demands by hyperventilation. The healthy infant who is cold stressed may double or triple the consumption of oxygen (James, 1973). In an infant with an elevated temperature, metabolic response may rise 10 percent for every degree of temperature elevation. The healthy infant may be able to compensate for increased oxygen demands, but the infant with respiratory or CNS compromise is unable to do so.

The very low birth weight infant, as the result of immaturity of the respiratory tract, may be unable to meet the metabolic demands. Without sufficient oxygenation, asphyxiated or hypoxic infants have a decreased ability to generate heat. The preterm infant is at risk for decreased oxygen intake even if distress is not apparent, because this infant may not be able to hyperventilate based on metabolic needs. Thermogenesis is directly dependent on tissue oxygenation to use heat energy.

Behavioral Instability

Body positioning is one's first attempt to respond to internal or environmental temperature changes. The term infant is able to assume a flexed body position to generate and retain body heat. The premature infant has a very limited ability to assume a flexed position and may indeed be incapable of changing position.

In the infant who is overheated, the body tends to achieve a more open or flaccid position to allow for a greater surface area for heat loss. Premature infants, unless assisted in achieving a flexed position, may remain in a heat-losing flaccid position even in a cool or neutral thermal environment.

In the infant who is cool, skin color may range from pale to cyanotic. Mottling in peripheral areas may also occur. The overheated infant may become slightly plethoric. Although the sweating mechanism is poorly developed in the infant, diaphoresis may occur.

The infant may have feeding difficulties. If energy is being utilized to generate heat, sufficient energy for sucking may not be available. The infant who is gavage fed may vomit feedings if the infant is too cool or overheated.

THERMAL MANAGEMENT

There is no true normal temperature for the infant. A normal range for an individual infant must be broad enough to allow for temperature variations that can occur during sleep or feedings. Premature infants are often stabilized at temperatures slightly lower than what is considered acceptable for term infants.

The healthy term infant is able to initiate heat production within a few hours after birth. The infant usually requires assistance in maintenance of body temperature during this time. After delivery, infants are often cared for in a warming bed until temperature stabilization has occurred. Once the infant has stabilized, a shirt and diaper may be put on and the infant wrapped in one or two cotton blankets. If the ambient temperature is cool, or if drafts occur in the immediate area, the head of the infant may be covered with a cotton stocking-knit cap.

Thermal management of the low birth weight or premature infant requires special attention (Table 6–1). There is no set temperature for which an infant is considered to be in a neutral thermal environment. For some low birth weight infants, a skin temperature of 36°C to 36.5°C may be acceptable. For others, a lower temperature range may be more appropriate as long as adequate calorie needs are being met, especially in the form of gastric feedings (Hey, 1994).

Environmental temperature is not the only factor in determining temperature stability. Use of humidity alters the need to increase the ambient temperature by as much as 1.5°C (Hey, 1994). Conversely, when humidity is lowered, the ambient temperature must be raised to provide for temperature stability in the infant.

Interventions

Thermal management can be controlled in a variety of ways. No single way works best for every infant under all conditions.

- Use of incubators is generally believed to be a safe and efficient method of providing for the heat needs (Boyd & Lenhart, 1996)
- Radiant and convective heat losses are kept to a minimum
- Air temperature is adjusted according to the infant's needs
- Portholes and doors must be kept closed unless a specific intervention is being carried out
- The temperature drops dramatically if the door is left open for any period of time. It may take from 10 to 20 minutes for an incubator's temperature to stabilize.

Premature infants who are having difficulty with thermoregulation inside an incubator may achieve better results in a double-walled incubator. The double wall serves as a barrier to radiative heat losses to the cool walls, because the inside wall is warmed by the ambient air temperature of the

---

TABLE 6–1. Protocols Used in the AWHONN Research Utilization Project: Transition to an Open Crib for the Very Low Birth Weight Infant

---

Insulating the Infant
Clothe infants as soon as they are considered medically stable.

Clothing the infant may occur several days or weeks before the infant is ready to be weaned to an open crib.

Clothing consists of double-thickness cap, cotton shirt, and diaper.

Decreasing Incubator Temperature
Establish that infant is eligible to begin weaning process:

- Approximately 1500 g
- Five days of consistent weight gain
- Stabilization of apnea and bradycardia episodes
- Enteral nutrition
- Medically stable
- Not requiring assisted ventilation

Once the above requirements are met, the second step of the transition process can begin:

1. Add two layers of blankets and place the incubator on manual control. (During the Research Utilization project, a Yellow Springs probe was placed on the abdomen. Although such a probe may be used to document temperature, it is not considered to be necessary during clinical use.)
2. The starting point of the incubator temperature should be the average temperature of the last 5 days minus 5% of the average temperature.
3. Record the temperature from the continuous monitor every 15 minutes for first hour after the incubator temperature has been decreased. Optimal infant abdominal skin temperature is between 36°C and 37°C.
4. If the infant's temperature is greater than 37°C, lower the incubator temperature another 0.5°.
5. If the infant's temperature is less than 36°C, increase incubator temperature 0.5°.
6. The goal is to have four stable temperature readings over a 1-hour time period. (Temperature monitoring every 15 minutes should be maintained until four stable temperature readings are obtained.)
7. After the infant's temperature is stable, temperature should be recorded q3–4h.

After 24 Hours, Each Day
1. Lower incubator 1.5°C. (There may be smaller decreases for the smaller infants and larger decreases for the larger infants.)
2. Continually monitor temperature, with q3–4h recording of values.

Once the Infant Has Reached a 28°C Incubator
1. Keep the infant in 28°C incubator for 8–24 hours.
2. If weight gain has remained stable over the entire weaning course, remove to open crib.

Open Crib—First Day
1. Place open crib in draft-free environment.
2. If temperature in nursery is greater than 3° different from the incubator temperature, add additional blanket on infant.
3. Recheck infant's temperature. If infant's temperature is less than 36°C, then add another blanket, for a total of two more layers from the incubator.
4. Record infant temperature every 15 minutes for first hour, then during routine vital signs (q3–4h).
5. Do not bathe the infant on the first day of the open crib.
6. Record daily weight.

Second and Third Day in an Open Crib
1. Record temperature every 3 to 4 hours.
2. Record daily weight.
3. If infant's temperature drops below 36°C, record temperature more frequently and take action to increase the temperature.

Transition Failure
1. If temperature is less than 36°C for more than 1 hour after a second blanket is added, return the infant to the incubator until temperature is stable. Record any identified problems. Try weaning again 72 hours later.
2. If there is a failure due to any other problems, document.

....

From Meier, P., Bliss-Holtz, J., Lund, C., et al. (1993). Transition of the preterm infant to an open crib. *AWHONN Voice, 1*(10), 10. Reprinted with permission.

incubator (Marks, Lee, Bolan, & Maisels, 1981). Double-walled incubators may lead to high convective heat losses in some infants, even though radiant heat losses may be lowered (Bell & Rios, 1983). Oxygen consumption is not significantly different in infants who are in radiant-heated incubators and those in conductive-heated incubators (LeBlanc, 1984).

A radiant warmer bed is efficient but allows more convective heat losses than other beds. In the delivery room, the infant can be more easily assessed. In the nursery, a radiant warmer bed meets the heat needs of those who require treatment or resuscitation and stabilization.

- An advantage is that it can be used for infants too large for standard incubators.
- Disadvantages are higher insensible water loss and higher oxygen intake than occur with incubators (LeBlanc, 1982; Marks, Gunther, Rossi, & Maisels, 1980).
- Evaporative heat losses can be decreased through the use of plastic blankets, which also play a role in convective losses (Baumgart, Engle, Fox, & Polin, 1981).

Many neonatal intensive care units (NICUs) use radiant warmers for all infants, regardless of size. These NICUs prefer compensating for the insensible water losses that are encountered even in the smallest of infants. Liberalization of fluids requires meticulous monitoring of intake and output to avoid fluid overload. Other NICUs would rather have the very low birth weight infants in incubators to reduce the difficulty in maintaining fluid balance.

HUMIDITY

Humidity lowers the evaporative losses.

- Greater than or equal to 50 percent humidity requires lower ambient temperature than if no humidity was used.
- Moisture or water reservoir serves as a potential source of infection.
- Above 50 percent humidity supports the growth of gram-negative microorganisms, which compromises the sick or premature infant (Nalepka, 1976). Addition of silver nitrate has been effective in controlling the growth of these organisms.
- Water should be drained from the reservoir every few days, and prewarmed water should be added.

Because heat is lost through the respiratory tract, humidity is always provided for the infant receiving oxygen therapy or assisted ventilation. Use of humidified air delivered to the infant through an endotracheal tube decreases the insensible water loss of the infant, although this humidification does not contribute to thermal equilibrium (Sosulski, Polin, & Baumgart, 1983).

HEAT SHIELDS

Plexiglas tents have been used as a method of shielding the infant within an incubator. Infants in radiant warmers have been shielded with plastic sheeting placed over the area of the infant. Effective heat loss shields may block the warming equipment from providing heat to the infant. In the cold-stressed infant, heat shields may be inappropriate.

WARMING PADS

Heated mattress pads are also effective in maintaining incubator heat in transport incubators before and during transport of the infant (Nielsen, Jung, & Atherton, 1976). A major concern is the effect of thermal burns on the skin of the infant. The skin of the preterm infant is extremely fragile and may suffer from thermal injury at lower temperatures than expected. Warming pads may best be used only if *no* other source of heat is available.

HEAD COVERINGS

The infant's head is the largest heat-losing body surface. In the delivery room, the infant is dried and wrapped in a prewarmed blanket. The infant's head is also covered at this time. The most common head covering used is a cotton stocking-knit cap (D'Apolito, 1994).

Once the infant is stabilized, the hat may continue to be used to prevent heat loss in drafty rooms or during periods of exposure for nursing care or examination. Some institutions use caps inside incubators as well. The premature infant may benefit from the addition of a plastic lining to the cap, which further insulates the head from evaporative and conductive heat losses (Greer, 1988; Rowe, Weinberg, & Andrews, 1983). If the infant has become cooled, use of a lined cap may prevent the infant from gaining heat through radiation or conduction (Templeman & Bell, 1986). In this case, the insulated cap should be removed and a plain cotton cap may be used. Some institutions prefer to use woolen caps, but this should be discontinued if skin irritation occurs.

PLASTIC WRAPS AND COVERINGS

Plastic wraps have been used on infants to decrease the amount of evaporative losses in the early postdelivery stage of life. Bubble plastic has also been shown to be an effective insulator, while allowing visualization of the infant (Besch, et al., 1971). In infants under radiant warmers, loosely fitting plastic wraps have been effective in decreasing insensible water loss and oxygen consumption as well as decreasing the heater output (Baumgart, 1984). Some professionals refer to this as "swamping" if humidity is also provided.

In the premature infant, the use of plastic wraps decreases insensible water and heat loss. Use of plastic wraps also assists in achieving thermal control in incubators at a lower ambient air temperature (Darnall & Ariagno, 1979).

SKIN PROTECTORS

Paraffin has been used with some success as a skin barrier in preventing evaporative heat losses (Brice, Rutter, & Hull, 1981). Skin irritations are possible and necessitate termination of treatment using this method.

Barrier creams have also been used, but the chemicals within the creams may be absorbed too much, related to the thin layer of skin of the preterm infant.

Skin protector treatments may need repeated applications, which disturb the infant. The skin of the infant must be assessed regularly for irritation. The contents of the products used must be analyzed to prevent complications for the infant.

SKIN-TO-SKIN CARE

Although not widely accepted as a means of thermal control, the skin-to-skin control method, or "kangaroo" care, as it is called, is a means of providing warmth to low birth weight infants who are stable when other methods of thermal control are unavailable or limited (Ludington-Hoe, Hadeed, & Anderson, 1991; Ludington-Hoe, Thompson, Swinth, Hadeed, & Anderson, 1994). This method of care involves the placement of the infant against the mother's skin in an upright position between her breasts. The infant is clothed only in a diaper and perhaps a hat.

The temperature of low birth weight infants who have been cared for in this manner for at least brief daily periods sometimes show either a slight decline in temperature readings of 0.2°C or a slight increase in maternal as well as infant temperature (Anderson, 1989; Bosque, Brady, Affonso, & Wahlberg, 1988; Whitelaw, Heisterkamp, Sleath, Acolet, & Richards, 1981).

THERMAL STRESS

Cold Stress

The effects of cold stress can be detected in all aspects of body functioning. The prevention of cold stress is essential in protecting the infant from multisystem stress.

The cardiorespiratory system manifests the most obvious symptoms:

- Peripheral vasoconstriction occurs to conserve heat.
- As central blood volume increases to compensate, pulse and blood pressure increase.
- Once central cooling has occurred, diuresis may result with a decline in pulse and blood pressure leading to decreased cardiac output.
- Arrhythmias may occur secondary to acidosis as fatty acids break down to generate heat.

The CNS can be affected by cold stress secondary to cardiovascular changes. With peripheral vasoconstriction, the following occur:

- Cerebral blood flow diminishes.
- Metabolic activity is compromised.
- Electroencephalographic activity may decline.
- Peripheral nerve conduction may also be delayed.
- Pupils may become fixed and dilated.

Metabolic response to cold stress encompasses fluid, electrolyte, and glucose aberrations.

- In the early stages, diuresis occurs.

- If cold stress continues, glomerular filtration declines along with the reabsorption of sodium, water, and glucose.
- Hypoglycemia occurs.
- Metabolic rate rises.
- Unstable glucose levels can lead to further acidosis and neurologic damage.
- As the release of nonesterified fatty acid increases, the liver slows metabolism of glucose, inhibiting thermogenesis.
- As liver function declines, drugs are metabolized and excreted more slowly.
- Acidosis: as tissue perfusion declines, lactic, pyruvic, and organic acids build.
- Enzymatic action within the kidneys is blocked, preventing acid–base regulation through a diminished excretion of hydrogen ions (Holdcroft, 1980).
- Fluid balance is further complicated by poor gastrointestinal absorption and decreased peristalsis.
- Acidosis continues with an increase in dissociation of the indirect bilirubin from albumin-binding sites.
- An increase in nonesterified fatty acids is caused by their high affinity for the albumin-binding sites.
- In the presence of high levels of nonesterified fatty acids, kernicterus can occur with relatively low bilirubin levels (Williams & Lancaster, 1976).
- There is a risk for bleeding and thrombocytopenia because clotting factors may be altered.
- An increase in hematocrit and viscosity of the blood, secondary to fluid shifts away from vascular space, may be noted.
- Lethargy may occur.
- Refusal to eat may be noted.
- Respirations become slow and shallow.
- Cry is weak.
- Response to painful stimuli is decreased.
- Ruddy coloring, secondary to the failure of dissociation of oxyhemoglobin, belies the seriousness of the infant's condition (Klaus, Martin, & Fanaroff, 1993).
- As the condition continues, edema or sclerema may occur.

METHODS OF REWARMING

- To keep oxygen consumption to a minimum during rewarming:
  - Incubator temperature should be adjusted 1°C to 1.5°C higher than the infant's temperature (Dodman, 1987).
  - Hourly, the incubator temperature may be adjusted upwardly by 1°C until the infant's temperature has been stabilized (Brueggemeyer, 1995).
- If the infant has been severely cold stressed, the temperature may continue to decline during the early stages of rewarming (Laburn & Laburn, 1985).

- Caps, plastic wrap, and heat shields should be removed to prevent them from interfering with heat gain.
- Feedings should always be warmed before being given to a premature or cold-stressed infant.
- Intravenous fluids may also be warmed by using blood-warming devices or by placing an extra length of tubing inside the incubator to allow the warmed environment to warm the fluids.
- High levels of serum sodium are associated with increased temperatures, whereas high levels of calcium indicate decreased temperatures. These findings may be related to the ratio of sodium to calcium and not isolated elevations of either electrolyte (Abels, 1986).
- Normal saline is administered intravenously during the rewarming process to assist in raising the body temperature (Klaus, Martin, & Fanaroff, 1993; Fanaroff & Martin, 1997).

Heat Stress

Heat stress, excluding the febrile state, should never occur in the neonate. When it does it is generally caused by improper use or monitoring of equipment to warm infants.

When core temperatures are elevated in febrile conditions, the skin temperatures of the distal extremities remain cool in comparison to the skin temperature of the trunk (Harpin, Chellappah, & Rutter, 1983). This difference may also be evident in very low birth weight infants if thermoregulation has not been satisfactorily achieved.

Overheating can lead to a variety of responses:

- Hypoactivity
- Restlessness
- Irritability
- Extended posture
- Flaccidity
- Tachycardia—eventually
- Tachypnea—eventually

The metabolic heat production should be kept to a minimum. The infant who assumes an extended position should be left in this position to encourage heat loss. Skin surfaces can be left exposed to enhance evaporative loss. Active temperature reduction methods should be used sparingly to prevent a dramatic loss of heat, potentially leading to cold stress and shock.

Apnea

Apnea is associated with sudden or dramatic temperature changes, especially in the premature infant (Fanaroff & Martin, 1997). Overheating can cause an increase in apneic spells in premature infants (Harpin, Chellappah, & Rutter, 1983).

REFERENCES

Abels, L. (1986). *Critical care nursing: A physiologic approach* (pp. 548–587). St. Louis: C. V. Mosby.

Anderson, G. C. (1989). Skin-to-skin: Kangaroo care in Western Europe. *American Journal of Nursing, 89,* 662–666.

Baumgart, S. (1984). Reduction of oxygen consumption, insensible water loss, and radiant heat demand with use of a plastic blanket for low-birth-weight infants under radiant warmers. *Pediatrics, 74,* 1022–1028.

Baumgart, S., Engle, W. D., Fox, W. W., & Polin, R. A. (1981). Effect of heat shielding on convective and evaporative heat losses and on radiant heat transfer in the premature infant. *Journal of Pediatrics, 99,* 948–956.

Bell, E. F., & Rios, G. R. (1983). A double-walled incubator alters the partition of body heat loss of premature infants. *Pediatric Research, 17,* 135–140.

Besch, N. J., Perlstein, P. H., Edwards, N. K., et al. (1971). The transparent baby bag. *New England Journal of Medicine, 284,* 121–124.

Bliss-Holtz, J. (1989). Comparison of rectal, axillary, and inguinal temperatures in full-term newborn infants. *Nursing Research, 38*(2), 85–87.

Bosque, E. M., Brady, J. P., Affonso, D. D., & Wahlberg, V. (1988). Continuous physiological measures of kangaroo versus incubator care in a tertiary level nursery. Abstract #1204. *Pediatric Research, 23,* 402A.

Boyd, H., & Lenhart, P. (1996). Temperature control: Servo versus nonservo—which is best? *Neonatal Network, 15*(2), 75–76.

Brice, J. E. H., Rutter, N., & Hull, D. (1981). Reduction of skin water loss in the newborn: Clinical trial of two methods in very low birthweight babies. *Archives of Disease in Childhood, 56,* 673–675.

Brueggemeyer, A. (1995). Thermoregulation. In L. P. Gunderson & C. Kenner (Eds.), *Care of the 24–25 week gestational age infant: Small baby protocol* (2nd. ed., pp. 27–42). Petaluma, CA: NICU Ink.

D'Apolito, K. (1994). Hats used to maintain body temperature. *Neonatal Network, 13*(5), 93–94.

Darnall, R. A., & Ariagno, R. L. (1979). Resting oxygen consumption of premature infants covered with a plastic thermal blanket. *Pediatrics, 63,* 547–551.

Dawes, G. (1968). *Foetal and neonatal physiology* (pp. 191–209). Chicago: Year Book Medical Publishers.

Dodman, N. (1987). Newborn temperature control. *Neonatal Network, 5*(6), 19–23.

Fanaroff, A. A., & Martin, R. J. (1997). *Neonatal-perinatal medicine: Diseases of the fetus and newborn* (6th ed.). St. Louis: C. V. Mosby.

Greer, P. S. (1988). Head coverings for newborns under radiant warmers. *Journal of Obstetric, Gynecologic, and Neonatal Nursing, 17,* 265–271.

Haddock, B., Vincent, P., & Merrow, D. (1986). Axillary and rectal temperatures of full-term neonates: Are they different? *Neonatal Network, 5*(1), 36–40.

Harpin, V. A., Chellappah, G., & Rutter, N. (1983). Responses of the newborn infant to overheating. *Biology of the Neonate, 44*(2), 65–75.

Hey, E. (1994). Thermoregulation. In G. B. Avery, M. A. Fletcher, & M. G. MacDonald (Eds.), *Neonatology: Pathophysiology and management in the newborn* (4th ed., pp. 357–365). Philadelphia: J. B. Lippincott.

Holdcroft, A. (1980). *Body temperature control in anesthesia, surgery & intensive care.* London: Bailliere Tindall.

James, L. S. (1973). Acid-base changes in the perinatal period. In R. W. Winters (Ed.), *The body fluids in pediatrics* (pp. 185–206). Boston: Little, Brown.

Klaus, M. H., Martin, R. J., & Fanaroff, A. A. (1993). The physical environment. In M. H. Klaus & A. A. Fanaroff (Eds.), *Care of the high-risk neonate* (34th ed., pp. 114–129). Philadelphia: W. B. Saunders.

Laburn, D. M., & Laburn, H. P. (1985). Pathophysiology of temperature regulation. *Physiologist, 28,* 507–517.

LeBlanc, M. H. (1982). Relative efficacy of an incubator and an open warmer in producing thermoneutrality for the small premature infant. *Pediatrics, 69,* 439–445.

LeBlanc, M. H. (1984). Relative efficacy of radiant and convective heat in incubators in producing thermoneutrality for the premature. *Pediatric Research, 18*, 425–428.

Ludington-Hoe, S. M., Hadeed, A. J., & Anderson, G. C. (1991). Physiologic responses to skin-to-skin contact in hospitalized premature infants. *Journal of Perinatology, 11*, 19–29.

Ludington-Hoe, S. M., Thompson, C., Swinth, J., et al. (1994). Kangaroo care: Research results, and practice implications and guidelines. *Neonatal Network, 13*(1), 19–37.

Maniscaleo, W. M., & Warshaw, J. B. (1978). Cellular energy metabolism during fetal and perinatal development. In J. Sinclair (Ed.), *Temperature regulation and energy metabolism in the newborn* (pp. 1–37). New York: Grune & Stratton.

Marks, K. H., Gunther, R. C., Rossi, J. A., & Maisels, M. J. (1980). Oxygen consumption and insensible water loss in premature infants under radiant heaters. *Pediatrics, 66*, 228–232.

Marks, K. H., Lee, C. A., Bolan, C. D., & Maisels, M. J. (1981). Oxygen consumption and temperature control of premature infants in a double-wall incubator. *Pediatrics, 68*, 93–98.

Meier, P., Bliss-Holtz, J., Lund, C., et al. (1993). Transition of the preterm infant to an open crib. *AWHONN Voice, 1*(10), 9–10.

Nalepka, C. D. (1976). Understanding thermoregulation in newborns. *Journal of Obstetric, Gynecologic, and Neonatal Nursing, 5*(6), 17–19.

Nielsen, H. C., Jung, A. L., & Atherton, S. O. (1976). Evaluation of the Porta-warm mattress as a source of heat for neonatal transport. *Pediatrics, 58*, 500–504.

Rowe, M. I., Weinberg, G., & Andrews, W. (1983). Reduction of neonatal heat loss by an insulated head cover. *Journal of Pediatric Surgery, 18*, 909–913.

Sosulski, R., Polin, R. A., & Baumgart, S. (1983). Respiratory water loss and heat balance in intubated infants receiving humidified air. *Journal of Pediatrics, 103*, 307–310.

Tappero, E., & Honeyfield, M. (1993). *Physical assessment of the newborn: A comprehensive approach to the art of physical examination.* Petaluma, CA: NICU Ink.

Templeman, M. C., & Bell, E. F. (1986). Head insulation for premature infants in servocontrolled incubators and radiant warmers. *American Journal of Diseases of Children, 140*, 940–942.

Williams, J. K., & Lancaster, J. (1976). Thermoregulation of the newborn. *MCN: American Journal of Maternal Child Nursing, 1*, 355–360.

Whitelaw, A., Heisterkamp, G., Sleath, K., et al. (1981). Skin to skin contact for very low birthweight infants and their mothers. *Archives of Disease in Childhood, 63*, 1377–1381.

Physiologic Adaptation of the Neonate

● ●

CHAPTER 7

Neonatal Assessment

GENERAL CONSIDERATIONS

Any measure possible must be used to alleviate stressors and conserve the newborn's limited energy stores. The admission process in itself may influence that adaptation in a negative way to an extent that a marginal transition newborn may require aggressive cardiorespiratory intervention.

Cardiorespiratory function is the sum of all of the processes that ultimately result in energy being supplied to all the cells of the body. A number of factors affect availability of oxygen to the cells:

- Reduced Pao_2, resulting in partially saturated hemoglobin
- Anemia
- Inadequate blood flow
- Reduced oxygen uptake by the cells

Maintaining an open airway for optimal air exchange and providing a necessary oxygen supply can be challenging during the admission procedure. Signs of increased work of breathing include the following:

- Retractions of the chest wall
- Tachypnea
- Nasal flaring

An accurate assessment requires a pulse oximeter (set at lowest interval time response) or a transcutaneous oxygen monitor followed by a correlating blood gas study. Positioning on the abdomen supports the chest wall and allows for greater lung excursion. However, according to the American Academy of Pediatrics (AAP), the prone position should not be used for most newborns owing to the possible link to sudden infant death syndrome (SIDS). If the prone position is used, the head should be turned to one side with the neck straight for maximum airway alignment. The infant's autonomic responses will provide clues to his or her optimal position: increase/decrease in heart rate; color changes; changes in quality and rate of respirations; jitteriness; body, face, and limb twitching; gagging; or spitting.

Maintenance of an optional thermal environment is necessary to minimize energy consumption for all neonates. Cold stress may be devastating to the small or ill individual. A hypoxic infant will undergo a greater than normal drop in core temperature as hypoxia blunts the normal response to cold (Fanaroff, Martin, & Miller, 1994). The infant with his or her large surface/mass ratio is extremely susceptible to cold stress from a cold delivery room. The delivery room should be draft free, and the dried newborn should be placed immediately in a preheated radiant warmer bed or prewarmed incubator for assessment and care. During subsequent examinations in the nursery, continued vigilance is necessary to prevent heat loss by radiation, conduction, evaporation, or convection. With the small premature infant, for example, modern double-walled isolettes improve insulation and much information can be obtained through observation and porthole access. Simply standing and looking at the infant without opening the portholes of the incubator, observing body position, quality and rate of breathing, and state, yield a great deal of information before actually laying on of hands. For the larger, stable infant who may be assessed in an examination room, a warm, draft-free environment, warm examination table, and warmed equipment not only help prevent heat loss but also avoid upsetting an otherwise quiet and cooperative infant.

Suggestions for supportive care are listed below:

- Warming hands and stethoscope
- Weighing infant on prewarmed scale or under an overhead heater
- Warming fluids
- Cleansing skin with water for attaching monitor leads
- Placing the infant in a flexed position with blanket rolls
- Decreasing sensory input from bright lights and environmental noise (Graven, 1996)

Maintenance of an optimal glucose level and hydration will support homeostasis. Individual nurseries vary in protocols but a generally acceptable serum glucose level is equal to or greater than 40 mg/dl.

- Obtain a Chemstrip/Dextrostrip to obtain glucose level using careful technique to prevent pain and bruising. Bundle and comfort when possible.
- Assess hydration and nutrition.
- Examine the skin for turgor and the anterior fontanelle for fullness. A sunken fontanelle may indicate dehydration. Nutritional status can be evaluated by such indicators as thin hair, narrow flat face, thin neck with wrinkles, accordion folding of the lower arm skin, skin loose and easily lifted from the scapular area, lack of gluteal fat and skin on the buttocks, prominent ribs, and loose skin, which is easily lifted on the abdomen (Metcoff, 1994).

Starting an intravenous infusion without stressing an infant is an art. A plan is needed: have all the necessary tools at hand, and bundle the infant evenly under a radiant warmer. It is comforting to have boundaries such as blanket rolls for nesting. A soft humming voice or music and a finger or pacifier are soothing. The infant should be observed for subtle clues and a minute or two break should be provided if needed to help the infant reorganize.

Attention must also be given to aseptic technique to avoid introducing infection to the neonate and possibly cross-infecting the nursery group. Handwashing remains one simple, effective, proven method of preventing infection in the nursery (Davenport, 1992; Kelly, 1994; Larson, 1987).

Should any laboratory specimens be obtained, each must without fail be taken and handled according to institutional infection control procedures and OSHA Universal Precautions Guidelines (1991) to avoid infecting the neonate, the nursery cohort, or the nursery or laboratory personnel.

ASSESSMENT

The examiner proceeds in an organized manner to obtain complete, accurate results (e.g., head-to-toe examination and least-to-most disturbing activities). To avoid tiring or otherwise stressing the infant, assessments should be done as quickly as is compatible with completeness and accuracy (and from the least to the most disturbing activities). If the infant becomes tired or irritable, portions of an assessment may be postponed to a more appropriate time.

MAJOR ASSESSMENTS IN THE NEONATAL PERIOD

There are three major assessments in the neonatal period: in the delivery room, on admission to the nursery, and before discharge (Olds, London, & Ladewig, 1988). Total neonatal assessment includes evaluating risk status based on review of pregnancy and delivery history, gestational age, physical parameters, laboratory reports (i.e., hematocrit, blood type, blood glucose, acid–base status), behavioral components, and parent–child interaction (Kenner, 1990; Volpe, 1995; Wong, 1995). Assessment begins at birth and is continued at every contact with the infant.

The assessment at birth is primarily a physical assessment, with the objective being the evaluation of adaptation to extrauterine life. The generally accepted instrument tool for this assessment is the Apgar score (Apgar, 1953), which measures heart rate, respiratory effort, color, muscle tone, and reflex response at 1 and 5 minutes. Scores range from 0 (cyanotic, bradycardic, unresponsive, little if any respiratory effort) to a "perfect 10." Values from 7 to 10 reflect a generally vigorous infant in little need of resuscitation. Scores that remain low on a repeat scoring at 10 to 15 minutes after birth may have traditionally been thought to be predictive of a poor outcome (Fanaroff, Martin, & Miller, 1994). Initial low Apgar scores may not be predictive of fetal asphyxia. Multiple factors other than a hypoxic-ischemic insult influence a low Apgar score.

The second major assessment is performed in the nursery, generally 1 to 4 hours after birth. For the well neonate, this consists of both a short physical examination to confirm a stable condition and a gestational assessment. The ill neonate also receives a gestational assessment as early as possible, as well as physical examinations as required for full clinical evaluation deferring to his or her organization and coping. The primary purpose of the gestational assessment is to anticipate problems related to development.

Battaglia and Lubchenco (1967) found that infants born before 38 weeks' gestation have a higher incidence of morbidity and mortality. They accepted 38 weeks as the dividing line between preterm and term births. Graphs show the distribution of birth weights at various gestational ages and define large for gestational age (LGA; weight greater than 90th percentile) and small for gestational age (SGA; weight less than 10th percentile) (Fig. 7–1). Infants who are appropriate for gestational age (AGA) and born at term are at least risk for neonatal difficulties. Other infants (preterm or postterm, SGA or LGA) are at greater risk, and the nature of probable neonatal

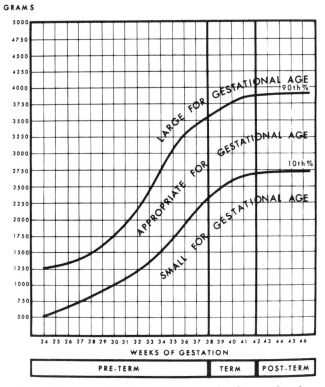

FIGURE 7–1. University of Colorado Medical Center classification of newborns by birth weight and gestational age. (From Battaglia, F. C., & Lubchenco, L. O. [1967]. A practical classification of newborn infants by weight and gestational age. *Journal of Pediatrics, 71*(2), 161. Reprinted with permission.)

morbidities has been identified as a function of birth weight and gestational age (Fig. 7–2).

Various tools have been developed to facilitate estimation of gestational age. In most widespread use are those of Lubchenco, Dubowitz, and Ballard (Figs. 7–3 and 7–4; Table 7–1). These assessments consist of an observation of external physical characteristics such as skin condition and ear development and an evaluation of neuromuscular development. The physical findings remain relatively unchanged in the immediate newborn period. By contrast, the neurologic system of the newborn is quite unstable. If results obtained in this portion of the gestational examination are grossly inconsistent with other findings, the examination may be repeated in 24 hours or, in the case of the Lubchenco evaluation, supplemented by a more detailed confirmatory examination on the second postnatal day.

A complete physical assessment performed by a physician or nurse practitioner will be on record for legal reasons before discharge. Various guides

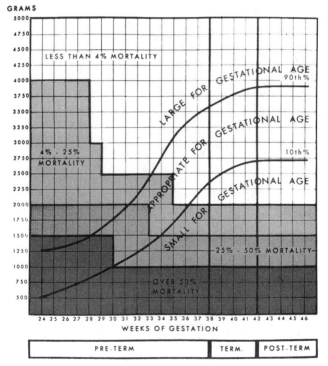

FIGURE 7–2. University of Colorado Medical Center classification of newborns by birth weight and gestational age and by neonatal mortality risk. (From Battaglia, F. C., & Lubchenco, L. O. [1967]. A practical classification of newborn infants by weight and gestational age. *Journal of Pediatrics, 71*(2), 161. Reprinted with permission.)

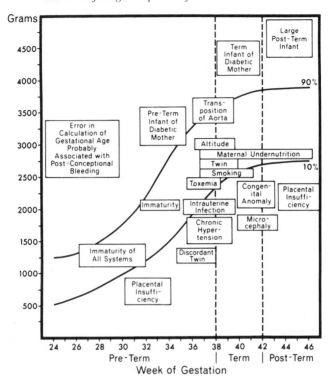

FIGURE 7–3. Deviations of intrauterine growth: neonatal morbidity by birth weight and gestational age. (From Lubchenco, L. O. [1967]. *The high risk infant* [p. 6]. Philadelphia: W. B. Saunders; as adapted from Lubchenco, L. O., Hansman, C., & Backstrom, L. [1968]. In J. H. P. Jonxis, H. K. A. Visser, & J. A. Troelstra [Eds.], *Aspects of prematurity and dysmaturity.* Springfield, IL: Charles C Thomas. Reprinted with permission.)

are in use to ensure completeness and accuracy of this evaluation, which will provide baseline data for well child care and any other follow-up required.

Gestational Assessment

The gestational assessment is a determination of the approximate duration of fetal development and a comparison against standardized norms of neonatal growth versus weeks of gestation. In clinical practice, the gestational assessment tools in common use are generally considered accurate within a range of ± 2 weeks (see Figs. 7–3 and 7–4 and Table 7–1).

CLINICAL ESTIMATION OF GESTATIONAL AGE (LUBCHENCO)

The Clinical Estimation of Gestational Age, developed by Lubchenco and colleagues at the University of Colorado (1970), is a scale designed for use

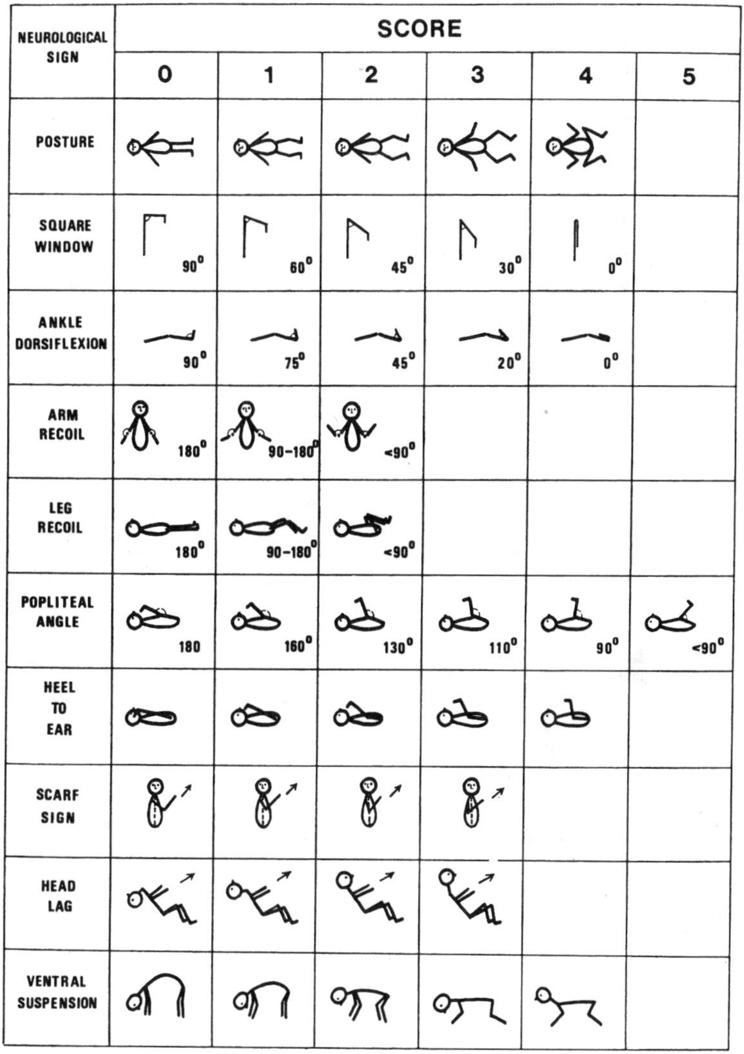

NEUROLOGICAL SIGN	SCORE					
	0	**1**	**2**	**3**	**4**	**5**
POSTURE						
SQUARE WINDOW	90°	60°	45°	30°	0°	
ANKLE DORSIFLEXION	90°	75°	45°	20°	0°	
ARM RECOIL	180°	90–180°	<90°			
LEG RECOIL	180°	90–180°	<90°			
POPLITEAL ANGLE	180	160°	130°	110°	90°	<90°
HEEL TO EAR						
SCARF SIGN						
HEAD LAG						
VENTRAL SUSPENSION						

FIGURE 7–4. Dubowitz scoring system for neurologic criteria. (From Dubowitz, L. M.., Dubowitz, V., & Goldberg, C. [1970]. Clinical assessment of gestational age in the newborn infant. *Journal of Pediatrics, 77*(1), 4. Reprinted with permission.)

TABLE 7-1. Dubowitz Scoring System for External Criteria

External Sign	Score*				
	0	1	2	3	4
Edema	Obvious edema of hands and feet; pitting over tibia	No obvious edema of hands and feet; pitting over tibia	No edema		
Skin texture	Very thin, gelatinous	Thin and smooth	Smooth; medium thickness; rash; superficial peeling	Slight thickening; superficial cracking and peeling, especially of hands and feet	Thick and parchment-like; superficial or deep cracking
Skin color	Dark red	Uniformly pink	Pale pink; variable over body	Pale; only pink over ears, lips, palms, or soles	
Skin opacity	Numerous veins and venules clearly seen, especially over abdomen	Veins and tributaries seen	A few large vessels clearly seen over abdomen	A few large vessels seen indistinctly over abdomen	No blood vessels
Lanugo	No lanugo	Abundant; long and thick over whole back	Hair thinning, especially over lower back	Small amount of lanugo and bald areas	At least half of back devoid of lanugo
Plantar creases	No skin creases	Faint red marks over anterior half of sole	Definite red marks over > anterior half; indentations over < anterior third	Indentations over > anterior third	Definite deep indentations over > anterior third

Nipple formation	Nipple barely visible, no areola	Nipple well defined; areola smooth and flat, diameter <0.75 cm	Areola stippled, edge not raised, diameter <0.75 cm	Areola stippled, edge raised, diameter >0.75 cm
Breast size	No breast tissue palpable	Breast tissue on one or both sides, <0.5 cm diameter	Breast tissue both sides; one or both 0.5–1.0 cm	Breast tissue both sides; one or both >1 cm
Ear form	Pinna flat and shapeless, little or no incurving of edge	Incurving of part of edge of pinna	Partial incurving whole of upper pinna	Well-defined incurving whole of upper pinna
Ear firmness	Pinna soft, easily folded, no recoil	Pinna soft, easily folded, slow recoil	Cartilage to edge of pinna but soft in places, ready recoil	Pinna firm, cartilage to edge, instant recoil
Genital, male	Neither testis in scrotum	At least one testis high in scrotum	At least one testis right down	
Genital, female (with hips half abducted)	Labia majora widely separated, labia minora protruding	Labia majora almost cover labia minora	Labia majora completely cover labia minora	

*If the score differs on the two sides, take the mean.

From Dubowitz, V., Dubowitz, L., & Goldberg, C. (1970). Clinical assessment of gestational age in the newborn infant. *Journal of Pediatrics, 77,* 7. As adapted from Farr, V., Mitchell, R. G., Neligan, G. A., et al. (1966). The definition of some external characteristics used in the assessment of gestational age in the newborn infant. *Developmental Medicine and Child Neurology, 8,* 507–511. Reprinted with permission.

in the first hours of life and requires little handling or exposure of the newborn. Completion of all items on this assessment form will yield a profile of the neonate's development and an estimation of gestational age.

CLINICAL ASSESSMENT OF GESTATIONAL AGE (DUBOWITZ)

Dubowitz, Dubowitz, and Goldberg (1970) developed a Clinical Assessment of Gestational Age, which assigns a score from 0 to 5 to each of 10 neurologic signs and from 0 to 4 to each of 11 external (physical) signs. The totals are added to give a composite score, which is correlated with weeks of gestation. This composite has a higher degree of correlation than does either the neurologic or the external portion considered separately ($\pm$ 2 weeks with 95 percent confidence). Furthermore, although SGA infants tend to under-score on external signs and overscore on neurologic signs, the composite is again reliable (Taylor, 1982).

NEWBORN MATURITY RATING (BALLARD)

Ballard, Novak, and Driver (1979) developed the Newborn Maturity Rating, a simplified version of the Dubowitz tool. This version was later modified by Ballard (1988) to assess neonates from 20 to 44 weeks of age (Fig. 7–5). As with the Dubowitz tool, the Ballard tool may be used from birth through the first 5 days and involves assigning a score from 0 to 5 to each of six neurologic and six physical criteria. However, it requires less time (3 to 4 minutes versus 10 to 15 minutes) and eliminates neurologic assessment signs requiring active muscle tone, which might be difficult if not impossible to assess in very ill newborns.

CLINICAL ASSESSMENT OF NUTRITIONAL STATUS AT BIRTH (CANSCORE)

Metcoff (1994) has looked at the Clinical Assessment of Nutritional Status at Birth (CANSCORE) as an assessment tool to further differentiate infants who may be classified as SGA, as having intrauterine growth retardation (IUGR), or even AGA but who have clinical characteristics indicative of fetal malnutrition. Fetal malnutrition affects body composition and impairs brain development. If maternal malnutrition is appropriately evaluated to predict the birth of small infants 20 weeks later and appropriate nutritional therapy is instituted, fetal malnutrition could be potentially corrected before birth.

INTERPRETATION OF RESULTS

The examination should be done as soon as is feasible after birth, when the infant is alert and not too hungry, so that an infant at risk may be promptly identified and given closer observation and prompt intervention as needed.

Test procedures should be followed exactly. Stick figures accompanying tools should be used as guides. Staff members not yet adept at gestational assessment should be given ample instruction and guidance by more experienced colleagues (Taylor, 1982). Gestational age is compared with infant weight, length, and head circumference to identify deviations from expected intrauterine growth.

If a significant discrepancy is found between maternal dates and the neonatal gestational assessment, several possibilities exist. The neonate should certainly be reevaluated after 24 hours, possibly using a more elaborate tool such as the Lubchenco Confirmatory Neurological Examination. The examination may be affected by neonatal or maternal conditions. If the infant is premature or postmature or has experienced IUGR, efforts should be made to identify the probable cause.

Physical Assessment

The first physical assessment is done immediately after birth. The skilled practitioner will readily apprehend much about the infant's condition from color, general vigor, responsiveness, and other factors well in advance of the 1-minute Apgar score. Results of this initial assessment will determine whether the newborn is admitted to the primary care nursery or to a secondary or tertiary care nursery (possibly requiring transport to another facility). A more complete physical examination is generally not performed until the infant is stable in the nursery.

Deterioration may be demonstrated by increased pallor or duskiness, increased respiratory rate and retractions, jitteriness, "strange" cry, or other deviations from the expected clinical course. The physician or neonatal nurse practitioner should be notified immediately of any problems.

Before the formal physical assessment, the practitioner should be familiar with the maternal and paternal medical histories; course of pregnancy; birth history (including type of delivery, medications received during labor and delivery, condition of the infant at birth, Apgar scores, and any resuscitative measures); any laboratory values available; and treatments, if any, in progress. The nurse may thus identify, in advance, many potential problems of a particular infant and plan the examination for efficiency and thoroughness.

The practitioner will obtain much valuable information by hands-off observation of the quiet infant (Bruno, 1995; Kenner, 1990). The term, healthy infant displays a flexed posture, indicating good muscle tone. Preterm infants often have a relaxed posture with less or little flexion. A head-to-toe approach is generally taken, but the areas most affected should the infant cry (e.g., color, heart and lung sounds) are evaluated first. Similarly, baseline measurements of body length and head circumference, for example, may be deferred to the end, because they are not affected by infant state. The following sections provide an overview of the elements of the physical assessment.

COLOR AND SKIN

Color is best evaluated in the quiet infant. Crying may cause cyanosis, resulting from generalized poor oxygenation or possibly a temporary reopening of the ductus arteriosus. Acrocyanosis (blue hands and feet) is common and generally insignificant in the transition period immediately after birth and reflects poor peripheral perfusion. However, it is also seen

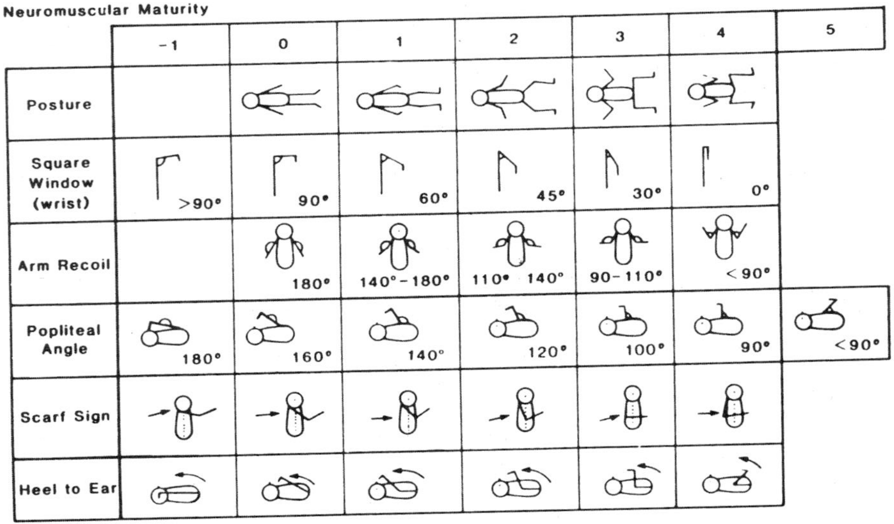

Neuromuscular Maturity

	-1	0	1	2	3	4	5
Posture							
Square Window (wrist)	>90°	90°	60°	45°	30°	0°	
Arm Recoil		180°	140°-180°	110°-140°	90°-110°	<90°	
Popliteal Angle	180°	160°	140°	120°	100°	90°	<90°
Scarf Sign							
Heel to Ear							

FIGURE 7–5.

Maturity Rating

score	weeks
-10	20
-5	22
0	24
5	26
10	28
15	30
20	32
25	34
30	36
35	38
40	40
45	42
50	44

Physical Maturity

	-1	0	1	2	3	4	5
Skin	sticky friable transparent	gelatinous red, translucent	smooth pink, visible veins	superficial peeling &/or rash, few veins	cracking pale areas rare veins	parchment deep cracking no vessels	leathery cracked wrinkled
Lanugo	none	sparse	abundant	thinning	bald areas	mostly bald	
Plantar Surface	heel-toe 40-50 mm: -1 <40 mm: -2	>50 mm no crease	faint red marks	anterior transverse crease only	creases ant. 2/3	creases over entire sole	
Breast	imperceptible	barely perceptible	flat areola no bud	stippled areola 1-2 mm bud	raised areola 3-4 mm bud	full areola 5-10 mm bud	
Eye/Ear	lids fused loosely: -1 tightly: -2	lids open pinna flat stays folded	sl. curved pinna; soft; slow recoil	well-curved pinna; soft but ready recoil	formed & firm instant recoil	thick cartilage ear stiff	
Genitals male	scrotum flat, smooth	scrotum empty faint rugae	testes in upper canal rare rugae	testes descending few rugae	testes down good rugae	testes pendulous deep rugae	
Genitals female	clitoris prominent labia flat	prominent clitoris small labia minora	prominent clitoris enlarging minora	majora & minora equally prominent	majora large minora small	majora cover clitoris & minora	

FIGURE 7-5. Maturational assessment of gestational age: Ballard score. (From Ballard, J. L., Khoury, J. C., Wedig, K., Wang, L., Eilers-Walsman, B. L., & Lipp, R. [1991]. New Ballard Score, expanded to include extremely premature infants. *Journal of Pediatrics, 119*(3), 417–423. Reprinted with permission.)

with cold stress and may improve as the infant is warmed. Generalized cyanosis may be present with serious cardiac or respiratory dysfunction. Evaluation of hypoxia without blood gas analysis can be difficult. Color is best interpreted in the context of the overall clinical assessment.

The neonate's skin indicates maturity. A full-term neonate has layers of subcutaneous fat, which provide for temperature regulation. The preterm infant lacks subcutaneous fat, and blood vessels are evident over the chest and abdomen.

The skin of white infants should be pink. The presence of pallor or plethora should be noted. These findings may reflect low or high hematocrit or vasoconstriction (shock, infection, and so on) versus vasodilatation and should be investigated for cause. Dark-skinned or Asian infants may be somewhat more difficult to assess, but the mucous membranes should be pink. These infants often have a mongolian spot over the buttocks—a dark, hyperpigmented area resembling a large bruise. Parents may need to be informed that this is a normal finding and will disappear with time. Mottling of the skin in response to chilling or stress is referred to as cutis marmorata. The harlequin sign is deep pink coloring on the dependent side of the body and paleness on the other side. This sign has no pathologic significance.

The skin should also be observed for petechiae, plethora, and jaundice. Petechiae, pinpoint-sized hemorrhagic spots on the skin that do not blanch with pressure, are usually related to birth trauma and generally disappear in a few days. Persistent petechiae warrant further evaluation because they indicate evaluation for platelet disorders. Similarly, ecchymoses of the presenting part are frequently noted as purplish blue irregular areas caused by blood outside the vessel. Milia (small white shiny nodules caused by sebaceous gland secretion) are often found on the nose and chin and disappear with treatment in a few days. Telangiectatic nevi ("stork bites") are localized areas of redness caused by capillary dilation and can be seen on the eyelids as well as the back of the neck and head and across the bridge of the nose. They generally disappear by 2 weeks of age. Excellent color plates of skin lesions can be found in *Physical Assessment of the Newborn: A Comprehensive Approach to the Art of Physical Examination* (Tappero & Honeyfield, 1993).

Jaundice is considered physiologic if it occurs after day 2 and is resolving by days 5 to 7. In the premature infant, this jaundice may peak slightly later, usually around day 5. Breast milk jaundice normally appears just as the physiologic jaundice is beginning to subside. It normally peaks around days 10 to 15. Jaundice may be difficult to evaluate in a plethoric or dusky newborn. Application of pressure to the skin will reveal jaundice, if present, in the blanched area. Cheesy vernix caseosa develops in the third trimester and continues to term. Lanugo first appears at 20 weeks, is most abundant at 28 to 30 weeks, and decreases as the infant matures. The distribution of vernix and lanugo, if present, is observed, and it is best evaluated on the newborn's upper back. The presence of both contributes to the gestational assessment.

CARDIOPULMONARY STATUS

The chest should be observed for overall symmetry. It is generally round and is 1 to 2 cm smaller in circumference than the head. Chest excursion should be observed during quiet respiration. Movement should be unlabored and equal bilaterally. The ribs are compliant, and therefore subcostal and intercostal retractions can be common even in healthy newborns. Infants breathe diaphragmatically in a paradoxical pattern: on inspiration, the lower thorax draws in and the abdomen protrudes; on expiration, the reverse occurs. With respiratory distress, a variety of signs are present. Flaring of the nostrils and mild retractions are seen in early or mild conditions. Severe retractions (substernal, supracostal, intracostal, supraclavicular), respiratory grunt, and stridor indicate serious distress. Suprasternal retractions are never normal.

Respirations should be counted for a full minute. The normal range for the quiet infant is 40 to 60 breaths/min. There can be considerable variability in rate and breathing pattern in the premature infant. Transient tachypnea may be present for the first few hours after birth, particularly for cesarean section births, because some lung fluid may be retained. Most infants with transient tachypnea develop difficulty within the first 30 min of life and are cyanotic. Rales and rhonchi are usually heard, and breath sounds are diminished bilaterally. Hyperexpansion of the lungs occurs along with a "barrel chest" presentation. Persistent or developing tachypnea may also indicate respiratory distress or sepsis. A work-up for sepsis including white blood cell count and chest radiograph along with an antenatal history may assist in the diagnosis of pneumonia. Periodic respiration (intermittent cessation of respiration for up to 10 sec) is a normal finding, especially among premature infants. Apneic episodes are of longer duration (>15–20 sec) and are accompanied by duskiness or cyanosis. These infants clearly require intervention (further respiratory assessment; septic work-up) and should be reported immediately. Any respiratory distress may result in retractions and requires further respiratory assessment in the sternum, clavicle area, and costal margins. Spontaneous pneumothoraces occur within the first 48 hours of life in 2 to 10 percent of full-term and post-term newborns (Merenstein & Gardner, 1993). Predisposing factors are intrapartum stressors or asphyxia and aspiration of meconium or amniotic fluid (Wyatt, 1995). Many of these factors may be asymptomatic and resolve without ever being noticed. Cardinal signs and symptoms include cyanosis, dyspnea, decreased breath sounds on the affected side, and a shift in the point of maximal impulse. Breath sounds may be diminished bilaterally because both lungs are compressed (Wyatt, 1995). A chest radiograph is needed for definitive diagnosis, but transillumination with a high-intensity fiberoptic light affords rapid diagnosis and emergency evaluation.

Auscultation of the chest should always be done with a warm stethoscope that has a small bell and diaphragm (neonatal stethoscope with a diaphragm no larger than 2.5 cm in diameter) (Bruno, 1995). Assessment of neonatal breath sounds is difficult for the novice, because sounds are readily transmitted in the small chest, making it difficult to localize their source. There may be considerable interference from heart sounds and gastric noises. Breath sounds should be clear anteriorly and posteriorly, with the possible exception of a few fine rales soon after birth in the otherwise asymptomatic neonate. Stridor, a high-pitched hoarse breath sound heard on inspiration or expiration, indicates partial obstruction of the airway and must immediately be evaluated (Simon, 1991). During the first period of reactivity (2 to 4 hours after birth), rates and rhythms may be irregular. Increased heart rate (up to 180 beats per minute) and respiratory rates (up to 80 breaths per minute) are usual (Kenner, 1990).

Diagnosis of pathologic conditions such as atelectasis, effusion, and pneumothorax is made on the basis of diminished or congested breath sounds or radiographic studies. Rhonchi and rales can often be heard together. Respirations are counted by looking at the upper abdomen for a full minute. As soon as the infant is touched, the rate and depth of breathing will change with arousal.

When assessing the heart, the chest should first be observed for pulsation. Chest pulsations are readily seen in preterm infants owing to thin skin and relative absence of subcutaneous tissue. The point of maximal impulse is usually found at the fourth or fifth intercostal space. It can shift if the newborn has a pneumothorax or other pulmonary pathologic process (Bruno, 1995). The heart rate is counted for a full minute by auscultation. Normal range is 100 to 160 beats per minute. Newborns are more likely to have abnormalities in rate and rhythm than older children. Premature infants frequently have marked sinus rhythms, sinus arrests, and premature ventricular contractions (Leppink, 1986). Murmurs are common in neonates. A slight murmur may be heard before complete closure of the ductus arteriosus. Bradycardia, tachycardia, and strong or persistent murmurs are abnormal findings requiring evaluation. Differential diagnoses include congenital heart defects, sepsis, prematurity (e.g., patent ductus arteriosus), and precipitating respiratory dysfunction.

Neonatal blood pressure must be assessed with an appropriately sized cuff (50 to 60 percent of upper arm length). Blood pressure should be approximately equal in all four extremities. Significant differences, particularly between upper and lower extremities, may indicate a cardiac defect. Normally, blood pressure increases with an increase in gestational age. Blood pressure can be measured either directly or indirectly (Kenner, 1990). The average systolic pressure at 28 to 32 weeks is 52, at 32 to 36 weeks it is 56 mm Hg, and at term it is 63 mm Hg (Cantu, Vaello, & Kenner, 1991; Kenner, Harjo, & Brueggemeyer, 1988). Infants weighing less than 1000 g have a range of 22 to 42 mm Hg, with the systolic range 30 to 60 mm Hg and the diastolic range 20 to 38 mm Hg (Gunderson, 1995). Infants whose mothers are hypertensive have higher blood pressures (Hegyi et al., 1994).

HEAD

The head of the infant should be observed for shape and symmetry. A vaginal delivery, vertex presentation, may cause the sutures to override, resulting in an irregularly shaped head "molding." This condition disappears spontaneously in the term infant within a few days but may persist for several weeks in the premature infant. Infants delivered by cesarean section generally have a well-rounded head.

Caput succedaneum, hemorrhage with edema external to the periosteum, presents as subcutaneous edema of the soft tissues of the scalp extending across suture lines and is caused by pressure on the head during labor and delivery in the vertex presentation. Similarly, edema or bruising may be noted in other areas, such as the buttocks or extremities, in the case of abnormal presentations. Caput is evident at birth and is gradually reabsorbed and disappears within a few days. Rarely is it problematic to the newborn.

Cephalhematoma, a collection of blood from ruptured blood vessels that forms between the skull and the periosteum, may also be caused by trauma to the head during the birth process. The hematoma does not cross suture lines. It may not become apparent for several hours and is not obvious in the delivery room. The cephalhematoma increases in size within 24 to 48 hours and may not be obvious at the time of birth. Reabsorption may take 2 to 3 weeks or longer. Cephalhematoma is associated with an underlying fracture in 10 percent of cases.

A *subgaleal hemorrhage* is rarely seen but is potentially serious. It is most commonly associated with vacuum extraction. Pallor and hypotonicity may be the first early clues, followed by increased heart rate and respiratory rate (Cavlovich, 1995). The scalp may present similar to caput succedaneum. Large volumes of fluid become redistributed and deplete total body volumes, leading to hypovolemic shock. The subgaleal hemorrhage may involve the entire scalp bilaterally and extend into the soft tissues of the neck and face, producing marked swelling of the forehead and eyelid closure. The hematocrit needs to be closely monitored along with signs and symptoms of anemia.

Further inspection may reveal bruising from forceps or bleeding or irritation from placement of an internal monitor electrode. The hair of a term newborn will have identifiable strands and will be predominantly over the top of the head. More generally dispersed "fuzz" indicates prematurity (Kenner, Harjo, & Brueggemeyer, 1988). Extreme hair unruliness with microcephaly, SGA, or unusual facies may indicate poor early fetal brain growth typically seen with Cornelia du Lange and Down syndromes (Avery, Fletcher, & MacDonald, 1994).

The skull is gently palpated to assess the fontanelles, the soft membranous spaces where the skull bones join. The anterior fontanelle is diamond shaped and lies between the sagittal and coronal sutures. It is usually 2 to 3 cm wide and 3 to 4 cm long and normally closes at 12 to 18 months of age. The posterior fontanelle is triangular and lies between the lambdoidal and sagittal sutures. It measures 1 to 2 cm and usually closes by 2 months. Either or both of the fontanelles may be difficult to palpate immediately after birth because of molding. The fontanelles should be assessed for fullness when the infant is quiet. Fullness is most readily assessed in the larger anterior fontanelle. Although some enlargement may be seen in the normal crying infant, a bulging fontanelle when the infant is at rest can indicate increased intracranial pressure. A depressed or sunken fontanelle is a sign of dehydration.

Head circumference is measured and plotted on a normal growth curve to determine whether head size is appropriate for age and body length (normocephalic). The presence of edema or molding may account for the head seeming large or small for age; therefore, the measurement should be repeated when these conditions have subsided. An unusually small head (microcephaly) is seen in a number of congenital syndromes and underdevelopment of the brain. A large head is seen with hydrocephalus, in which either the circulation of cerebrospinal fluid (CSF) is blocked or the CSF is produced in excess. In IUGR, the head may appear large owing to the relative thinness of the body, although it is actually within normal range on the growth curve.

EYES

Because the ophthalmic examination is frequently upsetting to the infant, it may be reserved until the latter part of the physical assessment. Assessment of the eyes in the initial head-to-toe examination may be confined to readily observed aspects.

The eyes should be clear with no redness, jaundice, or discharge. Swelling of the eyelids may occur from pressure during the delivery process or after instillation of silver nitrate to prevent gonorrheal conjunctivitis. The recent trend is to apply erythromycin ointment, which prevents gonorrheal conjunctivitis as well as chlamydial ophthalmia with no evidence of chemical conjunctivitis (Bryant, 1984). Frequently, subconjunctival hemorrhages can be seen in the sclera that result from pressure during delivery and are not pathologic. They disappear spontaneously in 1 to 3 weeks. Lagophthalmos describes the inability to close the eyes and results from facial nerve pressure from forceps (Fanaroff, Martin, & Miller, 1994). It usually resolves within a week but necessitates covering the exposed corneas and use of moisturizing eyedrops.

The iris should be evenly colored. The color will appear bluish in the white infant, although color may not be permanently established for several months. Dark-skinned or Asian infants usually have dark eyes at birth. The presence of small spots in the iris may be a sign of congenital abnormality (Brushfield's spots).

The corneas should be bright and shiny. The pupils should be equal, round, and reactive to light accommodation (PERRLA). Pupil reaction occurs consistently after 32 weeks' gestation but may be present as early as 28 weeks (Avery, Fletcher, & MacDonald, 1994). The lens should be observed for whiteness or opacity that could indicate congenital cataracts. Opacities are sometimes best visualized by cross illumination rather than by a light shined directly toward the eye. An opacity of the lens in early infancy is referred to as a cataract, and 1 in 250 infants will have some form of congenital cataract (Symanski, Newman, & Bachynski, 1994). The white pupillary reflex seen instead of a red reflex is called leukocoria. Cataracts of infancy and childhood may be hereditary, infectious, traumatic, or metabolic, and about one third have no clear cause. Before surgery, no special care is needed (Symanski, Newman, & Bachynski, 1994).

EARS

The development of the ears (cartilage formation, recoil) is an indication of maturity. It is also important to assess the position of the ears. The pinna of the ear should align with the inner canthus of the eye. Use of an otoscope to visualize ear canals is generally deferred unless indicated by the condition of the infant. Hearing can be assessed by observing the head turning to sound or the eye blink after sound. Hematomas of the external ear, usually caused by delivery trauma, liquefy slowly and may develop into a cauliflower ear and therefore need to be treated by evacuation (Fanaroff, Martin, & Miller, 1994).

NOSE

The nose of the newborn is generally slightly flattened. It should be midline, with both nares present and patent. A malpositioned or malformed nose may be seen with a variety of congenital syndromes. Because newborns are nose breathers, patency of the nares should be confirmed by passing a suction catheter into each nostril or by observing the infant breathe with the mouth shut and each nostril occluded one at a time. The nurse should take care to prevent nasal obstruction from developing (e.g., from mucus plugs). Nasal flaring, if present, may indicate developing respiratory distress from mucus plugs and edema from frequent irritation or suctioning. An infant who has experienced nasal trauma during delivery may demonstrate stridor and cyanosis. A nasal septal dislocation may be identified by finger pressure on the tip of the nose. Where the septum is dislocated the nostrils collapse and the septal deviation is more obvious. Early identification and surgical consultation are essential along with airway support as indicated.

MOUTH

Complete assessment of the mouth may be done toward the end of the examination, because it may upset the infant. Although crying may greatly facilitate the oral examination, it will hinder assessment of other areas, such as the abdomen.

The mouth should be midline and symmetrical in structure and movement, with lips fully formed and mouth, chin, and tongue in proportion. Micrognathia, or small lower jaw, may be seen in patients with some trisomies. Macroglossia, or large tongue, may be associated with Beckwith syndrome, hypothyroidism, or mucopolysaccharidosis (Tappero & Honeyfield, 1993). The mucous membranes should be pink and moist, indicating good hydration and oxygenation. Thrush, a candidal infection transmitted during the birth process, may be identified by white patches on the tongue and buccal mucosal that do not easily wipe off. Hard and soft palates are examined for cleft. Excessive salivation indicates possible tracheoesophageal fistula or esophageal atresia. Natal teeth are usually malformed and loose and are usually, therefore, removed.

Several reflexes may be demonstrated at this time. The term infant with normal neurologic function will have a gag reflex, a sucking reflex (sucking on a nipple or examiner's finger), and a rooting reflex (turning toward the cheek that is stroked). If a reflex is absent, an explanation is sought: prematurity and dysfunction of the nervous system are the most common causes.

If the infant is intubated with either an oral or a nasal endotracheal tube, the tube should be comfortably secured and marked such that displacement may be readily recognized. Breath sounds should be auscultated frequently. Presence of bilateral breath sounds helps confirm correct tube placement, whereas sounds unilaterally diminished or absent indicate poor ventilation on that side (possibly secondary to tube displacement).

NECK

The neck should be symmetrical and the head able to turn in full range of motion bilaterally. No lymph nodes or masses should be palpable. The clavicles should be symmetrical and even in appearance. Asymmetrical or "bumpy" clavicles indicate fracture secondary to birth trauma. Crepitus, if present, is easily palpable.

TRUNK

Much of this area was described previously in the section on cardiopulmonary status. The examiner will further assess the breast, abdomen, and back.

BREAST

Two nipples should be present and in normal alignment. The size of the areola depends on the gestational age. The term infant has a raised areola and breast tissue approximately 1 cm in diameter. A slight discharge ("witch's milk") may be present owing to the influence of maternal hormones.

ABDOMEN

The neonate's abdomen is soft, rounded, and slightly protuberant. Asymmetry, distention, weak musculature, visible peristaltic waves, masses, or herniations are clearly abnormal findings requiring prompt evaluation and possible intervention. Distention may be secondary to factors such as resuscitative measures, mechanical ventilation, enlargement of organs, or obstruction of the bowel.

The umbilical cord stump should be bluish, shiny, and moist, with no oozing or bleeding. Three vessels should be present (two arteries and one vein); a single artery is associated with congenital anomalies, most often renal. Meconium staining indicates stress before birth. Redness, discharge, or a foul odor are signs of infection. An arterial or venous line, if present, should be securely taped to prevent displacement and possible hemorrhage.

The bowel sounds are auscultated before palpation. The abdomen is palpated gently to locate vital organs as well as any abnormal masses.

Flexing the knees at the hips allows the abdominal muscles to relax. The liver margin is palpated inferior to the right costal margin, and the spleen tip can frequently be felt at the left costal margin. Both kidneys may be palpated, as well as the descending colon in the left lower quadrant.

BACK

The spinal column should be straight and flexible. There should be no visible defects. A meningocele presents as a soft rounded mass on the back and is usually skin covered. A meningomyelocele presents as a herniated sac containing meninges as well as neural tissue. It is usually flat at birth with spinal cord tissue lying exposed (e.g., mass, dimple, meningomyelocele) on the surface and surrounded by a bluish pink membrane. A spina bifida occulta is located in the lower lumbar and lumbosacral area and is a result of absence of one or more posterior arches of the spine. The meninges and spinal cord are normal. The defect is covered with skin, although there may be a dimple on the skin surface. The vertebrae should be palpable without pain.

ANOGENITAL AREA

The anus should be inspected for patency to rule out imperforate anus. Patency is indicated by the passage of meconium, and a closed anus can be diagnosed when it is impossible to insert a rectal thermometer. The latter practice, however, may be disappearing, because there is increasing controversy surrounding rectal temperatures in the neonate.

In both male and female preterm infants, the genitalia are useful in determining gestational age. The female genitalia consists of the labia majora, labia minora, and clitoris. In a full-term infant, the labia majora usually cover the labia minora, but in preterm infants, the labia minora and clitoris may be more prominent. A hymenal tag may be present and may protrude from the vagina. The labia may be engorged as a result of circulating maternal hormones. These hormones are also responsible for a milky vaginal discharge tinged with mucus or blood (pseudomenstruation).

The male genitalia consist of scrotum, testes, and penis. The external urinary meatus is usually covered by the prepuce. The foreskin should never be forced. The placement of the external meatus on the glans penis should be evaluated to rule out hypospadias (meatal opening on ventral portion of the penile shaft) or epispadias (meatal opening on the dorsal portion of the penile shaft). The scrotum should be inspected for size, amount of rugae, and presence of testes. In preterm infants, inguinal hernias are common. A chordee, ventral bowing of the penis, is often seen with hypospadias, and a malformed prepuce may represent a malformed urethra.

EXTREMITIES

The extremities are first observed in the resting state for symmetry, degree of flexion, and movement. Asymmetrical limbs are associated with trauma, maternal diabetes, drug use, and congenital syndromes.

There should be full range of joint motion in all extremities. Birth trauma resulting in damage to the fifth or sixth cervical nerves results in a paralysis of the upper portion of the arm called Erb-Duchenne paralysis. The grasp reflex is normal, but the Moro reflex is absent. Klumpke's palsy involves C8 through T1; and the hand and lower arm are paralyzed, and prognosis is poor. Brachial plexus palsy is a stretch injury and is serious from a functional standpoint. Neurologic function returns in a few days, and hemorrhage and edema resolve.

Flexion, however, is related to the gestational age of the infant. Flexion begins in the lower portion of the body and moves upward to the arms. The hands and feet should be observed for extra digits, clubbing, or webbing and for creases. The most common crease is the simian crease, a palmar crease associated with trisomy 21 or Down syndrome. Because this crease is found in the general population as well, its presence alone does not signify that the infant has Down syndrome.

The lower extremities are evaluated for congenital hip dislocation. Ortolani's maneuver is performed by placing the fingers on both trochanters while the thumbs grip the medial aspects of the femur. Both legs are flexed and abducted so that they nearly touch the examining table. If dislocation is present, a click may be felt or heard as the femoral head is reduced into the acetabulum. Conversely, Barlow's maneuver tests for ready dislocation of the femoral head from the acetabulum. With the examiner's hands placed as for Ortolani's maneuver, the infant's legs are adducted and pressed down gently. Dislocation, if present, will be palpable. Both Ortolani's and Barlow's tests should be performed to confirm presence or absence of abnormality.

The feet are examined for presence of clubfoot or rocker-bottom feet. Either of these conditions should be referred to an orthopedist or geneticist, or both, because both conditions require further assessment and intervention. The presence of rocker-bottom feet is often related to a chromosomally induced congenital syndrome such as trisomy 13 or 18.

INTERPRETATION OF RESULTS AND INTERVENTION

The physical assessment findings are recorded clearly, completely, concisely, and systematically. The health team may wish to collaborate on the development of a standardized form for this purpose if one is not already in use. Standardization facilitates both communication among team members and comparison of infants (or comparison of a given infant with normal findings). The examiner should list problems identified and recommendations for follow-up (e.g., request for chest radiograph or consultation with orthopedist). Problems requiring immediate attention, such as respiratory distress, are immediately reported to the physician in an appropriate manner.

PREDICTIVE VALUE OF NEWBORN ASSESSMENTS

The various elements of newborn assessment are designed not only to identify but also to anticipate, insofar as possible, those problems likely to develop hours, days, months, or possibly years later.

REFERENCES

Apgar, V. (1953). A proposal for a new method of evaluation of the newborn infant. *Current Researches in Anesthesia and Analgesia, 32,* 260–267.

Avery, G., Fletcher, M. & MacDonald, M. (1994). *Neonatology: Pathophysiology and management of the newborn* (4th ed.). Philadelphia: J. B. Lippincott.

Ballard, J. (1988). Maturational assessment of gestational age: Ballard score. Cincinnati: University of Cincinnati.

Ballard, J. L., Khoury, J. C., Wedig, K., et al. (1991). New Ballard Score, expanded to include extremely premature infants. *Journal of Pediatrics, 119,* 417–423.

Ballard, J. L., Novak, K. K., & Driver, M. (1979). A simplified score for assessment of fetal maturation of newly born infants. *Journal of Pediatrics, 95,* 769–774.

Battaglia, F. C., & Lubchenco, L. O. (1967). A practical classification of newborn infants by weight and gestational age. *Journal of Pediatrics, 71,* 159–163.

Bruno, J. (1995). Systematic neonatal assessment and intervention. *MCN: American Journal of Maternal Child Nursing, 20(1),* 21–24.

Bryant, B. G. (1984). Unit dose erythromycin ophthalmic ointment for neonatal ocular prophylaxis. *Journal of Obstetric, Gynecologic, and Neonatal Nursing, 13,* 83–87.

Cantu, D., Vaello, L., & Kenner, C. (1991). Neonatal assessment. In S. M. Cohen, C. A. Kenner, A. O. Hollingsworth (Eds.), *Maternal, neonatal, and women's health nursing* (pp. 832–870). Philadelphia: Springhouse.

Cavlovich, F. (1995). Subgaleal hemorrhage in the neonate. *Journal of Obstetric, Gynecologic, and Neonatal Nursing, 24,* 397–404.

Davenport, S. (1992). Frequency of handwashing by registered nurses caring for infants on radiant warmers and in incubators. *Neonatal Network, 11*(1), 21–25.

Dubowitz, L. M., Dubowitz, V., & Goldberg, C. (1970). Clinical assessment of gestational age in the newborn infant. *Journal of Pediatrics, 77,* 1–10.

Fanaroff, A., Martin, R., & Miller, M. (1994). Identification and management of high risk problems in the neonate. In R. Creasy & R. Resnick (Eds.), *Maternal–fetal medicine: Principles and practice* (3rd ed., pp. 1135–1172). Philadelphia: W. B. Saunders.

Graven, S. (1996). *The physical and developmental environment of the high risk neonate.* Conference and paper presentation at the Sheraton Sand Key, Clearwater Beach, FL, sponsored by the University of South Florida, Tampa.

Gunderson, L. (1995). Embryology and development of the infant born at 24–25 weeks of gestation. In L. P. Gunderson & C. Kenner (Eds.), *Care of the 24–25 week gestational age infant (small baby protocol)* (2nd ed., pp. 1–26). Petaluma, CA: NICU Ink.

Hegyi, T., Carbone, M. T., Anwar, M., et al. (1994). Blood pressure ranges in premature infants: I. The first hours of life. *Journal of Pediatrics, 124,* 627–633.

Kelly, J. (1994). General care. In Avery, G., Fletcher, M., & MacDonald, M. (1994). *Neonatology: Pathophysiology and management of the newborn* (4th ed., pp. 301–304). Philadelphia: J. B. Lippincott.

Kenner, C. (1990). Measuring neonatal assessment. *Neonatal Network, 9*(4), 17–22.

Kenner, C., Harjo, J., & Brueggemeyer, A. (1988). *Neonatal surgery: A nursing perspective.* Orlando, FL: Grune & Stratton.

Larson, E. (1987). Rituals in infection control: What works in the newborn nursery? Handwashing and gowning. *Journal of Obstetric, Gynecologic, and Neonatal Nursing, 16,* 411–416.

Leppink, M. A. (1986). Assessment of the newborn. In N. Streeter (Ed.), *High-risk neonatal care* (pp. 57–60). Rockville, MD: Aspen.

Lubchenco, L. O. (1970). Assessment of gestational age and development at birth. *Pediatric Clinics of North America, 17,* 125–145.

Lubchenco, L. O., Hansman, C., & Backstrom, L. (1968). In J. H. P. Jonxis, H. K. A. Visser, & J. A. Troelstra (Eds.), *Aspects of prematurity and dysmaturity.* Springfield, IL: Charles C Thomas.

Merenstein, G., & Gardner, S. (1993). *Handbook of neonatal intensive care* (3rd ed.). St. Louis: C. V. Mosby.

Metcoff, J. (1994). Clinical assessment of nutritional status at birth: Fetal malnutrition and SGA are not synonymous. *Pediatric Clinics of North America, 41,* 875–891.

Occupational Safety and Health Administration (OSHA) (1991). Occupational Exposure to Bloodborne Pathogens; Final Rule 29 CRF Part 1910, 1030. Washington, DC: Department of Labor

Olds, S. B., London, M. L., & Ladewig, P. A. (1988). *Maternal–newborn nursing: A family centered approach* (3rd ed.). Menlo Park, CA: Addison-Wesley.

Simon, N. (1991). Evaluation and management of stridor in the newborn. *Clinical Pediatrics, 30,* 211–216.

Symanski, M., Newman, C., & Bachynski, B. (1994). Treating congenital cataracts. *MCN: American Journal of Maternal Child Nursing, 19,* 335–338.

Tappero, E. & Honeyfield, M. (1993). *Physical assessment of the newborn: A comprehensive approach to the art of physical examination.* Petaluma, CA: NICU Ink.

Taylor, K.M. (1982). Gestational age assessment. In S. Humenick (Ed.), *Analysis of current assessment strategies in the health care of young children and childbearing families* (pp. 129–145). Norwalk, CT: Appleton-Century-Crofts.

Volpe, J. (1995). *Neurology of the newborn* (3rd ed.). Philadelphia: W. B. Saunders.

Wong, D. (1995). *Whaley & Wong's Nursing care of infants and children* (5th ed.). St. Louis: C. V. Mosby.

Wyatt, T. (1995). Pneumothorax in the neonate. *Journal of Obstetric, Gynecologic, and Neonatal Nursing, 24,* 211–216.

CHAPTER 8

Assessment and Management of Respiratory Dysfunction: New Care Technologies

NEWBORN PULMONARY PHYSIOLOGY AND THE ONSET OF BREATHING

The fetal lung is fluid-filled and underperfused, and its gas exchange is dormant. It receives only roughly 10 percent of the cardiac output. Because the placenta is the gas exchange organ in fetal life, a high blood flow is directed toward it rather than to the lungs. Consequently, the majority of the right ventricular output is shunted from the pulmonary artery across the ductus arteriosus into the aorta, bypassing the pulmonary circulation.

Within moments of clamping of the umbilical cord, the newborn begins extrauterine respirations, converting fetal circulation to the adult pattern. The lung fluid is absorbed and replaced with air, thus establishing lung volume and allowing for normal neonatal pulmonary function (Nelson, 1994; Ross Laboratories, 1978). The process of fetal lung fluid absorption actually begins before birth, when the rate of alveolar fluid secretion declines. Reabsorption speeds up during labor. With the onset of breathing and lung expansion, water moves rapidly from the air spaces into the interstitium and is removed from the lung by lymphatics and pulmonary blood vessels (Bland, 1988). Because a large portion of the clearance of lung fluid occurs during labor, neonates born after cesarean section without labor are at particularly high risk for delayed absorption of fetal lung fluid and thus for transient tachypnea.

With the onset of breathing, highly negative intrathoracic pressures are generated with inspiratory efforts, filling the alveoli with air. Replacing alveolar fluid with air causes a precipitous drop in hydrostatic pressure in the lung, and therefore pulmonary artery pressure drops, lowering pressure in the right atrium and causing an increase in pulmonary blood flow. These changes result in a rise in PaO_2, resulting in constriction of the ductus arteriosus, which normally shunts right ventricular blood away from the lungs. Cord clamping removes the large, low-resistance, placental surface area from the circulation. This change causes an abrupt rise in systemic arterial pressure. As left atrial pressure rises, the opening between the atria, known as the foramen ovale, is closed by its flap valve. This closure prevents blood from bypassing the lungs by eliminating the shunt across the foramen ovale from the right atrium to the left atrium. As a result of closure of fetal pathways and decreased pulmonary artery pressure, systemic pressure is greater than pulmonary artery pressure. Blood coming from the right ventricle now flows in its new path of least resistance (lower pressure) to the lungs instead of shunting across the foramen ovale to the left atrium or across the ductus arteriosus from the pulmonary artery to the aorta. The infant has now successfully converted to neonatal circulation.

The respiratory system is composed of the following (Harris, 1988):

- Pumping system (the chest wall muscles, diaphragm, and accessory muscles of respiration), which moves free gas into the lungs
- Bony rib cage, which provides structural support for respiratory muscles and limits lung deflation
- The conducting airways, which connect gas-exchanging units with the outside but offer resistance to gas flow
- An elastic element, which offers some resistance to gas flow but provides pumping force for moving stale air out of the system
- Air–liquid interfaces, which generate surface tension that opposes lung expansion on inspiration but supports lung deflation on expiration
- Abdominal muscles, which aid exhalation by active contraction

The newborn has particular limits on the respiratory system, thus increasing his or her susceptibility to respiratory difficulty:

- Circular, poorly ossified rib cage, with a flat instead of angular insertion of the diaphragm
- Small muscles and a relative paucity of type I muscle fibers
- Relatively low functional residual capacity (lung volume at the end of exhalation) because a comparatively floppy chest wall offers little resistance to collapse

Surface tension depends on alveolar diameter. According to Laplace's law, increasingly higher pressures are required to inflate the alveolus as its diameter decreases. The inflating pressure is also related to the surface tension. Pulmonary surfactant is a surface tension–reducing mixture of phospholipids and proteins found in mature alveoli. Surfactant is produced by an alveolar cell known as the type II pneumocyte. Surfactant coats alveoli, preventing alveolar collapse and loss of lung volume during expiration. Neonates with respiratory distress syndrome (RDS) have surfactant deficiency. In the absence of surfactant, surface tension is high and the tendency is toward collapse of alveoli at end expiration.

Compliance is the lung's elasticity or distensibility. It is expressed as the change in volume caused by a change in pressure. The higher the compliance, the larger the volume delivered to the alveoli per unit of applied inspiratory pressure.

Surface tension and compliance are particularly important in the preterm infant with RDS. Surface tension is a force that opposes lung expansion. Surfactant deficiency leads to increased surface tension in the alveoli. Clinically, the effects of this increased surface tension are manifested by the presence of retractions. When a preterm infant with RDS is intubated, a high peak inspiratory pressure (PIP) is required to expand the thorax (i.e., tidal volume is obtained only with a high change in pressure). After giving surfactant, the chest rise increases without changes in PIP. This PIP stability is due to a decrease in surface tension (i.e., a smaller force is now opposing lung distention). Thus, tidal volume obtained with the same PIP is increased.

Surface tension decreases, and it becomes easier to inflate the lung (i.e., compliance is improved).

Resistance is a term used to describe characteristics of gas flow through the airways and pulmonary tissues. Resistance can be thought of as the capacity of the lung to resist air flow. The principal component of resistance is determined by the small airway. Pressure is required to force gas through the airways (airway resistance) and to overcome the elasticity of the lung and chest wall, which work to deflate the respiratory system (tissue resistance). Because the infant has airways of relatively small radius, the resistance to gas flow through those airways is high.

The *time constant* is the time necessary for airway pressure to equilibrate throughout the respiratory system and equals the mathematical product of compliance and resistance. In other words, the time constant is a measure of how quickly the lungs can inhale or exhale. An infant with RDS has decreased compliance, so the time constant or the respiratory system is relatively short. In this type of infant, little time is required for pressure to equilibrate between the proximal airway and alveoli, so short inspiratory and expiratory times may be appropriate during mechanical ventilation. However, when compliance improves (increases), the time constant becomes longer. If sufficient time is not allowed for expiration, alveoli may become overdistended and an air leak may result (Carlo, Greenough, & Chatburn, 1994).

BLOOD GAS ANALYSIS AND ACID–BASE BALANCE

Oxygen diffuses across the alveolar-capillary membrane moved by the difference in oxygen pressure between the alveolus and the blood. In the blood, oxygen dissolves in the plasma and binds to hemoglobin. Thus, arterial oxygen content (CaO_2) is the sum of dissolved and hemoglobin bound oxygen, as described by the following equation:

$$CaO_2 = (1.37 \times Hb \times SaO_2) + (0.003 \times PaO_2)$$

where

CaO_2 = Arterial oxygen content (ml/100 ml of blood)
1.37 = Milliliters of oxygen bound to 1 g of hemoglobin at 100 percent saturation
Hb = Hemoglobin concentration (g/dl)
SaO_2 = % of hemoglobin bound to oxygen (%)
0.003 = Solubility factor of oxygen in plasma (ml/mm Hg)
PaO_2 = Oxygen partial pressure in arterial blood (mm Hg)

In the equation for arterial oxygen content, the first term ($1.37 \times Hb \times SaO_2$) is the amount of oxygen bound to hemoglobin. The second term ($0.003 \times PaO_2$) is the amount of oxygen dissolved in plasma. Most of the oxygen in the blood is carried by hemoglobin. For example, if a premature infant has a PaO_2 of 60 mm Hg, an SaO_2 of 92 percent, and a hemoglobin concentration of 14 g/dl, CaO_2 is the sum of oxygen bound to hemoglobin ($1.37 \times 14 \times 92/100$) = 17.6 ml, plus the oxygen dissolved in plasma (0.003×60) = 0.1 ml. In this example, only 1 percent of oxygen in blood is dissolved in plasma; 99 percent is carried by hemoglobin. If the infant has an intraventricular hemorrhage and hemoglobin concentration drops to 10.5 g/dl but Pa_{O_2} and Sa_{O_2} remain the same, Ca_{O_2}, as calculated by $(1.37 \times 10.5 \times 92/100) + (0.003 \times 600)$, equals 13.4 ml/dl of blood. Thus, without any change in Pa_{O_2} or Sa_{O_2} a 25 percent drop in hemoglobin concentration (from 14 to 10.5 g/dl) reduces the amount of oxygen in arterial blood by 24 percent (from 17.6 to 13.4 ml/dl of blood). This concept is an important one to remember when taking care of patients with respiratory disease. Pa_{O_2}, Sa_{O_2}, and hemoglobin should be monitored and, if low, corrected to keep an adequate level of tissue oxygenation.

The force that loads hemoglobin with oxygen in the lungs and unloads it in the tissues is the difference in partial pressure of oxygen. In the lungs, alveolar oxygen partial pressure is higher than capillary oxygen partial pressure so that oxygen moves to the capillaries and binds to the hemoglobin. Tissue partial pressure of oxygen is lower than that of the blood, so oxygen moves from hemoglobin to the tissues. The relationship between partial pressure of oxygen and hemoglobin is better understood with the oxyhemoglobin dissociation curve (Fig. 8–1). Several factors can affect the affinity of hemoglobin for oxygen. Alkalosis, hypothermia, hypocapnia, and decreased levels of 2,3-diphosphoglycerate (2,3 DPG) increase the affinity of hemoglobin for oxygen. Acidosis, hyperthermia, hypercapnia, and increased 2,3 DPG have the opposite effect, decreasing the affinity of hemoglobin for oxygen, so that the hemoglobin dissociation curve shifts to the right. This characteristic of hemoglobin facilitates oxygen loading in the lung and unloading in the

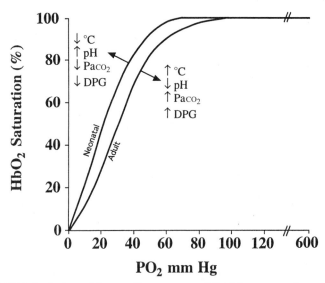

FIGURE 8–1. Oxyhemoglobin equilibrium curves of blood from term infants at birth and from adults (at pH 7.40).

tissue where the pH is lower and Pa_{CO_2} is higher. Fetal hemoglobin, which has a higher affinity for oxygen than adult hemoglobin, is more fully oxygen saturated at lower Pa_{O_2} values. This high affinity is represented by a left shift on the curve of dissociation of hemoglobin.

Once loaded with oxygen, the blood should reach the tissues to transfer oxygen to the cells. Oxygen delivery to the tissue depends on cardiac output (CO) and arterial oxygen content (Ca_{O_2}), as described in the following equation:

$$\text{Oxygen delivery} = \text{CO} \times Ca_{O_2}$$

The key concept is that when assessing a patient's oxygenation, more information than just Pa_{O_2} and Sa_{O_2} should be considered. Pa_{O_2} and Sa_{O_2} may be normal, but if hemoglobin concentration is low or cardiac output is decreased, oxygen delivery to the tissues is decreased.

The acid–base balance is maintained within narrow limits by complex interactions between the pulmonary system, which eliminates carbon dioxide, and the kidneys, which conserve carbon dioxide and eliminate metabolic acids. Acid–base balance is controlled by homeostatic mechanisms and is expressed as pH (the negative logarithm of the hydrogen ion concentration):

$$\text{pH} = 6.1 \log \frac{HCO_3^-}{0.03 \times P_{CO_2}}$$

It can be seen from this mathematical relationship that acid–base balance depends on the interplay of bicarbonate ion (HCO_3^-) and carbon dioxide. Serum pH is tightly regulated in the normal range. Low pH (acidosis) can contribute to vasoconstriction, resulting in worsening hypoxemia due to extrapulmonary shunt across the ductus and/or foramen ovale. pH below 7.0 is not well tolerated and is associated with poor survival:

- If Pa_{CO_2} rises above normal, as in hypoventilation, pH falls and the patient suffers from respiratory acidosis.
- Chronic respiratory acidosis may retain bicarbonate, self-inducing a compensatory metabolic alkalosis.
- A patient who is hyperventilated with a low Pa_{CO_2} has respiratory alkalosis.

Depressed HCO_3^- concentration (below approximately 20 mmol/L in plasma) is called metabolic acidosis and can be associated with any cause of anaerobic metabolism, such as poor cardiac output from congenital heart disease, extreme prematurity, and inborn errors of metabolism. With a knowledge of the accepted normal values and definitions of the simple blood gas disorders and their compensatory mechanisms, the clinician can examine data in light of the disease process and interpret blood gas values in a fairly straightforward manner. When pH is abnormal, an examination of Pa_{CO_2} and HCO_3^- will determine whether the process is respiratory, metabolic, or mixed. The clinician should determine which derangement occurred first. For example, an acidotic, acutely ill hypoxemic infant with a high Pa_{CO_2} and depressed HCO_3^- value is usually hypoventilating and suffering metabolic acidosis secondary to anaerobic metabolism. The infant with a low Pa_{CO_2} is hyperventilating, either spontaneously or secondary to overzealous mechanical ventilation. A concomitantly low pH and low HCO_3^- indicates that the infant is compensating for metabolic acidosis with hyperventilation in an effort to normalize the pH. A pure metabolic alkalosis with high pH is nearly always due to HCO_3^- administration. The infant with chronic lung disease has a compensated respiratory acidosis, with an elevated $PaCO_2$ and concomitantly elevated HCO_3^-. The pH may be in the normal range or slightly acidotic. A severely depressed pH indicates acute decompensation.

ASSESSMENT OF THE NEONATE WITH RESPIRATORY DISTRESS

History

The mother's prenatal record should be reviewed. The practitioner should look for the following:

- Maternal age, gravidity, parity, blood type, and Rh status
- Duration of rupture of membranes before delivery, maternal fever, and the presence of amnionitis
- Prenatal administration of corticosteroids to the mother
- Administration of narcotics to the mother close to delivery
- History of prior preterm births
- Obstetrician's/midwife's best estimate of gestational age and early ultrasonography that has contributed to dating of the pregnancy
- Prenatal detection of anomalies
- Adequate maternal weight gain; an excess weight gain may indicate diabetes, multiple gestation, or polyhydramnios
- Glucose tolerance screening results

PHYSICAL EXAMINATION OF THE RESPIRATORY SYSTEM

One or more of the major signs of respiratory difficulty, as listed here, may be noted:

- Cyanosis
- Tachypnea
- Grunting
- Retractions

Nasal flaring (cyanosis, tachypnea, grunting, retractions, and nasal flaring) is usually present in neonates with both pulmonary and nonpulmonary causes of respiratory distress. Observation of the distressed infant with the unaided eye and ear is the clinician's first step in the physical assessment.

Cyanosis may be central, as caused by pulmonary disease and cyanotic heart disease, or peripheral, as occurs in conditions with impaired cardiac output. *Tachypnea* typically presents in patients with decreased lung compliance such as RDS, whereas patients with high airway resistance (e.g., airway obstruction) usually have deep but slow breathing. *Grunting*, which helps maintain lung volume, is more typical of infants with decreased functional residual capacity. *Chest wall retractions* occur more frequently in very premature infants because of their highly compliant chest wall (Avery, 1994; Bueuvalas & Balisteri, 1995).

When the infant is intubated, careful observation of the chest gives important information. Close observation of chest wall excursions produced by the ventilator allows the clinician to adjust the magnitude of the ventilator pressure so that better gas exchange is achieved while risk of barotrauma is minimized. An overinflated thorax is a sign of gas trapping. In the intubated infant, this observation should prompt the clinician to adjust the positive end-expiratory pressure (PEEP) or expiratory time so that gas trapping and air leak are prevented. Signs of endotracheal tube obstruction include cyanosis and a gasping and anguished intubated infant.

Careful attention should be given to the various sounds emanating from the respiratory tract, because their quality often aids in localization of the source of respiratory distress. *Stridor* is common in neonates with upper airway and laryngeal lesions. *Inspiratory stridor* occurs most frequently with upper airway and laryngeal lesions, whereas w*heezing* commonly accompanies lower airway disorders. *Hoarseness* is a common sign of laryngeal disorders. *Forced inspiratory efforts* may indicate upper airway or laryngeal involvement, whereas *expiratory wheezes* suggest a lower airway disease.

Auscultation of the chest further aids the examiner. Because they have low lung volumes, infants with RDS have faint breath sounds, usually without *rales*. An infant with pneumonia may have rales, which indicate alveolar filling. Auscultation allows the clinician to detect the presence of secretion in the airway and to evaluate the response to physiotherapy and suctioning.

In infants with meconium aspiration and/or a pneumothorax the following may occur:

- Rhonchi may be heard in neonates with airway disease, such as meconium aspiration syndrome.
- Unequal breath sounds may be due to a pneumothorax or to one of the many causes of diminished ventilation to a lung lobe (e.g., atelectasis, mainstream bronchial intubation, pleural effusion).
- A shift of the apex of the heart can occur with a pneumothorax, diaphragmatic hernia, unilateral pulmonary interstitial emphysema, pleural effusion, or atelectasis.
- Transillumination of the chest may help to differentiate causes of chest abnormalities between the conditions.
- Dullness to percussion may be due to a pleural effusion or solid mass.
- Muffled heart tones suggest a pneumopericardium.
- Respiratory distress may occur in many chest wall disorders that restrict rib cage movements.
- Increased oral secretions and choking with feedings are common in neonates with a tracheoesophageal fistula.
- Because newborns are obligate nasal breathers, those with choanal atresia typically improve with crying and develop worsening respiratory distress with rest and feeding.
- Characteristic Potter facies and other compression deformities and contractures may be present in neonates with hypoplastic lungs secondary to oligohydramnios.

- Examination of the cardiovascular system and assessment of peripheral perfusion yields many clues toward arriving at a diagnosis.
- Pallor and poor perfusion may indicate anemia, hypotension, and/or hypovolemia.
- Polycythemia with plethora may also cause respiratory distress.
- Cardiovascular signs of congestive failure (e.g., hyperactive precordium, tachycardia, or hepatomegaly), poor cardiac output, pathologic murmurs, decreased femoral pulses, and nonsinus rhythm suggest a primary cardiac cause for the respiratory distress.
- When hypotonia, muscle weakness, or areflexia accompany respiratory distress, a neuromuscular cause should be considered. Often in such cases there is an accompanying history of decreased fetal movement. Sometimes there is a history of muscular disease in the family.
- Brachial plexus injury or fracture of a clavicle may accompany phrenic nerve injury and diaphragm paralysis.

Abnormalities of the abdominal examination will enlighten the examiner to other causes of respiratory difficulty. Abdominal distention due to causes such as ascites, necrotizing enterocolitis, abdominal mass, ileus, or tracheoesophageal fistula can cause respiratory distress, whereas scaphoid configuration of the abdomen suggests a diaphragmatic hernia.

Other nonpulmonary disorders such as sepsis, metabolic acidosis, hypothermia or hyperthermia, hypoglycemia, and methemoglobinemia may also cause respiratory distress in the neonate.

RADIOGRAPHIC AND LABORATORY INVESTIGATION

Radiographic examination is often the most useful part of the laboratory evaluation and may serve to narrow the differential diagnosis.

- A routine anteroposterior view is obtained.
- A lateral chest radiograph is taken if fluid, masses, or free air is suggested.
- Ultrasonography, fluoroscopy, computed tomography, or magnetic resonance imaging may be helpful in selected patients.
- Bronchoscopy allows direct visualization of the upper airway and is used to aid in differential diagnosis and treatment of obstructive lesions.
- Arterial blood is analyzed for pH and gas tensions. Blood chemistry and hematocrit can be performed on venous samples. Capillary blood samples can be used for all testing but are less accurate and, if used, the extremity used needs to be warmed and good blood flow established to reduce hemolysis of cells.
- Noninvasive methods to assess gas exchange, such as transcutaneous blood gas measurements or oxygen saturation, may also be used.

CONVENTIONAL MANAGEMENT OF NEONATAL HYPOXEMIA

The conventional management of neonatal hypoxemia includes the following:

- Administration of oxygen to the pregnant woman to increase fetal oxygenation; administration of oxygen and/or mechanical ventilation to the newborn after birth

- Intermittent blood transfusion or erythropoietin administration to optimize oxygen-carrying capacity of the blood
- Maintenance of neutral thermal environment by minimizing oxygen demand and subsequently reducing the risk of cell injury secondary to tissue hypoxia. Attempts to create a near-neutral thermal environment have been associated with improved survival of sick premature newborns, presumably by favorably affecting the balance between oxygen demand and oxygen supply (Perlstein, 1987).
- Maintenance of cardiac output delivers adequate blood flow to vital organs, reducing the risk of tissue hypoxia. Methods commonly employed for maintenance of adequate cardiac output include the following:
  - Volume expansion of the hypovolemic newborn and administration of inotropic drugs to stimulate the poorly contractile myocardium
  - Determination of the rate of capillary refill
  - Presence/absence of acrocyanosis
  - Skin mottling
  - Relative coolness of the extremities
  - Determination of pulse strength and blood pressure/serial hematocrit determination to diagnose acute blood loss
  - Echocardiography to evaluate cardiac contractility
  - Use of indwelling cardiac catheters for estimation of cardiac output, measuring mixed venous oxygen, pulmonary vascular resistance, and pulmonary capillary wedge pressure. These are not widely available for use in the newborn with evidence of low cardiac output.
  - Measuring transcutaneous PaO_2 and transcutaneous oxygen saturation. This nearly continuously provides fairly reliable estimations of blood oxygen levels in addition to intermittent arterial blood gas analysis.

COMMON DISORDERS OF THE RESPIRATORY SYSTEM

Respiratory distress syndrome, or hyaline membrane disease, is the most common cause of respiratory distress in premature neonates (Bueuvalas & Balisteri, 1995). It is estimated that there are more than 40,000 cases of RDS per year in the United States (Farrell & Wood, 1976).

RDS is progressively more common in infants of decreasing gestational age. Rarely, term infants born to diabetic mothers or term infants who have experienced asphyxia develop RDS. Characteristics of RDS include the following:

- Deficiency in pulmonary surfactant, a surface-tension reducing agent that prevents alveolar collapse at end expiration and loss of lung volume
- Progressive atelectasis leading to intrapulmonary shunting, owing to perfusion of unventilated lung, and subsequent hypoxemia. The radiograph displays a characteristic ground-glass, reticulogranular appearance with air bronchograms.

- Poor lung inflation
- Respiratory acidemia as well as hypoxemia as revealed by arterial blood gas analysis

Therapy is directed toward improving oxygenation as well as maintaining optimal lung volume by way of the following:

- Continuous positive airway pressure (CPAP), or positive end expiratory pressure (PEEP), applied to prevent volume loss during expiration
- Mechanical ventilation
- Administration of exogenous surfactants (artificial and natural)
- High-frequency ventilation for treatment of RDS. This has met with mixed results and should be considered experimental except in specific circumstances, such as in infants with air leaks and severe hypercapnia.
- Extracorporeal membrane oxygenation (ECMO). This has salvaged near-term infants with RDS and respiratory failure unresponsive to ventilatory management.

An experienced NICU nurse is invaluable in the ill newborn's recovery. Nursing measures are listed below:

- Monitor the quality of respirations, including the depth and the degree of difficulty the infant is experiencing as well as color and symmetry of breath sounds.
- Monitor serial arterial blood gas tensions and pH and continuous noninvasive monitoring of oxygenation to detect early gas exchange problems.
- Calm infants, including the appropriate use of analgesics. A crying newborn on nasal CPAP loses airway pressure when the mouth is open.
- Assess the intubated infant for appropriate endotracheal tube position and patency.
- Suction only when needed. Pass the suction catheter only as far as the end of the endotracheal tube, because overzealous suctioning can denude the tracheal epithelium (Bailey, Kattwinkel, Teja, & Buckley, 1988). Lung volume can be lost during prolonged disconnection from the ventilator, especially when high-frequency ventilation is being used. Rapid loss of lung volume can precipitate hypoxemia in these patients. Any sudden decompensation should alert the nurse to investigate for ventilator failure, pneumothorax, or tracheal tube plugging.

Bronchopulmonary Dysplasia

DEFINITION

There is little agreement on the precise definition of bronchopulmonary dysplasia (BPD) other than that BPD is associated with an increase in survival of very low birth weight (VLBW) infants. Significant variability in incidence exists from center to center, even within regions (Avery et al., 1987; Boynton, 1988), and may be due to any or all of the following (Boynton, 1988):

- Variability in diagnostic criteria
- Variability in criteria for identification of the at-risk population
- Differences in composition of patient population

- Temporal changes in survival rates of VLBW neonates
- Differences in clinical management of neonates with respiratory disease

The natural history of the disease is not well understood. Not all infants who meet some of the BPD criteria have had RDS at birth requiring oxygen therapy and mechanical ventilation, the two factors thought to trigger BPD, nor do all infants with BPD require supplemental oxygen therapy after discharge, even though they continue to have abnormalities in lung function and chest radiographs for years. Some therapies are effective for some infants but not for others.

However, after acknowledging how little is known, the following is a summary of common outcomes among infants with BPD (Boynton, 1988):

- Excessively high postnatal mortality rate occurs within the first year of life.
- Recurrent lower respiratory tract infections in the first few years of life often require hospitalization.
- Delays in growth and development, in spite of what may appear to be adequate or even excessive nutritional support, are found.
- Although pulmonary dysfunction does decrease with time, measurable abnormalities persist in pulmonary mechanics, even in the absence of an oxygen requirement or other clinical symptoms.

ETIOLOGY

The classic BPD formula of Philip (1975) could be altered to include this interaction:

$$Oxygen + pressure + time + susceptible\ host = BPD$$

Two commonly used respiratory treatments, oxygen therapy and mechanical ventilation, have been strongly implicated in initiating a cascade of events that lead to the development of BPD (Boynton, 1988).

Oxygen Toxicity

The mechanisms of oxygen toxicity are as follows:

- Free radicals are generated during breathing. The high level of free radicals is due to overproduction of free radicals associated with oxygen therapy/hypoxia and immature levels of functioning of protective systems that neutralize free radicals.
- Normally, enzyme and nonenzyme systems operate to scavenge and neutralize free radicals that can damage and kill tissue.
- Unscavenged radicals have a direct toxic effect on pulmonary epithelial cells, causing cell membrane injury, enzyme inactivation, and structural protein damage.
- Reaction of the free radicals with proteins may also generate byproducts that amplify the initial damage.
- Damage to the alveolar-capillary membrane causes the loss of the membrane's integrity as a barrier, resulting in a leak of fluids and proteins into the lung (e.g., "capillary leak syndrome") (Shannon & Epstein, 1986; Sinkin & Phelps, 1987).

- Fibronectin production associated with capillary leak syndrome may be responsible for the build-up of fibrinous tissue in the pulmonary tree, which is often associated with chronic lung changes in the neonate (Polin, 1990).
- An inflammatory response, together with an influx of polymorphonuclear cells and macrophages that release proteolytic enzymes further aggravates the damage. The influx of fluid, proteins, and enzymes causes an inactivation of any surfactant that is present (Merritt & Hallman, 1988), worsening the initial lung disease.
- Destruction of elastin causes disruption of alveolar septal development in the developing lung and may have long-term effects on the ability of the lung to grow and develop normally in infancy and childhood (Monin & Vert, 1987).
- All this damage, together with resulting alveolar and bronchiolar necrosis, causes regenerative efforts by the lung, that is, the growth of new alveolar lining cells with a fibroproliferative response.

This cycle of lung injury and necrosis followed by fibrotic repair mechanisms is typical of BPD and is also associated with the other iatrogenic trigger, barotrauma.

Barotrauma

Barotrauma, the damage done to lung structures (primarily small airways and alveoli) by mechanical stress, has been implicated as a major contributor to the incidence of BPD. Barotrauma occurs when lung volume exceeds physiologic limits, especially when tissue structures are "stiff" or noncompliant. Overdistention of the airways and alveoli in the premature infant is most often caused by the large and frequently oscillating pressure differences associated with mechanical ventilation (Thibeault, 1986). Mechanical stresses occur in all planes of the alveolar wall, but the strain is especially significant at the junction of the alveolus and the related bronchioles, where large excursions in diameter occur during ventilation (Monin & Vert, 1987; Thibeault, 1986.) Tissue breakdown, epithelial necrosis, and alveolar rupture occur as a consequence of these large, unbalanced stresses (Thibeault, 1986). In the bronchi and bronchioles, these stresses produce desquamation of epithelium and ciliary apparatus, an increase in goblet cells and smooth muscle, and necrotizing bronchiolitis that heals with fibrosis.

PATHOGENESIS

Alterations in Lung Mechanics

The following may occur:

- Protein leakage inhibits surfactant production and function, leading to increased surface tension, decreased dynamic compliance, and increased atelectasis (Obladen, 1988).
- Increase in pulmonary resistance from increased mucus production, decreased mucus transport due to damaged cilia, low lung volume, and airway occlusion are noted.
- Hypoxia and hypercapnia cause an elevation in minute ventilation,

respiratory rate, work of breathing, and oxygen consumption (Monin & Vert, 1987).

- Functional residual capacity is abnormal.

Further Complications

There may be additional complications:

- Lower respiratory tract infections recur.
- There is a seven times higher rate of sudden infant death in these infants (Boynton, 1988).
- Bronchial reactivity occurs (Monin & Vert, 1987).
- Pulmonary hypertension and cardiac failure BPD has inhibitory effects on future lung growth and development, preventing some of these infants from ever reaching fully normal capacity and function (Bonikos & Bensch, 1988).
- Delays and retardation of total growth and development are reported.
- Tracheobronchial injuries from prolonged respiratory treatments include partial to near-total airway occlusion by abnormal growth of granulation tissue, subglottic stenosis, tracheobronchiomalacia, tracheomegaly, necrotizing tracheobronchitis, vocal cord injuries, and inspissated secretions (Miller, Fanaroff, & Martin, 1992).
- Pulmonary air leaks are caused by rupture of the alveoli when the lung is overdistended by the oscillating pressures of mechanical ventilation (Thibeault, 1986). Most pulmonary air leaks are preceded by intrapulmonary interstitial emphysema.
- Interstitial emphysema is a common air leak in ventilated VLBW neonates and predisposes the infant to developing BPD.
- Congenital lobar emphysema is an overdistention of an abnormal lung lobe that occurs in utero (Lazar & Stolar, 1995). Mechanical ventilation distends the lobe, increases respiratory distress, and leads to circulatory collapse and chronic lung changes (Lazar & Stolar, 1995). The only treatment is removal of the cyst.
- A pneumomediastinum is a collection of air that collects anterior to the heart and is often benign. A pneumomediastinum that does not cause clinical symptoms of cardiac or respiratory embarrassment does not need treatment (Thibeault, 1986).
- A pneumothorax is preceded by rupture of the alveoli, with interstitial air traveling through fascial planes to the mediastinum, where it breaks through the mediastinal pleura to form collections of air outside the lung (Thibeault, 1986). Pneumothoraces are usually caused by positive-pressure ventilation, obstructive pulmonary pathology such as ball–valve air trapping, and/or rupture of subpleural blebs from interstitial emphysema or BPD.
- A pneumopericardium is a very rare complication of mechanical ventilation caused by lung overdistention with high peak inspiratory and positive end-expiratory pressures. A pneumopericardium is usually preceded by either interstitial emphysema or a pneumomediastinum, or both. The exact mechanism of air dissection into the pericardial space is unknown.

TREATMENT

Early Treatment Strategies

The most efficient way of preventing BPD is to identify those newborns at risk for its development and to prevent events that trigger the cascade of underlying pathogenic mechanisms in the development of the disease (e.g., prematurity) (Goetzman, 1986).

Prevention of Risk

Methods to prevent risk of BPD are presented below:

- Tocolysis is done to stop or delay preterm labor. Antenatal corticosteroids (betamethasone or dexamethasone) are administered at least 24 hours before or less than 7 days before delivery to enhance surfactant synthesis (National Institutes of Health, 1994).
- Antenatal corticosteroids given concomitantly with thyrotropin-releasing hormone reduces BPD more than if corticosteroids were used alone (National Institutes of Health, 1994).
- Postnatal surfactant therapy reduces the incidence of BPD (National Institutes of Health, 1994).

Limitation of Injury

If attempts to prevent prematurity/RDS have failed, the next strategy is to limit the iatrogenic tissue injury in the first few weeks of life that leads to the development of chronic BPD. This strategy includes the prevention of oxygen toxicity injury by the following measures:

- Intubation and mechanical ventilation should be limited.
  - Reducing the "acceptable" range of oxygenation (PaO_2) to a mid range (50 to 70 mm Hg). Considering the in utero PaO_2 of about 25 mm Hg, many authors advocate minimizing oxygenation (PaO_2, 35 to 40 mm Hg) as long as perfusion, hematocrit, blood pressure, and other parameters of tissue oxygenation are normal (Avery et al., 1987; Rhodes, et al. 1983; Usher, 1987).
  - Weaning, as soon as possible by altering one parameter at a time beginning with reducing positive inspiratory pressure or oxygen (Boynton & Jones, 1988)
  - Antioxidant therapy to neutralize and clear free oxygen radicals (Rosenfeld & Concepcion, 1988)
  - Stabilizing the endotracheal tube to avoid frequent reintubations resulting in trauma to airway and/or transient hypoxic episodes leading to need for increased respiratory support
- Extracorporeal membrane oxygenation (ECMO) and alternative ventilation techniques may be used.
- High-frequency ventilation (HFV), both jet and oscillation, is used to attempt to decrease barotrauma:
  - Decreasing airway pressures (Karp et al., 1986)
  - Changing the mechanics of air flow (Inwood, Finley, & Fitzhardinge, 1986; Karp et al., 1986; Karp, 1991)
  - Decreasing the development of hyaline membranes (Sinkin & Phelps, 1987)

- ECMO decreases barotrauma and oxygen toxicity by controlling oxygenation outside the lungs, thereby decreasing the need for mechanical ventilation and oxygen (Nugent, 1986).
- Nitric oxide inhalation is an experimental therapy for infants with persistent pulmonary hypertension of the newborn. It activates vasorelaxation, diminishes pulmonary vascular resistance (Southwell, 1995), and results in effective oxygenation and perfusion at lower mechanical ventilation pressures. Side effects include the following:
  - Methemoglobinemia (Methemoglobin is a breakdown product of nitric oxide that does not effectively carry oxygen.)
  - An increased susceptibility to lung injury due to increased permeability of the tissue and bleeding tendencies due to this change in permeability (Southwell, 1995)
- Developmental enhancement techniques can be used:
  - A developmental enhancement program based on individualized assessment may be helpful in decreasing morbidity in the VLBW neonate. If care is planned in response to the infant's tolerance to handling, the infant will experience fewer hypoxic episodes from adverse reactions to environmental stress and, thus, require less respiratory support and sustain less damage from barotrauma and oxygen toxicity.

Medical Treatment of Fixed Bronchopulmonary Dysplasia

Once BPD is present, treatment of the disease is focused on the twin goals of enhancing the natural healing process and controlling complications caused by the damaged lung tissue and abnormal lung mechanics of BPD. Treatment includes the following:

- Oxygen therapy ensures adequate and stable oxygenation for growth and healing and prevents recurrent hypoxemia during the fluctuating oxygen demands of exercise and stress.
- Diuretics counteract the increased interstitial fluid and pulmonary edema that play a role both in the etiology and in the ongoing complications of BPD.
- Bronchodilators modify hypoxemia caused by reactive airway disease (because of muscular hypertrophy and peribronchial edema) and peripheral airway closure (because of hypoventilation), which are common in infants with BPD.
- Corticosteroids promote weaning from ventilatory support and decrease inflammatory responses and promote improvement in pulmonary function test results.
- The infant's need for suctioning is evaluated to reduce unnecessary tracheal injury and hypoxemia (Miller, Woo, Kellman, & Slagle, 1987).
- Adequate nutrition is needed to restore a balance between lung injury and lung repair, to promote normal total and lung growth and development, and to compensate for increased oxygen and caloric consumption. Providing adequate nutrition is complicated by intolerance of increased fluid intake, inefficient substrate utilization, relative protein calorie malnutrition, gastroesophageal reflux, and disturbed feeding mechanics

such as uncoordinated suck and increased vomiting (Boyle, Baker, & Cassaday, 1995; Boynton & Jones, 1988; Kurzner et al., 1988a, 1988b).

- High caloric requirements, low fluid and stress tolerances, and maladaptive feeding behaviors are common.
- Individualized interventions such as increasing FIO_2, promoting nonnutritive sucking, reducing extraneous stimulation during feeding, swaddling, fortifying feedings, and individualizing a feeding schedule within overall caloric and fluid goals can promote maximum growth and development with fewer complications (Boynton & Jones, 1988). Usually 120 to 150 kcal/kg/day is adequate for growth, but some infants may need more (Kurzner et al., 1988a, 1988b). These infants are at risk for gastroesophageal reflux, feeding intolerances, and aspiration (Boyle, Baker, & Cassaday, 1995). Metoclopramide may be necessary to decrease the reflux (Boyle, Baker, & Cassaday, 1995).
- Continuity of care through consistent nursing care is important to detect subtle changes in the infant's condition.
- The environment of the infant needs to be carefully regulated to not overwhelm the infant.
- Frequent rest periods during intervention, accessing one sensory modality at a time, and detecting infant's "time out" cues are essential for the caregiver to recognize when the infant is becoming overstimulated.
- Complete parent teaching of any specialized care is necessary.

Air Leak

Pneumothorax is a frequent complication of RDS and other neonatal respiratory disorders. Pneumothorax is but one of a number of entities that compose the air leak syndromes, characterized by air in an ectopic location. Many air leak syndromes begin with at least some degree of *pulmonary interstitial emphysema,* which is the result of alveolar rupture from overdistention, usually concomitant with mechanical ventilation or continuous distending airway pressure. It occurs most commonly in preterm infants but may be seen in infants of any gestational age. Lung compliance is nonuniform, so that there are areas of poor aeration and alveolar collapse. Interspersed are alveoli of normal or near-normal compliance that become overdistended. The more normal lung units (those with better compliance) become overdistended and eventually rupture. Air is forced from the alveolus into the loose tissue of the interstitial space and dissects toward the hilum of the lung, where it may track into the mediastinum and cause a *pneumomediastinum,* or into the pericardium and cause a *pneumopericardium.* The astute nurse may notice an infant's chest becoming barrel shaped with overdistention and note that breath sounds become distant on the affected side. Typically, the infant who suffers a pneumothorax becomes unstable, developing cyanosis, oxygen desaturation, and carbon dioxide retention. The infant may become hypotensive and bradycardic as high intrathoracic pressure impedes cardiac output. A *tension pneumothorax,* in which free pleural air compresses the lung, is a medical emergency, and prompt relief by thoracentesis or tube thoracostomy is indicated.

Transient tachypnea of the newborn occurs typically in infants born by cesarean section, particularly in the absence of labor. The cause of the disorder is thought to be a transient pulmonary edema, which makes sense because it is known that the infant has "missed" the chance during labor to absorb pulmonary alveolar fluid (Avery, Gatewood, & Brumley, 1966). The chest radiograph may show increased perihilar interstitial markings and small pleural fluid collections, especially in the minor fissure. In contrast to the infant with RDS, arterial blood gas analysis usually reveals a relative normocarbia or hypocarbia, with normal pH. Oxygenation can usually be maintained by supplementing oxygen with a hood, although some infants will benefit from a short course of positive pressure support. The infant usually recovers in 24 to 48 hours.

Pneumonia

Pneumonia may be caused by bacteria, viruses, or other infectious agents. It may be transmitted transplacentally, as has been shown with group B *Streptococcus,* or by an ascending bacterial invasion associated with maternal amnionitis and prolonged rupture of the membranes. The usual organisms of active postamnionitis pneumonia are group B *Streptococcus, Escherichia coli, Haemophilus influenzae,* and, less commonly, *Streptococcus viridans, Listeria monocytogenes,* and anaerobes.

There is a strong association of bacterial pneumonias with premature birth, which may be due to a developmental deficiency of bacteriostatic factors in the amniotic fluid (Schlievert et al., 1975), or the infection may be a precipitating factor in preterm labor. Amnionitis can occur even in the presence of intact membranes (Naeye & Peters, 1978). Blood cultures and other diagnostic tests are necessary to help direct specific antimicrobial therapy. The nurse should be attuned to the labor history. Were membranes ruptured for more than 12 to 24 hours? Did the mother have fever before delivery? The term infant who remains tachypneic, has prolonged grunting or retractions, or develops temperature instability should be evaluated carefully. Blood cell counts may be helpful, and the neutropenic infant should be carefully monitored. Careful consideration of infection should be given to any newborn with respiratory distress and more than transient oxygen requirements. Tracheal aspirates obtained within 8 hours of birth that show both bacteria and white cells on Wright's stain are highly predictive of pneumonia (Brook, Martin, & Finegold, 1980).

Treatment is usually begun with broad-spectrum antibiotics, such as ampicillin and an aminoglycoside, pending culture results. Lumbar puncture may be undertaken or may be postponed until results of blood culture are obtained. When cultures result in the identification of the organism, the study of antibiotic sensitivity allows the clinician to choose the most effective antibiotic or combination of antibiotics for the causative agent. Antibiotic treatment for 10 to 14 days may be necessary.

Persistent Pulmonary Hypertension of the Newborn

Persistent pulmonary hypertension of the newborn (PPHN), or persistent fetal circulation, is a term applied to the combination of pulmonary hypertension (high pressure in the pulmonary artery), subsequent right-to-left shunting through fetal channels (the foramen ovale and/or ductus arteriosus) away from the pulmonary vascular bed, and a structurally normal heart. The syndrome may be idiopathic or more commonly secondary to another disorder such as meconium aspiration syndrome, congenital diaphragmatic hernia, RDS, asphyxia, sepsis, hyperviscosity of the blood, or hypoglycemia. Other factors that may cause PPHN include pulmonary hypoplasia as a primary event secondary to thoracic space-occupying masses such as diaphragmatic hernia, which is often complicated by increased pulmonary vascular resistance as a consequence of decreased pulmonary vascular cross-sectional area. A secondary cause may be maternal ingestion of prostaglandin synthesis inhibitors such as aspirin or indomethacin in the third trimester.

The neonatal pulmonary vasculature is sensitive to changes in PaO_2 and pH, and during stress it can become even hyperreactive, constricting to cause increased pressure against which the neonatal heart cannot force blood flow to the lungs. If the pulmonary artery pressure is higher than systemic pressure, blood flows through the path of least resistance, away from the lungs through the foramen ovale and the ductus arteriosus. The infant becomes progressively hypoxemic and acidemic, and the cycle perpetuates.

Collaborative management includes the following:

- Sedation and muscle paralysis are often necessary to prevent episodes of hypoxemia.
- Alkalosis, either with bicarbonate infusion or by hyperventilation, often relaxes the pulmonary vascular bed and allows better pulmonary perfusion and thus oxygenation. The approach to therapy should be directed toward preventing hypoxemia and acidosis, because the infant's condition may be stable with a PaO_2 around 100 mm Hg and a high pH (usually higher than 7.55) (Drummond, Gregory, Heymann, & Phibbs, 1981). The critical pH necessary for overcoming pulmonary vasoconstriction seems to be unique to the individual and may be referred to as a "set point."
- High applied ventilator pressures predispose the lung to air leak syndromes, further increasing the risk of sudden destabilization.
- Vasopressor therapy with dopamine and dobutamine are often used in conjunction with hyperventilation.
- When conventional therapies fail, high frequency ventilation may be attempted.
- Inhalation of nitric oxide has shown to be a promising therapy for PPHN (Roberts, Polaner, Lang, & Zapol, 1992; Kinsella, Neish, Shaffer, & Abman, 1992; Kinsella et al., 1993), but further studies are needed to determine which patients benefit from this therapy.
- ECMO has been shown to salvage approximately 80 percent of those patients with reversible causes of lung disease.

Meconium Aspiration Syndrome

Meconium aspiration syndrome is the most common aspiration syndrome that causes respiratory distress in neonates. The role of meconium in the pathophysiology of aspiration pneumonia has become controversial in the pediatric literature. It is unclear whether the material itself causes severe enough pneumonia to lead to hypoxemia, acidosis, and pulmonary hypertension or if the presence of meconium in the amniotic fluid is merely a marker for other events that may have predisposed the fetus to severe pulmonary disease. The severely ill infant with meconium aspiration pneumonia typically comes from a stressed labor and has depressed cord pH due to metabolic acidosis. Frequently, these infants are post mature and exhibit classic signs of weight loss, skin peeling, and deep staining of the nails and umbilical cord.

Pulmonary disease arises both from chemical pneumonitis, interstitial edema, and small airway obstruction and from concomitant persistent pulmonary hypertension. The infant may have uneven pulmonary ventilation with hyperinflation of some areas and atelectasis of others, leading to ventilation-perfusion mismatching and subsequent hypoxemia. The hypoxemia may then exacerbate pulmonary vasoconstriction, leading to deeper hypoxemia and acidosis. Infants with meconium aspiration syndrome may have evidence of lung overinflation with a barrel-chested appearance. Auscultation reveals rales and rhonchi. The radiograph shows patchy or streaky areas of atelectasis and other areas of overinflation.

There is debate among neonatologists as to whether infants born through thinly meconium-stained fluid should be intubated at delivery for suctioning, but most agree that the stressed infant with thick or particulate meconium may benefit from airway suctioning. Ideally, the nose, mouth, and pharynx are emptied before delivery of the shoulders; then the infant is rapidly intubated under direct laryngoscopy for suctioning of the airway. An endotracheal tube of adequate caliber to remove particulate matter should be used.

As with other cases of pulmonary hypertension, nursing care of these infants centers on maintenance of good oxygenation and acid–base balance and avoidance of cold stress (which contributes to acidosis). There is a high incidence of air leaks in these infants, and positive-pressure ventilation is best avoided if the patient can be adequately oxygenated, even at very high inspired oxygen concentrations. Use of antibiotics for these infants is also controversial. No studies have shown that infection is etiologic, but meconium itself may enhance bacterial growth as a culture medium. However, antibiotics are often used, particularly in desperately ill infants at least until a bacterial infection is ruled out. The infant is often exquisitely sensitive to environmental stimuli and should be nursed in as quiet an environment as possible (Langer, 1990). Interventions should be planned ahead to maximize efficiency of handling the neonate.

Less common than aspiration of meconium, aspiration of blood, amniotic fluid, or gastrointestinal contents may make a neonate symptomatic. The history is important in the differential diagnosis because radiographs are nondiagnostic.

Pulmonary Hemorrhage

Pulmonary hemorrhage is rarely an isolated condition and usually occurs in an otherwise sick infant. RDS, asphyxia, congenital heart disease, aspiration of gastric contents or maternal blood, and disseminated intravascular coagulation (DIC) and other bleeding disorders may play a role in the etiology of pulmonary hemorrhage. Pulmonary hemorrhage affects about 10 percent of infants who receive either natural or artificial surfactant (Horbar et al.,

1993). Massive bleeding may also occur as a complication of airway suction secondary to direct trauma of the respiratory epithelium.

Pulmonary hemorrhage is manifested by the presence of bloody fluid from the trachea. When massive, it may be heralded by a sudden deterioration with pallor, shock, cyanosis, or bradycardia. Attention has to be paid to maintenance of a patent airway because the tracheal tube may become obstructed and require emergent replacement. Suctioning must be done with great care to avoid precipitation of further bleeding. Clotting factors can become consumed rapidly, and the nurse should be alert to signs of generalized bleeding.

Pleural Effusions

Pleural effusions may be caused by accumulation of fluid between the parietal pleura of the chest wall and the visceral pleura enveloping the lung. A pleural effusion may also be due to chylothorax (lymphatic fluid) or hemothorax (blood). Lymphatics are responsible for drainage of fluid that filters into the pleural space. Fluid accumulates in the pleural space as a result of either increased filtration or decreased absorption. An increase in filtration pressure, as seen with increased venous pressure in hydrops fetalis or congestive heart failure, leads to pleural effusion. The rate of filtration into the pleural space also increases if the pleural membrane becomes more permeable to water and protein, as with infection.

Pleural effusion with high glucose content in an infant receiving parenteral nutrition through a central venous catheter should raise the suspicion of catheter perforation into the pleural space. If the infant is also receiving lipid infusion, the fluid may be milky, and, thus, effusion can be confused with chylothorax.

Chylothorax may be congenital or acquired and is associated with obstruction or perforation of the thoracic duct. It may also be a surgical complication of repair of diaphragmatic hernia, tracheoesophageal fistula, and congenital heart defects. Congenital chylothorax may be suspected in the infant who cannot be ventilated in the delivery room. Breath sounds are difficult to hear, and chest movement with ventilation is minimal. Bilateral thoracenteses may be lifesaving. The typical pleural fluid in a chylothorax—opalescent and rich in fat—is present only if the infant has been fed.

Pleural effusions that embarrass respiratory function typically require drainage, either by thoracentesis or by tube thoracostomy. Chest tubes placed for chylothorax and thoracic duct injury may have to remain in place for extended periods while the infant is treated with total parenteral nutrition, receiving nothing by mouth and minimizing thoracic duct flow.

Apnea

Apnea is the common end product of a myriad of neonatal physiologic events. Apnea can be caused by hypoxemia, infection, anemia, thermal instability, gastroesophageal reflux, metabolic derangement, drugs, and intracranial pathology (Kattwinkel, 1977). An infant with visible respiratory excursions but absent air entry should be investigated for obstructive causes of apnea. The presence of a cardiac murmur with bounding pulses should alert the nurse to patent ductus arteriosus as a possible contributor to worsening apnea in the small preterm infant. These causes should be ruled out before idiopathic apnea of prematurity is diagnosed.

Apnea is noted in more than half of surviving premature infants born weighing less than 1.5 kg. The respiratory control mechanism and central responsiveness to carbon dioxide is progressively less mature at decreasing gestational age. In contrast to adults, infants respond to hypoxemia with only a brief hyperpneic response, followed by hypoventilation and/or apnea. Hypoxemia should always be ruled out in any infant who has apnea before embarking on any other work-up or institution of therapy.

Care of the infant with apnea requires constant attentiveness. Obstructive apnea cannot be detected with the impedance respiratory monitor, because there are normal or pronounced respiratory excursions of the chest wall. Prompt tactile stimulation for mild "spells" is often sufficient to abort the episode of apnea, obviating the need for further therapy. The infant with spells accompanied by cyanosis and profound bradycardia needs prompt attention to his or her immediate needs as well as a more aggressive diagnostic and therapeutic intervention.

Sensory stimulation with water beds or other means sometimes manages these infants, particularly those with mild apnea. Many apneic neonates respond to nasal CPAP at low pressures, because the apnea may be due to airway obstruction or intermittent hypoxemia (Speidel & Dunn, 1976). Pressure support may also stimulate pulmonary stretch receptors, thus stimulating respiration. Excellent nursing care directed toward maintenance of the neutral thermal environment, normoxia, good pulmonary toilet, and prevention of aspiration is essential in the care of neonates at risk for apnea.

Use of methylxanthines, such as aminophylline, has markedly simplified the treatment of apnea in some premature infants. Xanthines appear to exert a central stimulatory effect on brain stem respiratory neurons and often markedly decrease the frequency and severity of apneic episodes (Calhoun, 1996). The nurse must be attuned to the toxicities of aminophylline, including tachycardia, excessive diuresis, and vomiting, which may precede neurologic toxicity at inadvertently high blood drug levels.

Congenital Anomalies Affecting Respiratory Function

Congenital diaphragmatic hernia occurs with some frequency (1 in 2500 live births), and it may be unsuspected until birth. Herniation of abdominal contents into the chest cavity early in gestation is accompanied by ipsilateral pulmonary hypoplasia. By mechanisms that are not well understood, there is often some degree of pulmonary hypoplasia on the contralateral side. The majority of infants are symptomatic at birth with severe respiratory distress in the delivery room. The abdomen is usually scaphoid, and breath sounds are absent on the side of the defect (a left-sided defect occurs in 90 percent of cases). Bowel sounds may be heard in the chest. Heart sounds may be heard on the right side because the herniated abdominal contents push the mediastinum to the right (Chernick & Kendig, 1990; Langston & Thurlbeck, 1986).

As soon as the diagnosis is suspected, one should consider the following:

- Bag and mask ventilation should be avoided because this fills the hernia contents with air and can compress the lungs and worsen ventilation.
- Orogastric tube should be placed to aid in decompression of the herniated abdominal viscera.
- Trachea should be intubated promptly.
- Mechanical ventilation should be begun.
- Ventilation should be attempted with a rapid rate and low inflation pressure.

Congenital heart disease frequently presents as signs of respiratory distress. Neonates with congenital heart disease demonstrating right-to-left shunting and decreased pulmonary blood flow (tetralogy of Fallot, pulmonary valve atresia, and tricuspid valve atresia or stenosis) usually present with profound cyanosis unresponsive to oxygen supplementation. Neonates with congenital heart disease demonstrating increased pulmonary blood flow or obstruction to the left outflow tract (transposition of the great vessels, total anomalous pulmonary venous return, atrioventricular canal, hypoplastic left heart syndrome, and critical coarctation of the aorta) may transiently improve with oxygen supplementation. Neonates with noncyanotic lesions such as patent ductus arteriosus and ventricular septal defect may present with signs of congestive heart failure.

Choanal atresia causes upper airway obstruction in the neonate. The choanae, or nasal passages, are separated from the nasopharynx by a structure known as the bucconasal membrane, which normally perforates during gestation. Failure of this developmental event results in an obstructed airway. This occurs bilaterally in 50 percent of cases. Most affected infants are female, and half have associated anomalies. Because newborns are obligate nasal breathers, these infants present with chest retractions and severe cyanosis particularly during feeding and paradoxically turn pink when crying. Emergency treatment consists of tracheal intubation or placement of an oral airway. Surgical correction is indicated (Hall, 1979).

Cystic Hygroma

A variety of space-occupying lesions can impose on the airway of the newborn. Most are derived from embryonic tissues. Cystic hygroma is the most common lateral neck mass in the newborn. It is a structure derived from lymphatic tissue and is multilobular and multicystic; when large, it obstructs the airway. Surgery is curative although sometimes technically difficult. The nurse must always be mindful of the airway and its patency. Many of these lesions are of great cosmetic concern and cause great distress in the parents. A care plan should address these parental concerns. It is sometimes helpful to facilitate contact with parents of other children with similar problems who can share their experiences.

Pierre-Robin Syndrome or Sequence

The major feature of Pierre-Robin syndrome or sequence is micrognathia, a small mandible. The tongue is posteriorly displaced into the oropharynx, obstructing the airway. Sixty percent of patients will also have a cleft palate.

Obstructive respiratory distress and cyanosis are common and may be severe. In an emergency, as with all airway obstructions, tracheal intubation should be undertaken. The infant should be nursed in the prone position to prevent the tongue from falling backward. Nasogastric tube feedings are usually required in the neonatal period. With good care the infant has a good prognosis for survival, and the mandible usually grows and the problem resolves by 6 to 12 months of age.

The newer terminology for this condition is Pierre-Robin sequence because there are a variety of ways this cluster of symptoms can occur. For example, it may be multifactorial inheritance, part of other conditions, or genetic, in which an actual gene or genes is responsible. So it is more than just an explainable, describable syndrome but rather a sequence of visible defects (Prows, 1996).

Extracorporeal Membrane Oxygenation

In the past 20 years, prolonged cardiopulmonary bypass, also known as extracorporeal membrane oxygenation (ECMO) or extracorporeal life support, has been used in thousands of newborns with hypoxemia that appears to be intractable to aggressive nonsurgical management. There are a variety of contraindications to the uses of ECMO, the most important of which is prematurity. Other contraindications to ECMO use include pre-existing intracranial hemorrhage and hypoxemia that is not potentially reversible.

ECMO is most commonly applied using a venoarterial approach. Blood is removed from the patient by gravity using a large-bore, jugular venous, multiholed catheter advanced into the right atrium. Oxygenated blood is returned to the infant's aortic arch by means of a large-bore, multiholed catheter advanced through the carotid artery from a point of introduction in the neck.

Because a large fraction of systemic venous return is drained from the right atrium, it is assumed that pulmonary blood flow is minimal during the first hours of bypass. If this is true, tissue oxygen delivery is provided almost entirely by the ECMO circuit. The activated clotting time is measured frequently while the infant is on ECMO. The heparin dosage is adjusted as necessary to maintain adequate anticoagulation. Fluids, nutrients, transfusions, volume expanders, and medications are delivered directly into the ECMO circuit. Blood gases and pH are measured frequently while the patient is on bypass. The bypass flow rate and membrane oxygenator oxygen and carbon dioxide concentrations are adjusted to maintain blood gas and acid–base homeostasis.

Weaning from ECMO is accomplished by periodic reductions in the bypass flow rate. As lung function improves, gas exchange may be gradually returned to the mechanically ventilated lungs. Periodic chest radiographs and estimates of pulmonary function can be used to determine the appropriate time for decreasing the bypass flow rate. Typically, ECMO may be required for 4 to 7 days.

The most frequently reported ECMO complication is hemorrhage secondary to continuous systemic anticoagulation. Hemorrhage may lead to acute asphyxia or death from blood loss or, as has been documented more frequently, from long-term neurologic sequelae as a consequence of intra-cranial hemorrhage.

In an effort to avoid permanent carotid artery ligation, two new approaches are being evaluated. Several ECMO centers are now reanastomosing the proximal and distal carotid artery segments after removal of the carotid artery catheter. Another approach is the use of venovenous bypass (Andrews et al., 1983).

TREATMENT OF NEONATAL LUNG DISEASE WITH EXOGENOUS SURFACTANT

Surfactant Biochemistry and Physiology

Surfactant is generally defined as the noncellular liquid found in the more distal airways and alveoli of normal lungs. Surfactant exerts its surface tension–decreasing activity by the movement of certain surfactant components from the hypophase to the gas–liquid interface.

Surfactant Replacement

Exogenous surfactant can be broadly classified into two types. Natural surfactants are derived from animal lungs or human amniotic fluid. Survanta is a bovine surfactant; Curosurf is a protein-depleted, organic solvent extract of minced porcine lung; and a third natural surfactant has been subjected to controlled clinical trials after extraction from human amniotic fluid collected at the time of cesarean section delivery. Artificial surfactants are composed of "off-the-shelf" chemical mixtures and lack surfactant-associated proteins.

Nursing Care—Surfactant Therapy

Nursing care before administration of surfactant includes the following:

- Accurate infant weight for use in dose calculations
- Confirmation of proper placement of the infant's endotracheal tubes
- Continuous cardiac and respiratory monitoring, including electrocardiogram monitoring/arterial catheters, and transcutaneous measurement of Po_2 and/or Pco_2 and pulse oximetry
- Sedation or increases in ventilator settings before dosing for an infant who does not tolerate handling or who becomes hypoxic quickly
- Endotracheal suctioning approximately 15 minutes before surfactant dosing to rid the infant of secretions that may inhibit the administration of the surfactant
- Assessment for signs that indicate the need to slow or stop the dosing momentarily to allow the infant to recover, including bradycardia, duskiness, decrease in $TcPo_2$ or O_2 saturation
- Optimal positioning of the infant specific to type of surfactant being administered. Survanta is administered in four aliquots, each in a different body position (head down, body turned to the right; head down, body turned to the left; head up, body turned to the right; and head up, body turned to the left) (Horbar et al., 1989). The infant is

held in each position for 30 seconds after the dose is administered into the EAT. Administration of Exosurf only requires turning the head from midline to the right and then midline to the left.

Nursing care after surfactant administration is as follows:

- Assessment of infant's skin color, respirations, oxygen saturation, and carbon dioxide levels
- Assessment of arterial blood gases as surfactant produces changes in pulmonary compliance, which may require rapid weaning of ventilator settings
- Monitoring for the possibility of respiratory distress immediately after dosing
- Delay in endotracheal suctioning after dosing of surfactant for at least 1 to 2 hours to prevent removal of the instilled surfactant (Miller & Armstrong, 1990)
- Continuous monitoring to observe for sudden fluctuations in oxygen saturation

Side effects include sudden changes in cerebral blood flow, making intraventricular hemorrhage a very real possibility, and changes in retinal blood flow, increasing the chances for retinopathy of prematurity.

CONVENTIONAL VENTILATION

Although much in respiratory care is focused on new technologies, it is important to understand standard ventilatory therapies. In general, the indications for mechanical ventilation are apnea, oxygenation deficit, and ventilatory failure. Therefore, the goals of mechanical ventilation are increased minute volume, improved distribution of gas, improved ventilatory perfusion ratio, decreased work of breathing, and normalization of arterial blood gases.

The ventilator type refers to how cycling from inspiration to expiration occurs. Time-cycled ventilators terminate respiration and change to expiration at a definite time, providing a constant inspiratory/expiratory ratio. Lung compliance, the stiffness of elasticity of the respiratory system, can cause the tidal volume and peak inspiratory pressure (PIP) delivered to vary slightly from breath to breath. Other factors that can cause variability are flow, resistance, leaks, and pressure limits. Time-cycled with pressure limits is the most common type of ventilator for neonatal ventilation.

Volume-cycled ventilators terminate inspiration and change the expiration when an ordered volume of gas is delivered into the breathing circuit. The volume is independent of flow, inspiratory time, or pressure. It is worthwhile to note these changes in the PIP may reflect changes in mean airway resistance or lung compliance. Also volumes may vary because of uncuffed endotracheal tubes. Caution must be used in neonates because of the potential to deliver high pressures, and safety measures are incorporated to prevent this.

The modes of ventilation are as follows:

- Conventional mechanical ventilation (CMV), which includes assist/control (A/C) ventilation

- Intermittent mandatory ventilation (IMV), which includes synchronous intermittent mandatory ventilation (SIMV)
- Continuous positive airway pressure (CPAP)

In A/C ventilation both the neonate and the ventilator can initiate inspiration, delivering uniform breaths with a guaranteed controlled back-up rate if apnea occurs. The trigger sensitivity must be adjusted properly to enable the neonate to take the assist breath. The neonate can control his or her own rate and carbon dioxide levels.

IMV provides a continuous flow of gas through the breathing circuit for spontaneous breathing to occur between the mandatory breaths initiated by the ventilator. The IMV mode is more physiologic than CMV, allowing the neonate to control the rate and pattern of breathing, decreasing the need for sedation, and reducing the risk of barotrauma. IMV is the mode of choice for ventilating neonates and for weaning as well. Some ventilators offer synchronization (SIMV), which allows the neonate to breathe in synchrony with the ventilator, avoiding stacked breaths.

CPAP allows spontaneous breathing while a continuous gas flow is being delivered through the breathing circuit without any machine rate. This continuous pressure inflates the lung and makes breathing easier and facilitates alveolar gas exchange by maintaining the functional residual capacity of the lung. This type of support is often all that is needed if compliance is not the underlying problem. CPAP is used for weaning purposes. It is often administered by an endotracheal tube that allows for a quick return to a normal rate by CMV or IMV if necessary. It may also be delivered by nasal prongs or a nasopharyngeal tube.

Ventilatory adjustments must be based on thorough assessments of the pulmonary system. This assessment includes physical assessment and laboratory tests. It must be done with full consideration of the total clinical case situation of the neonate. PIP is based on the lowest level that will maintain an acceptable tidal volume. Tidal volumes are gauged at 6 to 15 ml/kg (Hargett, 1995). When adjustments are made of 1 to 2 cm of H_2O, the expected change is in the arterial oxygen. It should always be started at a low level and increased based on the clinical picture.

Positive end-expiratory pressure (PEEP) is used to distend the alveolar tissue, which has a tendency in the neonate to collapse with each breath. If PEEP is not maintained, then the neonate is always taking the first breath and expending a tremendous amount of energy. Levels, like PIP, should be started low at 2 to 6 cm H_2O and adjusted in relationship to the PIP so that the tidal volume is affected. It is the difference between these two values that determines the tidal volume.

Ventilatory adjustments must be based on thorough assessments of the pulmonary system, including physical assessment and laboratory tests. They must be done with full consideration of the total clinical case situation of the neonate. PIP is based on the lowest level that will maintain an acceptable tidal volume. Tidal volumes are gauged at 6 to 15 ml/kg (Hargett, 1995). When adjustments are made of 1 to 2 cm of H_2O, the expected change is in the arterial oxygen. It should always be started at a low level and increased based on the clinical picture.

Oxygen levels are aimed at keeping arterial blood gases within normal ranges of 80 to 100 mm Hg. The lowest level that maintains normal ranges should be sought. An FIO_2 of 0.4 to 0.6 is usually considered an acceptable safe level (Hargett, 1995).

Rate is set based on the neonate's alveolar ventilation needs. A conservative approach is to set a low rate of about half the expected respiratory rate (i.e., 30 breaths per minute). The PIP in this case would generally be set slightly higher than normal to maintain a normal tidal volume. If a higher rate is used more in the range of 40 to 60 breaths per minute, less PIP will generally be needed to maintain the tidal volume.

Inspiratory time is generally set in relationship to the expiratory time. The less compliant the lungs, the shorter the inspiratory time, because lungs are not expanding easily. Long inspiratory times have been associated with barotrauma due to overdistention of the lungs (Hargett, 1995). Longer inspiratory times, however, are needed when there are mechanical obstructions of gas flow, such as in meconium aspiration.

Adjustments of inspiratory time result in changes in arterial oxygen levels. An inspiratory time of 0.25 to 0.4 second is acceptable in most cases (Hargett, 1995). Inspiratory/expiratory ratios are normally maintained at 1:2 or 1:3.

Flow rates of the ventilatory circuit are calculated as twice the minute volume of the infant (Hargett, 1995). This is usually between 3 and 10 ml/min.

These are just a few of the conventional respiratory supports that are commonly used in neonatal care. They give a framework for understanding the new technologies such as high-frequency ventilation.

HIGH-FREQUENCY VENTILATION

In contrast to HFV, CMV uses ventilator rates and tidal volumes that correspond to the spontaneous ventilation patterns of newborns. High mean and peak airway pressures may be required during CMV to adequately ventilate noncompliant lungs (Carlo & Chatburn, 1988). Exposure to high inflating pressures may lead to lung and airway injury, including pulmonary interstitial emphysema, pneumothoraces, bronchopleural fistulas, and BPD. HFV attempts to avoid these complications by delivering low tidal volumes at high frequencies. It may be used as a "rescue" technique to prevent further damage in infants who have developed complications secondary to CMV. HFV allows severely ill infants to be adequately ventilated at lower volumes than with CMV while improving gas exchange (Merenstein & Gardner, 1989). HFV may be used perioperatively and postoperatively to reduce movement of the airway and thoracic cavity (Carlo & Chatburn, 1988). This type of ventilation may be beneficial to infants who have preexisting pneumothoraces or bronchopleural fistulas. One study showed that when these infants were treated with HFV there was a decrease in air flow through the pneumothorax and the fistula. They were also able to wean the peak and mean airway pressures of these infants while maintaining adequate gas exchange (Gonzalez, Harris, Black, & Richardson, 1987).

Modes of High-Frequency Ventilation

HIGH-FREQUENCY POSITIVE-PRESSURE VENTILATION

High-frequency positive-pressure ventilation (HFPPV) may be referred to as CMV with increased frequencies of 60 to 150 breaths per minute. In HFPPV, the tidal volume is greater than anatomic dead space but is less than is commonly used during CMV and is delivered with very short inspiratory times (Carlo & Chatburn, 1988). HFPPV comes from the Sjöstrand technique and employs passive expiration. HFPPV may be used for airway surgeries because of its open system design (Gordin, 1989).

HIGH-FREQUENCY FLOW INTERRUPTION

High-frequency flow interruption (HFFI) ventilation delivers tidal volumes that may be less than or greater than anatomic dead space at frequencies of 300 to 900 breaths per minute. HFFI works by interrupting the flow of gas with a motor-driven valve. The gas flows through the humidifier, flows through the interrupting valve, and is propelled down the endotracheal tube (Carlo & Chatburn, 1988). There is an expiratory limb through which passive expiration occurs. This is sometimes classified as a type of high-frequency oscillatory ventilation.

HIGH-FREQUENCY OSCILLATORY VENTILATION

High-frequency oscillatory ventilation (HFOV) delivers very low tidal volumes, less than anatomic dead space, at very high frequencies of 300 to 3000 breaths per minute. Expiration is active and is achieved by a piston pump or acoustic speaker. Active expiration decreases the risk of air trapping and may explain the minimal air trapping with HFOV (HIFI Study Group, 1989). HFOV consists of a fresh gas source to provide oxygen and remove carbon dioxide, an exit port, an oscillator to direct the pressurized gas down the airway, and an airway adapter. The oscillator, which may be a vibrating loudspeaker or a piston and flywheel combination, generates air movement toward the patient (Wetzel & Gioia, 1987). HFOV may also be delivered by pressure to the external chest wall. This delivery method can be achieved with "a thoracoabdominal chamber connected to a vacuum source that maintains lung volume by controlling the negative pressure" (Carlo & Chatburn, 1988, p. 372).

HIGH-FREQUENCY JET VENTILATION

High-frequency jet ventilation (HFJV) delivers tidal volumes that may be less than or greater then anatomic dead space at frequencies of 60 to 600 breaths per minute. HFJV operates similarly to constant-flow time-cycled ventilation with passive expiration (Carlo & Chatburn, 1988). Adequate humidification is needed with HFJV to prevent tracheal injury. In HFJV, a high-pressure gas source is connected to a small airway cannula using a high-frequency flow interrupter valve. This valve opens and closes rapidly, propelling the pressurized gas into the airway. As much as 50 percent of the tidal volume gases are entrained from a continuous gas flow circuit (Gordin, 1989; Wetzel & Gioia, 1987). Gas entrainment is the addition of gas from areas surrounding the airway cannula to the gas flow being delivered by the jet ventilator (Carlo & Chatburn, 1988). This important aspect of jet ventilation is needed to force the nonmoving gas into the moving stream of gases. HFJV requires a specific endotracheal tube with a lumen for the jet gas flow and a lumen for the fresh gas flow. The fresh gas flow allows for entrainment of gases and addition of PEEP. There is a port, near the jet gas flow lumen, for the instillation of nebulized saline to prevent tracheal erosion (Wetzel & Gioia, 1987). A conventional ventilator may be used with a jet ventilator to provide "background" ventilation or sighs at a low rate. Background ventilation may decrease the risk of microatelectasis that may occur with long-term HFJV (Gordin, 1989).

Complications Associated with High-Frequency Ventilation

Although HFV can provide adequate ventilation to infants, it is not without the possibility of the following complications:

- Fluid overload, hypothermia, and necrotizing tracheobronchitis from cold inspired air (Carlo & Chatburn, 1988).
- Tracheal inflammation and copious secretions unless there is proper humidification of gas. Use of nebulized saline in the stream of gases appears to prevent tracheal inflammation (Wetzel & Gioia, 1987). Regardless of the type of ventilation, decreased humidification will lead to the presence of thick secretions that can impair gas exchange and plug an endotracheal tube. This plugging will require frequent reintubations and thus further trauma to the airway.
- Gas trapping from decreased inspiratory and expiratory times associated with high ventilatory frequencies. Gas trapping occurs less frequently during HFOV because it is the only form of HFV in which expiration is active. Gas trapping can lead to decreased lung compliance and retention of carbon dioxide.
- Microatelectasis may occur with HFV but can be combated by using a low-rate conventional mechanical ventilator for "background" breaths to provide PEEP and extra gas flow for entrainment (Gordin, 1989).

Nursing Care—High-Frequency Ventilation

Nursing care for the newborn on HFV is as follows:

- Heightened physical assessment skills are needed to recognize subtle changes in the degree of chest wall vibration, an indicator of tidal volume. Decreased chest vibration may indicate pneumothorax, endotracheal secretions, and mechanical malfunction (Avila, Mazza, & Morgan-Trujillo, 1994).
- Breath sounds, heart tones, and bowel sounds are difficult to hear while an infant is connected to the ventilator so auscultation is best done when the infant is momentarily removed from the ventilator (for routine circuit changes) or when the ventilator is in standby (interruption

of oscillation but not from ventilator mean airway pressure). Disconnection from HFV is discouraged owing to possible alveolar collapse. Therefore, when necessary, disconnection from HFV should be limited to short periods of time. If the infant is on HFOV, it is also important to auscultate breath sounds while being oscillated to assess the symmetry of oscillatory intensity (Avila, Mazza, & Morgan-Trujillo, 1994).

- Airway management of an infant on HFV includes using two people to suction: one person to suction and the other person to either manually ventilate or return the infant to HFV. Disconnection from HFV may lead to alveolar collapse, so the infant may need to be manually ventilated or the mean airway pressure may need to be increased after suctioning. The need for manual ventilation or increase in mean airway pressure is individually based. It is a generally accepted practice to suction infants while off of HFOV and HFJV. With HFOV, there exists a possibility of air trapping during rapid-rate ventilation (Avila, Mazza, & Morgan-Trujillo, 1994). With HFJV, a possible shearing force on the airway exists, resulting from the combination of negative pressure suction and high-frequency positive pressure occurring simultaneously (Gordin, 1989). Therefore, use of closed tracheal suction systems with HFV is discouraged.
- Positioning and comfort of infants on HFV are also important facets of care.
- Two caregivers should be used when repositioning: one to turn the infant and stabilize the endotracheal tube, and one to reposition the circuit and ventilator (Avila, Mazza, & Morgan-Trujillo, 1994). Although water mattresses are not recommended, sheepskins, lambswool, and eggcrates may be used to provide comfort and prevent skin breakdown.
- Sedatives, paralytic agents, and analgesics may be necessary to facilitate comfort for an infant while on HFV. However, the necessity of pharmacologic agents is influenced by the infant's condition rather than by the mode of ventilation.
- Interventions such as bundling and soothing music may decrease the need for pharmacologic agents.

INHALED NITRIC OXIDE

In the past 20 years it has become apparent that vascular endothelium plays an important role in the regulation of vascular smooth muscle tone as well as other important physiologic functions. Relaxation of vascular smooth muscle in response to acetylcholine requires an intact endothelium (Furchgott & Zawadski, 1980). Nitric oxide is believed to be the molecule released from the endothelium that is responsible for vascular smooth muscle relaxation (Ignarro et al., 1987). These findings were the catalyst for additional investigations of the biologic effects of nitric oxide.

Nitric oxide has an unpaired electron and therefore rapidly combines with other free radicals. The biologic half-life of the molecule is estimated to be 110 to 130 msec (Lunn, 1995). In vivo, biologic activity of nitric oxide is limited because it is rapidly inactivated within the vessel lumen. Inactivation occurs because nitric oxide has a very high affinity for hemoglobin and avidly binds to the iron of heme proteins to form a biologically inactive compound, nitrosyl hemoglobin. Nitrosyl hemoglobin is then oxidized to form methemoglobin and nitrate.

The nitric oxide molecule is synthesized from the amino acid L-arginine in a reaction catalyzed by a group of enzymes called the nitric oxide synthases. The by-product of this reaction is L-citrulline:

$$\text{L-Arginine} + \text{molecular } O_2 > \text{Nitric oxide} + \text{L-citrulline}$$

There are three major types or isoforms of nitric oxide synthases.

- The first isoform is the endothelial or constitutive type, which is located in the vascular endothelial cell wall, endocardium, myocardium, and platelets.
- Neuronal nitric oxide synthase is the isoform located in both the peripheral and central nervous systems.
- The third isoform, called inducible nitric oxide synthase, is not present under normal physiologic conditions but is produced in response to various inflammatory stimuli. Excitation of the inducible nitric oxide synthase causes production of much greater quantities of nitric oxide than activation of other isoforms. Activation of inducible nitric oxide synthase during sepsis plays a major part in producing vasodilation and consequent hypotension.

The biologic actions of nitric oxide are mediated through the guanylate cyclase/cyclic guanosine monophosphate (GMP) system. After formation from L-arginine in the endothelial cell, nitric oxide readily diffuses into the cytosol of smooth muscle because it is a very small, lipophilic molecule. Once inside the smooth muscle cell, nitric oxide binds soluble guanylate cyclase, which in turn catalyzes the formation of cyclic GMP from guanosine triphosphate (GTP). Increases in cyclic GMP lead to activation of cyclic GMP–dependent protein kinase, which triggers a reduction in intracellular calcium concentration through extrusion and sequestration. The decreased calcium concentration causes smooth muscle relaxation.

Nitric oxide is a biologic mediator of a variety of physiologic responses in numerous systems in the body. In the healthy state, the arterial circulation is partially dilated by basal production of nitric oxide in the endothelium. At birth, production of endogenous nitric oxide in response to rhythmic distention of the lung, shear stress, and acetylcholine release plays a major role in mediating a decrease in pulmonary vascular resistance (Cornfield et al., 1992). In addition to being an important determinant of basal tone in small arteries and arterioles, nitric oxide inhibits platelet aggregation and adherence and may alter vascular permeability (Moncada & Higgs, 1993). In the nervous system, nitric oxide may have a role in memory formation, pain perception, and electrocortical activation. In the gastrointestinal and genitourinary tracts, nitric oxide participates in control of signals regulating smooth muscle relaxation. It is produced in large quantities in response to various immunologic stimuli. It may also have a role in nonspecific immunity because it is generated when macrophages are activated.

A particularly frustrating problem for caregivers in the NICU is the treatment of acute hypoxic respiratory failure due to pulmonary arterial vasoconstriction. When pulmonary vascular resistance remains elevated postnatally, blood is shunted right to left across the ductus arteriosus and foramen ovale and away from the lungs, causing hypoxemia and PPHN. The ideal agent for the treatment of pulmonary hypertension would be one that causes pulmonary vasodilation without decreasing systemic vascular resistance.

Beginning in the early 1990s, it was theorized that inhaled nitric oxide would diffuse from the alveolar space across the epithelium to directly mediate vascular smooth muscle relaxation. Ultimately, it would diffuse into the lumen of the pulmonary blood vessels and be inactivated on binding hemoglobin, thus avoiding effects on the systemic circulation. Theoretically, inhaled nitric oxide could increase systemic oxygenation by two mechanisms: global pulmonary arterial vasodilation with increased pulmonary blood flow and cardiac output and/or improved matching of ventilation and perfusion in the lung.

There is concern, however, with potential toxicities that might be associated with the use of inhaled nitric oxide. One potential problem is the formation of excess amounts of methemoglobin causing the clinical condition known as methemoglobinemia. This condition is serious and associated with hypoxemia owing to the inability of methemoglobin to carry oxygen. The body's defense mechanism against the formation of methemoglobin is the enzyme methemoglobin reductase, which readily converts methemoglobin back to hemoglobin. If the rate of accumulation of methemoglobin is slow, this enzyme will limit increases in methemoglobin. To date, significant methemoglobin levels have not been reported when low concentrations of inhaled nitric oxide are used in neonates.

Another possible problem is the production of nitrogen dioxide and higher oxides of nitrogen such as peroxynitrite when nitric oxide is used with high concentrations of oxygen. Nitrogen dioxide and peroxynitrite in high concentration have been shown to directly damage the lung (Haddad et al., 1993). By using low concentrations of nitric oxide and limiting the time of mixing of nitric oxide and oxygen, the formation of these toxic molecules is minimized.

Several multicenter, double-masked, randomized, placebo control studies are being conducted to further delineate the benefits and toxicities of inhaled nitric oxide.

LIQUID VENTILATION

Respiratory function in preterm infants is characterized by stiff lungs, increased work of breathing, uneven ventilation, and ventilation/perfusion mismatch. One way to decrease alveolar surface tension is to eliminate the air–liquid interface in the alveolus by filling it with liquid (Cox, Wolfson, & Shaffer, 1996). This could improve alveolar compliance, reverse ventilation/perfusion abnormalities, and, if the liquid contains oxygen, increase oxygen uptake.

Nursing Care—Liquid Ventilation

Because of the complexity of the delivery systems, a specialized team, similar to that of an ECMO team, is required to care for these infants. A two-person team will manage these infants. One team member would care for the infant while a second team member would be responsible for the breathing device. These specialists will need to be trained in fluid mechanics and liquid breathing techniques.

Acknowledgment

Thank you to Sharon Sapienz for her assistance with this chapter.

REFERENCES

Andrews, A. F., Klein, M. D., Toomasian, J. M., et al. (1983). Venovenous extracorporeal membrane oxygenation in neonates with respiratory failure. *Journal of Pediatric Surgery, 18*(4), 339–346.

Avery, G. B. (1994). *Neonatology: Pathophysiology and management of the newborn* (4th ed.). Philadelphia: J. B. Lippincott.

Avery, M. E., Gatewood, O. B., & Brumley, G. (1966). Transient tachypnea of the newborn: Possible delayed resorption of fluid at birth. *American Journal of Diseases in Childhood, 111*(4), 380–385.

Avery, M. E., Tooley, W. A., Keller, J. B., et al. (1987). Is chronic lung disease in low birth weight infants preventable? A survey of eight centers. *Pediatrics, 79*(1), 26–30.

Avila, K., Mazza, L., & Morgan-Trujillo, L. (1994). High-frequency oscillatory ventilation: A nursing approach to bedside care. *Neonatal Network, 13*(5), 23–30.

Bailey, C., Kattwinkel, J., Teja, K., & Buckley, T. (1988). Shallow versus deep endotracheal suctioning in young rabbits: Pathologic effects on the tracheobronchial wall. *Pediatrics, 82*(5), 746–751.

Bland, R. D. (1988). Lung liquid clearance before and after birth. [Review]. *Seminars in Perinatology, 12*(2), 124–133.

Bonikos, D. S., & Bensch, K. G. (1988). Pathogenesis of bronchopulmonary dysplasia. In T. A. Merritt, W. H. Northway, Jr., & B. R. Boynton (Eds.), *Bronchopulmonary dysplasia* (pp. 33–58). Boston: Blackwell Scientific Publications.

Boyle, K. M., Baker, V. L., & Cassaday, C. J. (1995). Neonatal pulmonary disorders. In S. L. Barnhart & M. P. Czervinske (Eds.), *Perinatal and pediatric respiratory care* (pp. 445–479). Philadelphia: W. B. Saunders.

Boynton, B. R. (1988). Epidemiology of BPD. In T. A. Merritt, W. H. Northway, Jr., & B. R. Boynton (Eds.), *Bronchopulmonary dysplasia* (pp. 19–32). Boston: Blackwell Scientific Publications.

Boynton, C. A., & Jones, B. (1988). Nursing care of the infant with bronchopulmonary dysplasia. In T. A. Merritt, W. H. Northway, Jr., & B. R. Boynton (Eds.), *Bronchopulmonary dysplasia* (pp. 313–330). Boston: Blackwell Scientific Publications.

Brook, I., Martin, W. J., & Finegold, S. M. (1980). Bacteriology of tracheal aspirates in intubated newborn. *Chest 78*(6), 785–877.

Bueuvalas, J. C., & Balisteri, W. F. (1995). The neonatal gastrointestinal tract: Development. In A. A. Fanaroff & R. Martin (Eds.), *Neonatal-perinatal medicine: diseases of the fetus and infant* (15th ed., pp. 1019–1023). St. Louis: C. V. Mosby.

Calhoun, L. K. (1996). Pharmacologic management of apnea of prematurity. *Journal of Perinatal & Neonatal Nursing, 9*(4), 56–62.

Carlo, W. A., & Chatburn, R. L. (1988). *Neonatal respiratory care.* Chicago: Year Book Medical Publishers.

Carlo, W. A., Greenough, A., & Chatburn, R. L. (1994). Advances in conventional mechanical ventilation. In B. R. Boynton, W. A. Carlo, & A. H. Jobe (Eds.), *New therapies for neonatal respiratory failure.* New York: Cambridge University Press.

Chernick, V., & Kendig, E. L. (1990). *Kendig's disorders of the respiratory tract in children.* Philadelphia: W. B. Saunders.

Cornfield, D. N., Chatfield, B. A., McQueston, J. A., et al. (1992). Effects of birth-related stimuli on L-arginine-dependent pulmonary vasodilation in ovine fetus. *American Journal of Physiology, 262,* H1474–H1481.

Cox, C. A., Wolfson, M. R., & Shaffer, T. H. (1996). Liquid ventilation: A comprehensive overview. *Neonatal Network, 15*(3), 31–43.

Drummond, W. H., Gregory, G. A., Heymann, M. A., & Phibbs, R. A. (1981). The independent effects of hyperventilation, tolazoline and dopamine on infants with persistent pulmonary hypertension. *Journal of Pediatrics, 98,* 603–611.

Farrell, P. M., & Wood, R. E. (1976). Epidemiology of hyaline membrane disease in the United States: Analysis of national mortality statistics. *Pediatrics, 58,* 167–176.

Furchgott, R. F., & Zawadski, J. W. (1980). The obligatory role of endothelial cells in the relaxation of arterial smooth muscle by acetylcholine. *Nature, 288,* 373–376.

Goetzman, B. W. (1986). Understanding bronchopulmonary dysplasia [Review]. *American Journal of Diseases of Children, 140,* 332–334.

Gonzalez, F., Harris, T., Black, P., & Richardson, P. (1987). Decreased gas flow through pneumothoraces in neonates receiving high-frequency jet versus conventional ventilation. *Journal of Pediatrics, 110,* 464–466.

Gordin, P. (1989). High-frequency jet ventilation for severe respiratory failure. *Pediatric Nursing, 15,* 625–629.

Hack, M., Wright, L. L., Shankaran, S., et al. (1995). Very-low-birth weight outcomes of the National Institute of Child Health and Human Development Neonatal Network, November 1989 to October 1990. *American Journal of Obstetrics and Gynecology, 172,* 457–464.

Haddad, I. Y., Ischiropoulus, H., Holm, B. A., et al. (1993). Mechanisms of peroxynitrite-induced injury to pulmonary surfactants. *American Journal of Physiology, 265,* L555–564.

Hall, B. D. (1979). Choanal atresia and associated multiple anomalies. *Journal of Pediatrics, 95,* 395–398.

Hargett, K. D. (1995). Mechanical ventilation of the neonate. In S. L. Barnhart & M. P. Czervinske (Eds.), *Perinatal and pediatric respiratory care* (pp. 294–312). Philadelphia: W. B. Saunders.

Harris, T. R. (1988). *Physiologic principles.* In J. P. Goldsmith & E. H. Karotkin (Eds.), Philadelphia: W. B. Saunders.

HIFI Study Group. (1989). High-frequency oscillatory ventilation compared with conventional mechanical ventilation in the treatment of respiratory failure in preterm infants. *New England Journal of Medicine, 320,* 88–93.

Horbar, J. D., Soll, R. F., Sutherland, J. M., et al. (1989). A multicenter randomized, placebo-controlled trial of surfactant therapy for respiratory distress syndrome. *New England Journal of Medicine, 320,* 959–965.

Horbar, J. D., Wright, L. L., Soll, R. F., et al. (1993). A multicenter randomized trial comparing two surfactants for the treatment of neonatal respiratory distress syndrome. *Journal of Pediatrics, 123,* 757–766.

Ignarro, L. J., Buga, G. M., Wood, K. S., et al. (1987). Endothelium derived relaxing factor produced and released from artery and vein is nitric oxide. *Procedures in the National Academy of Science, 84,* 9265–9269.

Inwood, S., Finley, G. A., & Fitzhardinge, P. M. (1986). High-frequency oscillation: A new mode of ventilation for the neonate. *Neonatal Network, 4*(5), 53–58.

Karp, T. B. (1991). High-frequency jet ventilation: Impact on neonatal nursing. In J. Nugent (Ed.), *Acute respiratory care of the neonate* (pp. 147–170). Petaluma, CA: NICU Ink.

Karp, T. B., Solon, J. F., Olson, D. L., et al. (1986). High frequency jet ventilation: A neonatal nursing perspective. *Neonatal Network, 4*(5), 42–50.

Kattwinkel, J. (1977). Neonatal apnea: Pathogenesis and therapy. *Journal of Pediatrics, 90*(3), 342–347.

Kinsella, J. P., Neish, S. R., Ivy, D. D., et al. (1993). Clinical responses to prolonged treatment of persistent pulmonary hypertension of the newborn with low doses of inhaled nitric oxide. *Journal of Pediatrics, 123*(1), 103–108.

Kinsella, J. P., Neish, S. R., Shaffer, E., & Abman, S. H. (1992). Low-dose inhalation nitric oxide in persistent pulmonary hypertension of the newborn. *Lancet, 340,* 819–820.

Kurzner, S. J., Garg, M., Bautista, D. B., et al. (1988a). Growth failure in infants with bronchopulmonary dysplasia: Nutrition and elevated resting metabolic expenditure. *Journal of Pediatrics, 81*(3), 379–384.

Kurzner, S. J., Garg, M., Bautista, D. B., et al. (1988b). Growth failure in bronchopulmonary dysplasia: Elevated metabolic rates and pulmonary mechanics. *Journal of Pediatrics, 112,* 73–80.

Langer, V. S. (1990). Minimal handling protocol for the intensive care nursery. *Neonatal Network, 9*(3), 23–27.

Langston, C. J., & Thurlbeck, W. (1986). Conditions altering normal lung growth & development. In D. Thibeault & G. Gregory (Eds.), *Neonatal pulmonary care* (2nd ed.). Norwalk, CT: Appleton-Century-Crofts.

Lazar, E. L., & Stolar, C. J. H. (1995). Congenital pulmonary and chest wall malformations. In S. L. Barnhart & M. P. Czervinske (Eds.). *Perinatal and pediatric respiratory care* (pp. 526–536). Philadelphia: W. B. Saunders.

Lunn, R. J. (1995). Inhaled nitric oxide therapy. *Mayo Clinical Proceedings, 70,* 247–255.

Merenstein, G. B., & Gardner, S. L. (1989). *Handbook of neonatal intensive care.* St. Louis: C. V. Mosby.

Merritt, J. A., & Hallman, M. (1988). Interactions in the immature lung: Protease-antiprotease mechanisms of lung injury. In T. A. Merritt, W. H. Northway, Jr., & B. R. Boynton (Eds.), *Bronchopulmonary dysplasia* (pp. 117–130). Boston: Blackwell Scientific Publications.

Miller, E. D., & Armstrong, C. L. (1990). Surfactant replacement therapy: Innovative care for the premature infant. *Journal of Obstetric, Gynecologic, and Neonatal Nursing, 19,* 14–17.

Miller, M. J., Fanaroff, A. A., & Martin, R. J. (1992). Respiratory disorders in preterm and term infants. In A. A. Fanaroff & R. J. Martin (Eds.), *Neonatal–perinatal medicine: Diseases of the fetus and infant* (6th ed., pp. 1040–1064). St. Louis: C. V. Mosby.

Miller, R. W., Woo, P., Kellman, R. K., & Slagle, T. S. (1987). Tracheobronchial abnormalities in infants with bronchopulmonary dysplasia. *Journal of Pediatrics, 111,* 779–782.

Moncada, S., & Higgs, A. (1993). The L-arginine-nitric oxide pathway [Review]. *New England Journal of Medicine, 329,* 2002–2011.

Monin, P., & Vert, P. (1987). The management of bronchopulmonary dysplasia [Review]. *Clinics in Perinatology, 14,* 531–549.

Naeye, R. L., & Peters, E. C. (1978). Amniotic fluid infections with intact membranes leading to perinatal death: A prospective study. *Pediatrics, 61,* 171–177.

National Institutes of Health (NIH). (1994). NIH consensus statement: Effect of corticosteriods for fetal maturation on perinatal outcomes. Rockville, MD: National Institutes of Health.

Nelson, N. (1994). Physiology of transition. In G. B. Avery, M. A. Fletcher, & M. G. MacDonald. (Eds.), *Neonatology, pathophysiology and management of the newborn* (4th ed., pp. 223–247). Philadelphia: J. B. Lippincott.

Nugent, J. (1986). Extracorporeal membrane oxygenation in the neonate. *Neonatal Network, 4*(5), 27–38.

Obladen, M. (1988). Alterations in surfactant composition. In T. A. Merritt, W. H. Northway, Jr., & B. R. Boynton (Eds.), *Bronchopulmonary dysplasia* (pp. 131–142). Boston: Blackwell Scientific Publications.

Perlstein, P. (1987). Physical environment. In A. A. Fanaroff & R. J. Martin (Eds.),

Neonatal–perinatal medicine: Diseases of the fetus and infant (5th ed., pp. 401–419). St. Louis: C. V. Mosby.

Philip, A. G. S. (1975). Oxygen plus pressure plus time: The etiology of bronchopulmonary dysplasia. *Pediatrics, 55,* 44–50.

Polin, R. A. (1990). Role of fibronectin in disease of newborn infants and children. *Reviews of Infectious Diseases, 12*(Suppl. 4), S428–S438.

Prows, C. (1996). Craniofacial defects. Presentation at Cincinnati, Ohio: University of Cincinnati.

Rhodes, P. G., Graves, G. R., Patel, D. M., et al. (1983). Minimizing pneumothorax and bronchopulmonary dysplasia in ventilated infants with hyaline membrane disease. *Journal of Pediatrics, 103,* 634–637.

Roberts, J. D., Jr., Polaner, D. M., Lang, P., & Zapol, W. M. (1992). Inhaled nitric oxide (NO) in persistent pulmonary hypertension of the newborn. *Lancet, 340,* 818–819.

Rosenfeld, W., & Concepcion, L. (1988). Pharmacologic intervention: Use of the antioxidant superoxide dismutase. In T. A. Merritt, W. H. Northway, Jr., & B. R. Boynton (Eds.), *Bronchopulmonary dysplasia* (pp. 365–374). Boston: Blackwell Scientific Publications.

Ross Laboratories. (1978). *Clinical education aid #1: Fetal circulation.* Columbus, OH: Author.

Schlievert, P., Larsen, B., Johnson, W., & Galask, R. P. (1975). Bacterial growth inhibition by amniotic fluid. Studies on the nature of bacterial inhibition with the use of plate-count determinations. *American Journal of Obstetrics and Gynecology, 122,* 814–819.

Shannon, D. C., & Epstein, M. (1986). Bronchopulmonary dysplasia. In D. W. Thibeault & G. A. Gregory (Eds.), *Neonatal pulmonary care* (2nd ed., pp. 697–707). Norwalk, CT: Appleton-Century-Crofts.

Sinkin, R. A., & Phelps, D. L. (1987). New strategies for the prevention of bronchopulmonary dysplasia [Review]. *Clinics in Perinatology, 14,* 599–620.

Southwell, S. M. (1995). Respiratory management. In L. P. Gunderson & C. Kenner (Eds.). *Care of the 24-25 week gestational age infant: A small baby protocol* (2nd ed., pp. 43–68). Petaluma, CA: NICU Ink.

Speidel, B. D., & Dunn, P. M. (1976). Use of nasal continuous positive airway pressure to treat severe recurrent apnea in very preterm infants. *Lancet, 2,* 658–660.

Thibeault, D. W. (1986). Pulmonary barotrauma: Interstitial emphysema, pneumomediastinum, and pneumothorax. In D. W. Thibeault & G. A. Gregory (Eds.), *Neonatal pulmonary care* (2nd ed., pp. 499–517). Norwalk, CT: Appleton-Century-Crofts.

Usher, R. (1987). Extreme prematurity. In G. B. Avery (Ed.), *Neonatology: Pathophysiology management of the newborn* (pp. 264–298). Philadelphia: J. B. Lippincott.

Wetzel, R. C., & Gioia, F. R. (1987). Extracorporeal membrane oxygenation: Its use in neonatal respiratory failure. *AORN Journal, 45,* 725–739.

CHAPTER 9

Assessment and Management of Cardiovascular Dysfunction

CARDIOVASCULAR ADAPTATION AT BIRTH

Fetal Circulation

Knowledge of the normal route of fetal blood flow is essential for understanding the circulatory changes that occur at delivery. The pattern of fetal circulation is illustrated in Figure 9–1. Fetal circulation involves unique anatomic features. The placenta is the exchange organ for oxygen and carbon dioxide and nutrients and wastes. The *ductus venosus* permits the majority of blood from the placenta to bypass the liver and enter the inferior vena cava. The *foramen ovale* is the opening in the interatrial septum that permits a portion of the blood to flow from the right atrium directly to the left atrium. The *patent ductus arteriosus (PDA)* is a tubular communication between the pulmonary artery and the descending aorta that allows blood to flow from the pulmonary artery to the aorta, bypassing the fetal lungs (Moller, 1987). Fetal circulation can be described as *two parallel circuits* rather than the serial circuit present in extrauterine life (Avery, Fletcher, & MacDonald, 1994).

Neonatal Circulation

Clamping of the umbilical cord and subsequent removal of the placenta cause immediate circulatory changes in the neonate. With the first breath and occlusion of the umbilical cord, systemic resistance is elevated, which reduces blood flow through the ductus arteriosus (Brook & Heymann, 1995; Heymann, 1995). Cord occlusion causes a prompt rise in blood pressure and a corresponding stimulation of the aortic baroreceptors and the sympathetic nervous system. The onset of respirations and lung expansion causes a decrease in pulmonary vascular resistance secondary to the direct effect of oxygen and carbon dioxide on the blood vessels. Resistance decreases as arterial oxygen increases and arterial carbon dioxide decreases (Sacksteder, 1978).

The major portion of the right ventricular output flows through the lungs and increases the pulmonary venous return to the left atrium. The increased amount of blood in the lungs and the heart causes increased pressure in the left atrium. The increased pressure in the left atrium, combined with the increased systemic resistance, functionally closes the foramen ovale.

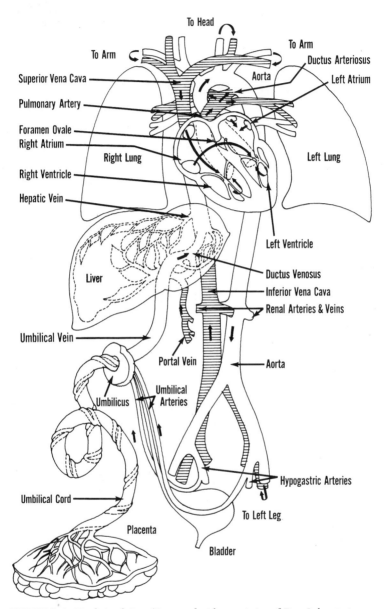

FIGURE 9–1. Fetal circulation. (Reprinted with permission of Ross Laboratories, Columbus, OH 43216, Clinical Education Aid, ©1985, Ross Laboratories.)

NORMAL CARDIAC FUNCTION

Heart Valves

Blood flow through the heart is directed through two sets of one-way valves. The *semilunar valves* comprise the pulmonary valve and the aortic valve. The pulmonary valve connects the right ventricle and the pulmonary artery. The aortic valve connects the left ventricle and the aorta. The *atrioventricular (AV) valves* consist of the tricuspid valve and the mitral valve. The tricuspid valve connects the right atrium and the right ventricle. The mitral valve connects the left atrium and the left ventricle.

Cardiac Cycle

Normal cardiac function involves two stages: systole and diastole. During systole, contraction of the ventricle causes the pressure inside the ventricle to increase to approximately 70 mm Hg in neonates (approximately 120 mm Hg in adults). When sufficient pressure is generated, the aortic and pulmonary valves open and blood is ejected from the ventricles. As the blood flows from the ventricles, the pressure decreases, causing the aortic and pulmonary valves to close (Conover, 1988).

During diastole, the mitral and tricuspid valves open and 70 percent of the blood in the atria flows into the ventricles. A small portion of the blood flows back into the aorta and enters the coronary arteries for perfusion of the heart. At the end of diastole, a small atrial contraction occurs (4 to 6 mm Hg on the right side; 7 to 8 mm Hg on the left side), and the mitral and tricuspid valves close. Metabolism of the heart is decreased during diastole. The average neonate's cardiac cycle is approximately 0.4 second, with 0.2 second for diastole and 0.2 second for systole (based on a heart rate of about 150 beats per minute) (Conover, 1988).

Cardiac Output

Cardiac output is the amount of blood pumped by the left ventricle in 1 minute. It is equal to the stroke volume times the heart rate (CO = SV × HR). The stroke volume is the volume of blood pumped per beat from each ventricle. The greater the stroke volume, the larger the amount of blood in the systemic circulation. An increase in cardiac output increases systole and decreases diastole. Cardiac output is influenced by changes in heart rate, pulmonary vascular resistance, and systemic resistance to flow.

Cardiac output is also influenced by the amount of blood returned to the heart. Venous return is determined by the passive movement of blood through the veins, the thoracic pump, and the venous muscle pump. Normally, when increased volume enters the heart, contractility is increased as a response to stimulation of stretch receptors in the heart muscle. The newborn's heart has fewer fibers and is unable to stretch sufficiently to accommodate increased volume; therefore, increased heart rate is the only effective mechanism by which the newborn can respond to increased volume (Braunwald, Sonnenblick, & Ross, 1988; Smith & Kampine, 1984; Talner, 1995).

When the volume exceeds the heart's ability to pump, cardiac failure results. Local factors that affect venous return to the heart include hypoxia, acidosis, hypercarbia, hyperthermia, increased metabolic demand, and increased metabolites (potassium, adenosine triphosphate, and lactic acid) (Conover, 1988).

Other factors that influence cardiac output include pressure and resistance. Pressure and resistance are inversely related; if pressure in the arterial bed is increased, resistance is decreased and flow is improved. The size (radius) of vessels influences resistance: the greater the radius of a vessel, the lower the resistance. Vessels obstructed by thromboses or constriction have greater resistance to vascular flow (Heymann, 1995).

Autonomic Cardiac Control

Cardiovascular function is modulated by the autonomic nervous system. Baroreceptors and chemoreceptors in the aorta and carotid sinus provide feedback to the autonomic nervous system. Feedback from these receptors stimulates the parasympathetic or sympathetic nervous system (Hazinski, 1984).

The parasympathetic nervous system is less powerful than the sympathetic system. Stimulation of the parasympathetic and sympathetic nervous systems results in vagal nerve stimulation and a decrease in heart rate. The majority of parasympathetic and sympathetic nervous system effects are on the atria, but decreased ventricular contractility may also occur. Right vagal stimulation affects the sinoatrial (SA) node, and left vagal stimulation affects the AV node. Acetylcholine is the active neurotransmitter for the parasympathetic and sympathetic nervous systems (Braunwald, Sonnenblick, & Ross, 1988; Smith & Kampine, 1984; Talner, 1995).

Stimulation of the sympathetic nervous system through the ganglionic chain releases norepinephrine and epinephrine, which act on the SA node, the AV node, the atria, and the ventricles. Maximal stimulation of the sympathetic nervous system can increase heart rate to 250 to 300 beats per minute. Contractility can be improved by approximately 100 percent. Alpha- and beta-adrenergic receptors are stimulated. Alpha-adrenergic receptors cause increased contractility (inotropic) and increased heart rate (chronotropic). Beta$_2$ receptors cause vasodilation, bronchodilation, and smooth muscle relaxation.

Term newborns have a decreased number of receptors but are capable of normal cardiovascular system function. The preterm infant is not able to smoothly maintain autonomic function, and energy expenditure is increased. Hence, the cardiovascular signs such as color changes and bradycardia may occur as a result of an excessive demand for autonomic nervous system function.

CARDIAC ASSESSMENT

Review of the maternal, fetal, and neonatal history is helpful in cardiac evaluation of the newborn. The following are associated with congenital heart defects:

- Maternal infections, especially viral and protozoal infections, early in pregnancy
- Maternal use of tobacco, alcohol, or drugs
- Maternal diseases
- Positive family history of hereditary disease, congenital heart disease, or rheumatic fever
- Neonatal history:
  - Cyanosis
  - Tachypnea without pulmonary disease
  - Sweating
  - Poor feeding
  - Edema

Incidence

The overall incidence of congenital heart defects is about 1 percent, or 8 per 1000 live births, excluding persistent PDA in preterm infants.

Physical Assessment

INSPECTION

The nurse should perform the following:

- Evaluate the newborn's activity: sleeping or awake, alert or lethargic, anxious or relaxed.
- Check respiratory effort, including the presence of signs of respiratory distress such as nasal flaring, expiratory grunting, stridor, retractions, or paradoxical respirations.
- Note color.
  - Cyanosis is the bluish color of the skin, mucous membranes, and nailbeds that occurs when there is at least 5 g/dl of deoxygenated hemoglobin in the circulation.
  - If cyanosis is present, one must differentiate between peripheral and central cyanosis and whether it improves with crying, does not change, or becomes worse with crying.
  - Pallor may indicate vasoconstriction.
  - Physiologic jaundice may be prolonged.
  - The infant is ruddy or plethoric, which is often seen in polycythemia.
- Check for presence of sweating.
- Assess for precordial bulging or precordial activity without bulging.
- Check for pectus excavatum, which may cause a pulmonary systolic ejection murmur or a large cardiac silhouette on an anteroposterior chest radiograph because of the decreased anteroposterior chest diameter.

PALPATION

During palpation the nurse should do the following:

- Note any hyperactivity.

- Check for thrill.
- Determine the point of maximal impulse (PMI).
- Count the peripheral pulse rate, noting any irregularities or inequalities of rate or volume.
- Evaluate the carotid, brachial, femoral, and pedal pulses to detect differences between sides and upper and lower extremities. If pulses are unequal, obtain four extremity blood pressures.
- Assess for bounding pulses.
- Palpate the abdomen to determine the size, consistency, and location of the liver and spleen.

AUSCULTATION

Identification of Heart Sounds

There are four individual heart sounds: S_1, S_2, S_3, and S_4. S_3 and S_4 are rarely heard in the newborn. S_1 is the sound resulting from closure of the mitral and tricuspid valves after atrial systole. It is best heard at the apex or lower left sternal border. S_1 is the beginning of ventricular systole. Splitting of S_1 is infrequently noted in newborns. Wide splitting of S_1 is heard in a newborn with right bundle branch block or Ebstein's anomaly (McNamara, 1990; Park, 1988).

S_2 is the sound created by closure of the aortic and pulmonary valves, which marks the end of systole and the beginning of ventricular diastole. It is best heard in the upper left sternal border or pulmonic area. Evaluation of the splitting of S_2 is important diagnostically. The timing of the closure of the aortic and pulmonary valves is determined by the volume of blood ejected from the aorta and pulmonary artery and the resistance against which the ventricles must pump (McNamara, 1990).

In the immediate newborn period, there may be no appreciable splitting of S_2. Because the right and left ventricles pump similar quantities of blood and the pulmonary pressure is close to the aortic pressure, these valves close almost simultaneously. Thus, S_2 is heard as a single sound. As the pulmonary vascular resistance falls, the pulmonary resistance decreases and becomes lower than the aortic pressure, causing a splitting of S_2 as the valve leaflets on the left side of the heart (aortic valve) close before those on the right (pulmonary valve).

By 72 hours of life, S_2 should be split. The absence of a split S_2 or a widely split S_2 usually indicates an abnormality. A fixed, widely split S_2 occurs in conditions that prolong right ventricular ejection time or shorten left ventricular ejection time.

A narrowly split S_2 occurs in conditions in which there is early closure of the pulmonary valve (pulmonary hypertension) or a delay in aortic closure. A single S_2 is significant because it could represent the presence of only one semilunar valve (aortic or pulmonary atresia, truncus arteriosus).

The relative intensity of the aortic and pulmonary components of S_2 must be assessed. In the pulmonary area (upper left sternal border), the aortic component is usually louder than the pulmonary component. Increased intensity of the pulmonary component, compared with the aortic component, occurs with pulmonary hypertension. Conditions that cause decreased diastolic pressure of the pulmonary artery (critical pulmonary stenosis, tetralogy of Fallot (TOF), tricuspid atresia) may cause decreased intensity of the pulmonary component.

As mentioned, S_3 and S_4 are rarely heard in the neonatal period; their presence denotes a pathologic process. Likewise, a gallop rhythm, the result of a loud S_3 and S_4, and tachycardia are abnormal.

After evaluation of individual heart sounds, the systolic and diastolic sounds are evaluated. The ejection sound or click occurs after S_1 and may sound like splitting of S_1. The *ejection click* is best heard at the upper left or right sternal border or base. The *pulmonary click* can best be heard at the second or third left intercostal space and is louder with expiration. The *aortic click,* best heard at the second right intercostal space, does not change in intensity with change in respiration.

CARDIAC MURMURS

Cardiac murmurs should be evaluated as to intensity (grades 1 to 6), timing (systolic or diastolic), location, transmission, and quality (musical, vibratory, or blowing):

Grade 1: barely audible
Grade 2: soft but easily audible
Grade 3: moderately loud; no thrill
Grade 4: loud; thrill present
Grade 5: loud; audible with stethoscope barely on chest
Grade 6: loud; audible with stethoscope near chest

The murmur grade is recorded as 1/6 and so on. The next step in evaluating a murmur is its classification in relation to S_1 and S_2. The three types of murmurs are systolic, diastolic, and continuous.

Systolic Murmurs

Most heart murmurs are systolic, occurring between S_1 and S_2. Systolic murmurs are either ejection or regurgitation murmurs. Ejection murmurs occur after S_1 and end before S_2. Ejection murmurs are caused by flow of blood through stenotic or deformed semilunar valves or increased flow through normal semilunar valves (Smith & Kampine, 1984; Talner, 1995). Systolic ejection murmurs are best heard at the second left or right intercostal space. Regurgitant systolic murmurs begin with S_1, with no interval between S_1 and the beginning of the murmur. Regurgitation murmurs generally continue throughout systole (pansystolic or holosystolic). Regurgitation systolic murmurs are caused by flow of blood from a chamber at a higher pressure throughout systole than the receiving chamber. Regurgitation systolic murmurs are associated with only three conditions: (1) ventricular septal defects (VSDs), (2) mitral regurgitation, and (3) tricuspid regurgitation (Park, 1988).

LOCATION

The location of the maximal intensity of the murmur is helpful in evaluation of the cardiac murmur. Figure 9–2 shows the locations at which various systolic murmurs can be heard.

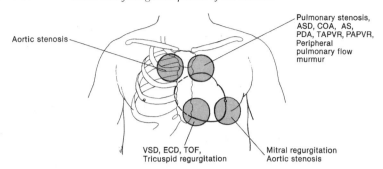

FIGURE 9–2. Location of systolic murmurs. AS, aortic stenosis; ASD, atrial septal defect; COA, coarctation of the aorta; ECD, endocardial cushion defect; PAPVR, partial anomalous pulmonary venous return; PDA, patent ductus arteriosus; TAPVR, total anomalous pulmonary venous return; TOF, tetralogy of Fallot; VSD, ventricular septal defect.

QUALITY

Murmurs are described as musical, vibratory, or blowing (Park, 1988). VSDs or mitral regurgitation murmurs have a high-pitched, blowing quality. Aortic stenosis and pulmonary valve stenosis murmurs have a rough, grating quality.

Diastolic Murmurs

Diastolic murmurs occur between S_1 and S_2. Diastolic murmurs are classified according to their timing in relation to heart sounds as early diastolic, mid-diastolic, or presystolic.

Early diastolic (protodiastolic) murmurs occur early in diastole, right after S_2, owing to incompetence of the aortic or pulmonary valve. Aortic regurgitation murmurs are high pitched and are best heard with the diaphragm at the third left intercostal space. This murmur radiates to the apex. Bounding pulses are present with significant regurgitation. Aortic regurgitation murmurs occur with bicuspid aortic valve, subaortic stenosis, and subarterial infundibular VSD. Pulmonary regurgitation murmurs are medium pitched unless pulmonary hypertension is present, in which case they are high pitched. Diastolic regurgitation murmurs are heard best at the second left intercostal space, radiating along the left sternal border. Pulmonary regurgitation murmurs occur with postoperative TOF, pulmonary hypertension, postoperative pulmonary valvotomy for pulmonary stenosis, or other deformity of the pulmonary valve (Park, 1988).

Mid-diastolic murmurs result from abnormal ventricular filling. These murmurs are low pitched and can best be heard with the bell of the stethoscope placed lightly on the chest wall. The murmur results from turbulent flow through the tricuspid or mitral valve due to stenosis. Mitral mid-diastolic murmurs are best heard at the apex and are referred to as apical rumbles. They are associated with mitral stenosis or large left-to-right shunt VSD or PDA, producing relative mitral stenosis secondary to increased flow across the normal-sized mitral valve. Tricuspid mid-diastolic murmurs can best be heard along the lower left sternal border and are associated with atrial septal defect (ASD), total or partial anomalous pulmonary venous return (TAPVR, PAPVR), endocardial cushion defects, or abnormal stenosis of the tricuspid valve.

Presystolic or late diastolic murmurs result from flow through AV valves during ventricular diastole as a result of active atrial contraction ejecting blood into the ventricle. These are low-frequency murmurs found with true mitral or tricuspid valve stenosis.

Continuous murmurs begin in systole and continue throughout S_2 into all or part of diastole.

Functional or innocent cardiac murmurs are common in children and can occur in newborns. These murmurs occur in the absence of abnormal cardiac structures. Functional murmurs are asymptomatic. The presence of any unusual or abnormal finding warrants consultation. Findings such as cyanosis, enlarged heart size on examination or cardiac silhouette on radiograph, abnormal electrocardiogram (ECG), diastolic murmur, grade 3/6 systolic murmur or a less intense murmur with a thrill, weak or bounding pulses, or other abnormal heart sounds are pathologic and must be investigated.

CONGENITAL HEART DEFECTS

Etiology

Cardiac development occurs during the first 7 weeks of gestation. Causes of congenital heart defects are classified as chromosomal (10 to 12 percent), genetic (1 to 2 percent), maternal or environmental (1 to 2 percent), or multifactorial (85 percent) (Moller, 1987). The vast majority are considered to be of multifactorial origin. These defects are probably the result of an interaction effect of the other causes.

Acyanotic Heart Defects

Acyanotic heart defects are those that produce a left-to-right shunt. Typically, these defects do not produce cyanosis because there is sufficient oxygenated blood in the circulation. The left-to-right or right-to-left shunts produce increased pulmonary blood flow and increased workload on the heart. The acyanotic heart defects discussed here are PDA, VSD, ASD, endocardial cushion defects, and aortic stenosis.

PATENT DUCTUS ARTERIOSUS

The *ductus arteriosus* is a wide muscular connection between the pulmonary artery and the aorta. The ductus arteriosus originates from the left pulmonary artery and enters the aorta below the subclavian artery. The ductus arteriosus allows oxygenated blood from the placenta to bypass the lungs and enter the circulation (Friedman, 1988; Hazinski, 1984; Moller, 1987).

The ductus arteriosus closes functionally by about 15 hours of life. During the first 24 hours of life, there may be some shunting of blood but the ductal opening must be greater than 2 mm for significant shunting to occur.

Closure of the ductus arteriosus occurs in response to increased arterial oxygen concentration after the initiation of pulmonary function. Other factors that contribute to closure of the ductus arteriosus include a decrease in prostaglandin E and an increase in acetylcholine and bradykinin (Park, 1988). The persistence of the ductus arteriosus beyond 24 hours of life is considered a PDA in the term newborn. PDA in the preterm neonate presents a different clinical problem and is discussed separately from PDA in the term newborn.

PATENT DUCTUS ARTERIOSUS IN THE TERM NEWBORN

Incidence. PDA accounts for 5 to 10 percent of all congenital heart defects, excluding preterm neonates. There is a higher ratio of PDA in females (about 3:1) (Park, 1988).

Hemodynamics. In extrauterine life, the flow of blood through the ductus arteriosus is reversed. The PDA allows blood to flow from left-to-right, thereby re-entering the pulmonary circuit and increasing pulmonary blood flow.

The amount of blood flow through the PDA and the effects of the ductal flow depend on the following:

- Difference between systemic and pulmonary vascular resistance
- Diameter of the ductus
- Length of the ductus

High pulmonary blood flow causes increased pulmonary vascular resistance, pulmonary hypertension, and right ventricular hypertrophy.

Manifestations. A small PDA may be asymptomatic. A large PDA with significant shunting may cause signs of congestive heart failure with tachypnea, dyspnea, hoarse cry, frequent lower respiratory tract infections, and coughing. Poor weight gain is common.

Diagnosis. The diagnosis of PDA is based on history and physical examination, radiograph, ECG, and echocardiogram. On physical examination, there may be bounding peripheral pulses, widened pulse pressure, and a hyperactive precordium. A systolic thrill may be felt at the upper left sternal border. A grade 1 to 4/6 continuous "machinery" murmur is audible at the upper left sternal border or left infraclavicular area. The murmur is heard throughout the entire cardiac cycle because of the pressure gradient between the aorta and the pulmonary artery in both systole and diastole. In severe PDA with large shunt, the S_2 is accentuated because of pulmonary hypertension (Brook & Heymann, 1995; Heymann, 1995; Park, 1988).

A small PDA may not be distinguishable on radiograph. With more severe shunting there may be cardiomegaly and increased pulmonary vascularity. The ECG may show left atrial and ventricular enlargement and an abnormal QRS axis for age. The definitive diagnosis is made with an echocardiogram. With two-dimensional echocardiography, PDA can be directly visualized. A ductus is considered to be hemodynamically significant if the left atrium to aortic root ratio (LA:AO) is greater than 1:3 in term newborns or greater than 1:0 in preterm newborns (Brook & Heymann, 1995; Friedman, 1988; Park, 1988).

Management. Medical management includes prophylactic antibiotics against bacterial endocarditis. Definitive treatment is surgical ligation through a posterolateral thoracotomy. The surgery is performed between 1 and 2 years of age, unless there is congestive heart failure, recurrent pneumonia, or pulmonary hypertension. The mortality rate is less than 1 percent (excluding preterm newborns). The prognosis is excellent, and complications are rare (Brook & Heymann, 1995; Heymann, 1995; Park, 1988).

PATENT DUCTUS ARTERIOSUS IN THE PRETERM NEWBORN

The ductus in the preterm newborn is not as responsive to increased oxygen content as that in the term newborn and does not close. The decreased pulmonary vascular resistance causes blood to shunt from left to right and re-enter the pulmonary circuit. This shunting causes increased pulmonary venous congestion, which decreases lung compliance, making the lungs stiff (Kirsten, 1996). Large shunts result in symptoms of congestive heart failure and an inability to wean ventilatory support or an increased oxygen requirement (Avery, Fletcher, & MacDonald, 1994).

Clinical findings of PDA are as follows:

- Bounding peripheral pulses
- Hyperactive precordium
- Widened pulse pressures (greater than 25 mm Hg)
- Continuous murmur, best heard at the upper left and middle sternal border

Radiographic findings include increased pulmonary vascularity and cardiomegaly.

Management. PDA is managed with the following:

- Fluid restriction
- Diuretic therapy
- Use of cardiac glycosides (controversial)

The preterm newborn's myocardium has a higher amount of connective tissue and water, which may decrease the left ventricular distensibility; thus, digitalis would have no effect. Digitalis toxicity may occur because of poor elimination of the drug. If digitalis is used, the dose should be decreased and monitored carefully (Park, 1988).

Indomethacin, a prostaglandin synthetase inhibitor, may be used to close the ductus. Prostaglandin E_2 is produced in the walls of the ductus arteriosus to prevent closure during fetal life. Indomethacin inhibits the production of prostaglandin E_2 and promotes ductal closure. Smaller infants may require a higher dose to obtain effective plasma levels. Indomethacin works best if used with newborns younger than 13 days of life; it is not effective after 4 to 6 weeks of life. The dosage for indomethacin is 0.2 mg/kg intravenously every 12 hours for three doses. Indomethacin is highly nephrotoxic, so the blood urea nitrogen and creatinine levels must be monitored.

Contraindications to the use of indomethacin are as follows (Avery, Fletcher, & MacDonald, 1994; Park, 1988):

- Renal failure
- Low platelet count

- Bleeding disorders
- Necrotizing enterocolitis
- Hyperbilirubinemia

Surgical ligation is reserved for those cases in which indomethacin failed or was contraindicated. The mortality rate for ligation is slightly less than 2 percent. Mortality is highest in the more preterm, sicker infants, especially if pulmonary hypertension has developed.

VENTRICULAR SEPTAL DEFECT

A VSD is a defect or opening in the ventricular septum that results from imperfect ventricular division during early fetal development. The defect can occur anywhere in the muscular or membranous ventricular septum. The size of the defect and the degree of pulmonary vascular resistance are more important in determining the severity than the location. With a small defect, there is a large resistance to the left-to-right shunt at the defect and the shunt is not dependent on the pulmonary vascular resistance. With a large VSD, there is little resistance at the defect and the amount of left-to-right shunt is dependent on the level of pulmonary vascular resistance (Graham & Getgesell, 1995).

Incidence. VSD is the most common congenital heart defect, accounting for 20 to 25 percent of all congenital heart defects.

Hemodynamics. The hemodynamic consequences of a VSD depend on its size; thus, this discussion of hemodynamics is divided into small, moderate, and large defects.

SMALL VSD. Small VSDs produce minimal shunting and may not be symptomatic. The chest radiograph and ECG are also normal. There is usually a loud, harsh pansystolic heart murmur, best heard in the third and fourth left intercostal space at the sternal border.

MODERATE VSD. With moderate-sized VSDs, the blood is shunted from the left to right ventricle because of higher pressure in the left ventricle and higher systemic vascular resistance. The shunt of VSD occurs during systole, when the right ventricle contracts so that the blood enters the pulmonary artery rather than remaining in the right ventricle. This prevents the development of right ventricular hypertrophy.

LARGE VSD. With large VSDs, blood is shunted from the left-to-right ventricle. The larger the VSD, the greater the shunt and the higher the pressure in the right ventricle and pulmonary artery. If pulmonary artery pressure is increased, thickening of the walls of the pulmonary arterioles may develop and the increased resistance may decrease the left-to-right shunt. Pulmonary vascular disease can lead to right-to-left shunting and cyanosis (Graham & Getgesell, 1995).

Manifestations. Manifestations of VSD depend on the degree of shunting. Small VSDs may produce no hemodynamic compromise and be asymptomatic. Larger defects are associated with decreased exertional tolerance, recurrent pulmonary infections, poor growth, and symptoms of congestive heart failure. With severe VSD, there may be pulmonary hypertension and cyanosis.

Diagnosis. A systolic thrill may be palpated at the lower left sternal border. There may be a precordial bulge with very large VSDs. A grade 2 to 5/6 regurgitant systolic murmur is heard at the lower left sternal border. There may also be an apical diastolic rumble. The pulmonary heart sound may be loud.

Radiographs show cardiomegaly involving the left atrium, left ventricle, and possibly the right ventricle. There is also increased pulmonary vascularity. ECG may reveal left ventricular hypertrophy. Right ventricular hypertrophy may also be present in severe cases. Echocardiogram shows a large left atrium (M-mode). Two-dimensional echocardiogram shows the presence or absence of other defects and the diagnosis of the size and location of the VSD (Avery, Fletcher, & MacDonald, 1994; Park, 1988).

Physical examination of infants with a large VSD, not detected in the neonatal period, may reveal inadequate weight gain, cyanosis, and clubbing of the digits.

Management. Management of VSD is as follows:

- Monitoring for signs of congestive heart failure (CHF)
- Prompt initiation of therapy for CHF if present. Congestive heart failure is treated with diuretics and digitalis.
- Unless pulmonary hypertension, no activity restriction
- Prophylaxis against bacterial endocarditis

Surgical management involves direct closure of the VSD. Cardiopulmonary bypass is required for the surgical correction. The timing of the surgery depends on the severity of the circulatory and pulmonary compromise. Infants with significant left-to-right shunting with evidence of severe compromise require surgery. Signs of congestive heart failure that do not respond to conservative medical management or increasing pulmonary vascular resistance are indications for surgical correction. Asymptomatic children with a moderate VSD usually have surgical correction between 2 and 4 years of age.

The mortality rate for VSD correction is approximately 5 percent. Mortality is higher among smaller infants, those with other defects, and those with multiple VSDs (Graham & Getgesell, 1995).

ATRIAL SEPTAL DEFECT

An ASD is a defect or opening in the atrial septum that develops as a result of improper septal formation early in fetal cardiac development. There are three types of ASDs (Park, 1988): (1) ostium secundum, commonly associated with mitral valve; (2) ostium primum, an endocardial cushion defect associated with anomalies of one or both AV valves; and (3) sinus venosus, often associated with partial anomalous pulmonary venous connection.

Incidence. ASDs account for 5 to 10 percent of all congenital heart defects.

Hemodynamics. An ASD usually does not produce symptoms until pulmonary vascular resistance begins to fall and right ventricular end-diastolic and right atrial pressures fall. All types of ASDs produce some blood flow alterations (Feldt et al., 1995; Porter et al., 1995).

With an ASD, blood shunts from left-to-right across the defect because the right ventricle, being more compliant than the left, offers less resistance to filling. Any factors that decrease right ventricular distensibility or obstruct flow into the right ventricle (pulmonary stenosis, tricuspid stenosis) can reduce or reverse the shunt direction. The left-to-right shunt increases right ventricular volume, but pulmonary vascular resistance decreases, so pulmonary artery pressure is almost normal. The large pulmonary blood flow will eventually lead to increased pulmonary artery pressures. These changes are gradual (Feldt et al., 1995).

Manifestations. The findings of ASD are listed below:

- It is usually asymptomatic.
- There may be a grade 2 to 3/6 systolic ejection murmur, which can best be heard at the upper left sternal border.
- S_2 may be widely split and fixed.
- With a large ASD, a mid-diastolic rumble may be present caused by the relative tricuspid stenosis audible at the lower left sternal border (Park, 1988).
- Cardiomegaly is noted, with prominent main pulmonary artery segment.
- Pulmonary vascularity is increased.
- ECG shows right-axis deviation and mild right ventricular hypertrophy.
- There may be incomplete right bundle branch block.
- Echocardiogram by M-mode shows increased right ventricular dimension and paradoxical movement of the ventricular septum.
- Thinness is evident.
- Easy fatigability is noted.
- Precordial bulge occurs by late infancy.

Diagnosis. Diagnosis can be made by two-dimensional echocardiography, which shows the location and size of the defect.

Management. Untreated ASD can lead to congestive heart failure, pulmonary hypertension, and atrial arrhythmias in adults. Spontaneous closure of ASDs occurs in the first 5 years of age in up to 40 percent of children (Park, 1988).

Medical management of ASDs includes prevention or treatment of congestive heart failure. Activity is not restricted. Surgical correction is accomplished by a simple patch or with direct closure during open heart surgery using cardiopulmonary bypass. Timing of surgery depends on the severity of the defect. The presence of a significant left-to-right shunt is an indication for surgical correction. Surgery is performed between 2 and 5 years of age. The surgery is not performed in infancy unless there is congestive heart failure that is unresponsive to medical management. The mortality rate of the surgery is less than 1 percent. The highest risk is for small infants with congestive heart failure or increased pulmonary vascular resistance.

ENDOCARDIAL CUSHION DEFECTS

Endocardial cushion defects are lesions that result from inappropriate fusion of the endocardial cushions during fetal development. They produce abnormalities of the atrial septum (ostium primum), ventricular septum, and

AV valves. Endocardial cushion defects take many forms, characterized by downward displacement of the AV valves as a result of deficiency in ventricular septal tissue and an elongation of the left ventricular outflow tract. The term *complete AV canal* is used to describe the large opening in the center of the heart between the atria and the ventricles. An AV canal consists of the following defects (Feldt et al., 1995; Park, 1988):

- An ostium primum ASD
- A VSD in the inlet portion of the ventricular septum
- A cleft in the anterior mitral valve leaflet
- A cleft in the septal leaflet of the tricuspid valve, which results in common anterior and posterior cusps of the AV valve

Incidence. Endocardial cushion defects account for 2 percent of all congenital heart defects.

Hemodynamics. The hemodynamic consequences depend on the type and severity of the endocardial cushion defect. There may be interatrial and interventricular shunts, left ventricle to right atrium shunts, or AV valve regurgitation (Hazinski, 1984).

Manifestations. The manifestations of this defect result from the increased pulmonary blood flow caused by the abnormal connection between both ventricles and the atria and by absent or malformed AV valves.

- Respiratory distress
- Signs of congestive heart failure
- Tachycardia
- Cardiac murmur
- Mitral regurgitation: grade 3 to 4/6 holosystolic regurgitant murmur audible at the lower left sternal border, which transmits to the left back and may be audible at the apex
- Mid-diastolic rumble at the lower left sternal border or at apex
- Accentuated S_1
- Narrowly split S_2
- Pulmonary closure sound increased in intensity (Feldt et al., 1995; Hazinski, 1984; Park, 1988).
- Cardiomegaly
- Increased pulmonary vascularity
- Prominent main pulmonary artery segment
- Left-axis deviation with a prolonged PR interval, right and left atrial enlargement, right ventricular hypertrophy, and incomplete right bundle branch block
- Recurrent respiratory infections
- Failure to thrive

Management. The management of endocardial cushion defects is presented below:

- Preventing or treating congestive heart failure with diuretics and digitalis
- Prophylaxis against bacterial endocarditis
- Surgical closure of the ASD and VSD, with reconstruction of AV valves under cardiopulmonary bypass, or deep hypothermia, or both

In some cases, pulmonary artery banding may be performed as a palliative procedure if there is not significant mitral regurgitation. This procedure carries a slightly higher mortality risk than when primary surgical repair is performed.

Surgery is indicated when there is congestive heart failure that is unresponsive to medical therapy, recurrent pneumonia, failure to thrive, or a large shunt with development of pulmonary hypertension and increasing pulmonary vascular resistance. The repair is performed from approximately 6 months to 2 years of age. The mortality rate has declined in recent years to 5 to 10 percent. The mortality rate for those who undergo pulmonary banding is approximately 15 percent. Factors that increase risks are as follows (Feldt et al., 1995; Park, 1988):

- Very young infant
- Severe AV valve incompetence
- Hypoplastic left ventricle
- Severe symptoms before surgery

AORTIC STENOSIS

Aortic stenosis is one of a group of defects that produce obstruction to ventricular outflow. Aortic stenosis may be valvular, subvalvular, or supravalvular. Valvular stenosis is the most common, and supravalvular is the least common (Park, 1988).

In valvular stenosis, there is usually a bicuspid valve. Subvalvular stenosis can involve either a simple diaphragm or a long tunnel-like ventricular outflow tract. Idiopathic hypertrophic subaortic stenosis (IHSS) is a form of subvalvular stenosis that presents as a cardiomyopathy. Supravalvular stenosis is associated with Williams' syndrome, or elfin facies, characterized by mental retardation, short palpebral fissures, and thick lips (Park, 1988).

Incidence. Aortic stenosis accounts for 5 percent of all congenital heart defects. It is four times more common in males.

Hemodynamics. Aortic stenosis causes increased pressure load on the left ventricle, leading to left ventricular hypertrophy. The resistance to blood flow through the stenosis gradually causes a pressure gradient between the ventricle and the aorta. Eventually, coronary blood flow decreases.

Manifestations. Symptoms depend on the severity of the defect. Mild aortic stenosis may not cause symptoms. With more severe defects, there is activity intolerance, chest pain, or syncope. With severe defects, congestive heart failure develops (Friedman, 1988).

Diagnosis. The diagnosis of aortic stenosis is based on the following features:

- Normal development
- Acyanosis
- Narrow pulse pressure
- Higher systolic pressure in the right arm with severe supravalvular aortic stenosis
- Systolic murmur of about grade 2 to 4/6, best heard at the second right or left intercostal space with transmission to the neck

- With valvular aortic stenosis: ejection click
- With severe aortic stenosis: paradoxical splitting of S$_2$
- Aortic insufficiency: high-pitched
- Bicuspid aortic valve or subvalvular stenosis: early diastolic decrescendo murmur (Friedman, 1995; Hazinski, 1984; Park, 1988)
- Radiograph: normal or may show a dilated ascending aorta or, in the case of valvular stenosis, a prominent aortic "knob" caused by poststenotic dilation (Park, 1988)
- Cardiomegaly
- ECG: normal or may show mild left ventricular hypertrophy and inverted T waves
- Echocardiogram: prominent thickening of the septum and abnormal mitral valve motions

Management. Management of aortic stenosis is as follows:
- Preventing or treating the congestive heart failure with fluid restriction, diuretics, and digitalis
- Restricting activity to prevent increased demand on the heart (in moderate to severe cases)
- Performance of balloon valvuloplasty sometimes at the time of cardiac catheterization to improve circulation
- In critical aortic stenosis, maintenance of the patency of the ductus arteriosus with prostaglandin E$_1$ to prevent hypoxia (Avery, Fletcher, & MacDonald, 1994)

The type of surgical correction depends on the exact location and severity of the defect. The procedure may consist of aortic valve commissurotomy or valve replacement with a prosthetic valve or a graft. The placement of prosthetic valves is usually deferred until adult-sized prosthetic valves can be inserted. The timing of the surgery is dependent on the severity of the defect. Infants with critical aortic stenosis with congestive heart failure must have corrective surgery. Surgery is performed on children when there is a peak systolic pressure gradient greater than 80 mm Hg or when there are symptoms of chest pain (Friedman, 1988).

The mortality risk for infants and small children is 15 to 20 percent.

Cyanotic Heart Defects

Cyanotic heart defects are those defects with a right-to-left shunt with either reduced or increased pulmonary blood flow.

TETRALOGY OF FALLOT

Tetralogy of Fallot consists of a large VSD, pulmonary stenosis or other right ventricular outflow tract obstruction, overriding aorta, and hypertrophied right ventricle. The right ventricle may not be hypertrophied initially. In the most severe form, there is pulmonary valve atresia (Zuberbuhler, 1995).

Incidence. Tetralogy of Fallot accounts for 10 percent of all congenital heart defects. It is the most common cyanotic heart defect beyond infancy.

Hemodynamics. The VSD causes equalization of pressure in the ventricles. Unsaturated blood flows through the VSD into the aorta because of the obstruction to blood flow from the right ventricle into the pulmonary artery.

Manifestations. Cardinal signs include the following:

- Cyanosis
- Hypoxia
- Dyspnea

Newborns can present with just a loud murmur, or they may be cyanotic. Severe decompensation or "tet" spells are common in infants or children but can also occur in neonates. Children instinctively assume a squatting position, which traps venous blood in the legs and decreases systemic venous return to the heart.

Chronic arterial desaturation stimulates erythropoiesis, causing polycythemia.

The following may occur:

- Increased blood viscosity
  - Microcytic anemia
  - Cerebrovascular accident (stroke)
- Brain abscesses
- Chronic hypoxemia and polycythemia:
  - Increased risk of hemorrhagic diathesis because of thrombocytopenia due to decreased platelet survival time and reduced platelet aggregation
  - Impaired synthesis of vitamin K–dependent clotting factors (Hazinski, 1984; Park, 1988; Pinsky & Arciniegas, 1990; Zuberbuhler, 1995)

Diagnosis. The diagnosis of TOF is based on the following:

- Varying degrees of cyanosis
- Long, loud, grade 3 to 5/6 systolic ejection murmur heard at the middle and upper left sternal border
- Ventricular tap along the lower left sternal border
- Systolic thrill at the lower and middle left sternal border
- PDA murmur possibly present in severe disease (Park, 1988).
- Chest radiograph: decreased or normal heart size
  - Decreased pulmonary vascularity
  - Typical boot shape caused by the concave main pulmonary artery segment with upturned apex
  - Right atrial enlargement and a right aortic arch
- Echocardiography: large VSD and overriding aorta

Management. The definitive therapy for TOF is surgical repair under cardiopulmonary bypass. Medical management is as listed below:

- Prevention or treatment of the following:
  - Hypoxemia
  - Polycythemia
  - Infection
  - Microcytic hypochromic anemia
- Avoidance of dehydration to prevent increased risk of cerebral infarcts because of hemoconcentration
- Education of parents in signs of decompensation

• Education of parents to recognize and treat hypercyanotic or "tet" spells

Surgical management can be either palliative or corrective. Palliative procedures are undertaken to improve pulmonary blood flow by creating a pathway between the systemic and pulmonary circulation. They are indicated for infants with TOF and pulmonary atresia, severely cyanotic infants younger than 6 months old, infants with medically unmanageable "tet" spells, or children with a hypoplastic pulmonary artery in whom corrective surgery is difficult (Park, 1988; Zuberbuhler, 1995). Common surgical procedures are listed in Table 9–1.

Surgical correction is performed under cardiopulmonary bypass after the infant is 6 months old. Surgery may be delayed until 2 to 4 years in asymptomatic children or in those who have had a palliative procedure. The defect is repaired by patch closure of the VSD and resection and widening of the right ventricular outflow tract (Pinsky & Arciniegas, 1990). The mortality rate for TOF varies with the severity of the circulatory compromise caused by the defect. The postoperative mortality rate is 5 to 10 percent in the first 2 years for uncomplicated TOF. More severe cases have a higher mortality rate, exhibit residual pulmonary outflow tract obstruction, and may require further surgery (Hazinski, 1984). Because these infants have the potential of myocardial damage from the restriction of the right ventricular blood flow during the surgery, cardiac support is needed to ensure adequate myocardial perfusion. Extracorporeal membrane oxygenation (ECMO) is being used by some centers to support the cardiovascular perfusion (Suddaby & O'Brien, 1993).

PULMONARY ATRESIA

Pulmonary atresia results in the absence of communication between the right ventricle and the pulmonary artery at the level of the main pulmonary artery or the pulmonary valve. Atresia of the pulmonary valve, with a diaphragm-like membrane, is the most common type. The right ventricle is usually hypoplastic, with thick ventricular walls. Less frequently, the right ventricle is of normal size with tricuspid regurgitation. The presence of a PDA, ASD, or patent foramen ovale to allow mixing of blood is crucial for survival (Mair et al., 1995a).

Incidence. Pulmonary atresia accounts for less than 1 percent of all congenital heart defects (Park, 1988).

Hemodynamics. Pulmonary atresia with VSD results in a small, hypoplastic right heart. The absence of a right ventricular outflow tract results in high right ventricular end-diastolic pressures. Tricuspid insufficiency occurs and right atrial pressures increase, causing systemic venous blood to shunt from the right to the left atrium through the patent foramen ovale or ASD. Mixed venous blood flows into the left ventricle and aorta. The PDA produces the only pulmonary blood flow. Closure of the PDA causes severe cyanosis, hypoxemia, and acidosis.

In the presence of a VSD, right ventricular size is usually adequate. Systemic venous blood shunts from the right ventricle through the VSD to the left ventricle and enters the aorta. The PDA still provides the only pulmonary blood flow.

TABLE 9–1. Common Cardiac Surgical Procedure

Procedure	Type	Defect	Description
Blalock-Hanlon	Palliative	TGA	Surgical creation of an ASD; rarely used; still useful for complex TGA or mitral atresia and single ventricle
Blalock-Taussig	Palliative	TOF, PA, PS, VSD	Anastomosis of the subclavian artery and pulmonary artery to improve pulmonary blood flow
Brock	Corrective	PVA	Blind pulmonary valvotomy incision of PV
Fontan	Corrective	HLHS (stage 2), tricuspid atresia, tricuspid stenosis	Bypass of the right ventricle by connection of the right atrium to pulmonary artery
Gore-Tex shunt	Palliative	TOF	Interposition of Gore-Tex between subclavian artery and ipsilateral pulmonary artery
Jatene	Corrective	TGA	Switching of transposed great arteries to their anatomically correct position
Mustard	Corrective	TGA	Use of a pericardial or synthetic baffle in the atria so that venous blood is shunted across the right atrium to the left ventricle and into the pulmonary artery. Systemic blood is shunted across the left atrium to the right ventricle, which delivers blood to the aorta.
Norwood	Palliative	HLHS (stage 1)	1. Main pulmonary artery is divided, and the proximal stump is anastomosed to the descending aorta; distal main pulmonary artery is closed. 2. Right-sided Gore-Tex shunt is performed to increase pulmonary blood flow. 3. Excision of atrial septum to allow interatrial mixing.
Potts	Palliative	TOF	Surgical creation of a window between descending aorta and left pulmonary artery; difficult to take down; rarely used
Pulmonary artery banding	Palliative	VSD, single ventricle	Placement of a band around the pulmonary artery to decrease the blood flow to the lungs
Rashkind	Corrective	PA, TGA	Atrial septostomy created at cardiac catheterization by passing a balloon-tipped catheter through the patent foramen ovale, inflating the balloon, and snapping it back through the patent foramen
Rastelli	Corrective	TGA, TOF, PA, TA	Commonly applied to all valved conduits from the right ventricle to pulmonary artery
Senning	Corrective	TGA	Creation of an intra-atrial baffle, using atrial tissue, to shunt blood from the vena cava to the left ventricle and from the pulmonary veins to the right ventricle
Waterston	Palliative	TOF	Window created between the ascending aorta and the pulmonary artery, improving oxygenation of systemic blood; rarely used because of the distortion and/or obstruction of pulmonary artery

ASD, atrial septal defect; HLHS, hypoplastic left heart syndrome; PA, pulmonary artery; PS, pulmonary stenosis; PV, pulmonary valve; PVA, pulmonary valve atresia; TA, truncus arteriosus; TGA, transposition of the great arteries; TOF, tetralogy of Fallot; VSD, ventricular septal defect.

Manifestations. The manifestations of pulmonary atresia include the following:

- Cyanosis at birth
- Tachypnea
- No obvious respiratory distress
- Single S_2
- Soft systolic PDA murmur: upper left sternal border
- Tricuspid insufficiency: harsh systolic murmur along the lower right and left sternal border (Hazinski, 1984; Mair et al., 1995a; Park, 1988).
- Heart size: normal or enlarged
- Concave main pulmonary artery segment similar to tricuspid atresia
- Pulmonary vascular markings: decreased
- ECG: normal QRS axis, left ventricular hypertrophy (type I) or, less frequently, right ventricular hypertrophy (type II)
- Right atrial hypertrophy in about 70 percent of cases (Park, 1988)
- Two-dimensional echocardiogram: shows atretic pulmonary valve and the hypoplastic right ventricular cavity and tricuspid valve

Management. Pulmonary atresia is managed as follows:

- Prostaglandin to maintain ductal patency
  - Prostaglandin E_1 (Prostin) given as a continuous intravenous infusion
  - Initial dose: 0.1 μg/kg/min
  - Dose incrementally decreased to a maintenance of 0.01 μg/kg/min
- Balloon atrial septostomy performed at cardiac catheterization to promote better mixing of systemic and pulmonary venous blood in the atria
- Surgical correction: a systemic–pulmonary artery shunt using Gore-Tex between the left subclavian artery and the left pulmonary artery (Blalock-Taussig procedure)
- Performance of a closed heart pulmonary valvotomy if pulmonary valve atresia is present (Brock's procedure)

The mortality rate for these procedures is 10 to 25 percent.

If the initial systemic-pulmonary shunt is not effective, a second shunt is attempted in another location. Right ventricular outflow tract reconstruction can be attempted if the right ventricle size is adequate; this procedure has a mortality rate of 25 percent. The Fontan procedure is attempted in the presence of a hypoplastic right ventricle in late childhood; the mortality rate for this procedure can be as high as 40 percent.

The prognosis of pulmonary atresia depends on the size of the pulmonary outflow tract established through surgery and the degree of fibrosis of the right ventricle. If there is severe fibrosis and significant outflow tract obstruction, there is an increased risk of development of dysrhythmias and right ventricular dysfunction (Hazinski, 1984; Mair et al., 1995a; Park, 1988).

PULMONARY STENOSIS

Pulmonary stenosis is caused by abnormal formation of the pulmonary valve leaflets during fetal cardiac development. Pulmonary stenosis can be valvular, subvalvular (infundibular), or supravalvular. Valvular pulmonary stenosis is the most common, accounting for 90 percent of cases.

Incidence. Pulmonary stenosis makes up 5 to 8 percent of all congenital heart defects. It is often associated with other defects.

Hemodynamics. Pulmonary stenosis results in obstruction to blood flow from the right ventricle to the pulmonary artery. The right ventricle hypertrophies in response to the increased pressure caused by the obstruction to outflow. Pulmonary blood flow volume is normal in the absence of intracardiac shunting (Rocchini & Emmanouilides, 1995).

Manifestations. Pulmonary stenosis may be asymptomatic if it is mild. Moderate pulmonary stenosis may cause easy tiring. Severe or critical pulmonary stenosis will cause congestive heart failure.

Diagnosis. The diagnosis is determined from the following:
- Pulmonary systolic ejection click at upper left sternal border
- Widely split S_2 and soft or delayed pulmonary component
- Systolic ejection murmur (grade 2 to 5/6), upper left sternal border and transmits across the back
  - Severity directly related to loudness and duration of the murmur
- Systolic thrill: upper left sternal border
- Hepatosplenomegaly
- Congestive heart failure
- ECG normal in mild pulmonary stenosis
- Right-axis deviation and right ventricular hypertrophy within the moderate stenosis
- Right atrial hypertrophy and right ventricular strain with severe pulmonary stenosis
- Normal heart size
- Prominent main pulmonary artery segment
- Pulmonary markings normal in mild to moderate stenosis
- Critical type: decreased pulmonary markings
- Echocardiogram: decreased motion of the pulmonary valve leaflets and poststenotic dilation of the main pulmonary artery segment (Park, 1988; Rocchini & Emmanouilides, 1995).

Management. This disorder is managed as follows:
- Treatment determined by the severity of the obstruction to flow
- Mild type: generally requires no therapy except antimicrobial prophylaxis against subacute infective endocarditis
- Moderate pulmonary stenosis: balloon valvuloplasty

Surgical correction is performed in children when the right ventricular pressure measures 80 to 100 mm Hg and balloon valvuloplasty is not successful or if the pulmonary stenosis is infundibular in origin. Infants with critical pulmonary stenosis and congestive heart failure require prostaglandin E_1 infusion to maintain ductal patency until surgery is performed (Park, 1988; Rocchini & Emmanouilides, 1995).

Prognosis for pulmonary stenosis is excellent. The mortality rate is less than 1 percent in older infants. The mortality rate is higher in newborns with critical pulmonary stenosis and congestive heart failure (Park, 1988).

TRUNCUS ARTERIOSUS

Truncus arteriosus is a large vessel located in front of the developing fetal heart. The truncus arteriosus gives rise to the coronary and pulmonary arteries and the aorta. The persistence of the truncus arteriosus results from inadequate division of the common great vessel into a separate aorta and pulmonary artery during fetal cardiac development. A single, large great vessel arises from the ventricles and gives rise to the systemic, pulmonary, and coronary circulations. Inadequate closure of the conal ventricular septum results in a VSD.

Incidence. Persistent truncus arteriosus accounts for less than 1 percent of all congenital heart defects.

Hemodynamics. Desaturated blood from the right ventricle and oxygenated blood from the left ventricle are received in the truncus arteriosus. The pressures of both ventricles are equal. The truncus arteriosus supplies blood to the systemic and pulmonary circuits. The amount of flow depends on the resistance of the two circulations. Pulmonary vascular resistance is high at birth, so pulmonary and systemic flow is relatively equal initially. Pulmonary resistance gradually decreases, causing increased pulmonary blood flow. Congestive heart failure may develop as a result of increased pulmonary blood flow. If not corrected, pulmonary vascular disease develops in response to high pressure and increased pulmonary blood flow; this decreases pulmonary blood flow. These changes, although compensatory initially, complicate the hemodynamics after surgical correction. Frequently, the volume overload is compounded by incompetent truncal valves, allowing regurgitation of blood into the ventricles (Mair et al., 1995b).

Manifestations. The signs and symptoms of truncus arteriosus are as follows:

- Cyanosis absent or present
- Congestive heart failure
- Systolic click at the apex and upper left sternal border
- Harsh, grade 2 to 4/6 systolic murmur along the lower sternal border
- Increased pulmonary blood flow: atrial rumble
- Truncal valve insufficiency: high-pitched, early diastolic decrescendo murmur
- Bounding arterial pulses
- Widened pulse pressure
- Single S_2
- If truncus arteriosus is not detected in the newborn period:
  - Poor feeding
  - Failure to thrive
  - Frequent respiratory infections
  - Signs of congestive heart failure

Diagnosis. Truncus arteriosus is diagnosed by the following:

- Increased heart size
- Possibly increased pulmonary blood flow
- Fifty percent of truncus arteriosus: right aortic arch (Park, 1988)
- ECG: normal QRS axis and ventricular hypertrophy

- Echocardiography: truncus arteriosus overriding a VSD and the absence of the pulmonary valve (Mair et al., 1995a; Park, 1988)

Management. This defect is treated as follows:

- Treatment of congestive heart failure
- Prophylaxis with antimicrobial agents
- Pulmonary artery banding, performed as a palliative measure, in small infants with increased pulmonary blood flow and congestive heart failure unresponsive to medical management

The mortality rate for this group of infants is close to 30 percent (Park, 1988).

The definitive surgical correction is Rastelli's procedure. Surgery is performed during infancy because of the high mortality rate of uncorrected truncus arteriosus. The mortality rate associated with surgery is also high, ranging from 20 to 60 percent. Reoperation may be required to enlarge the conduit as growth occurs (Moller, 1987; Park, 1988).

COMPLETE TRANSPOSITION OF THE GREAT ARTERIES OR VESSELS

Transposition of the great arteries (TGA) is the result of inappropriate septation and migration of the truncus arteriosus during fetal cardiac development. It may be dextrotransposition of the great arteries (D-TGA) or levotransposition of the great arteries (L-TGA). In D-TGA, the aorta arises from the right ventricle and the pulmonary artery arises from the left ventricle. The aorta receives unoxygenated systemic venous blood and returns it to the systemic arterial circuit. The pulmonary artery receives oxygenated pulmonary venous blood and returns it to the pulmonary circulation.

In L-TGA, the great vessels are transposed, with the aorta arising from the right ventricle and the pulmonary artery arising from the left ventricle. The aorta is to the left and anterior to the pulmonary artery. This type of transposition is called *corrected* because functionally the hemodynamics are normal. The oxygenated blood comes into the left atrium, enters the right ventricle, and goes through the aorta to the systemic circulation. However, frequently there are other associated cardiac defects (Park, 1988; Paul, 1995).

Incidence. TGA accounts for 5 percent of all congenital heart defects. It is more common in males (3:1). D-TGA is the most common cyanotic heart defect in newborns.

Hemodynamics. Hemodynamically, two separate parallel circulations result from complete D-TGA. Oxygenated blood from the lungs is returned to the left atrium, enters the left ventricle, and goes through the pulmonary artery to the lungs again. Desaturated blood from the systemic circulation enters the right atrium, goes to the right ventricle, enters the aorta, and is directed back into the systemic circulation. The end result is that the heart and brain and other vital tissues are perfused with desaturated blood. This defect is incompatible with life. A communication between the two circulations must exist to allow mixing of the oxygenated and desaturated blood.

This communication can be at the ductal, atrial, or ventricular level. The best mixing occurs with a large VSD.

Manifestations. The signs of transposition include the following:

- Marked cyanosis: prominent sign
  - Degree of cyanosis varies with amount of communication between the two circulations
- Congestive heart failure
- Loud and single S_2
- If a VSD is present: loud, harsh systolic murmur of variable intensity
- Hypoglycemia
- Hypocalcemia
- Metabolic acidosis

Diagnosis. The diagnosis is based on the following findings:

- Cardiomegaly
- Heart with narrow base: egg shaped
- Pulmonary blood flow: increased
- ECG: right-axis deviation of the QRS and right ventricular hypertrophy
- Echocardiography: abnormal origin of the great arteries from the ventricles

Management. TGA is a cardiac emergency. Immediate management includes the following:

- Correction of acidosis
- Correction of hypoglycemia
- Correction of hypocalcemia
- Administration of oxygen
- Administration of prostaglandin E_1
- Treatment of congestive heart failure
- Cardiac catheterization: balloon atrial septostomy
- Surgical excision of the posterior aspect of the atrial septum (Blalock-Hanlon procedure): performed without cardiopulmonary bypass as a palliative measure if the septostomy and prostaglandin E_1 infusion do not sufficiently improve oxygenation and has a 10 to 25 percent mortality rate (Park, 1988)
- Definitive surgical correction: switching the right- and left-sided structures at the ventricular level (Rastelli's procedure), the artery level (Jatene's procedure), or the atrial level (Senning's or Mustard's procedure)

The prognosis for TGA without surgical intervention is poor; 90 percent of infants die within the first year. The surgical procedures have high mortality rates and a high rate of postoperative complications (dysrhythmias, obstruction to systemic or pulmonary venous return, and right ventricular dysfunction).

COARCTATION OF THE AORTA

Coarctation is a narrowing or constriction of the aorta in the aortic arch segment. The most common location is below the origin of the left subclavian artery. Coarctation may occur as a single lesion owing to improper development of the aorta or may occur secondary to constriction of the ductus arteriosus. The severity of the circulatory compromise depends on the location and the degree of constriction. Coarctation proximal to the ductus arteriosus (preductal coarctation) has associated defects in 40 percent of cases. Associated defects include VSD, TGA, and PDA. Collateral circulation is poorly developed with preductal coarctation. Postductal coarctation is usually not associated with other defects, and collateral circulation is more effective. Infants with postductal coarctation may not be symptomatic. Over half of infants with coarctation have a bicuspid aortic valve (Beekman, 1995; Gersony, 1989; Park, 1988).

Incidence. Coarctation of the aorta accounts for 8 percent of all congenital heart defects. It occurs twice as often in males and is found in 30 percent of infants with Turner's syndrome (Park, 1988).

Hemodynamics. Coarctation causes obstruction to flow, which leads to varying pressure across the aortic segment. The portion of aorta proximal to the constriction has an elevated pressure, which leads to increased left ventricular pressure. The increased left ventricular pressure results in left ventricular hypertrophy and dilation. Collateral circulation develops from the proximal to distal arteries, bypassing the constricted segment of the aorta. This is a compensatory mechanism to increase flow to the lower extremities and abdomen, producing lower pulses in the lower extremities.

Manifestations. The features of coarctation of the aorta include the following:

- Congestive heart failure
- Absent, weak, or delayed pulses in the lower extremities
- Bounding pulses in the upper extremities
- Weak pulses if congestive heart failure is present
- Loud and single S_2 with severe coarctation
- Systolic thrill: suprasternal notch
- Ejection click: at apex if there is a bicuspid aortic valve or if systemic hypertension is present
- Systolic ejection murmur: grade 2 to 3/6: upper right and middle or lower left sternal border and at the left interscapular area in the infant's back
- No murmur heard in over half of sick infants
- Murmur possibly resulting from correction of congestive heart failure (Beekman, 1995; Gersony, 1989; Hazinski, 1984; Park, 1988).

Diagnosis. In asymptomatic infants, radiographs may show the following:

- Normal or slightly enlarged heart
- Dilation of the ascending aorta
- Characteristic "E" sign on barium swallow that is usually not evident until at least 4 months of age
- "E" due to the large proximal aortic segment or prominent subclavian artery above and the poststenotic dilation of the descending aorta below, the constricted segment (Park, 1988).

In symptomatic infants, radiographic findings are as follows:

- Cardiomegaly
- Increased pulmonary venous congestion

Other findings may include the following:

- ECG of asymptomatic infant: left-axis deviation of the QRS and left ventricular hypertrophy
- ECG of symptomatic infant: normal or right-axis deviation of the QRS
- Right ventricular hypertrophy or right bundle branch block present in infants
- Left ventricular hypertrophy present in older children (Park, 1988)

Management. Surgery is performed at 3 to 5 years of age if signs and symptoms can be medically controlled. Earlier surgery is indicated if medical management is not successful.

MEDICAL MANAGEMENT

- Provide adequate oxygenation.
- Prevent or treat congestive heart failure.
- Prevent subacute infective endocarditis.
- Prostaglandin E_1 may be needed to maintain ductal patency if the constricted segment is at the level of the ductus arteriosus (Park, 1988).

SURGICAL MANAGEMENT

- Surgical intervention involves excision of the constricted segment of the aorta with end-to-end anastomosis, patch graft, bypass tube graft, or Dacron graft (Park, 1988).
- Alternatively, a subclavian flap aortoplasty may be performed.
- Surgery is indicated in the presence of congestive heart failure with or without circulatory shock.
- With large VSD, pulmonary artery banding is done to reduce pulmonary blood flow to prevent pulmonary hypertension.
- Pulmonary artery banding is removed and the VSD is repaired at 6 months to 2 years of age.

The mortality rate for surgical corrections is less than 5 percent. Postoperative complications include renal failure and recoarctation.

HYPOPLASTIC LEFT HEART SYNDROME

Hypoplastic left heart syndrome (HLHS) consists of a group of cardiac defects, including a small aorta, aortic and mitral valve stenosis or atresia, and a small left atrium and ventricle. The great vessels are usually normally related.

Incidence. HLHS accounts for 1 to 2 percent of all congenital heart defects, but it accounts for 7 to 8 percent of heart defects producing symptoms in the first year of life (Bailey & Gundry, 1990), making it the leading cause of death from congenital heart defects in the first month of life (Norwood, Lang, & Hansen, 1983). HLHS is not associated with abnormalities in other organ systems.

Hemodynamics. Left ventricular output is greatly reduced or eliminated secondary to the valvular obstruction and small size of the left ventricle. Left atrial and pulmonary venous pressures are elevated, and there is pulmonary edema and pulmonary hypertension. With a PDA, blood shunts from the pulmonary artery into the aorta. The PDA provides the *only* cardiac output because there is little or no flow across the aortic valve. Retrograde flow through the aortic arch supplies the head, upper extremities, and coronary arteries (Freedom & Benson, 1995).

Although circulation is abnormal in utero, the high pulmonary vascular resistance and the low systemic vascular resistance make survival possible. The right ventricle maintains normal perfusion pressure in the descending aorta by a right-to-left ductal shunt. At birth, the onset of pulmonary ventilation causes the pulmonary vascular resistance to fall. The systemic vascular resistance rises because of the elimination of the placenta. Closure of the ductus arteriosus further decreases systemic cardiac output and aortic pressure, leading to metabolic acidosis and circulatory shock. Increased pulmonary blood flow causes increased left atrial pressure and pulmonary edema.

Manifestations. Presenting symptoms include the following:

- Progressive cyanosis
- Pallor
- Mottling

Other symptoms are as follows:

- Tachycardia
- Tachypnea
- Dyspnea
- Pulmonary rales
- Loud and single S_2
- Poor peripheral pulses
- Vasoconstriction of the extremities
- Cardiac murmur: absent or a grade 1 to 3/6 nonspecific systolic murmur (Park, 1988)

Diagnosis. The diagnosis is based on the following findings:

- Mild to moderate cardiomegaly
- Pulmonary venous congestion
- Pulmonary edema
- Metabolic acidosis
- Right ventricular hypertrophy: usually diagnostic
- Small left-sided heart structures
  - Small left ventricle
  - Small ascending aorta
  - Small aortic root
  - Absent or abnormal mitral valve
- Dilated or hypertrophied right-sided heart structures
  - Enlarged right ventricle
- Abnormal left ventricle to right ventricle end-diastolic ratio (Freedom & Benson, 1995; Park, 1988)

Management. The following therapy is recommended:

- Prevention of hypoxemia
- Correction of metabolic acidosis

- Administration of prostaglandin E_1: continuous infusion to maintain ductal patency
- Balloon atrial septostomy to decompress the left atrium

Surgical correction of the HLHS is experimental and has a high mortality rate. However, this defect was once considered 100 percent fatal. Surgical correction is performed in stages. The first stage, the modified Norwood procedure, is performed in the neonatal period to maintain pulmonary blood flow and create interatrial mixing of blood. The second stage, a modified Fontan procedure, is performed at 6 months to 2 years of age. This procedure closes the Gore-Tex shunt, closes the atrial communication, and forms a direct anastomosis of the right atrium and pulmonary artery.

Mortality for this defect remains very high. The first-stage surgical repair has a mortality rate of nearly 75 percent. For the survivors, there is a 50 percent mortality rate with the second-stage operation (Freedom & Benson, 1995; Park, 1988).

Nursing care is critical after the first-stage repair. Callow (1992) outlines this management as twofold, assessing for changes in homeostasis and pulmonary blood flow as well as nutritional status:

- Closely monitor vital signs for symptoms of blood loss.
- Check chest tube outputs greater than 10 percent of the total blood volume per hour, lasting over a period of several hours.
- Evaluate platelet counts, which may require treatments with fresh-frozen plasma, platelets, or cryoprecipitate at 10 ml/kg until stable.
- Evaluate need for daily liver function studies, which may require vitamin K treatment.
- Obtain guaiac testing of body fluids such as stool and gastric drainage.
- Maintain ventilatory status with a mean airway pressure of less than 10 cm H_2O or peak inspiratory pressure of less than 25 cm H_2O.
- Assess blood gases for persistent acidosis or systemic hypotension, as evidenced by arterial oxygen pressures greater than 45 mm Hg or saturations greater than 85 percent.
- Assess the need for dopamine at 5 to 10 µg/kg/min to decrease pulmonary vasoconstriction (Callow, 1992).
- Know that use of dobutamine or isoproterenol may only dilate the pulmonary arterioles, thus making the situation worse.
- Assess need for fentanyl, which may be advantageous to keep pulmonary vascular resistance balanced (Callow, 1992).
- Assess need for diuretic or peritoneal dialysis to maintain a fluid balance.
- Use high-frequency jet ventilation to support pulmonary function in the face of acidosis and stiffening lungs.
- Consider use of ECMO with these infants.
- Provide nutritional support.
- Monitor daily weights.
- Order urine tests for ketones, glucose, and protein.
- Determine levels of serum electrolytes and trace minerals to adjust the parenteral fluids (Callow, 1992).
- Start enteral feedings in the first 2 weeks postoperatively if the infant is stable and when the greatest danger of necrotizing enterocolitis is past.

Another complication of this surgery is pericardial effusion. This effusion may not occur until several days or weeks after the Fontan procedure. Alterations in tissue perfusion and changes in system blood flow return indicate this effusion (Smith & Vernon-Levett, 1993).

TOTAL ANOMALOUS PULMONARY VENOUS RETURN

With TAPVR the pulmonary veins drain into the right atrium (rather than the left atrium) directly or through connection with the systemic veins. There is no direct connection between the pulmonary veins and the left atrium.

Incidence. TAPVR accounts for 1 percent of all congenital heart defects. There is a 1:1 male:female ratio of occurrence.

Hemodynamics. If there is an ASD or patent foramen ovale, a portion of the mixed blood from the right atrium can cross into the left atrium, into the left ventricle, and on into the systemic circulation. Direction of the blood flow and the amount that crosses the atrial communication into the left atrium or that enters the left ventricle are determined by the ventricular compliance.

Two clinical hemodynamic states exist with TAPVR. If there is no obstruction to pulmonary blood flow, this flow is greatly increased. The result is highly saturated blood in the right atrium and mild cyanosis. If there is obstruction to pulmonary blood flow, the volume of flow is decreased and cyanosis is severe. Pulmonary edema often occurs secondary to elevated pulmonary venous pressure. Obstruction to pulmonary blood flow is a common occurrence when the TAPVR is below the diaphragm (Lucas & Krabill, 1990; Park, 1988).

Manifestations. The manifestations of TAPVR depend on the absence or presence of pulmonary venous obstruction.

TAPVR WITHOUT PULMONARY VENOUS OBSTRUCTION

- Mild cyanosis
- Frequent pulmonary infections
- Poor growth
- Congestive heart failure

TAPVR WITH PULMONARY VENOUS OBSTRUCTION

- Severe cyanosis
- Respiratory distress
- Progressive growth failure
- Increased cyanosis associated with feeding secondary to the compression of the common pulmonary vein by the filled esophagus (Park, 1988)
- Congestive heart failure

Diagnosis

TAPVR WITHOUT PULMONARY VENOUS OBSTRUCTION

- Precordial bulge
- Hyperactive right ventricular impulse

- Point of maximal impulse: xiphoid process or lower left sternal border
- Widely split and fixed S_2
- Pulmonic sound: may be pronounced
- Grade 2 to 3/6 systolic ejection murmur: upper left sternal border
- Mid-diastolic rumble: lower left sternal border
- Quadruple or quintuple gallop rhythm
- ECG: right-axis deviation of the QRS complex; right atrial hypertrophy
- Mild to moderate cardiomegaly
- Increased pulmonary markings
- "Snowman" sign: anatomic appearance of the left superior vena cava, the left innominate vein, and the right superior vena cava. Seldom visible before 4 months of age
- Echocardiography: pulmonary veins draining into a common chamber *posterior* to the left atrium
- Visualization of ASD and small left atrium and left ventricle
- Visualization of dilated coronary sinus protruding into the left atrium or a dilated innominate vein and superior vena cava, if present

TAPVR WITH PULMONARY VENOUS OBSTRUCTION

- Minimal cardiac findings
- Loud and single S_2
- Gallop rhythm
- Faint systolic ejection murmur: upper left sternal border
- Audible pulmonary rales
- Right-axis deviation for age
- Right ventricular hypertrophy in the form of tall R waves in the right precordial leads
- Heart size: normal
- Pulmonary edema
- Echocardiography: small left atrium and left ventricle
- Visualization of anomalous pulmonary venous return below the diaphragm

Management. Management of TAPVR is surgical. However, the surgery is emergent with TAPVR with pulmonary venous obstruction below the diaphragm. Medical management includes the following:

- Preventing or treating congestive heart failure
- Preventing hypoxemia
- Diuretics: pulmonary edema
- Balloon atrial septostomy to enlarge the interatrial communication and promote better mixing of blood
- Delay in surgery if response to medical management is good but surgery usually performed in infancy (Park, 1988)

The surgical procedure depends on the site of the anomalous drainage. Cardiopulmonary bypass is required. Surgery involves the anastomosis of the pulmonary veins to the left atrium, closure of the ASD, and division of the anomalous connection. The surgical mortality rate is high, 10 to 25 percent, but it is lower than with medical management alone. The highest mortality is with the infracardiac type.

Complications of Congenital Heart Defects

CONGESTIVE HEART FAILURE

Congestive heart failure (CHF) is a condition in which the blood supply to the body is insufficient to meet the metabolic requirements of the organs. It is a manifestation of an underlying disease or defect rather than a disease itself:

- Volume is increased from fluid overload or fluid retention.
  - In the normally functioning myocardium, fluid retention does not cause CHF.
  - Fluid retention complicates CHF from other causes.
  - In neonates, the most common cause of increased volume is congenital heart defects or altered hemodynamics, as in PDA.

CHF due to obstruction to outflow occurs if the normal myocardium must pump against increased resistance, as noted in the following:

- Structural defects such as valvular stenosis or coarctation of the aorta
- Pulmonary disease
- Cor pulmonale
- Pulmonary hypertension
- Abnormal stresses placed on the heart
- Electrolyte imbalances
- Acidosis
- Myocardial ischemia
- Rheumatic fever
- Infectious myocarditis
- Kawasaki disease
- Anomalous origin of the left coronary artery
- Dysrhythmias:
  - Complete AV block: bradycardia that prohibits adequate circulation of blood
  - Sustained primary tachycardia: insufficient time for ventricular filling; decreasing cardiac output
- Severe anemia: excessive demand for cardiac output
  - Oxygen-carrying capacity diminished; heart pumps more blood per minute to meet tissue oxygenation requirements.

Compensatory mechanisms function to meet the body's increased demand for cardiac output. These mechanisms are regulated by the sympathetic nervous system and mechanical factors. The compensatory mechanisms can sustain adequate cardiac output for only a short period of time. If the underlying condition is not corrected, congestive heart failure develops.

SYMPATHETIC NERVOUS SYSTEM COMPENSATORY MECHANISMS

Decreased blood pressure stimulates vascular stretch receptors and baroreceptors in the aorta and carotid arteries, which trigger the sympathetic nervous system. Decreased systemic blood pressure inactivates baroreceptors, resulting in the following:

- Increased sympathetic stimulation
- Increased heart rate
- Increased cardiac contractility
- Increased arterial blood pressure
- Increased catecholamine release and beta-receptor stimulation:
  - Increased rate and force of myocardial contraction
  - Increased venous tone, so that blood is returned to the heart more effectively
- Decreased circulation to the skin, kidneys, extremities, and splanchnic bed
- Increased circulation to brain, heart, and lungs
- Decreased renal blood flow, stimulating the release of renin, angiotensin, and aldosterone
- Retention of sodium and fluid, resulting in increased circulating volume and putting additional work on the heart (Hazinski, 1984)

MECHANICAL COMPENSATORY MECHANISMS

The heart muscle thickens to increase myocardial pressure. The hypertrophy is effective in the early stages; but as soon as the muscle mass increases, the compliance decreases. This change in compliance requires greater filling pressure for adequate cardiac output. The hypertrophied heart eventually becomes ischemic because it does not receive adequate circulation to meet its metabolic needs. Ventricular dilation occurs as myocardial fibers stretch to accommodate heart volume. Initially, this increases the contraction force, but it too fails after a point.

Effects of congestive heart failure include the following:

- Right ventricle unable to pump blood into the pulmonary artery
- Less blood oxygenated by the lungs
- Increased pressure in the right atrium and systemic venous circulation
- Edema in the extremities and viscera
- Left ventricle unable to pump blood into the systemic circulation
  - Increased pressure in the left atrium and pulmonary veins
  - Lungs become congested with blood
  - Elevated pulmonary pressures and pulmonary edema

The end effects of congestive heart failure are listed below:

- Decreased cardiac output
- Stimulation of sympathetic nervous system:
  - Tachycardia
  - Increased contractility
  - Increased vasomotor tone
  - Peripheral vasoconstriction
  - Diaphoresis
- Decreased renal perfusion
  - Stimulation of renin–angiotensin/aldosterone mechanism:
  - Sodium and water retention
- Systemic venous engorgement
  - Hepatomegaly
  - Jugular venous distention

- Periorbital and facial edema
- Ascites
- Dependent edema
- Pulmonary venous engorgement
  - Tachypnea
  - Decreased tidal volume
  - Increased respiratory effort
  - Grunting
  - Rales
  - Decreased lung compliance
  - Increased airway resistance
  - Early closure of the small airways with air trapping
  - Increased work of breathing
- Stimulation of the J-receptors in the lung, causing the infant to become apprehensive (Talner, 1995)

Diagnosis

The diagnosis of congestive heart failure is based on the following findings:

- Significant respiratory distress
- Tachypnea
- Grunting
- Retractions
- Peripheral pallor, appearing to be ashen or gray in color
- Active precordium
- Loud murmurs heard throughout systole and diastole
- Pulses usually full
- May be a pulse pressure difference between upper and lower extremities
- Hepatomegaly
- Irritability
- Arterial blood gases: metabolic acidosis and hypoxemia
- If CHF is severe, concurrent presence of respiratory acidosis because of the pulmonary edema caused by left-sided heart failure
- Pulmonary ventilation/perfusion mismatch, which may cause hypoxemia
- Hypocalcemia: inappropriate response to stress
- Hypoglycemia
- Enlarged heart
- Increased pulmonary congestion
- ECG: not generally diagnostic unless arrhythmia
  - Nonspecific changes in the T waves
  - Changes in the ST segment
  - Increase in the height of the P wave
- Electrolyte imbalances: hyponatremia, hypochloremia, and increased bicarbonate
- Hyperkalemia resulting from the release of intracellular cations, related to poor tissue perfusion
- Elevated lactic acid levels indicative of tissue hypoxia (Talner, 1995)
- Atrial natriuretic factor (ANF), a peptide hormone, may be important

in the regulation of volume and blood pressure. ANF release causes natriuresis, diuresis, and vasodilation. ANF acts with other volume regulators, such as renin, aldosterone, and vasopressin. An increased ANF level may be found when there is increased pulmonary blood flow, increased left atrial pressure, or pulmonary hypertension (Talner, 1995).

Treatment

The goal is to improve cardiac function while identifying and correcting the underlying cause.

General Measures

General measures to improve cardiac function include the following:

- Administer oxygen to improve ventilation/perfusion at the alveolar level.
- Ventilate with positive end-expiratory pressure at 6 to 10 cm H_2O, which may relieve the effects of congestive heart failure by reduction of pulmonary edema.
- Restrict fluid intake.
- Carefully monitor serum electrolyte levels.
- Monitor intake and output.
- Monitor weight.
- Count *all* fluid in the total daily fluid volume.
- Know that infant does not usually feed well and may require caloric supplementation with hyperalimentation or gavage feedings (Park, 1988).
- Provide sedation with continuous infusions of morphine sulfate or fentanyl to improve the infant's comfort and oxygenation. Cautious use may reduce anxiety and agitation, increasing comfort and decreasing the demand for oxygen.
- Assess for maintenance of a normal hematocrit.
- Maintain thermoneutral environment.
- Provide minimal stimulation.

Pharmacologic Interventions

Table 9–2 lists the medications most commonly used in the management of cardiac conditions. The mainstay of management of congestive heart failure beyond the neonatal period is *digitalis* (digoxin). Digoxin slows conduction through the AV node, prolongs the refractory period, and slows the heart rate through vagal effects on the SA node.

Use of digoxin in preterm or term neonates is controversial. The preterm newborn is at risk for digitalis toxicity because of the narrow range between therapeutic and toxic drug levels. The preterm infant requires a lower maintenance dose because of limited renal excretion of the drug (Table 9–3). If digoxin is used, the neonate must be carefully monitored for signs and symptoms of digitalis toxicity. Lead II ECGs should be obtained before each dose for the first 3 days; the dose should be withheld if the PR interval is greater than 0.16 second or if an arrhythmia is present. Digoxin levels should be monitored and should be less than 2.0 ng/ml (Avery, Fletcher, & MacDonald 1994; Beckman & Brent, 1994; Giacoia & Yaffe, 1987; Park,

TABLE 9–2. Drugs Used in the Management of Congenital Heart Defects

Drug	Dosage	Action	Onset	Comments
Diuretics				
Furosemide (Lasix)	1 mg/kg/dose IV 1–3 mg/kg/dose	Loop diuretic; inhibits sodium and chloride reabsorption in proximal tubule	15–30 min 30–60 min	Associated with increased PDA; calcium loss
Spironolactone (Aldactone)	1.5–3.0 mg/kg/day PO	Competitive antagonist of aldosterone	3–5 days	Potassium sparing
Chlorothiazide	20–40 mg/kg/day PO	Inhibits sodium and chloride reabsorption along the distal tubules	1–2 hr	
Inotropic Agents				
Dopamine	Low: 2–5 µg/kg/min	Increased renal blood flow; beta-adrenergic effects		Monitor ECG; BP
	Mod: 5–10 µg/kg/min	Increased renal blood flow; heart rate, BP, and contractility		
	High: 10–20 µg/kg/min	Peripheral vasoconstriction, increased heart rate, and contractility		
Dobutamine	2–10 µg/kg/min	Increased renal blood flow; increased contractility	Rapid	Decreased systemic vascular resistance; increased pulmonary wedge pressure
Isoproterenol	0.05–0.5 mg/kg/min	Increased venous return to heart and decreased pulmonary vascular resistance		Tachycardia, dysrhythmias, decreased renal perfusion

Drug	Dose	Action	Onset	Nursing Considerations
Vasodilators				
Sodium nitroprusside (Nipride)	0.5–6 μg/kg/min	Directly relaxes smooth muscles in arteriolar and venous walls; increases cardiac output if the decrease is secondary to myocardial dysfunction	Seconds	Monitor BP and thiocyanate levels; light sensitive; monitor heart rate
Prostaglandins				
PGE$_1$	0.05–0.1 mg/kg/min	Produces vasodilation and smooth muscle relaxation of ductus arteriosus and pulmonary and systemic circulations; increased arterial saturation by 25%–100%	Rapid	Monitor BP; vasopressors may be required; apnea, flush, fever, seizure-like activity; decreased heart rate
Prostaglandin Synthetase Inhibitors				
Indomethacin	0.2 mg/kg IV (1st) q24h 0.1 mg/kg IV (2nd & 3rd) >48 hr & <14 days: 0.3 mg/kg IV & 3 doses q24h >14 days & <6 wk: 0.2–0.3 mg/kg q12h	Promotes ductal closure by inhibition of PGE$_2$ in the walls of the ductus	12–24 hr	Monitor renal function, bilirubin, electrolytes, glucose, platelets, bleeding

....

PDA, patent ductus arteriosus.

TABLE 9–3. Digoxin Prescription Information

Total Digitalizing Dose (TDD)	Maintenance Dose
Preterm	
0.025–0.05 mg/kg	0.008–0.012 mg/kg/day
Term	
0.04–0.08 mg/kg	0.01–0.02 mg/kg/day
	($\frac{1}{8}$ TDD)

To digitalize:
1. Give $\frac{1}{2}$ TDD.
2. Six to 8 hr later, give $\frac{1}{4}$ TDD.
3. Six to 8 hr later, get a rhythm strip; if normal, give $\frac{1}{4}$ TDD.
4. Give maintenance dose ($\frac{1}{8}$ TDD) 12 hr after last digitalizing dose and then every 12 hr.

Slow digitalization, with decreased risk of toxicity, can be achieved by starting with the maintenance dose.

1988; Smith, Braunwald, & Kelly, 1988; Talner, 1995). Blood samples for digoxin levels should be drawn after the drug has achieved equilibrium in the body, 6 to 8 hours after administration (Yeh, 1985).

Other inotropic agents can be used to improve cardiac output. *Dopamine,* a norepinephrine precursor, has direct and indirect beta-adrenergic effects that are dose dependent. At low doses (2 to 5 μg/kg/min), there is increased renal blood flow with minimal effect on heart rate, blood pressure, or contractility. Medium doses (5 to 10 μg/kg/min) increase renal blood flow, heart rate, blood pressure, and contractility. Pulmonary artery pressure may be increased; peripheral resistance is not affected. High doses (10 to 20 μg/kg/min) cause alpha effects, resulting in peripheral vasoconstriction, increased cardiac rate, and contractility (Park, 1988).

Dobutamine is a synthetic catecholamine that acts on beta- and alpha-adrenergic receptors. Dobutamine (2 to 10 μg/kg/min) has decreased effects on the heart rate and rhythm and causes less peripheral vasoconstriction.

Isoproterenol (Isuprel), a synthetic epinephrine-like substance, has beta$_1$- and beta$_2$-adrenergic effects. Isuprel's usefulness in the neonate is limited because it produces increased heart rate, arrhythmias, and decreased systemic vascular resistance, which may make the hypotension worse (Park, 1988; Talner, 1995).

The primary goal is to increase renal perfusion (with inotropic agents or vasodilators) and to increase sodium delivery to distal diluting sites of the renal tubules. Diuretic agents increase the renal excretion of sodium and other anions by inhibition of tubular reabsorption of sodium (Park, 1988).

Furosemide (Lasix), a loop diuretic, blocks sodium and chloride reabsorption in the ascending limb of the loop of Henle. Loop diuretics interfere with the formation of free water and free water reabsorption by preventing the transport of sodium, potassium, and chloride into the medullary interstitium. Loop diuretics cause increased excretion of potassium by delivering increased quantities of sodium to sites in the distal nephron where potassium can be excreted. Furosemide also increases excretion of calcium but does not affect the kidney's ability to regulate acid–base balance (Oh, 1985).

An aldosterone antagonist such as *spironolactone* (Aldactone) may be useful because it is a potassium-sparing diuretic. Spironolactone works by binding to the cytoplasmic receptor sites and blocking aldosterone action, thus impairing the reabsorption of sodium and the secretion of potassium and hydrogen ion. Spironolactone has no effect on free water production and absorption. *Thiazide diuretics* (chlorothiazide and hydrochlorothiazide) inhibit sodium and chloride reabsorption along the distal tubules. They are not as effective as the loop diuretics and are infrequently used (Park, 1988).

Complications of Diuretic Therapy. The complications of diuretic therapy include the following:

- Volume contraction
- Hyponatremia
- Metabolic alkalemia or acidemia
- Hypokalemia or hyperkalemia (Hazinski, 1984; Talner, 1995).

When using diuretics, fluid and electrolyte balance must be maintained by administration of water and electrolytes. The adequacy of the volume can be determined by monitoring serum electrolytes, blood urea nitrogen, creatinine, urinary output, weight, specific gravity, and skin turgor.

The increased renal losses of sodium can lead to hyponatremia, if adequate sodium is not supplied. There may also be increased antidiuretic hormone release secondary to changes in the osmoreceptors or inhibition of antidiuretic hormone action. This can best be managed by decreasing the amount of total water and improving the cardiac output, thus increasing renal perfusion.

Metabolic alkalosis can result from administration of loop diuretics that interfere with sodium- and potassium-dependent chloride reabsorption. Hypochloremia results in a greater aldosterone production and an increase in bicarbonate concentration. Hypokalemia is a frequent complication of loop diuretic therapy. An increased ratio of intracellular to extracellular potassium results in the clinical signs and symptoms of hypokalemia. Hypokalemia increases the risk for digoxin toxicity. In contrast, hyperkalemia may result when the cardiac output is low and tissue perfusion is severely compromised. Other complications of diuretic therapy include increased calcium excretion, hyperuricemia, and glucose intolerance (Talner, 1995).

Vasodilators may be used in severe congestive heart failure to reduce the right and left ventricular preload and afterload to improve cardiac function (Hazinski, 1983). Vasodilators cause arterial and venous dilation, resulting in decreased systemic and pulmonary vascular resistance. Sodium nitroprusside (Nipride) is a smooth muscle relaxant that decreases ventricular afterload, by decreasing pulmonary and systemic vascular resistance, and decreases venous return and ventricular preload. This leads to decreased ventricular end-diastolic volume, increased ejection fraction, increased heart rate and cardiac index, and decreased pulmonary and systemic resistance. Sodium nitroprusside is sensitive to light and must be stored in dark containers. Side effects are cyanide toxicity and decreased platelet function (Hazinski, 1984; Park, 1988).

The prognosis of congestive heart failure depends on the severity of the underlying condition and on the degree of congestive heart failure.

SUBACUTE INFECTIVE ENDOCARDITIS

Subacute infective endocarditis (SAIE) can be a complication of congenital heart defects. Two factors are important in the development of SAIE: (1) structural abnormalities that create turbulent flow or pressure gradients and (2) bacteremia. All cardiac defects that produce turbulent flow or have a significant pressure gradient predispose to bacterial invasion of the cardiac endothelium. The turbulent flow causes damage to the endothelial lining and platelet–fibrin thrombus formation. Prevention of bacterial SAIE requires scrupulous daily oral care as well as prophylactic antimicrobial agents for dental procedures (Park, 1988). All congenital heart defects, except secundum-type ASDs, predispose to SAIE. VSDs, TOF, and aortic stenosis are the congenital heart defects most commonly associated with SAIE (Park, 1988).

Vegetation of SAIE is usually on the low pressure side of the defect, where endothelial damage is established by the jet effect of the defect. More than 90 percent of SAIE cases are caused by *Streptococcus viridans, S. faecalis* (enterococcus), and *Staphylococcus aureus.* Other organisms include *Haemophilus influenzae, Pseudomonas, Escherichia coli, Proteus, Aerobacter,* and *Listeria. Candida* may be the organism in infants who have been on long-term antimicrobial or corticosteroid therapy (Dajani & Taubert, 1995; Kaplan & Shulman, 1989).

Procedures for which SAIE prophylaxis is indicated include the following:

- All dental procedures
- Tonsillectomy or adenoidectomy
- Surgical procedures involving the respiratory mucosa
- Bronchoscopy
- Incision and drainage of infected tissue
- Gastrointestinal or genitourinary procedures

REFERENCES

Avery, G. B., Fletcher, M. A., & MacDonald, M. G. (Eds.). (1994). *Neonatology: Pathophysiology and management of the newborn* (4th ed.). Philadelphia: J. B. Lippincott.

Bailey, L. L., & Gundry, S. R. (1990). Hypoplastic left heart syndrome [Review]. *Pediatric Clinics of North America, 37,* 137–151.

Beckman, D. A., & Brent, R. L. (1994). Effects of prescribed and self-administered drugs during the second and third trimesters. In G. B. Avery, M. A. Fletcher, & M. G. MacDonald (Eds.), *Neonatology: Pathophysiology and management of the newborn* (4th ed., pp. 197–206) Philadelphia: J. B. Lippincott.

Beekman, R. H. (1995). Coarctation of the aorta. In G. C. Emmanouilides, H. Allen, T. Riemenschneider, & H. Gutgesell (Eds.), *Moss and Adams heart disease in infants, children, and adolescents including the fetus and young adult* (5th ed., pp. 1111–1132). Baltimore: Williams & Wilkins.

Braunwald, E., Sonnenblick, E. H., & Ross, J. (1988). Mechanisms of cardiac contraction and relaxation. In E. Braunwald (Ed.), *Heart disease: A textbook of cardiovascular medicine* (pp. 383–425). Philadelphia: W. B. Saunders.

Brook, M. M. & Heymann, M. A. (1995). Patent ductus arteriosus. In G. C. Emmanou-

ventricular septal defects. In G. C. Emmanouilides, H. Allen, T. Riemensch-neider, & H. Gutgesell (Eds.), *Moss and Adams heart disease in infants, children, and adolescents including the fetus and young adult* (5th ed., pp. 983–997). Baltimore: Williams & Wilkins.

Mair, D. D., Edwards, W. D., Julsrud, P. R., et al. (1995b). Truncus arteriosus. In G. C. Emmanouilides, H. Allen, T. Riemenschneider, & H. Gutgesell (Eds.), *Moss and Adams heart disease in infants, children, and adolescents including the fetus and young adult* (5th ed., pp. 1026–1041). Baltimore: Williams & Wilkins.

McNamara, D. G. (1990). Value and limitations of auscultation in the management of congenital heart disease. *Pediatric Clinics of North America, 37,* 93–113.

Moller, J. H. (1987). Clinical education aid: Congenital heart anomalies. Columbus, OH: Ross Laboratories.

Norwood, W. I., Lang, P., & Hansen, D. D. (1983). Physiologic repair of aortic atresia—hypoplastic left heart syndrome. *New England Journal of Medicine, 308,* 23–26.

Oh, W. (1985). Diuretic therapy. In T. F. Yeh (Ed.), *Drug therapy in the neonate and small infant* (pp. 299–304). Chicago: Year Book Medical Publishers.

Park, M. K. (1988). *Pediatric cardiology for practitioners.* Chicago: Mosby–Year Book.

Paul, M. H. (1995). Complete transposition of the great arteries. In G. C. Emmanoui-lides, H. Allen, T. Riemenschneider, & H. Gutgesell (Eds.), *Moss and Adams heart disease in infants, children, and adolescents including the fetus and young adult* (5th ed., pp. 1154–1224). Baltimore: Williams & Wilkins.

Pinsky, W. W., & Arciniegas, E. (1990). Tetralogy of Fallot [Review]. *Pediatric Clinics of North America, 37,* 179–192.

Porter, C. J., Feldt, R. H., Edwards, W. D., et al. (1995). Atrial septal defects. In G. C. Emmanouilides, H. Allen, T. Riemenschneider, & H. Gutgesell (Eds.), *Moss and Adams heart disease in infants, children, and adolescents including the fetus and young adult* (5th ed., pp. 687–703). Baltimore: Williams & Wilkins.

Rocchini, A. P., & Emmanouilides, G. C. (1995). Pulmonic stenosis. In G. C. Emma-nouilides, H. Allen, T. Riemenschneider, & H. Gutgesell (Eds.), *Moss and Adams heart disease in infants, children, and adolescents including the fetus and young adult* (5th ed., pp. 930–961). Baltimore: Williams & Wilkins.

Sacksteder, S. (1978). Congenital cardiac defects: Embryology and fetal circulation. *American Journal of Nursing, 78,* 262–264.

Smith, J. B., & Vernon-Levett, P. (1993). Care of infants with hypoplastic left heart syndrome. *AACN Clinical Issues, 4,* 329–339.

Smith, J. J., & Kampine, J. P. (1984). *Circulatory physiology.* Baltimore: Williams & Wilkins.

Smith, T. W., Braunwald, E., & Kelly, R. A. (1988). The management of heart failure. In E. Braunwald (Ed.), *Heart disease: A textbook of cardiovascular medicine.* Philadelphia: W. B. Saunders.

Suddaby, E. C., & O'Brien, A. M. (1993). ECMO for cardiac support in children. *Heart & Lung, 22,* 401–407.

Talner, N. S. (1995). Heart failure. In G. C. Emmanouilides, H. Allen, T. Riemen-schneider, & H. Gutgesell (Eds.), *Moss and Adams heart disease in infants, children, and adolescents including the fetus and young adult* (5th ed., 1746–1772). Baltimore: Williams & Wilkins.

Yeh, T. F. (1985). Congestive heart failure. In T. F. Yeh (Ed.), *Drug therapy in the neonate and small infant* (pp. 139–160). Chicago: Year Book Medical Publishers.

Zuberbuhler, J. R. (1995). Tetralogy of Fallot. In G. C. Emmanouilides, H. Allen, T. Riemenschneider, & H. Gutgesell (Eds.), *Moss and Adams heart disease in infants, children, and adolescents including the fetus and young adult* (5th ed., pp. 998–1017). Baltimore: Williams & Wilkins.

ilides, H. Allen, T. Riemenschneider, & H. Gutgesell (Eds.). *Moss and Adar heart disease in infants, children, and adolescents including the fetus and you adult* (5th ed., pp. 746–763). Baltimore: Williams & Wilkins.

Callow, L. B. (1992). Current strategies in the nursing care of infants with hypoplas left-heart syndrome undergoing first-stage palliation with the Norwood operatic *Heart & Lung, 21,* 463–470.

Conover, M. B. (1988). Anatomy and physiology of the heart. In M. B. Conover (E *Understanding electrocardiography: Arrhythmias and the 12-lead EKG* (pp. 1–1 St. Louis: C. V. Mosby.

Dajani, A. S. & Taubert, K. A. (1995). Infective endocarditis. In G. C. Emmanouilid H. Allen, T. Riemenschneider, & H. Gutgesell (Eds.), *Moss and Adams he disease in infants, children, and adolescents including the fetus and young ad* (5th ed., pp. 1541–1554). Baltimore: Williams & Wilkins.

Feldt, R. H., Porter, C. J., Edwards, W. D., et al. (1995). Atrioventricular se defects. In G. C. Emmanouilides, H. Allen, T. Riemenschneider, & H. Gutge (Eds.), *Moss and Adams heart disease in infants, children, and adolescents incl ing the fetus and young adult* (5th ed., pp. 704–723). Baltimore: Williams & V kins.

Freedom, R. M., & Benson, L. (1995). Hypoplastic left heart syndrome. In G. Emmanouilides, H. Allen, T. Riemenschneider, & H. Gutgesell (Eds.), *Moss Adams heart disease in infants, children, and adolescents including the fetus young adult* (5th ed., pp. 1133–1153). Baltimore: Williams & Wilkins.

Friedman, W. F. (1988). Congenital heart disease in infancy and childhood. In Braunwald (Ed.), *Heart disease: A textbook of cardiovascular medicine* (pp. 8 975). Philadelphia: W. B. Saunders.

Friedman, W. F. (1995). Aortic stenosis. In G. C. Emmanouilides, H. Allen Riemenschneider, & H. Gutgesell (Eds.), *Moss and Adams heart disease in infa children, and adolescents including the fetus and young adult* (5th ed., pp. 10 1110). Baltimore: Williams & Wilkins.

Gersony, W. M. (1989). Coarctation of the aorta. In F. H. Adams, G. C. Emman lides, & T. A. Riemenschneider (Eds.), *Heart disease in infants, children, adolescents* (pp. 243–255). Baltimore: Williams & Wilkins.

Giacoia, G. P., & Yaffe, S. J. (1987). Drugs and the perinatal patient. In G Avery (Ed.), *Neonatology: Pathophysiology and management of the newborn* 1317–1349). Philadelphia: J. B. Lippincott.

Graham, T. P., & Getgesell, H. P. (1995). Ventricular septal defects. In G. C. Em nouilides, H. Allen, T. Riemenschneider, & H. Gutgesell (Eds.), *Moss and Ad heart disease in infants, children, and adolescents including the fetus and yc adult* (5th ed., pp. 724–745). Baltimore: Williams & Wilkins.

Hazinski, M. F. (1983). Congenital heart disease in the neonate (part III): Conge heart failure. *Neonatal Network, 1*(6), 8–17.

Hazinski, M. F. (1984). Cardiovascular disorders. In M. F. Hazinski (Ed.), *Nur care of the critically ill child* (pp. 63–252). St. Louis: C. V. Mosby.

Heymann, M. A. (1995). Fetal and postnatal circulations: Pulmonary circulation G. C. Emmanouilides, H. Allen, & T.A. Riemenschneider, & H. Gutgesell (E *Moss and Adams heart disease in infants, children, and adolescents including fetus and young adult* (5th ed., pp. 209–223). Baltimore: Williams & Wilkins.

Kaplan, E. L., & Shulman, S. T. (1989). Endocarditis. In F. H. Adams, G Emmanouilides, & T. A. Riemenschneider (Eds.), *Heart disease in infants, dren, and adolescents* (pp. 718–730). Baltimore: Williams & Wilkins.

Kirsten, D. (1996). Patent ductus arteriosus in the preterm infant. *Neonatal Netu 15*(2), 19–28.

Lucas, R. V., & Krabill, K. A. (1990). Anomalous venous connections, pulmonary systemic. *Pediatric Clinics of North America, 37,* 580–616.

Mair, D. D., Edwards, W. D., Julsrud, P. R., et al. (1995a). Pulmonary artresia

Fluids, Electrolytes, Vitamins, and Trace Minerals: Basis of Ingestion, Digestion, Elimination, and Metabolism

ASSESSMENT AND EVALUATION OF FLUID AND ELECTROLYTE THERAPY

Estimating fluid needs depends on the infant's age, weight, and disease process. Fluid needs can be calculated by using body weight, body surface area, or caloric expenditure (Behrman, Kliegman, & Arvin, 1995). An easily used method is that of caloric expenditure, whereby caloric needs are calculated and fluid and electrolyte requirements are related to it.

To begin these calculations, it must be remembered that 1 kcal is the amount of heat needed to raise 1 L of water 1°C. "Caloric expenditures up to 10 kilograms = 100 calories/kilogram/24 hours" (Donler, 1990). For example, a 1700-g infant would expend 170 calories in 24 hours, whereas a 460-g infant would expend 46 calories in 24 hours. Caloric expenditures can be modified by an increase or decrease in body temperature as well as by specific disease states and can be used to determine water needs, because every 100 calories metabolized requires 100 ml of fluid (Behrman, Kliegman, & Arvin, 1995; Donler, 1990). Water needs are determined based on calculated insensible losses from the skin and pulmonary system and actual losses from urine, stool, and sweat (Table 10–1).

Insensible water loss can be affected by skin integrity and the degree of that integrity. An example of this is the newborn with a large gastroschisis. This midline abdominal wall defect predisposes to large amounts of insensible water loss because of the exposed abdominal organs with an absent omentum or peritoneum. Another example is the 23-week, 400-g infant with the typical "translucent" skin that has not yet formed a protective keratin layer, thus predisposing the infant to dehydration secondary to large insensible water losses.

Also affecting insensible water loss are environmental factors:

- Presence or absence of humidity
- Increased or decreased ambient temperature
- Use of radiant warmers

....

Much of the content of this chapter is based on a study funded in part by the National Institutes of Health (NIH) with the following grants: HD 11725, Diabetes in Pregnancy Program Project; NIHL-T32-HD07200, Research Training in Perinatology; and NIH-HD20748, Perinatal Emphasis Research Center.

TABLE 10–1. Fluid Intake and Output

	Range (ml/100 cal/24 hr)	Average (ml/100 cal/24 hr)
Output		
Insensible water losses		
Pulmonary	10–20	15
Skin	25–35	30
Urine	50–70	60
Stool	5–10	7
Sweat	0–20	0
Intake		112
Water of oxidation		−12
		100 ml/100 cal/day average maintenance requirements

- Phototherapy
- Increased metabolic rate
- Increased body temperature
- Activity

Fluids are usually calculated on a daily basis, taking into consideration past losses, projected losses, and maintenance requirements. However, depending on the disease process, fluids may need to be calculated as often as every 4 hours, to keep up with ongoing losses and to make appropriate adjustments in fluid therapy. A general estimate of fluid requirements can be calculated based on the following guidelines (for normal, term newborns):

Day 1: 80 ml/kg/day
Day 2: 100 ml/kg/day
Day 3: 120 ml/kg/day
Day 4: 135 ml/kg/day
Day 5: 150 ml/kg/day

Again, these are just guidelines, and requirements may be different based on the gestational age and disease process. A premature, low birth weight infant may require as much as 150 to 200 ml/kg/day during the first 24 hours of life, whereas a term, asphyxiated infant may be restricted to no more than 40 to 50 ml/kg/day for the first 72 hours of life.

Electrolyte requirements are usually calculated on the basis of 100 calories metabolized:

Sodium: 2 to 3 mEq/100 cal/24 hr (or 2 to 3 mEq/kg/day)
Potassium: 1 to 2 mEq/100 cal/24 hr (or 1 to 2 mEq/kg/day)

Standard intravenous solutions containing a predetermined quantity of sodium are routinely used in neonatal intensive care units (e.g., 5 percent dextrose in 0.45 percent NaCl) with potassium chloride added as indicated (Table 10–2).

TABLE 10–2. Electrolyte Components of Intravenous Fluids

Solution	mEq Na/1000 ml	mEq Na/100 ml
D5 1/2 NS	77	7.7
D5 1/4 NS	38.5	3.8

Caloric requirements cannot be met solely by the intravenous solutions commonly used in neonatal intensive care units (i.e., 5 or 10 percent dextrose). These solutions are relatively low in calories; there are only 4 calories per gram of glucose (carbohydrate), and the number of calories in intravenous solutions is calculated on a percent solution and based on grams per deciliter. Therefore, 5 percent dextrose in water (D_5W) contains 5 g/dl ml of fluid, and 10 percent dextrose in water ($D_{10}W$) contains 10 g/dl. To carry this calculation further, D_5W and $D_{10}W$ intravenous solutions contain 20 and 40 calories, respectively (e.g., D_5W = 5 g/dl at 4 cal/g = 20 cal).

The amount of dextrose concentration administered to the infant also depends on the infant's gestational age and renal function. Glucose excretion may be altered by the ability of the premature kidney to concentrate urine and conserve electrolytes and glucose, thus "spilling sugar" into the urine. An essential test of the infant's response to intravenous glucose therapy can easily be done at the bedside with the urine dipstick. This test requires only a few drops of urine on a dipstick to determine the presence of glucose, protein, ketones, and blood and the pH level, an important indicator of acid–base balance.

Specific gravity is normally between 1.008 and 1.012, an early indicator of hydration status (Korones, 1986). Urine dipstick and specific gravity tests should be performed at least every shift, and more often as the infant's condition warrants. Along with these two parameters, fluid intake and output should be strictly monitored to ensure adequate hydration status. Urine output is monitored and calculated on an hourly basis over a 24-hour period. It should be *no less than 1 ml/kg/hr/day.* For example, for a 2-kg infant:

$$\text{Urine output} = 240 \text{ ml/24 hr} = 10 \text{ ml/2 kg} = 5 \text{ ml/kg/hr}$$

To promote improved nutritional status for infants requiring long-term intravenous therapy, total parenteral nutrition is used and may be started within the first 24 to 72 hours of life. Total parenteral nutrition spares protein, increases calories, and, when used in conjunction with intralipids, further increases caloric intake. When infused through a peripheral vein, glucose concentration is limited to no more than 12.5 percent because of the risks of tissue irritation and sloughing with infiltration; however, when it is infused through central lines, higher concentrations may be used. In addition to the increased glucose concentrations (thus increasing calories), higher concentrations of protein, fat,° and other essential minerals and trace elements may be infused.

· · · · · · · · · · · · · · · · · · · ·

°Fat calories should not exceed 50 percent of the total caloric intake.

Caloric supplementation with total parenteral nutrition can be shown as follows:

Protein (4 cal/g): 1 to 2.5 g/kg/day; 4 to 10 cal/kg/day

Fat (9 cal/g): up to 4 g/kg/day; 10 percent emulsion = 1.1 cal/ml; 20 percent emulsion = 2.0 cal/ml

Fluid orders should always be double checked to ensure that the ordered rate and solution are appropriate for that infant.

Weight is an important indicator of overall fluid status. Infants are usually weighed on a daily basis; infants with extremely low birth weight and infants with excessive fluid losses and needs may be weighed more often, on an every-12-hour schedule or even on an every-6-hour schedule, with ongoing fluid needs recalculated based on weight changes. Care must be used when weighing infants because inaccuracies that show extreme weight fluctuations can have a detrimental impact on therapy. For example, an inaccurate weight showing an increase of 100 g in a 12-hour period for an infant with severe respiratory distress syndrome may result in an unnecessary dose of furosemide. The infant should be weighed without clothing, with as much equipment removed as possible (e.g., ECG leads, probes) at the same time each day and on the same scale. Newer, in-bed scales are now available that give a constant weight read-out, simplifying the weighing process (Kavanaugh, Engstrom, Meier, & Lysakowski, 1990).

The physical examination can reveal changes in the infant's fluid status and should be used in conjunction with laboratory data to plan interventions in fluid and electrolyte therapy. A general assessment will include the infant's color, skin turgor, activity, mucous membranes, fontanelles, and vital signs.

Color: pink and well-perfused versus pale and mottled

Activity: active with good tone versus lethargic and hypotonic

Mucous membranes: pink and moist versus dry and gray

Fontanelles: soft and flat versus depressed or full and tense

Vital signs: bradycardia/tachycardia, slowed respirations/tachypnea, normotensive versus hypotensive or hypertensive, hypothermia versus hyperthermia, or temperature instability

Urine output: normal versus excessive, decreased, or absent

For more information on normal ranges for serum and urine chemistries the reader is referred to Chapter 25, Diagnostic Test and Laboratory Values.

REFERENCES

Behrman, R. E., Kliegman, R. M., & Arvin, A. M. (Eds.). (1995). *Nelson textbook of pediatrics* (15th ed.). Philadelphia: W. B. Saunders.

Donler, J. (1990). Fluid and electrolyte balance. In *Neonatal intensive care nursing review* (p. 137). Washington, DC: Nurses Association of the American Association of Obstetrics and Gynecology.

Kavanaugh, K., Engstrom, J. L., Meier, P. P., & Lysakowski, T. Y. (1990). How reliable are scales for weighing preterm infants? *Neonatal Network, 9*(3), 29–32.

Korones, S. (1986). *High-risk newborn infants: The basis for intensive nursing care* (4th ed., p. 199). St. Louis: C. V. Mosby

Nutrition: Physiologic Basis of Metabolism and Management of Enteral and Parenteral Nutrition

BASIC NEEDS

Many controversies exist about what infants need nutritionally. It is generally accepted that infants require at least 50 cal/kg/day to meet the basic metabolic requirement (BMR). Intravenously administered calories are the most efficiently used, so providing only 50 cal/kg/day even by this route will almost assuredly only meet BMR in the most stable infants. If these calories are given enterally, the loss of calories by means of inefficient absorption must be considered. Once the BMR is met, calories and protein are increased to allow for positive nitrogen balance and protein sparing and, ultimately, to meet growth requirements. The recommendations for target calories vary from 80 to 110 cal/kg/day intravenously.

Intravenous nutrient delivery must be balanced and provide for maintenance as well as growth needs. Recommended intravenous protein intake is as follows (Kerner, 1991; Pereira, 1995; Schulman, Buffone, & Wise, 1985):

- 3 g/kg/day for term infants
- 3.5 g/kg/day for preterm infants

Whereas third-trimester accretion is 2 to 3 g/kg/day, certain postnatal events such as surgery, respiratory disease, and/or necrotizing enterocolitis increase the protein needs and deplete the protein stores very rapidly.

- Fats should make up 40 to 50 percent of total caloric intake and therefore are a large contributor to total required calories.
  - Intravenous fat intake should not exceed 3 to 4 g/kg/day.
  - If intravenously administered fats exceed this range, fat overload can occur, affecting oxygen diffusion and increasing triglyceride and cholesterol levels (Kerner, 1991).
- All infants should have their triglyceride and cholesterol levels monitored at least weekly (Kerner, 1983, 1991).
- Carbohydrate intake should be 40 to 50 percent of total caloric intake.

METHODS OF DELIVERY AND TECHNICAL PROBLEMS

Parenteral nutrients can be delivered in many ways in today's neonatal intensive care unit (NICU). Table 11–1 lists the methods and the risks and

TABLE 11–1. Methods of Intravenous Access Techniques and the Risks and Benefits of Each

Pros/Benefits	Cons/Risks
Peripheral	
Reduced risk of systemic infection	Limited % glucose and % protein
Multiple team members have skill for insertion	High fluid volumes required to meet energy and protein needs of sick infants (150–200 ml/kg)
No central venous access risks	
Low cost per device	Intermittent pain, hypoxia, cold stress, and hypoglycemia with restarts
	Possible tissue damage with infiltration
	Restriction of positioning and motion when extremities used
	Limited veins in very small infants and infants with long-term IV needs
Central	
Nutrient needs met with limited fluids (high caloric density possible)	Central access risks effusion, thrombus, and infection
Staff time minimal once inserted (no need for restarts)	If surgical access used, vein loss, cost increased for device and surgeon fee
No positional restraints	Need for radiograph to determine tip and follow-over time
Percutaneous access can be done with no vein loss, no surgical incision; small size reduces thrombus, embolus, and effusion risks of central access	Increased nursing skill required for patient monitoring and troubleshooting device
No intermittent loss of therapy (glucose and fluids) due to infiltration	

benefits of each. Two to 3 weeks of some form of intravenously administered nutrition is common.

There are two major nutritional constraints to peripheral intravenous nutrient delivery: the amount of glucose (energy) and the amount of protein that can be administered. The maximum amount of carbohydrate (glucose) concentration that can be delivered is 10 to 12.5 percent and that of protein is 2 g/dl. The higher the osmolality, the more likely infiltration and tissue damage will occur. Considering most sick infants require fluid limitations, it is almost impossible to administer 80 cal/kg/day and 3 g of protein/kg/day by this method.

Other major issues of peripheral administration are listed below:

- Adequacy of peripheral veins
- Pain of intermittent restarts
- Hypoxia from crying
- Cost of personnel time
- Poor subsequent growth if nutrient delivery is low or frequently interrupted

To avoid some of these issues, use of percutaneous central venous catheters (PCVCs) has become widespread. All PCVCs are made of Silastic, silicone, or polyurethane, and all go through needles that break away or are threaded out of the system. There are now double-lumen devices and devices small enough to thread through a 24-gauge break-away needle.

PCVC administration guidelines are as follows:

- Vein of choice is the cephalic or basilic vein of the arm, at the hand or the antecubital fossa.
- Saphenous veins at the ankle or knee are also safe sites of insertion.
- Tips of PCVCs are usually threaded to the superior vena cava (SVC) or inferior vena cava (IVC) or IVC–right atrial junction to provide the highest flow area, which minimizes the risk of infiltration and extravasation and reduces the possibility of arrhythmia. The position of the PCVC tip should be confirmed by a radiograph with contrast medium enhancement.
- Conray in a volume of 0.5 ml is adequate to fill and visualize the catheter even if the long lines are used.
- One should document that there is good blood return and that flushing meets no resistance.

Broviac catheters, which are surgically placed, are reserved for infants who need months of parenteral nutrition.

Other issues: All NICUs that use peripheral alimentation must have a procedure or protocol for initial treatment of the site. Hyaluronidase (Wydase) reduces the extent of tissue necrosis dramatically by breaking down the cell membrane and dissipating the chemical irritant (the total parenteral nutrition [TPN]) (Pettit & Hughes, 1993; Zenk, Dungy, & Greene, 1981). A dose of 15 units given in three to four subcutaneous injections around the perimeter of the edema within an hour will give best results (Pettit & Hughes, 1993).

- Common risks of central access are infiltration, infection, and loss of device due to technical difficulties such as occlusion. Infiltration risks can all but be eliminated when the tips of the catheters are left at the SVC or IVC or the IVC–right atrial junction.

For catheter tips in the innominate, subclavian, auxiliary, or jugular vein, swelling can usually be detected with regular inspection of the neck or chest wall. When the patient has generalized edema, asymmetrical swelling that does not disappear with position change may be detected.

Careful radiographic review for the presence of differential edema may be helpful. Certain resistant bacterial strains and fungi are present on the skin of these infants within a few days after admission to an NICU (Evans et al., 1988). Any loss of skin integrity, tracheal trauma, or skin puncture can introduce the flora into the blood stream. Fungal infection remains a problem, because the intravenous presence of fat in the system provides an ideal culture medium not only for *Candida albicans* but also for all yeasts, including *Malassezia furfur*, which will also occlude the line (Aschner, Punsalang, Maniscalco, & Menegus, 1987; Azimi et al., 1988; Powell et al., 1984). Occlusion with this fungus requires that the line be pulled, because there is no pharmacologic treatment for *M. furfur* fungal infection.

If fungal infections are suspected, the contents of the catheters need to be antiseptically flushed into a container and sent to the laboratory for identification, with specific instructions to examine the specimen for fungus.

Complications related to patient intolerance of solution components include metabolic imbalances, such as hyperglycemia or hyponatremia, and clinically significant deficiency states if essential nutrients, minerals, or vitamins are omitted. All NICUs should have system checks in place that aid in the comprehensive ordering of these solutions. Systems include standardized order sheets, computer programs that calculate solution additives based on target orders per kilogram per day, or manual pharmacist checks to determine safety and completeness (Ball, Candy, Puntis, & McNeish, 1985; Yamamoto, Gainsley, & Witek, 1986). Metabolic problems should be avoided by the systematic advancing of the fluid constituents and regular monitoring through weekly laboratory tests, growth graphs, and daily screens such as bedside serum glucose testing or bedside glucose testing. Hyperglycemia and hypoglycemia are probably the most common ongoing problems associated with the use of TPN. One way to reduce these is through a system that requires a calculation of grams of glucose per kilogram per day or milligrams per kilogram per minute when the TPN rate is ordered. Using the traditional incremental increase by glucose percentage, a preterm infant may not be able to metabolize such an increase and exhibit hyperglycemia. For example, a 1-kg infant may receive 7.5 percent glucose on day 3 of life with a stable blood glucose level; on day 4 the percentage is increased to 10 percent with additional increase in amount of glucose delivered because the fluid rate was increased too, as fluids liberalize. Thus the infant's glucose level is increased from 8 to 12 g/kg/day. Hyperglycemia sometimes occurs under the best of circumstances in very low birth weight infants. With the mandate of providing calories to meet the BMR as soon as possible, it is sometimes necessary to add insulin to the TPN solution. It has been shown that this practice is feasible and can improve the glucose tolerance in very low birth weight infants and therefore can provide better caloric intake early in hospitalization (Binder, Raschko, Benda, & Reynolds, 1989; Ostertag, Jovanovic, Lewis, & Auld, 1986; Simeon, Geffner, Levin, & Lindsey, 1994; Vaucher, Waltson, & Morrow, 1982).

Parenteral therapy is collaborative: the therapy is ordered by the physician, the enteral solution is checked and mixed by the pharmacist, and the administration of the solution is monitored by the nurse.

ENTERAL NUTRITION

Preterm infants require approximately 120 cal/kg/day for tissue repair and growth. Term infants who have some disease state may require as many calories but usually will grow on 100 to 110 cal/kg/day, owing to more efficient digestion and absorption.

Growth charts allow clinicians to plot weight, length, and head circumference of infants as immature as 24 weeks and compare individual infants with standardized norms. The graphs that should be used are those that show intrauterine growth.

Although it is clear that the caloric intake should be higher when enteral nutrition is started, this caloric intake should be gradually increased as parenteral nutrition is gradually reduced. Intravenously administered calories should not be withdrawn until infants are receiving target calories of 100 to 120 cal/kg/day for at least 1 or 2 days.

- Fluid intake should not be less than 100 ml/kg/day to provide basic hydration, and the upper limits need to be determined based on each infant's assessment.
- Infants with lung disease may need moderate restriction of 140 to 150 ml/kg/day or conservative restriction of 120 ml/kg/day.
- If there are no fluid constraints owing to disease or inability of intake, premature infants have been observed to take in as much as 250 ml/kg/day of formula during the recovery phase of illness with no ill effects.
- If fluid restraints are ongoing, the caloric density of the formula needs to be adjusted to allow for target caloric intake (Darby & Loughead, 1996).

Nutrient needs should not be a major issue if fortified human milk or premature formulas are used. These diets provide the premature infant with the additional protein, vitamins, and minerals needed when target caloric intake is achieved. Standard infant formulas should not be used in this population, because of the following:

- They are too low in protein.
- Vitamin and mineral content is inadequate for the growing preterm infant (Anderson, 1987). When an elemental diet is needed, Pregestimil is recommended.
- Alimentum is being used by some.

See Table 11–2 for a comparison of standard formulas.

Methods of Enteral Feeding

GAVAGE FEEDINGS

Gavage feedings, either by the orogastric or the nasogastric route, are indicated for preterm infants who are unable to feed orally.

Continuous Versus Intermittent Gavage or Bolus Feedings

Prior to the 1970s, preterm infants received gavage or bolus feedings intermittently, in 1- to 4-hour intervals. In the 1970s, an alternative was referred to as transpyloric continuous nasojejunal (CNJ) alimentation (Cheek & Staub, 1973; Rhea & Kilby, 1970). Theoretically, preterm infants could receive larger daily volumes of milk with minimal physiologic and biochemical alterations. The continuous milk flow minimized gastric disten-

TABLE 11–2. Comparison of Human Milk, Soy Protein Formulas, and Cow's Milk

	Mother's Milk	SMA*	Similac with Iron	Gerber with Iron*	Enfamil with Iron*	Good Start	Whole Cow's Milk
Protein (%) (weight/volume)	1.1	1.5	1.5	1.5	1.5	—	3.6
Casein (%)	40	40	82	82	40	—	82
Whey Protein (%)	60	60	18	18	60	100§	18
Fat (%) (weight/volume)	3.9	3.6	3.6	3.7	3.8	3.5	3.7
Monounsaturated (%)	41.6	41.3	17.6	17.6	16.0	25.6	30.4
Polyunsaturated (%)	14.2	14.5	37.3	37.3	29.0	31.9	3.8
Saturated (%)	44.2	44.2	45.1	45.1	55.0	42.5	65.8
Oils							
Soy (%)	—	15	60	60	45	—	—
Coconut (%)	—	27	40	40	55	18	—
High oleic safflower/sunflower (%)	—	25	—	—	—	22	—
Palmolein (%)	—	—	—	—	—	60	—
Oleo (%)	—	33	—	—	—	—	—
Minerals (milligrams/liter)							
Total (ash)	2000	2500	3300	NA	3000	NA	7200
Sodium	150	150	190	225	180	162	520
Potassium	550	560	730	730	720	662	1480
Calcium	340	420	510	510	460	433	1220
Phosphorus	140	280	390	390	320	243	960
Chloride	360–480	375	450	475	420	400	960
Iron	0.5	12†	12†	12†	13†	10	0.6
Zinc	3	5	5	5	5	5	5

Selected Vitamins (per liter)

Vitamin A (IU)	2000	2000	2030	2030	2100	2030	1400
Contains beta-carotene	Yes	Yes	No‡	No‡	No‡	No‡	Yes
Vitamin C (mg)	40	55	60	60	54	54	10
Vitamin D (IU)	22	400	410	406	420	406	20
Carbohydrate (%) (weight/volume)	7.2 lactose	7.2 lactose	7.2 lactose	7.2 lactose	6.9 lactose	7.4 lactose, maltodextrin	4.8 lactose
Nucleotides	Yes	Yes	No‡	No‡	No‡	No‡	Not‡

NOTE: All data for competitive products are derived from product labels, *Physicians' Desk Reference*, or analyses.

*Concentrated liquid with iron (standard dilution).

†SMA Lo-iron and Similac contain 1.5 mg of iron per liter. Enfamil low-iron and Gerber low-iron contain 1.1 mg of iron per liter. Infants fed these formulas should receive supplemental dietary iron from an outside source to meet daily requirements.

‡Trace amounts only.

§Partially hydrolyzed whey protein.

NA, not available.

Courtesy of Wyeth-Ayerst Laboratories, Philadelphia, Pa.

tion and consequent circulatory and respiratory changes. Additionally, the milk was delivered into the jejunum, bypassing both the cardiac and the pyloric sphincters, so the probability of regurgitation and aspiration was reduced.

CNJ feedings were gradually replaced with continuous nasogastric (CNG) feedings (Landwirth, 1974). CNG feedings were administered by very slow infusion rates into the stomach, so that rapid distention of the stomach was avoided.

Gavage Feedings of Expressed Mother's Milk

Milk expressed by mothers of preterm infants can be fed to the infants by gavage until the infant is able to suckle at the breast, provided that certain safeguards are observed. Two outcomes preclude administration of expressed mother's milk (EMM) by the CNG route when traditional infusion tubing is used: (1) nutrient loss due to its adherence to the tubing (Brennan-Behm, Carlson, Meier, & Engstrom, 1994; Brooke & Barley, 1978; Greer, McCormick, & Loker, 1984; Lemons et al., 1983; Narayanan, Singh, & Harvey, 1984; Stocks, Davies, Allen, & Sewell, 1985); and (2) bacterial growth in EMM that has been previously colonized (Botsford et al., 1986; Lemons et al., 1983; Meier & Wilks, 1987; Wilks & Meier, 1988).

EMM is allowed to remain at room temperature, often for several hours, before being used. The warm temperature permits further bacterial growth, so the infant may receive a sizable inoculate of bacteria.

Continuous infusion of EMM by syringe pump may circumvent problems with bacterial growth (McCoy et al., 1988), in that the syringe pump and infusion tubing can be changed very frequently (e.g., every 2 hours), with minimal wasting of EMM.

Orogastric and Nasogastric Routes for Intermittent Gavage or Bolus Feedings

A clinical dilemma concerning intermittent gavage or bolus feedings is whether orogastric or nasogastric intubation should be used for milk administration. Clinically, nasogastric tubes are simpler to insert and maintain in position than are orogastric tubes. Determining the correct insertion length is essential for both methods (Gallaher et al., 1993).

Type of Gavage Tube

Ideally, the tube used for gavage feedings should have the smallest bore to deliver the feeding. For nasally placed tubes, a 5 French is desirable. However, the 5 French has a very small end hole and may occlude during feeding. An 8 French may be used for orogastric intubation because occlusion of the nare is not a consideration.

Tubes made of polyvinyl chloride should be used for a single feeding or left in place for no more than 1 day. Thus, if these tubes are used routinely, nurses need to develop a mechanism whereby the tubes are changed on a daily basis. For gavage tubes that will remain in place for longer than 1 day, a tube made of a softer, more biocompatible plastic, such as Silastic or polyurethane, should be used. Small-bore polyurethane feeding tubes with weighted tips are also available and should be considered for infants with reflux.

Selected Nursing Interventions During Intermittent Gavage or Bolus Feedings

Selected nursing interventions can be categorized as follows:

- Controlling the rate of milk flow
- Warming the milk to body temperature
- Optimizing infant position
- Using intermittently placed gavage tubes rather than indwelling gavage tubes
- Providing nonnutritive sucking opportunities

Administration Rate. Clinical protocols for intermittent gavage or bolus feedings should reflect an infusion rate (in milliliters per kilogram of body weight per minute) rather than an infusion time.

Milk Temperature. Preterm infants receive formula that may be as much as 25°F to 30°F lower than body temperature.

Infant Position. Infant position may influence oxygenation during gavage feeding. For those infants who demonstrate hypoxemia, modification of position may promote improved oxygenation.

Nonnutritive Sucking. The beneficial long-term effects of administering nonnutritive sucking with a pacifier during intermittent gavage feeding include the following:

- Accelerated maturation of the sucking reflex
- Earlier initiation of bottle feedings
- Greater daily weight gain
- Shorter hospital stay
- Hospital cost savings

Oral Feedings. Feeding orally requires the integration of three functions: sucking, swallowing, and breathing.

SCHEDULED VERSUS CUE-BASED FEEDINGS

Many NICUs still use scheduled feedings. Self-regulatory or cue-based feedings involve feeding the infant based on caregiver interpretation of infant hunger versus feeding the infant every 3 or 4 hours independent of the presence or absence of behaviors that suggest hunger. Demand feedings generally refer to an infant's being fed when crying commences, whereas cue-based feedings refer to an infant's being fed based on demonstrated hunger cues, that is, alert state, hand-to-mouth movement, and rooting reflex, which precede the onset of crying (Gill, White, & Anderson, 1984).

BOTTLE FEEDING

The process of feeding by bottle results in significant physiologic and biochemical alterations for many term infants (Bodefeld et al., 1979; Durand et al., 1981; Mathew & Bathia, 1989; Mathew, Clark, & Pronske, 1985; Mathew et al., 1985; Rosen, Glaze, & Frost, 1984) and preterm infants (Guilleminault & Coons, 1984; Meier, 1988; Rosen, Glaze, & Frost, 1984; Shivpuri, Martin, Carlo, & Fanaroff, 1983). The general consensus of these studies is that hypoxemia, hypercarbia, decreased minute ventilation, and more extreme manifestations of distress (that is, apnea, bradycardia, and cyanosis) occur owing to immaturity in the integration of sucking, swallowing, and breathing.

In general, as the infant begins to suck with the bottle, minute ventilation falls from a combination of decreases in respiratory frequency and tidal volume. Consequently, oxygenation declines and carbon dioxide levels increase. A more exaggerated response includes apnea, bradycardia, and cyanosis.

Nursing Interventions

Traditionally, nurses have not identified bottle feeding as an intervention that requires professional attention. Consequently, convalescing preterm infants have been referred to as "feeders" or "growers," suggesting that persons other than professional nurses can provide their care. Given the documented frequency of hypoxemia during bottle feeding, nurses should refocus professional care on the assessment and management of feeding-related hypoxemia.

Bottle feeding necessitates more frequent swallowing. Because swallowing interrupts respiration, more frequent swallowing might compromise ventilatory function for the preterm infant. However, Dowling (1995) reported that selected preterm infants were able to maintain regular breathing patterns, and, consequently, oxygenation, during bottle feeding with Nuk-type nipple. Another nursing intervention, related to controlling the rate of milk flow, is to allow the infant to set the pace of the feeding. Preterm infants may require more time to complete a feeding than do term infants, and the ability to pace the bottle feeding may be a protective mechanism, allowing the infant to expend less energy while feeding.

A related intervention is the avoidance of force feeding for preterm infants. In the clinical setting it is not unusual to see nurses manipulating infants' faces, mouths, and the bottle, forcing an already fatigued infant to complete the remainder of a feeding. Stimulating an infant to suck has potential for interfering with the infant's self-regulation of sucking and breathing, which, especially for a fatigued infant, may precipitate hypoxemia.

BREASTFEEDING

Preterm infants are seldom allowed to breastfeed until bottle feedings have been well established and an arbitrary weight criterion is achieved. However, delay in initial breastfeeding is associated with undesirable outcomes for mothers and preterm infants (Ehrenkranz, Ackerman, Mezger, & Bracken, 1985; McCoy et al., 1988; Measel, Neu, & Anderson, 1987; Meberg, Willgraff, & Sande, 1982; Meier, 1988; Meier & Pugh, 1985; Pereira, Schwartz, Gould, & Grim, 1984). The most important of these is breastfeeding failure, defined as the cessation of breastfeeding during the infant's hospitalization, or in the early postdischarge period, before the mother's intended weaning.

The breastfeeding failure rate for mothers of preterm infants may exceed 50 percent of those mothers who try to breastfeed by the time infants are discharged from the hospital nursery (Pereira et al., 1984).

Significance of Breastfeeding for Preterm Infants and Mothers

Infants receive the unique immunologic and nutritional properties of human milk, which cannot be reproduced in commercial formulas (American Academy of Pediatrics, 1980; World Health Organization, 1981). Breastfeeding is associated with lower rates of postneonatal morbidity than is formula feeding in the United States (Kovar, Serdula, Marks, & Fraser, 1984) and with lower rates of postneonatal mortality and morbidity in developing countries (Jason, Nieburg, & Marks, 1984). Also, preterm infants subjected to painful procedures and separation from their mothers after birth would experience the pleasurable sensations and closeness of breastfeeding (Meberg, Willgraff, & Sande, 1982). Physiologically, pilot research has demonstrated that contrary to popular assumption, breastfeeding is less stressful than bottle feeding, especially when infants are smallest and least mature (Meier, 1988). For mothers, breastfeeding may facilitate mother–infant attachment (Alberts, Kalverboer, & Hopkins, 1983; Newton & Newton, 1967) and provide a sense that they are contributing something to the care of their infant that no one else can (Ehrenkranz & Ackerman, 1986; Measel, Neu, & Anderson, 1987).

REFERENCES

Alberts, E., Kalverboer, A. F., & Hopkins, B. (1983). Mother-infant dialogue in the first days of life: An observational study during breastfeeding. *Journal of Child Psychology and Psychiatry and Applied Disciplines, 24,* 145–161.

American Academy of Pediatrics. (1980). Encouraging breast-feeding. *Pediatrics, 65,* 657–658.

Anderson, D. M. (1987). Nutrition care for the premature infant. *Topics in Clinical Nutrition, 2,* 1–9.

Aschner, J. L., Punsalang, A. Jr., Maniscalco, W. M., & Menegus, M. A. (1987). Percutaneous central venous catheter colonization with *Malassezia furfur:* Incidence and clinical significance. *Pediatrics, 80,* 535–539.

Azimi, P. H., Levernier, K., Lefrak, L. M., et al. (1988). *Malassezia furfur:* A cause of occlusion of percutaneous central venous catheters in infants in the intensive care nursery. *Pediatric Infectious Disease Journal, 7,* 100–103.

Ball, P. A., Candy, D. C. A., Puntis, J. W. L., & McNeish, A. S. (1985). Portable bedside microcomputer system for management of parenteral nutrition in all age groups. *Archives of Disease in Childhood, 60,* 435–439.

Binder, N. D., Raschko, P. K., Benda, G. I., & Reynolds, J. W. (1989). Insulin infusion with parenteral nutrition in extremely low birth weight infants with hyperglycemia. *Journal of Pediatrics, 114,* 273–280.

Bodefeld, E., Schachinger, H., Huch, A., et al. (1979). Continuous $tcPO_2$ monitoring in healthy and sick newborn infants during and after feeding. In A. Huch, R. Huch, & J. F. Lucey (Eds.), *Continuous transcutaneous blood gas monitoring* (pp. 503–508). New York: Alan R. Liss.

Botsford, K. B., Weinstein, R. A., Boyer, K. M., et al. (1986). Gram-negative bacilli in human milk feedings: Quantitation and clinical consequences for premature infants. *Journal of Pediatrics, 109,* 707–710.

Brennan-Behm, M., Carlson, E., Meier, P., & Engstrom, J. (1994). Caloric loss from expressed mother's milk during continuous gavage infusion. *Neonatal Network, 13*(2), 27–32.

Brooke, O. G., & Barley, J. (1978). Loss of energy during continuous infusions of breast milk. *Archives of Disease in Childhood, 53,* 344–345.

Cheek, J. A. Jr., & Staub, G. F. (1973). Nasojejunal alimentation for premature and full-term newborn infants. *Journal of Pediatrics, 82,* 955–962.

Darby, M. K., & Loughead, J. L. (1996). Neonatal nutritional requirements and formula composition: A review. *JOGNN, Journal of Obstetric, Gynecologic, and Neonatal Nursing, 25,* 209–217.

Dowling, D. A. (1995). *Responses of preterm infants to enteral feedng.* Unpublished doctoral dissertation, University of Illinois, Chicago.

Durand, M., Leahy, F. N., MacCallum, M., et al. (1981). Effect of feeding on the chemical control of breathing in the newborn infant. *Pediatric Research, 15,* 1509–1512.

Ehrenkranz, R. A., & Ackerman, B. A. (1986). Metoclopramide effect on faltering milk production by mothers of premature infants. *Pediatrics, 78,* 614–620.

Ehrenkranz, R. A., Ackerman, B. A., Mezger, J., & Bracken, M. B. (1985). Breastfeeding and premature infant: Incidence and success. *Pediatric Research, 19,* 99A (Abstract 530).

Evans, M. E., Schaffner, W., Federspiel, C. F., et al. (1988). Sensitivity, specitivity, and predictive value of body surface cultures in a neonatal intensive care unit. *Journal of the American Medical Association, 259,* 248–252.

Gallaher, K. J., Cashwell, S., Hall, V., et al. (1993). Orogastric tube insertion length in very low birth weight infants. *Journal of Perinatology, 13,* 128–131.

Gill, N. E., White, M. A., & Anderson, G. C. (1984). Transitional newborn infants in a hospital nursery: From first oral cue to first sustained cry. *Nursing Research, 33,* 213–217.

Greer, F. R., McCormick, A., & Loker, J. (1984). Changes in fat concentration of human milk during delivery by intermittent bolus and continuous mechanical pump infusion. *Journal of Pediatrics, 105,* 745–749.

Guilleminault, C., & Coons, S. (1984). Apnea and bradycardia during feeding in infants weighing > 2000 grams. *Journal of Pediatrics, 104,* 932–935.

Jason, J. M., Nieburg, P., & Marks, J. S. (1984). Mortality and infectious disease associated with infant-feeding practices in developing countries [Review]. *Pediatrics, 74*(4 pt 2)S, 702–727.

Kerner, J. A. (1983). *Manual of pediatric parenteral nutrition* (pp. 63–68, 117–217) New York: John Wiley.

Kerner, J. A. (1991). Parenteral nutrition. In W. A. Walker, P. Durie, R. Hamilton, et al. (Eds.), *Pediatric gastrointestinal diseases* (Vol. 2). Philadelphia: B. C. Decker.

Kovar, M. G., Serdula, M. K., Marks, J. S., & Fraser, D. W. (1984). Review of the epidemiologic evidence for an association between infant feeding and infant health. *Pediatrics, 74*(4 pt. 2)S, 615–638.

Landwirth, J. (1974). Continuous nasogastric infusion feedings of infants of low birth weight. *Clinical Pediatrics, 13,* 603–608.

Lemons, P. M., Miller, K., Eitzen, H., et al. (1983). Bacterial growth in human milk during continuous feeding. *American Journal of Perinatology, 1,* 76–80.

Mathew, O. P., & Bhatia, J. (1989). Sucking and breathing patterns during breast- and bottle-feeding in term neonates: Effects of nutrient delivery and composition. *American Journal of Diseases of Children, 143,* 588–592.

Mathew, O. P., Clark, M. L., & Pronske, M. H. (1985). Apnea, bradycardia, and cyanosis during oral feeding in term neonates [Letter]. *Journal of Pediatrics, 10,* 857.

Mathew, O. P., Clark, M. L., Pronske, M. L., et al. (1985). Breathing pattern and ventilation during oral feeding in term newborn infants. *Journal of Pediatrics, 106,* 810–813.

McCoy, R., Kadowaki, C., Wilks, S., et al. (1988). Nursing management of breastfeeding for preterm infants. *Journal of Perinatal and Neonatal Nursing, 2,* 42–55.

Measel, C. P., Neu, J., & Anderson, G. C. (1987). *Establishing and maintaining lactation: Experiences of mothers of very low birth weight infants.* Unpublished manuscript.

Meberg, A., Willgraff, S., & Sande, H. A. (1982). High potential for breastfeeding among mothers giving birth to pre-term infants. *Acta Paediatrica Scandinavica, 71,* 661–662.

Meier, P. P. (1988). Bottle and breastfeeding: Effects on transcutaneous oxygen pressure and temperature in preterm infants. *Nursing Research, 37,* 36–41.

Meier, P. P., & Pugh, E. J. (1985). Breast-feeding behavior of small preterm infants. *MCN: American Journal of Maternal Child Nursing, 10,* 396–401.

Meier, P. P., & Wilks, S. O. (1987). The bacteria in expressed mothers milk. *MCN: American Journal of Maternal Child Nursing, 12,* 420–423.

Narayanan, I., Singh, B., & Harvey, D. (1984). Fat loss during feeding of human milk. *Archives of Disease in Childhood, 59,* 475–477.

Newton, N., & Newton, M. (1967). Psychologic aspects of lactation [Review]. *New England Journal of Medicine, 277,* 1179–1188.

Ostertag, S. G., Jovanovic, L., Lewis, B., & Auld, P. A. M. (1986). Insulin pump therapy in the very low birth weight infant. *Pediatrics, 78,* 625–630.

Pereira, G. R. (1995). Nutritional care of the extremely premature infant [Review]. *Clinics in Perinatology, 22,* 61–75.

Pereira, G. R., Schwartz, D., Gould, P., & Grim, N. (1984). Breastfeeding in neonatal intensive care: Beneficial effects of maternal counseling. *Perinatology/Neonatology, 8,* 35–42.

Pettit, J. D. & Hughes, K. (1993). Intravenous extravasation: Mechanisms, management and prevention. *The Journal of Perinatal and Neonatal Nursing, 6*(4), 74–85.

Powell, D. A., Aungst, J., Snedden, S., et al. (1984). Broviac catheter–related *Malassezia furfur* sepsis in five infants receiving intravenous fat emulsions. *Journal of Pediatrics, 105,* 987–990.

Rhea, J. W., & Kilby, J. O. (1970). A nasojejunal tube for infant feeding. *Pediatrics, 46,* 36–40.

Rosen, C. L., Glaze, D. G., & Frost, J. D. Jr. (1984). Hypoxemia associated with feeding in the preterm and full-term neonate. *American Journal of Diseases of Children, 138,* 623–628.

Schulman, R. J., Buffone, G., & Wise, L. (1985). Enteric protein loss in necrotizing enterocolitis as measured by fecal 1-antitrypsin excretion. *Journal of Pediatrics, 107,* 287–289.

Shivpuri, C. R., Martin, R. J., Carlo, W. A., & Fanaroff, A. A. (1983). Decreased ventilation in preterm infants during oral feeding. *Journal of Pediatrics, 103,* 285–289.

Simeon, P. S., Geffner, M. E., Levin, S. R. & Lindsey, A. M. (1994). Continuous insulin infusions in neonates: Pharmacologic availability of insulin in intravenous solutions. *Journal of Pediatrics 124,* 818–820.

Stocks, R. J., Davies, D. P., Allen, F., & Sewell, D. (1985). Loss of breast milk nutrients during tube feeding. *Archives of Disease in Childhood, 60,* 164–166.

Vaucher, Y. E., Walson, P. D., & Morrow, G. III. (1982). Continuous insulin infusion in hyperglycemic, very low birth weight infants. *Journal of Pediatric Gastroenterology and Nutrition, 1,* 211–217.

Wilks, S. O., & Meierp, P. P. (1988). Helping mothers express milk suitable for preterm and high-risk infant feeding. *MCN: American Journal of Maternal Child Nursing, 13,* 121–123.

World Health Organization. (1981). *Contemporary patterns of breast-feeding: Report on the WHO collaborative study of breast-feeding.* Geneva: Author.

Yamamoto, L. G., Gainsley, G. J., & Witek, J. E. (1986). Pediatric parenteral nutrition management using a comprehensive user-friendly computer program designed for personal computers. *Journal of Parenteral and Enteral Nutrition, 10,* 535–539.

Zenk, K. E., Dungy, C. I., & Greene, G. R. (1981). Nafcillin extravasation injury: Use of hyaluronidase as an antidote. *American Journal of Diseases of Children, 135,* 1113–1114.

CHAPTER 12

Assessment and Management of Gastrointestinal Dysfunction

PHYSIOLOGY OF THE GASTROINTESTINAL TRACT

The major function of the gastrointestinal tract is to transfer food and water from the external to the internal environment, where they can be digested, absorbed, and distributed to the cells of the body by the circulatory system. While these processes are occurring, contractions of the smooth muscle lining the walls of the intestines move the contents through the lumen, releasing any material not digested and absorbed during transit.

MATURATION OF GASTROINTESTINAL FUNCTION

The supporting structures of the gastrointestinal tract are relatively thinner in the newborn, especially in the prematurely born, than in the adult. The following characterize the neonate's gut:

- Supporting musculature is relatively deficient.
- Immature motor mechanisms, particularly in the prematurely born, at best allow for only irregular peristaltic activity that occurs in disorganized patterns.
- Infrequent and irregular activity tends toward distention in the infant and in the ill or prematurely born, increasing the likelihood of delayed transit and stooling.
- Antenatal corticosteroid treatment to initiate production of pulmonary surfactant seems to promote gut maturation, but maturation appears to be delayed in infants affected with significant central nervous system insult or abnormality, such as asphyxia and hydrocephalus.
- Decreased peristalsis among premature infants can be seen by comparing passage of meconium among infants of various weights by 48 hours of age.
- Further delay in maturation occurs in low birth weight infants who are ill, especially those with severe respiratory distress syndrome, in whom enteral feedings are consequently delayed.
- Even in the absence of congenital gastrointestinal problems, very low birth weight infants might not be expected to pass their first stool until as late as 7 to 12 days of age.

ASSESSMENT OF THE GASTROINTESTINAL TRACT

History

A careful history is obtained:

- The prenatal history is checked, and any maternal illness or drugs (legal

197

and illegal substances), family history of anomalies, and presence of polyhydramnios is noted.

- Most cases of isolated abdominal and gastrointestinal defects occur sporadically.
- Cleft lip and/or palate and pyloric stenosis may exhibit familial recurrence patterns, suggesting at least some degree of genetic influence mediated by environmental factors (McCormack, 1979).
- The best evidence ·of fetal gastrointestinal anomalies is obtained through prenatal ultrasonography. The fetal abdomen can be identified as early as 10 weeks from the last menstrual period. However, embryogenesis is continuing, so reliable visualization becomes possible during the second and third trimesters, when the gastrointestinal structures are established.
- Polyhydramnios may indicate high gastrointestinal defects. If there is a gastrointestinal obstruction, the fetus is unable to effectively swallow amniotic fluid, resulting in polyhydramnios.
- Postnatally, three cardinal signs of gastrointestinal obstruction include (1) persistent vomiting, especially if it is bile stained; (2) abdominal distention; and (3) failure to pass meconium within the first 48 hours of birth (Chang, 1980b; Ghory & Sheldon, 1985):
  - Vomiting is an indicator of high gastrointestinal defects. Bilious vomiting indicates obstruction is distal to the ampulla of Vater, where bile is emptied from the common bile duct into the duodenum. Conversely, nonbilious vomiting would be noted if obstruction were proximal to the ampulla (Ricketts, 1984).
  - Abdominal distention occurs with obstruction as swallowed air and fluid collect in the bowel, digestive fluids accumulate, and electrolytes and proteins are lost from the circulation into the lumen of bowel, which becomes progressively edematous (Guyton, 1996).
  - Failure to pass meconium within the first 2 days of life may indicate obstruction of the large intestine. Stooling is variable in premature, sedated, debilitated, or hypoxic infants.

Physical Assessment

INSPECTION

Many of the gastrointestinal defects are grossly apparent. A systematic head-to-toe method of inspection is necessary for complete examination.

Mouth

- Observe position, shape, size, and symmetry of mouth.
- Evaluate lips, palate, and uvula for clefting.
- Inspect for any niche in the lip that might easily be overlooked. Abundant oral secretions or saliva provides an early clue to esophageal atresia, particularly when a history of polyhydramnios has been reported (Johnson, 1993; Scanlon, Nelson, Grylack, & Smith, 1979).

Abdomen

- Inspect for contour, symmetry, and integrity.
- Be aware that distention as opposed to a characteristic rounded appearance serves as a hallmark of obstruction.
- Observe for visible peristalsis in premature infants owing to decreased abdominal muscle tone. When peristalsis is accompanied by vomiting or distention, obstruction is suggested.
- Assess character of umbilical cord and site of insertion. Although most cases of omphalocele are obvious, an abnormal thickness of the stump or cord should raise suspicion of a single herniated loop of intestine. Any such enlargement must be differentiated from a Wharton's jelly cyst or umbilical hernia through the lax rectus muscles.

Anus

- Examine anus for position and perineal area for fistulas.
- Assess muscle tone of the anal sphincter by stroking anal area with a gloved finger and observing for the contraction "wink" that normally occurs around the anal opening.
- If clinically indicated, check anal patency by digital examination using the gloved little finger (Conner, 1993; Kiernan & Scoloveno, 1986; Scanlon, Nelson, Grylack, & Smith, 1979).
- Do not take the infant's temperature rectally because this risks perforating the rectum (Merenstein, 1970).

AUSCULTATION

- Bowel sounds are audible within the first 15 to 30 minutes of life, as the bowel fills with swallowed air and peristaltic activity is activated by the parasympathetic nervous system (Desmond & Rudolph, 1965; Lepley, 1980).
- A metallic tinkling sound occurs two to five times per minute (Roberts, 1977).
- Hyperactive, absent, or even normal bowel sounds are noted with intestinal obstruction (Sunshine, Sinatra, Mitchell, & Santulli, 1983).
- Sounds should be interpreted in relationship to other pertinent historical and clinical findings.
- Often the abdomen is misleadingly silent (Flake & Ryckman, 1992).

PALPATION

Abdominal palpation is performed with the infant in a supine position and is best carried out when the infant is quiet and preferably during the first 24 hours of life, when the abdominal musculature is lax. Holding the infant's knees and hips in a flexed position also helps to relax the abdominal musculature. The pads of the fingers of a warm hand are used to feel the liver, spleen, and kidneys using slow, gentle pressure. Taking care to perform abdominal palpation in as gentle a manner as possible cannot be overemphasized. Not only are the multiple maneuvers often distressing to the newborn, but also the pressure applied even during a routine examination may result in significant although transient elevations in both systolic and diastolic blood pressures (Conner, 1993; Sinkin, Phillips, & Adelman, 1985).

Palpation of Liver

The liver is found by placing the index finger just above and to the right of the groin and slowly advancing upward until the edge of the liver can be felt to slip beneath the pad of the finger. Normally the organ is firm (but not hard) with a sharp edge that extends 1 to 2 cm below the right costal margin and can be followed across the abdomen into the left upper quadrant.

Palpation of Spleen

The spleen is found on the left side in a similar manner, but generally only the tip of the organ is felt at the left costal margin, or it may be entirely unpalpable.

Palpation of Kidneys

The kidneys are located in the flank areas above the level of the umbilicus and are normally 4.5 to 5.0 cm in length in the term infant. Palpation may be performed bimanually with one hand supporting and stabilizing the flanks posteriorly, while the thumb or a finger of the free hand is moved anteriorly over the same area. Alternatively, they may be found using a single hand with the fingers of the hand supporting the flank posteriorly while the free thumb of the same hand explores the flank anteriorly. Although the upper position of the right kidney may be obscured by the overlying liver, the entire left kidney should easily be felt.

Palpation for Masses

The remainder of the abdominal examination consists of a gentle search for pathologic masses. Although most masses found are of renal origin, it may be possible to detect stool-filled bowel, particularly in the case of meconium ileus (Conner, 1993; Scanlon, Nelson, Grylack, & Smith, 1979).

RELATED FINDINGS

History of maternal polyhydramnios, vomiting, distention, and failure to pass stool are most indicative of gastrointestinal dysfunction. Other relatively subtle and often nonspecific signs may also be noted (Ghory & Sheldon, 1985).

Respiratory Difficulty

- The infant may not be able to handle the abundant oral secretions commonly found in esophageal atresia.
- Gastric contents may be aspirated because of an associated tracheo-esophageal fistula.
- Abdominal distention may impede diaphragmatic excursions and therefore decrease ventilation.

- Frank airway obstruction may even occur in the case of cleft palate if the negative inspiratory pressure pulls the tongue into the hypopharynx (Avery, Fletcher, & Williams, 1981).
- Jaundice may occur if the removal of bilirubin is hampered. With biliary atresia, the conjugated bilirubin, which is a normal component of bile, is unable to pass into the duodenum for excretion in the stool. In the case of intestinal atresia, meconium ileus, and Hirschsprung's disease, the enterohepatic circulation becomes exaggerated because stasis of the luminal contents promotes intestinal reabsorption of the bilirubin that is present (Poland & Ostrea, 1993).
- Systemic hypertension may be an additional, although rarely noted, subtle sign, and usually occurs in situations in which masses or distention significantly increase intra-abdominal pressure (Sinkin, Phillips, & Adelman, 1985).

RISK FACTORS

Maternal, neonatal, and other risk factors associated with gastrointestinal dysfunction may be found in Table 12–1. These factors are discussed under sections outlining the management of specific problems.

NURSING MANAGEMENT

General Principles

Early recognition accompanied by medical or surgical intervention for infants with gastrointestinal obstructions or alterations is necessary to decrease the likelihood of a poor outcome. The general considerations that guide nursing care in alteration of the gastrointestinal system include gastrointestinal decompression, fluid and electrolyte balance, thermoregulation, positioning, prevention of infection, and nutrition.

GASTRIC DECOMPRESSION

- Gastric decompression prevents aspiration, respiratory compromise, or gastric perforation. Unrelieved intestinal obstruction with abdominal distention may exert upward pressure on the diaphragm, which compromises respirations.
- Orogastric tube (10 French soft-vinyl double-lumen sump) to low intermittent suction provides sufficient decompression for most infants.
- Tube patency is essential if gastric decompression is to be maintained.
- Tube placement should be assessed periodically.
- Irrigating the tube every 2 hours with 2 ml of air ensures that the tube remains open and functioning.

FLUID AND ELECTROLYTE BALANCE

- In intestinal obstruction, the fluids that are normally reabsorbed by the intestine become trapped.

TABLE 12–1. **Risk Factors Associated with Gastrointestinal Dysfunction**

Risk Factor	Gastrointestinal Dysfunction
Maternal	
Cigarette smoking	Cleft lip with or without cleft palate
Diabetes	Small left colon syndrome
Hypovitaminosis	Cleft lip with or without cleft palate
Influenza with fever	Cleft lip with or without cleft palate
Ionizing radiation exposure	Biliary atresia
Polyhydramnios	Esophageal atresia with or without TE fistula, duodenal atresia, meconium ileus
Stress and anxiety	Pyloric stenosis
Medications:	
Doxylamine succinate–pyridoxine hydrochloride	Pyloric stenosis
Benzodiazepines	Cleft lip with or without cleft palate
Cortisone	Cleft lip with or without cleft palate
Dilantin	Cleft lip with or without cleft palate
Magnesium sulfate	Meconium plug syndrome
Opiates	Cleft lip with or without cleft palate
Penicillin	Cleft lip with or without cleft palate
Salicylates	Cleft lip with or without cleft palate
Positive family history:	
"Apple peel" type of jejunoileal atresia	Similar anomaly
Cleft lip with or without cleft palate	Similar anomaly
Cystic fibrosis	Meconium ileus
Hirschsprung's disease	Similar anomaly
Neonatal	
Apnea	Necrotizing enterocolitis
Aseptic environment	Necrotizing enterocolitis
Asphyxia or ischemic episodes	Biliary atresia, necrotizing enterocolitis
Cyanotic spells	Necrotizing enterocolitis
Exchange transfusion	Necrotizing enterocolitis
Feeding practices	Pyloric stenosis, necrotizing enterocolitis
Hyperbilirubinemia	Duodenal atresia, jejunoileal atresia
Polycythemia	Necrotizing enterocolitis
Respiratory distress	Necrotizing enterocolitis
Vascular catheterization	Necrotizing enterocolitis
Infections:	
Cytomegalovirus	Biliary atresia
Gastroenteritis	Intussusception
Hepatitis A and B	Biliary atresia
Reovirus type 3	Biliary atresia
Respiratory infection	Intussusception
Rubella	Biliary atresia
Viral infection	Pyloric stenosis
Medications:	
Hyperosmolar medications	Necrotizing enterocolitis
Xanthines	Gastroesophageal reflux

TABLE 12–1. Risk Factors Associated with Gastrointestinal Dysfunction
Continued

Risk Factor	Gastrointestinal Dysfunction
Other	
Congenital deafness	Hirschsprung's disease
Congenital heart disease	Esophageal atresia with or without TE fistula, duodenal atresia, biliary atresia, omphalocele, anorectal atresia
Diaphragmatic hernia	Malrotation
Genitourinary anomalies	Esophageal atresia with or without TE fistula, duodenal atresia, biliary atresia, omphalocele, Hirschsprung's disease, malrotation, anorectal atresia
Imperforate anus	Esophageal atresia with or without TE fistula, duodenal atresia
Intestinal atresia or obstruction	Gastroesophageal reflux, esophageal atresia with or without TE fistula, biliary atresia, omphalocele, gastroschisis, malrotation
Malrotation	Duodenal atresia, jejunoileal atresia
Meckel's diverticulum	Malrotation, intussusception
Meconium ileus	Jejunoileal atresia
Neurologic abnormalities	Hirschsprung's disease, meconium plug syndrome
Ocular neurocristopathies	Hirschsprung's disease
Pancreatic defects	Meconium ileus
Tracheoesophageal anomalies	Duodenal atresia, anorectal atresia
Vertebral malformations	Esophageal atresia with or without TE fistula

TE, tracheoesophageal.

- Intravascular fluid shifts into the interstitial compartment, called "third spacing" or capillary leak syndrome. If severe, this loss of intravascular volume can result in relative hypovolemia and hypoperfusion, leading to shock.
- Vomiting, diarrhea, and gastric suction can cause excessive volume depletion and electrolyte abnormalities, especially losses of sodium, potassium, and chloride.
- Fluid maintenance: 60 to 80 ml/kg for the first 24 hours of life and then 120 to 160 ml/kg/day (Kenner, Harjo, & Brueggemeyer, 1988). A rate should be maintained such that urine output is at least 1 ml/kg/hr and maintains a specific gravity of 1.005 to 1.012.
- Sodium is provided at a rate 2 to 3 mEq/kg/day and potassium at 2 mEq/kg/day, as serum electrolytes indicate.
- Gastric loss is measured from orogastric tube every 4 to 8 hours. The amount of gastric output should be replaced milliliter for milliliter every 4 to 8 hours with 5 percent dextrose in 0.9 percent NaCl with 10 mEq KCl per liter (Kenner, Harjo, & Brueggemeyer, 1988). This amount of fluid is given in addition to maintenance fluids. Fluid volume

deficit and electrolyte imbalances may occur if replacement therapy is inadequate. The adequacy for fluid replacement is assessed by changes in vital signs, amount of urinary output, urine specific gravity, levels of electrolytes and blood urea nitrogen, and hematocrit.

Acid-Base Imbalance

- Metabolic alkalosis may occur with pyloric stenosis or high jejunal obstruction because of loss of acidic gastric juice. In obstructions in the distal segment of the small intestine, larger quantities of alkaline fluids may be lost than acidic fluids, resulting in metabolic acidosis. If the obstruction is below the proximal colon, acid-base balance may be maintained because most of the gastrointestinal fluids are absorbed before reaching the obstruction.
- Respiratory acidosis may develop in patients with abdominal distention owing to carbon dioxide retention from hypoventilation (Methany, 1987).
- Correction of acid-base imbalances would be made in the instance of a pH less than 7.35 or greater than 7.45 or for base excess below -4 or above $+4$ (Merenstein & Gardner, 1989).

THERMOREGULATION

Thermoregulation is vital in the care of all newborns and becomes more critical for the stressed neonate.

- Cold stress dramatically increases oxygen requirements and predisposes to hypoglycemia and metabolic acidosis.
- Appropriate heat source such as Isolette or radiant warmer should be used.
- The infant's head should be covered.
- Temperature monitoring (ambient air and infant) should be done hourly.
- Profound heat loss is associated with gastroschisis and omphalocele from exposed bowel.
  - A bowel bag is used from the feet to the axillae.
  - Use of plastic wrap helps decrease evaporative losses.

POSITIONING

The infant is positioned head up for the following reasons:

- To minimize pressure that a distended bowel places on the diaphragm
- To minimize gastric reflux. A 30-degree prone position has been shown to be the most effective position to decrease reflux (Meyers & Herbst, 1982).

PREVENTION OF INFECTION

- Broad-spectrum antibiotics are administered immediately in neonates with presumed infections.

- Antibiotics are administered preoperatively to prevent infection.
- Good handwashing is essential.
- Assessment for early signs of infection should be ongoing.

NUTRITION

Postoperative caloric and metabolic needs of infant with gastrointestinal dysfunction include the following:

- Hyperalimentation is provided to meet nutritional needs until feedings can be resumed after surgery.
- Enteral feedings are begun with clear liquids, progressing to elemental feedings such as Pregestimil, gradually increasing from one-quarter to one-half to full strength.
- Initial feedings are small, frequent, or continuous drip, are supplemented with intravenous hyperalimentation, and are gradually advanced.
- Advancement of feeding should be stopped if there are signs of intolerance, such as diarrhea, vomiting, abdominal distention, or presence of reducing substances in stool (Kenner, Harjo, & Brueggemeyer, 1988).

General Preoperative Management

All the principles of preoperative management revolve around the prevention or minimization of identified stressors:

- Correct all fluid losses.
- Decompress the distended bowel.
- Support failing organ systems.

General Postoperative Management

General postoperative management involves the following:

- Hydration
- Maintenance of electrolyte balance
- Continued gastric decompression
- Respiratory and other therapy that the individual case warrants
- Assessment of pain and administration of nonpharmacologic and pharmacologic interventions. Some drugs slow peristalsis so the choice of drug intervention must be individually determined for infants recovering from surgery on their bowel.
- Institution of total parenteral nutrition if enteral feedings are delayed beyond 3 to 5 days, to prevent excessive catabolism
- Initiation of feedings when bowel sounds are present, stools are being passed normally, and the gastric drainage clears and lessens in amount (Pereira & Ziegler, 1989)

OSTOMY CARE

- Skin care is provided to prevent frequent problems associated with excoriation and fungal and other infections.

- Skin appliances are used to maximally protect skin from contact with effluent, and the stoma appliance should be changed if the seal is broken. Allergic reaction to the products used for stoma appliances occurs less than 1 percent of the time.
- Hydration is assessed and urine and stool output, gastric drainage, and stomal drainage should be monitored (Harrell-Bean & Klell, 1983).
- The stoma is assessed. Healthy stomas appear dark pink to red, with a smooth, moist surface that slightly protrudes. Any deviation or change in appearance should be reported immediately.

SHORT-BOWEL (SHORT-GUT) SYNDROME

Short-bowel syndrome is a complication of many neonatal surgeries involving extensive resection of the gastrointestinal tract:

- Loss of considerable absorptive surface results in a complex, malabsorptive problem with episodic diarrhea, steatorrhea, and dehydration, which if allowed to progress may cause metabolic derangements and ultimately poor growth and development.
- A 1- to 2-year hospitalization may not be unusual (Leape, 1987). The duration of initial hospitalization and length of dependence on parenteral nutrition are both inversely related to the length of remaining bowel (Chaet, Farrell, Ziegler, & Warner, 1994).
  - Absorptive area increases through intestinal growth and hypertrophy of mucosal wall; villi become hyperplastic (Swaniker et al., 1995).
  - In cases of extensive resection, in which less than 75 cm remains of the bowel (the approximate length of the small intestine in the normal newborn is 200 cm), particularly when the ileocecal valve has also been removed, completely normal absorption may never be achieved.
  - General survival is considered possible with as little as 11 cm of residual jejunoileum if the ileocecal valve is intact and with as little as 25 cm when the valve is removed (Dorney et al., 1985).
  - Recently, perhaps owing to improved techniques and advances in enteral nutrition to stimulate the adaptation response, one case has been reported of a survivor with 12 cm of jejunum without an ileocecal valve (Surana, Quinn, & Puri, 1994).
  - Infants with massive resection and those demonstrating no spontaneous adaptation after 6 to 12 months (refractory short-bowel syndrome) may require radical surgical treatment to slow intestinal transit (eg, intestinal valves, reversed segment, colon interposition, intestinal pacing) or increase mucosal surface area (eg, intestinal lengthening, tapering enteroplasty, neomucosa, small bowel transplantation) and thus increase absorption (Warner & Ziegler, 1993).
  - Prevention of skin breakdown (due to diarrhea) and of infection is critical.
  - Parents must be involved in their infant's care and every effort made to stimulate normal growth and development (Gantt & Thompson, 1985).

MANAGEMENT OF PROBLEMS WITH INGESTION

Cleft Palate and Lip

PATHOPHYSIOLOGY

Although cleft lip and cleft palate are often associated, these defects are embryologically distinct disorders. Cleft lip occurs when the maxillary process fails to merge with the medial nasal elevation on one or both sides. Cleft palate occurs when the lateral palatine processes fail to meet and fuse with each other, the primary palate, or the nasal septum (Moore & Persaud, 1993). Studies indicate that when both cleft lip and cleft palate occur, the failure of the secondary palate to close may be a developmental consequence of the abnormalities in the primary palate associated with the cleft lip, rather than an intrinsic defect in the secondary palate. It is possible, therefore, that isolated cleft lip and cleft lip with an associated cleft palate represent varying degrees of the same embryologic defect (Fraser, 1970; Habib, 1978a).

INCIDENCE

Cleft lip with or without an associated cleft palate affects 14 of every 10,000 newborns, with rates higher in males than in females and in Asians than in whites. In contrast, isolated cleft palate has a lower incidence rate of 4 in 10,000 infants, occurs more frequently in females, and has no clear racial variation (Habib, 1978a, 1978b; Oka, 1979). Although rates of recurrence risks indicate that genetic factors are often involved, environmental factors also appear to contribute in some way, indicating a multifactorial mode of inheritance.

RISK FACTORS

- First-trimester maternal ingestion of benzodiazepines, phenytoin, opiates, penicillin, salicylates, and cortisone has been associated with clefting.
- Fever and influenza during the first trimester have been associated; however, it is questionable as to whether the viral agent or the therapeutic drugs are the causative factors.
- Threatened abortion in the first and second trimesters and premature delivery of children with clefts have also been reported as risk factors, but it is uncertain whether these indicate an unfavorable intrauterine environment or simply an already malformed fetus (eg, Pierre Robin syndrome).
- Maternal smoking, hypovitaminosis, and hypervitaminosis, especially of vitamin A, have also been supported as risk factors.

CLINICAL MANIFESTATIONS

Generally defined, *cleft lip* is the term that signifies a congenital fissure in the upper lip, whereas *cleft palate* indicates a congenital fissure either in the soft palate alone or in both the hard and soft palates. The two conditions may occur in isolation or together. Isolated cleft lip may be either unilateral or bilateral and may range in severity from a slight notch in the lip to a complete cleft into the nostril. Isolated cleft palate may also be unilateral or bilateral and may be as mild as a submucous cleft characterized by a notch at the posterior edge of the hard palate, an imperfect muscle union across the palate, a thin mucosal surface, and a bifid uvula. In this mild form, diagnosis may never be made. Combined clefts of the lip and palate are the most severe form of the defect, particularly if bilateral (Shah & Wong, 1980).

DIFFERENTIAL DIAGNOSIS

The major condition requiring differential diagnosis is van der Woude syndrome, which is inherited as an autosomal dominant trait. This syndrome ranges in appearance from a single, barely visible lower lip depression to frank pits or fistulas usually occurring in pairs on the vermilion of the lower lip, with clefting of the lip with or without palate involvement (Bowers, 1970; Jones, 1988; Schneider, 1973).

PROGNOSIS

Although an excellent prognosis for survival can be expected, an individual born with a cleft defect is faced with more than just a cosmetic problem. The following are associated complications:

- Language and speech tend to be retarded in affected individuals. This is further compounded by the fact that hearing impairment is more frequent in these individuals (Bergstrom, 1978; Krogman, 1979; Shah & Wong, 1980).
- Olfactory defects have also been demonstrated in males with cleft palate; however, females appear to be less frequently affected (Richman et al., 1988).
- Dental problems, such as malocclusion, irregularity of the teeth, and increased frequency of caries, may also be encountered by affected individuals (Shah & Wong, 1980).
- There are more than 154 syndromes that include cleft lip and/or palate as a feature (Cohen, 1978).

COLLABORATIVE MANAGEMENT

Management includes a multidisciplinary team approach: pediatrician, plastic surgeon, audiologist, speech pathologist, dental specialist, geneticist, social worker, and nursing personnel at various levels.

Surgical Repair

- The defect is closed to minimize maxillary growth retardation, to limit dental deformity, and to allow for normal speech development.
- Cleft lip repair is done at about 3 months of age among healthy infants.
- Repair of an associated cleft palate is generally postponed until some later time to allow for medial movement of the palatal shelves, which appears to be initiated by lip closure. Depending on the involvement, palate closure may occur as a two-step process, with the hard palate

being corrected at 14 to 16 months, followed by soft palate repair at 18 to 20 months.

- Additional repair of the lip or nose may be required for aesthetic purposes and is postponed until sufficient structural growth has been achieved, generally after 12 years of age (Krogman, 1979; Shah & Wong, 1980).

Feeding

Feeding requires a great deal of patience and attention to technique. Nurses need to teach parents appropriate feeding techniques:

- The bottle should be held securely and the cheeks grasped so that the cleft is pushed closed to help the infant create a vacuum necessary for adequate sucking.
- Frequent burping is required.
- The infant is held in an upright or semi-upright position, and the flow of milk directed to the side of the mouth.
- Use of a preemie nipple or a special cleft palate nipple may also be helpful.
- Frequent, small feedings help in preventing fatigue and frustration.
- Breastfeeding is possible, although considerable creativity may be required.
- A pillow placed between the infant's back and the mother's arm can maintain an upright position.
- The clefted area is cleaned with sterile water or a small amount of sterile water is offered after each feeding because the area becomes easily encrusted with milk and is prone to excoriation and infection (Pate, 1987; Styer & Freeh, 1981).

Esophageal Atresia and Tracheoesophageal Fistula

PATHOPHYSIOLOGY

Esophageal atresia and tracheoesophageal (TE) fistula occur when the trachea fails to differentiate and separate from the esophagus. The atresia appears most likely to be the result of either a spontaneous posterior deviation of the esophagotracheal septum or some mechanical force that pushes the dorsal wall of the foregut in an anterior direction. A fistula occurs when the lateral ridges of the septum fail to completely close in their normal, zipper-like fashion so that a communication is left between the foregut and the primitive respiratory tree (Moore & Persaud, 1993; Sadler, 1985).

INCIDENCE

Esophageal atresia with or without TE fistula occurs approximately once in every 3000 live births. Although rare cases of familial occurrence have been reported, most represent an accident of embryology.

RISK FACTORS

- Polyhydramnios
- Associated malformations (present in 30 to 70 percent):

- Congenital heart disease: ventricular and atrial septal defects
- Vertebral malformations (25 to 30 percent)
- Atresias of the small intestine (5 percent)
- Imperforate anus (10 to 20 percent)
- Genitourinary anomalies (10 to 21 percent)
- VATER association, the acronym representing a complex of vertebral and ventricular septal defects, anal atresia, TE fistula with esophageal atresia, and radial and renal anomalies (approximately 15 percent)
- VACTERL association, used by some experts to describe the same cluster of symptoms as VATER association with the addition of congenital heart defects and limb deformities.
- Prematurity. Overall, 20 to 30 percent are premature or small for gestational age; but in the case of isolated esophageal atresia, the incidence of prematurity approaches 50 percent.

CLINICAL MANIFESTATIONS

Although the infant may appear well at birth, because effective swallowing is not possible, oral secretions and saliva collect in the upper esophageal pouch and appear in the mouth and about the lips. The typical description of "excessive" secretions, however, is a misnomer. The body does not produce greater amounts of secretions. They simply cannot be handled properly and thus become more visible. Respiratory difficulty may be encountered if the secretions and mucus fill the esophageal pouch and overflow into the upper airway or find their way into the trachea through a proximal fistula. Any attempts at feeding are generally accompanied by coughing, choking, and cyanosis. If a distal fistula is present, crying may force air into the stomach, where it collects and causes progressive distention. This gastric distention may impede diaphragmatic excursions, leading to worsening respiratory status or a reflux of gastric contents through the fistula into the trachea. If there is no distal fistula, the abdomen is more likely to appear scaphoid owing to the lack of swallowed air. True vomiting is not possible (except in the case of an isolated TE fistula) because the esophagus and stomach are not connected. This triad of "excessive" secretions, reflux, and respiratory distress, particularly in association with a maternal history of polyhydramnios, indicates esophageal atresia until proved otherwise (Chang, 1979; Gryboski & Walker, 1983; Holder & Ashcraft, 1981). However, the clinical presentation may vary slightly, depending on the specific type of anomaly found (Fig. 12–1). Whereas there are five major pathologic types of esophageal atresia with or without TE fistula, approximately 100 subtypes have been described (Kluth, 1976; Lambrecht & Kluth, 1994).

DIFFERENTIAL DIAGNOSIS

Diagnosis of esophageal atresia is confirmed by attempting to pass a radiopaque catheter from the nares through the esophagus into the stomach. If the esophagus is atretic, the catheter cannot be advanced farther than a depth of 9 to 12 cm before meeting resistance, and any aspirated contents is alkaline rather than acidic. A chest radiograph will show the tube ending or coiling in the upper esophageal pouch. Air in the bowel indicates the

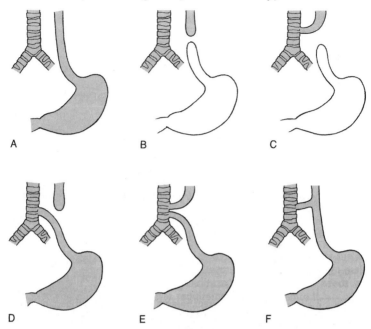

A, Normal. B   C

D   E   F

FIGURE 12–1. Esophageal atresia and transesophageal (TE) fistula. Shading represents areas of lucency typically found on radiographs. Percentages reflect relative occurrence. *A*, Normal. *B*, Isolated esophageal atresia (8 percent), characterized by excessive salivation. *C*, Esophageal atresia with proximal TE fistula (1 percent), characterized by respiratory distress, especially with feeding. *D*, Esophageal atresia with distal TE fistula (86 percent), characterized by excessive salivation, respiratory distress, and reflux. *E*, Esophageal atresia with both proximal and distal TE fistulas (1 percent), characterized by respiratory distress, especially with feeding, and reflux. *F*, Isolated (H-type) TE fistula (4 percent), characterized by respiratory distress, especially with feeding, and reflux. (Data from Cassani, V. L. [1984]. Tracheoesophageal anomalies. *Neonatal Network,* 3[2], 20–27; Desjardins, J. G.. [1987]. Esophageal atresia. In L. Stern & P. Vert [Eds.], *Neonatal medicine* [pp. 1036–1042]. New York: Masson Publishing; and Sunshine, P., Sinatra, F. R., Mitchell, C. H., & Santulli, T. V. [1983]. The gastrointestinal system. In A. A. Fanaroff & R. J. Martin [Eds.], *Behrman's neonatal-perinatal medicine: Diseases of the fetus and infant* [3rd ed., pp. 477–535]. St. Louis: C. V. Mosby.)

presence of a distal TE fistula. If the abdomen is airless, no such fistula is present. Contrast studies are generally contraindicated, owing to the danger of aspiration, but may become necessary in the diagnosis of an isolated or H-type TE fistula. In these cases that are more difficult to diagnose, bronchoscopy or endoscopy may be required to allow direct visualization of the fistulous site (Chan & Saing, 1995; Chang, 1979; Holder & Ashcraft, 1981; Martin & Alexander, 1985; Ryckman, Flake, & Balistreri, 1992).

PROGNOSIS

With early diagnosis and efforts to prevent aspiration pneumonia, most full-term infants do well, with a survival rate of 97 percent. However, mortality dramatically increases in the presence of prematurity or associated major anomalies, particularly cardiac disease. When birth weight is less than 1500 g or major cardiac disease is present, survival is approximately 60 percent. When both conditions are present, survival falls to 22 percent (Holder & Ashcraft, 1981; Spitz, Kiely, Morecroft, & Drake, 1994).

COLLABORATIVE MANAGEMENT

Surgical Correction

- Esophageal anastomosis (esophagoesophagostomy) is performed with obliteration of any fistula present.
- If a great distance separates the two ends of the esophagus, the repair is more difficult and must often be staged. The ends may be brought into closer approximation either preoperatively by stretching the upper esophageal pouch daily with a bougie to produce progressive elongation or intraoperatively by performing multiple circular myotomies so that the upper esophageal segment can be lengthened in a telescoping fashion; or a combination of the two methods may be used.
- If these procedures are not effective, or if the gap is particularly large, a segment of the small or large intestine or an inverted tube of gastric tissue may be used for esophageal replacement (Cusick, Batchelor, & Spicer, 1993). Such a dramatic procedure is generally delayed until 1 year of age.
- If the gap makes primary repair impossible, the upper esophageal pouch can be brought to the surface as a cervical esophagostomy ("spit fistula") to allow for the drainage of saliva, with gastrostomy performed for feeding. In these protracted cases, sham feeding may be attempted in which orally fed milk is collected with saliva in the ostomy bag attached to the esophagostomy stoma and refed through the gastrostomy tube into the stomach (Chang, 1979; Holder & Ashcraft, 1981; Kimura & Soper, 1994; Martin & Alexander, 1985).
- Generally, repair is performed through an incision at the base of the neck, but if the lesion is located exceptionally low within the chest, a thoracic approach may be used, necessitating chest tube placement. A gastrostomy may also be performed to allow for feeding during healing (Ashcraft & Holder, 1981; Holder & Ashcraft, 1981; Kemmotsu, Joe, Nakamura, & Yamashita, 1995).

Preoperative Care

- Overflow of secretions must be prevented. A sump catheter (Replogle tube) is placed into the upper esophageal pouch and connected to low intermittent suction. The tube lumen becomes easily occluded by tenacious secretions and should therefore be changed daily. Catheter irrigation is potentially dangerous and is not recommended.
- Humidified air helps to liquefy tenacious secretions for easier removal.

- Elevating the head 30 to 40 degrees helps avoid reflux of gastric secretions into the trachea via a distal fistula.
- Comfort measures to prevent crying reduce the amount of air swallowed through the fistula, thus limiting gastric distention and further reducing risk of reflux.
- If no TE fistula is present, a flat or head-down position may be preferable to avoid gravity drainage of saliva from an overflowing esophageal pouch.
- Fluids and electrolytes are given intravenously.
- Supplemental oxygen and intubation may be needed if respiratory distress occurs. However, use of positive-pressure ventilation increases the propensity for gastric distention and may even necessitate preoperative gastrostomy for decompression (Cassani, 1984; Chang, 1979; Dienno, 1987; Martin & Alexander, 1985).

Postoperative Care

- Vital signs are monitored.
- The anastomotic site is assessed frequently for leaking. If a chest tube has been placed, such leakage presents as persistent or increased drainage.
- The endotracheal tube is generally left in place for at least 24 hours to allow full recovery from anesthesia and relaxants. When suctioning the airway, the catheter should be well marked and inserted to a predetermined depth above the site to avoid disruption or trauma.
- The quantity and appearance of secretions are assessed and respiratory difficulties reported.
- Gastrostomy feedings may be started within 48 hours, with oral feedings generally withheld for 5 to 10 days to ensure healing.
- Gastroesophageal reflux is a common complication because of the upward pull on the lower esophageal pouch and stomach and generally poor peristalsis, occurring in 50 to 75 percent of infants, and should be managed as described in the next section.
- Long-term postoperative complications include stricture of the anastomosis (40 to 50 percent) and recurrence of the fistula (5 to 12 percent).
- Support and communication are the cornerstones of parental care throughout hospitalization.

Gastroesophageal Reflux

PATHOPHYSIOLOGY

Gastroesophageal reflux (GER) is the spontaneous passage of acidic gastric contents from the stomach into the esophagus. Berenberg and Neuhauser (1950) described the classic and radiologic findings of GER in infants. They suggested the term *chalasia,* referring to an abnormal relaxation of the gastroesophageal junction.

The distal esophagus possesses a physiologic sphincter, approximately 0.5 cm long in the infant, called the esophageal vestibule, which has a higher pressure than that of the stomach below or the esophagus above and helps prevent retrograde flow of gastric contents into the esophagus.

RISK FACTORS

- Prematurity
- Infants with high bowel obstructions have delayed maturation of the valve mechanism and are at risk for chalasia due to structural weakness.
- Twelve percent of infants with congenital diaphragmatic hernia experience reflux after repair, most likely due to deviation of the esophagus to the affected side, malposition of the stomach, increased intra-abdominal pressure, and/or gastric dysmotility (Nagaya, Akatsuka, & Kato, 1994; Sigalet et al., 1994).

A high percentage of infants with neurologic damage exhibit GER, possibly due to reduced swallowing frequency and weaker esophageal sphincter control (Hlusko & McMurray, 1991).

CLINICAL MANIFESTATIONS

The primary symptoms of gastroesophageal reflux in infants are vomiting, growth retardation, aspiration pneumonia, apneic spells, and esophagitis (Guzzetta et al., 1994). Persistent vomiting due to GER often leads to failure to thrive. Such infants tend to be pale, thin, hypoactive, listless, and underweight and are often misdiagnosed as having a nutritional deficiency. Infants with growth retardation due to reflux usually improve promptly and dramatically after corrective surgery.

The most commonly recognized pulmonary symptom associated with GER is recurrent aspiration pneumonia. It is characterized by fever, cough, poor appetite, and typical findings on radiography.

Apneic spells, most commonly seen in the early weeks of life, may be caused by reflux. GER is capable of causing laryngospasm, with cardiac slowing or arrest, apnea, and death if this sequence is not halted (Avery & Taeusch, 1984). Well-documented recurrent apneic spells have been completely eliminated in many cases after antireflux surgery. Asthma or asthma-like symptoms related to reflux are rare during the first year of life but have been seen occasionally in infants.

Esophagitis is generally not seen in the early months of life. Infants suffering from esophagitis caused by GER are usually fussy, irritable, and colicky. Frank bleeding is rare but may be present with anemia and guaiac-positive stools.

DIFFERENTIAL DIAGNOSIS

Differential diagnosis includes other causes of vomiting (distal outlet obstruction as in pyloric stenosis or neurologic or metabolic disease). Newborns with cystic fibrosis or bronchitis may present with a similar clinical picture.

PROGNOSIS AND TREATMENT

- First-line treatment is medical management for 3 months; 75 percent recover, 10 to 15 percent require prolonged medical management, and 10 to 15 percent require surgery.

- If medical management of reflux symptoms is successful, it is continued for 15 months.

Medical Management

- Positioning: A 30-degree prone position after feedings is better than upright and supine, both awake and asleep (Lynn, 1986; Meyers & Herbst, 1982; Orenstein, 1992). Contrary to popular thinking, infants placed in infant seats had 50 percent more reflux episodes that lasted twice as long than when they were in the prone position.
- Thickening feedings: with rice cereal (at a ratio of 15 ml cereal to 30 ml formula), which is then fed by nipple with an enlarged hole, has been found to decrease vomiting, decrease crying time, and increase sleep in the postprandial period (Orenstein, 1992; Orenstein, Magill, & Brooks, 1987).
- Respirations should be monitored.
- Apneic episodes and recurrent aspiration pneumonia have been associated with GER.
- Xanthines are used to improve respiratory function and reduce apnea, but they also increase gastric acid secretion and decrease lower esophageal sphincter pressure, which may further increase GER (Young & Mangum, 1997).
- Medications include the following:
  - Antacids and H2-receptor antagonists (cimetidine, famotidine, or ranitidine) are used to treat esophagitis.
  - Bethanechol increases lower esophageal sphincter pressure, decreases vomiting, and increases weight gain in reflux patients with failure to thrive. Because of its cholinergic effect, it must be used with care in infants with chronic lung disease (Herbst, 1983; Orenstein, 1992).
  - Metoclopramide increases tone and amplitude of gastric contractions, relaxes the pyloric sphincter and duodenal bulb, increases peristalsis of the duodenum and jejunum, and increases the resisting tone of the lower esophageal sphincter. Once medication is begun, the infant must still be monitored carefully for apnea and regurgitation.
  - Cisapride acts by selectively stimulating release of acetylcholine from neurons within the myenteric plexus.

Surgical Intervention

- Nissen fundoplication: the proximal stomach is wrapped around the distal esophagus, creating a junction that is very effective in preventing reflux. Most infants have a gastrostomy placed temporarily postoperatively to vent swallowed air and decrease bloating. The tube is usually removed after 3 to 6 weeks. Associated problems usually improve promptly with corrective surgery.
- Surgical intervention is 95 percent effective when assessed at checkups after 10 years or more (Bettex & Oesch, 1983; Herbst, 1983). Approximately one third of surgically treated patients experience mild gas, bloating, slow eating, inability to burp, or vomiting.

Pyloric Stenosis

PATHOPHYSIOLOGY

Although many cases are believed to be acquired postnatally, this disorder is properly referred to as congenital hypertrophic pyloric stenosis. The pathologic picture consists of marked hypertrophy of the pylorus with spasm of the muscular coat, creating a tumor-like nodule constricting the lumen of the pyloric canal. The etiology is poorly understood but probably has a genetic basis with a polygenic mode of inheritance, modified by gender (Jedd et al., 1988).

INCIDENCE

The prevalence rate typically ranges from 1.5 to 4 per 1000, with higher rates in whites than blacks (Mitchell & Risch, 1993). More males, especially first-born males, have the disease than do females, and approximately 5 percent of affected infants are born to women who have the disease (Merenstein & Gardner, 1989).

RISK FACTORS

Associated factors include maternal stress and anxiety, feeding practices, and antenatal exposure to doxylamine succinate–pyridoxine hydrochloride. Seasonal factors such as infection have also been reported (Jedd et al., 1988).

CLINICAL MANIFESTATIONS

- The infant is healthy for the first 2 weeks of life and then begins to vomit (nonbilious), which worsens to frequent projectile vomiting.
- Anxiety and irritability are present.
- Excessive hunger is noted, with decreased frequency of stools and weight loss.
- Vomiting may cause dehydration, metabolic alkalosis, hypochloremia, and hypokalemia.
- Level of indirect bilirubin is significantly elevated in 5 percent.

DIFFERENTIAL DIAGNOSIS

Most cases (89 percent) of pyloric stenosis may be clinically diagnosed by palpation of a small, olive-sized mass below the liver. However, if the mass cannot be felt, a barium swallow or ultrasound examination is indicated (Breaux, Georgeson, Royal, & Curnow, 1988). Differential diagnosis for nonbilious vomiting includes sepsis, withdrawal syndromes, gastroesophageal reflux, and metabolic diseases such as organic acidemias, hyperammonemia, galactosemias, and adrenogenital syndrome.

PROGNOSIS

Once diagnosed and surgically treated, the prognosis is excellent, with complete relief of symptoms. The mortality rate is less than 1 percent, provided the infant has not become too dehydrated and malnourished (Mitchell & Risch, 1993).

COLLABORATIVE MANAGEMENT

- There is no effective medical treatment.
- Surgical correction is the treatment of choice. Pyloromyotomy involves making a simple incision in the hypertrophied longitudinal and circular muscles of the pylorus, thus releasing the obstruction (Leape, 1987).
- Fluid and electrolyte management is paramount.
- Nasogastric tube connected to low continuous suction is maintained to prevent distention and vomiting and to decrease the risk of aspiration.
- Vital signs are monitored every 2 to 4 hours.
- Thermoregulation is maintained to prevent exacerbation of symptoms.

Postoperative Care

- Intravenous hydration and electrolyte balance must be maintained.
- Nasogastric suction is continued for 4 to 24 hours. The tube may be discontinued when the infant is fully awake and bowel sounds are present.
- The suture line is assessed for signs of infection or skin breakdown.
- Feedings are done at 6 to 24 hours postoperatively, beginning with clear liquids and progressing slowly with formula administration. Full feedings should be implemented in 3 to 5 days (Kenner, Harjo, & Brueggemeyer, 1988).

MANAGEMENT OF PROBLEMS WITH DIGESTION

Biliary Atresia

PATHOPHYSIOLOGY AND INCIDENCE

Biliary atresia is the complete obstruction of bile flow due to fibrosis of the extrahepatic ducts. It is the most common form of ductal cholestasis, occurring in approximately 1 of every 10,000 births; there is a female predominance. The etiology remains unclear. Pathologically, the obstruction of the common bile duct prevents bile from entering the duodenum. Consequently, digestion and absorption of fat are impaired, leading to deficiencies in fat-soluble vitamins and vitamin K, which impact on bleeding tendencies. Because of the obstruction, bile accumulates in the ducts and gallbladder and causes distention of these structures. The atresia appears to progress to the intrahepatic ducts, leading to biliary cirrhosis and ultimately death if the bile flow is not established.

RISK FACTORS

Associated congenital defects, found in 15 percent of reported cases, include congenital heart disease, polysplenic syndrome, small bowel atresia, bronchobiliary atresia, and trisomies 17 and 18. Teratogenic factors include ionizing radiation, drugs, ischemic episode, and viruses such as reovirus type

3, cytomegalovirus, rubella virus, and hepatitis viruses types A and B (Oell-rich & Cusumano, 1987).

CLINICAL MANIFESTATIONS

- The infant is normal at birth and passes stools with appropriate pigmentation.
- Clinical signs are subtle:
  - Jaundice persists after the first week of life.
  - Direct bilirubin level slowly increases.
  - Skin appears greenish bronze.
- Gradually stools become clay colored to pale to yellowish tan.
- Urine becomes dark as the result of bile excretion.
- Over a 2- to 3-month period, the liver becomes cirrhotic.
- Portal hypertension is noted.
- Esophageal, umbilical, and rectal veins are enlarged.
- Splenomegaly is evident.
- Hemorrhoids are noted.
- Abdominal veins are enlarged.
- Ascites is present.
- Blood is present in the stools.
- Additional complications include the following:
  - Decreased clotting ability
  - Anemia
  - Ineffective metabolism of nutrients
- End-stage liver disease may lead to rupture of veins in the esophagus and stomach, hepatic coma, and eventual death from liver failure (Oellrich & Cusumano, 1987).

DIFFERENTIAL DIAGNOSIS

Differential diagnosis includes neonatal hepatitis, choledochal cyst, inborn errors of metabolism, trisomies 18 and 21, α_1-antitrypsin deficiency, neonatal hypopituitarism, cystic fibrosis, TORCH infectious agents (*Toxoplasma,* rubella, cytomegalovirus, and herpesvirus, with the "O" standing for other agents such as syphilis), or bacterial sepsis, drug-induced cholestasis, and cholestasis associated with parenteral nutrition (Sinatra & Rosenthal, 1987).

PROGNOSIS

Survival in untreated cases of biliary atresia is less than 2 years. Success rates for surgical intervention range from 45 to 85 percent with satisfactory bile drainage. The risk of cholangitis is very high.

Many children grow naturally and lead normal lives. Prognosis is best when the original surgery takes place before the child is 2 months old, when there is minimal hepatocellular damage, there are ducts in the porta hepatis, and postoperative complications are minimal (Zink, 1985).

When portoenterostomy is unsuccessful, liver transplantation is an acceptable alternative therapy, with 1-year survival rates ranging from 57 to 70 percent and 4-year survival rates from 28 to 69 percent (Oellrich & Cusumano, 1987; Zink, 1985).

COLLABORATIVE MANAGEMENT

Medical, surgical, and nursing staff must strive diligently in the diagnostic work-up and ultimate treatment.

Surgical Intervention
- Hepatic portoenterostomy, called the Kasai procedure, consists of dissection and resection of the extrahepatic bile duct. The porta hepatis, where the ducts normally occur, is cut, and a loop of bowel is brought up to permit bile drainage from the liver surface to the gastrointestinal tract.
- If the Kasai procedure is unsuccessful, the only alternative for treatment is transplantation.

Diagnostic Work-Up
- Careful monitoring is done of vital signs and blood pressure.
- Multiple blood samples are collected for study of the following: levels of bilirubin, serum aspartate aminotransferase, serum alanine aminotransferase, alkaline phosphatase, albumin, protein, and cholesterol; prothrombin time; complete blood cell count; reticulocyte count; Coombs' test; measurement of platelets; red blood cell morphology; thyroxine; thyroid-stimulating hormone; glucose; cultures; and TORCH titers.
- Urine samples are collected for urinalysis, culture, and metabolic screening.
- Radiography, ultrasonography, and liver biopsy may be performed.

Nutritional Needs
- It is difficult to meet nutritional requirements.
- Metabolism is accelerated so the infant needs one and one-half to two times the normal caloric requirements.
- Ascites and pressure on the stomach make it difficult for the infant to eat.
- Formulas need to contain medium-chain triglycerides for easier absorption.
- Supplementation with fat-soluble vitamins is required because of impaired absorption.
- Parenteral nutrition is given to provide adequate calories.
- Phenobarbital may be an ongoing therapy to stimulate bile flow (Haber & Lake, 1990).

Duodenal Atresia

PATHOPHYSIOLOGY

Duodenal atresia occurs as the result of incomplete recanalization of the lumen. The mechanism by which recanalization is prevented is not known but most likely occurs when the proliferative villi abnormally adhere to one another. The result is the formation of a transverse diaphragm of tissue that completely obstructs the lumen (Davis, 1985; Gryboski & Walker, 1983; Moore & Persaud, 1993; Sadler, 1985).

INCIDENCE

Overall occurrence is approximately 1 in every 6000 to 10,000 live births (Avery & Tausch, 1984; Chang, 1980b; Davis, 1985).

RISK FACTORS

- Polyhydramnios is present.
- Associated anomalies are present in 60 to 70 percent and include trisomy 21, malrotation, tracheoesophageal anomalies, imperforate anus, congenital heart disease, VATER or VACTERL association, and renal anomalies. An annular pancreas, due to the failure of the two pancreatic buds to fuse normally, allowing the deformed pancreas to encircle the duodenum, is found in approximately 20 percent of patients.
- Nearly half of all infants are premature or of low birth weight.
- Forty percent develop hyperbilirubinemia.

CLINICAL MANIFESTATIONS

- Polyhydramnios has been previously noted.
- In the absence of polyhydramnios, a large amount of gastric aspirate (more than 10 to 15 ml) may be obtained on routine delivery room screening. Normal amounts of gastric aspirate equal 4 to 7 ml. (Gryboski & Walker, 1983; James, 1987; Pickering & Adcock, 1980).
- Although atresia may be located at any point along the duodenum, most obstructions (80 to 90 percent) are situated below the ampulla of Vater. Bilious vomiting is a common presenting sign.
- There is a 70 percent failure to pass meconium.
- Both the onset of vomiting and the ability to pass stool are related to the site of obstruction. Proximal duodenal obstructions tend to present as vomiting within a few hours of birth, although stool may be normally passed. Distal obstructions tend to present as later-onset vomiting and failure to pass stool. Abdominal distention is generally not noted; but when present, it is confined to the upper abdomen, giving the lower abdomen an almost scaphoid appearance (Avery & Tausch, 1984; Davis, 1985; Leape, 1987; Ricketts, 1984; Touloukian, 1978).

DIFFERENTIAL DIAGNOSIS

Radiographic examination provides confirmation of duodenal atresia with the classic finding of a "double bubble." These bubbles reflect the localization of swallowed air in the stomach and in the distended portion of the duodenum lying above the obstruction; the remainder of the bowel is totally airless. If gas is present elsewhere, other anomalies causing partial obstruction must be presumed. An upper gastrointestinal series may be helpful in identifying such incomplete obstructions as duodenal stenosis, duodenal web, or annular pancreas or in ruling out associated malrotation (Davis, 1985; Gryboski & Walker, 1983; Ricketts, 1984).

PROGNOSIS

A 65 to 84 percent survival rate is reported, with deaths attributed to associated cardiac or renal anomalies or to infectious or respiratory complications (Chang, 1980b; Davis, 1985; Ghory & Sheldon, 1985).

COLLABORATIVE MANAGEMENT

Surgical Treatment

- The atretic site is excised (unless the area so closely approximates the pancreatic and bile ducts that injury to these structures is risked) and side-to-side anastomosis done of the free ends.
- Level of the obstruction determines whether a duodenoduodenostomy or a duodenojejunostomy is carried out.
- Gastrostomy is performed for decompression, so as to avoid trauma to the anastomotic site (Chang, 1980b; Davis, 1985; Ghory & Sheldon, 1985; Gryboski & Walker, 1983; Touloukian, 1978).

Preoperative Care

- Further decompression with intermittent gastric suction by use of a sump tube reduces the risk of aspiration or perforation due to overdistention.
- Vital signs are taken frequently, at least every 2 to 4 hours.
- Hydration status is monitored by recording fluid intake and output, urine specific gravity, and serum electrolyte levels.
- Intravenous administration of fluids, electrolytes, and crystalloid is provided as needed.
- Antibiotics may be given for preoperative prophylaxis or when perforation or sepsis is suggested (Chang, 1980b; Davis, 1985; Touloukian, 1978).

Postoperative Care

- Decompression is continued.
- Nutritional support is with total parenteral nutrition.
- Oral feedings are generally begun at 10 to 14 days with an oral electrolyte solution such as Lytren, advancing to such low osmolality formulas as Nutramigen or Pregestimil before instituting regular formula (Chang, 1980b; Davis, 1985; Touloukian, 1978).

Jejunoileal Atresia

PATHOPHYSIOLOGY

Atresias of the jejunum and ileum are thought to be the result of a mesenteric vascular compromise, with necrosis and eventual resorption of the involved area. The presence of bile, meconium, epithelial cells, and lanugo distal to the atresia indicates that this ischemic injury occurs relatively late in utero, possibly as late as 3 to 6 months' gestation (Bishop, 1976; Chang, 1980b; Flake & Ryckman, 1992; Touloukian, 1978).

INCIDENCE

The occurrence rate is 1 in 20,000 live births, with an apparently equal distribution of atresias between the jejunum and the ileum (Gryboski & Walker, 1983).

RISK FACTORS

Maternal polyhydramnios does not generally present as a risk factor as it does in the higher atresias of the esophagus and duodenum (Chang, 1980b). Associated anomalies are rare; and when they do occur, they are primarily restricted to the gastrointestinal tract, with malrotation and meconium ileus being most common (Sunshine et al., 1983; Touloukian, 1978). Between 25 and 30 percent experience hyperbilirubinemia, and 25 to 38 percent are born prematurely. Of the four types of jejunoileal atresia that have been identified (Fig. 12–2), only the "apple peel" or "Christmas tree" type is typically familial, indicating that this one form alone may involve some autosomal recessive or multifactorial type of inheritance (Gryboski & Walker, 1983). Although it is the rarest form of jejunoileal atresia, it carries the highest mortality rate (54 percent) and higher rates of prematurity and malrotation in comparison with the more conventional types (Seashore, Collins, Markowitz, & Seashore, 1987).

CLINICAL MANIFESTATIONS

Signs are present at 1 or 2 days of age and are virtually the same for all four types of jejunoileal atresia. Presentation includes the following:

- Bilious vomiting
- Failure to pass stool
- Generalized abdominal distention

DIFFERENTIAL DIAGNOSIS

- Abdominal radiographs show multiple bubbles, reflecting dilatation and collection of swallowed air proximal to the obstruction.
- Intraperitoneal calcifications are present in 10 percent of patients, which indicates antenatal intestinal perforation with resultant meconium peritonitis. The peritonitis in this case is due to chemical irritation (there is no infection because the bowel and meconium are sterile before birth), causing fibrosis, granuloma formation, and ultimately calcifications.
- Perforated site usually heals spontaneously before delivery, leaving no evidence of what occurred other than the residual calcifications.

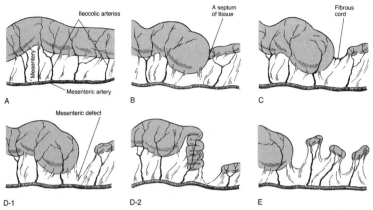

FIGURE 12–2. Jejunoileal obstruction. Percentages reflect relative occurrence. *A,* Normal anatomy. *B,* Type I or diaphragmatic form (20 percent): single atresia in which the integrity of the bowel wall is preserved but its lumen is obstructed by a septum of tissue; the mesentery is intact. *C,* Type II or cord anomaly (30 to 35 percent): single but discontinuous atresia with opposing ends connected by a long, fibrous cord; the mesentery is intact. *D-1,* Type IIIa or mesenteric defect (35 to 45 percent): single but discontinuous atresia with a V-shaped defect in the intervening mesentery. *D-2,* Type IIIb or "apple peel" (< 1 percent): single but discontinuous atresia with a V-shaped defect in the intervening mesentery; the intestine coils around a single ileocolic artery, which is its sole source of circulation. *E,* Type IV or multiple atresias (5 to 10 percent): multiple discontinuous atresias with intervening V-shaped mesenteric defects giving it the appearance of sausage links. (Data from Gryboski, J., & Walker, W. A. [1983]. *Gastrointestinal problems in the infant* [2nd ed.]. Philadelphia: W. B. Saunders; Leape, L. L. [1987]. *Patient care in pediatric surgery.* Boston: Little, Brown; and Touloukian, R. J. [1978]. Intestinal atresia. *Clinics in Perinatology,* 5[1], 3–18.)

- An airless, unused distal portion of the gut is generally contracted and of a much smaller caliber than normal.
- Visualization of this distal "microcolon" by barium or Gastrografin enema may be necessary to rule out malrotation and meconium ileus.

PROGNOSIS

Survival rates have risen to as high as 84 to 96 percent. Deaths are generally the result of prematurity, postoperative short gut or bowel syndrome, or infectious complications (Avery & Taeusch, 1984; Ghory & Sheldon, 1985; Touloukian, 1978).

COLLABORATIVE MANAGEMENT

Surgical Management

- The dilated proximal gut and atretic, bulbous ending are resected and a search made for multiple distal atresias.

- Three types of closures are as follows:
  - Primary closure by end-to-end or side-to-end anastomosis generally follows.
  - Preliminary tapering of the distended distal segment may be required.
  - End-to-oblique closure may be performed.
- When there is considerable discrepancy (more than 2:1) between the dilated proximal portion and the distal microcolon, an ostomy (either double-barrel or single) will be created (Bishop, 1976; Chang, 1980b; Ghory & Sheldon, 1985).

Preoperative Care

- Bowel decompression is done.
- Intravenous hydration is provided with the correction of any electrolyte imbalance that may occur as the result of vomiting or third spacing.
- Antibiotics may be given prophylactically but certainly should be used in the case of peritonitis (Touloukian, 1978).

Postoperative Care

- Parenteral nutrition is used until bowel peristalsis and enzymatic integrity resume.
- Initial feedings are of Lytren, progressing serially to elemental formulas such as Nutramigen or Pregestimil until standard formula can be tolerated.
- Assessment is done for evidence of short-bowel syndrome, commonly seen with atresias that are multiple or of the "apple peel" variety, necessitating excision of an extensive length of bowel (Chang, 1980b; Leape, 1987; Touloukian, 1978).

Omphalocele

PATHOPHYSIOLOGY

Omphalocele results from the failure of the intestines to return from the umbilical cord into the abdominal cavity. Because some defects can be sufficiently large to also contain the liver and other organs that do not normally participate in the migratory process, it has been further proposed that their passage can only be accommodated when there is incomplete folding of the embryonic disk so that the future abdominal wall cannot completely close, resulting in an unusually large umbilical ring.

INCIDENCE

Omphalocele occurs in roughly 1 of every 5000 to 6000 live births, with a male predominance.

RISK FACTORS

Multiple and often life-threatening syndromes and anomalies occur with an unusually high frequency (50 to 77 percent) and include trisomy 13, trisomy

18, Beckwith-Wiedemann syndrome, pentalogy syndrome, congenital heart defects, diaphragmatic and upper midline defects, malrotation, intestinal atresia, and genitourinary anomalies. Additionally, 30 to 33 percent of affected infants are premature, and approximately 19 percent are small for gestational age.

CLINICAL MANIFESTATIONS

Omphalocele is generally an immediately apparent anomaly, ranging between 2 and 15 cm. However, the very small defects involving perhaps a single loop of intestine may be easily overlooked unless the physical examination is carried out in an unhurried fashion and the umbilical ring is clearly absent on palpation. The larger defects generally contain the intestine and possibly the liver, spleen, stomach, bladder, ovaries and tubes, or testes. These two extremes most likely reflect the difference in the time at which normal embryogenesis is interrupted. If the interruption is early, around the 3- to 4-week window, when infolding is in its last stages, the defect is large. If the interruption occurs later, at 9 to 10 weeks, when migration is generally completed, the defect is smaller. However, in both cases, the intestine, and possibly other abdominal organs, herniate into the umbilical cord. The viscera are covered by a thin, transparent membrane composed of peritoneum and amnion, and the visible bowel has a normal appearance. The abdominal cavity is often relatively small and underdeveloped, having never held the growing intestine (Avery & Taeusch, 1984; Frentner, 1987; Gryboski & Walker, 1983; Kim, 1976; Richey, 1990).

DIFFERENTIAL DIAGNOSIS

Although omphaloceles are generally covered by a membrane, intrauterine rupture of that membrane occurs in 11 to 23 percent of patients (Seashore, 1978; Yazbeck & Bensoussan, 1987). As a consequence of prolonged exposure to the amniotic fluid, the bowel becomes matted and edematous and difficult to differentiate from gastroschisis. Closer examination may reveal the sac remnants, but if none are noted, one need only look to the base of the cord. In gastroschisis, the umbilical cord is intact, inserted normally at the abdominal wall and separated from the defect by a small amount of skin (Frentner, 1987).

PROGNOSIS

Overall mortality rate is 30 percent and is primarily dependent on the size of the defect, associated chromosomal and other anomalies, and coincidental prematurity or low birth weight (Frentner, 1987; Gryboski & Walker, 1983; Richey, 1990). Malrotation with the resultant danger of volvulus, ischemia, and necrosis is common. Antenatal membrane rupture may also add the dimension of potential sepsis.

COLLABORATIVE MANAGEMENT

Medical Treatment

If surgery is contraindicated because of coexisting chromosomal or other syndromes, the defect may be treated medically by repeatedly painting the sac with silver nitrate solution, Mercurochrome, or alcohol. These topical agents promote eschar formation and epithelization with complete coverage by skin within 6 to 8 weeks. Should the patient survive, a later repair of the muscle wall will become necessary. Biologic dressings have also been used to provide temporary protection (Avery & Taeusch, 1984; Frentner, 1987; Kim, 1976; Leape, 1987; Seashore, 1978).

Preoperative Care

Protection of the eviscerated organs includes the following:

- Loose application of sterile, warmed, saline-soaked gauze in a turban style around the defect, wrapping the ends around the body and covering with a dry gauze or sterile bowel bags
- Avoidance of trauma and infection and limitation of the loss of fluids and body heat

If the defect is small, the infant may then be positioned on the back; but if the defect is large, it may be best to place the infant on the side. In the side-lying position a small blanket or diaper may be slipped between the covered viscera and the bed surface so that no traction is placed on the bowel that might cause physical injury to the gut or impede circulation.

Standard interventions include those previously discussed:

- Decompression of the gut
- Thermoregulation
- Antibiotics
- Comfort measures to reduce or prevent crying with concomitant air swallowing
- Intravenous fluids
- Assessment of hydration status
- Intake and output determination every 2 to 4 hours
- Close monitoring of vital signs for hypovolemia, tachycardia, thready pulses, hypotension, poor perfusion, and decreased output of urine with increased specific gravity

Umbilical catheterization for venous access is contraindicated because of the nature and site of the defect. Poor venous return from the lower extremities indicates the potential for vena caval compression.

Surgical Treatment

The definitive surgical treatment is return of the viscera into the abdominal cavity and closure of the defect. Primary closure is preferred.

- Large defects (greater than 5 cm) may require a staged repair.
  - Silastic pouch or chimney (silo) is used to suspend the viscera above the patient.
    - Daily reduction maneuvers are used to return the suspended organs

into the relatively small abdominal cavity. Complete return of organs into the abdominal cavity is generally achieved over 7 to 10 days, and the infant is returned to surgery for closure of the abdomen.

- Gradual reduction minimizes compression of the inferior vena cava, with reduced filling of the heart and decreased cardiac output and impedance of the diaphragmatic excursions, resulting in respiratory compromise.
- A gastrostomy provides decompression.
- An appendectomy avoids atypically presenting appendicitis later in life (Frentner, 1987; Kim, 1976; Leape, 1987; Meller, Reyes, & Loeff, 1989; Yazbeck & Bensoussan, 1987).

Postoperative Management

- Aggressive respiratory management with increased pressures may be required to achieve adequate ventilation if diaphragmatic movements are hampered.
- Third-spacing, or capillary leak syndrome, may occur as a result of the bowel being exposed to the air and manipulated surgically.
- Assessment for signs of hypovolemia should be documented.
- Serum electrolytes, albumin, and total serum protein values should also be followed, with fluid and other replacements as necessary.
- Ileus and cholestasis are common after repair, so enteral feedings may be considerably delayed while the infant is supported on parenteral nutrition.
- Decompression by gastric tube or gastrostomy is generally required for a considerable period of time until peristaltic activity returns.
- When feedings are begun, an elemental formula is used initially.
- Inspection of the lower extremities and palpation of pedal pulses are helpful in assessing for impaired circulation. Elevating the extremities may promote venous return to the heart.
- Silo provides an open port for bacterial invasion. Povidone-iodine or Silvadene ointment may be applied with dressing changes, and most certainly antibiotic therapy is continued postoperatively (Frentner, 1987).
- Pain management appropriate for the infant should be instituted.
- Thermoregulation is essential.
- Early psychosocial support should be given to the parents.
- Genetic counseling may also be required.

Gastroschisis

PATHOPHYSIOLOGY

Gastroschisis is a full-thickness defect in the abdominal wall through which the uncovered intestines protrude. The defect is generally thought to arise as the result of incomplete lateral infolding of the embryonic disk. As a result of this primary failure, the abdominal wall is incompletely formed, allowing herniation of the gut (Frentner, 1987; Meller, Reyes, & Loeff, 1989; Richey, 1990; Seashore, 1978).

INCIDENCE

The overall incidence is approximately 1 per 30,000 to 50,000 live births (Frentner, 1987).

RISK FACTORS

Prematurity (58 percent) and low birth weight (92 percent) are extremely common. Malrotation is found in all affected infants, and a few may exhibit intestinal atresia, but anomalies of systems other than the gastrointestinal tract are infrequent and relatively minor (Seashore, 1978).

CLINICAL MANIFESTATIONS

Gastroschisis is an immediately apparent defect in the abdominal wall through which the intestine and possibly portions of the colon protrude. The liver and other solid organs generally remain in the abdominal cavity, although evisceration is possible. The defect is usually small (2 to 5 cm) and located to the right of the umbilicus, from which it is separated by a narrow margin of skin. The bowel is uncovered and, as a consequence of chemical peritonitis caused by long exposure to the amniotic fluid, appears as an edematous and matted mass with no identifiable loops. The abdominal cavity is small and underdeveloped (Frentner, 1987; Meller, Reyes, & Loeff, 1989; Richey, 1990).

DIFFERENTIAL DIAGNOSIS

Although it is often confused with a ruptured omphalocele, with gastroschisis the umbilical cord is normally inserted. The defect is *next to*, rather than in, the umbilical cord and there is no protective sac or remnants thereof (Leape, 1987; Richey, 1990).

PROGNOSIS

A 13 to 28 percent mortality rate is reported for gastroschisis, with all deaths directly related to the defect. Early deaths are largely attributable to a combination of shock, sepsis (associated with perforation or contamination of the exposed bowel), and hypothermia. Profound hypothermia (temperature lower than 35°C [95.0°F]) is reported to occur in 67 percent of affected infants. Late deaths come as a result of sepsis, respiratory failure, and the inability of the bowel to sustain nutrition (Seashore, 1978; Yazbeck & Bensoussan, 1987).

COLLABORATIVE MANAGEMENT

Although a primary closure may be possible in gastroschisis, the majority are closed by staged repair using the Silastic pouch as described in the case of omphalocele. Although gastroschisis is a smaller defect than omphalocele, the distortion of the viscera with typical thickening and edema of the bowel make primary closure more difficult. Often the defect must be surgically enlarged to allow thorough inspection of the entire length of the gastrointestinal tract and so as not to restrict passage of the eviscerated intestine back into the abdominal cavity. All have some degree of malrotation, predisposing them to both intestinal atresias and infarction. Bowel resection and anastomosis are frequently necessary; however, primary anastomosis is contraindicated in the face of peritonitis or inflammation. In such situations, an enterostomy is performed away from the defect, with anastomosis delayed until final closure of the abdominal wall. The visceral mass is returned to the abdominal cavity as a whole. Because of the potential for bowel injury and blood loss, no attempt is made to unravel the adherent loops of bowel (Meller, Reyes, & Loeff, 1989; Seashore, 1978).

The care of patients with gastroschisis is much like that for omphalocele, focusing on prevention of infection, maintenance of hydration/fluid resuscitation, and provision of respiratory support, thermoregulation, gastric decompression, and nutrition (Frentner, 1987).

Total parenteral nutrition is generally continued for several weeks until intestinal function returns. Feedings are begun with elemental formula, eventually progressing to standard formula, with diligent assessment for evidence of intestinal obstruction during the process (Frentner, 1987; Leape, 1987).

MANAGEMENT OF PROBLEMS WITH ELIMINATION

Hirschsprung's Disease

PATHOPHYSIOLOGY

Hirschsprung's disease (also known as congenital megacolon or aganglionic megacolon) is an abnormality of the colon marked by the congenital absence of ganglion cells (aganglionosis). Failure of the neural crest cells to migrate in their usual craniocaudal fashion results in aberrant bowel innervation and interrupted neuromuscular conduction of the messages promoting peristalsis of the anal sphincters. This local failure of relaxation results in functional intestinal obstruction. Fecal matter accumulates in the normally innervated proximal bowel, producing dilation (megacolon) and hypertrophy of the muscular wall as normal peristaltic activity works against the obstruction. The distal, aganglionic segment is unused and in relation to the proximal dilation may appear narrowed, but it is in fact of a normal caliber. Between the ganglionic proximal section and the distal aganglionic section lies a "transition zone" of tapered bowel (Boley, Dinari, & Cohen, 1978; Kenner & Brueggemeyer, 1984; Martin & Torres, 1985; Ricketts, 1984; Flake & Ryckman, 1992; Sadler, 1985).

The rectum is always involved, and most cases (85 percent) involve the sigmoid colon as well. Rarely, aganglionosis may also be found in the upper portion of the colon or throughout the entire intestine (Chang, 1980b; Stringer et al., 1994). Atypical forms of Hirschsprung's disease have also been described in which areas of normal innervation are found between aganglionic areas, but the presence of such "skip areas" is extremely rare (Martin & Torres, 1985).

INCIDENCE

Hirschsprung's disease occurs in 1 in 2000 to 5000 live births.

RISK FACTORS

- Trisomy 21 and asymptomatic urologic anomalies are associated infrequently.
- A limited number of infants may also exhibit congenital deafness and ocular neurocristopathies (Meire, Standaert, deLaey, & Zeng, 1987).
- Five percent have associated neurologic abnormalities (e.g., developmental delay, mental retardation, cerebral palsy).
- A positive family history in 17 to 30 percent of cases rises to 50 percent when total colonic aganglionosis is present (Boley, Dinari, & Cohen, 1978; Kenner & Brueggemeyer, 1984; Marty et al., 1995a).
- Higher incidence among males may suggest that a form of X-linked recessive transmission is occurring (Reyna, 1994).

CLINICAL MANIFESTATIONS

The signs and symptoms of Hirschsprung's disease in the newborn are primarily those of intestinal obstruction:

- Bilious vomiting occurs.
- Distention is evident.
- Failure to pass meconium is noted.
- If the disease goes undiagnosed, fecal stagnation may lead to increased intraluminal pressures, reduced colonic blood flow, and bacterial overgrowth with resultant enterocolitis.
- The disease may cause "overflow" diarrhea, with complicating dehydration, hypoproteinemia, electrolyte imbalance, and sometimes perforation and shock.

DIFFERENTIAL DIAGNOSIS

- It may be clinically indistinguishable from jejunoileal atresia, meconium ileus, meconium plug syndrome, and small left colon syndrome (Quinn & Shannon, 1996; Ricketts, 1984; Stringer et al., 1994).
- Plain radiographic examination offers little help.
- Barium contrast studies are indicated to determine the caliber of the distal colon. Occasionally, barium enema will demonstrate the "pigtail" or "funnel" sign characteristic of Hirschsprung's disease. Retention of barium noted by follow-up film 24 hours later is suggestive of Hirschsprung's disease but may also be noted in its absence.
- Anorectal manometry is done to determine the ability of the internal sphincter to relax, but results are generally unreliable in the neonate.
- Final diagnosis can only be made with suction or punch rectal biopsy through the anus and histologic examination of the specimen obtained.
- Should questions regarding diagnosis persist, a full-thickness operative biopsy under general anesthesia may be performed to collect deeper

nerve plexuses, but this is rarely needed (Boley, Dinari, & Cohen, 1978).

PROGNOSIS

The mortality rate is generally less than 5 percent but may be as high as 15 to 20 percent in the neonatal period. Good surgical results can be expected in the vast majority of patients (90 percent), but diarrhea, constipation with distention, and intermittent colitis may occur in 2 to 34 percent of patients as the result of residual aganglionosis, postoperative stricture formation, overactivity of the sphincter, or motility disorders.

COLLABORATIVE MANAGEMENT

- Daily enemas are contraindicated during the neonatal period owing to the risk of fatal enterocolitis with perforation, peritonitis, and septicemia.
- Surgical intervention includes temporary colostomy, placed proximal to the aganglionic segment, to decompress the bowel and divert the fecal contents. Definitive repair is done between 6 and 12 months of age with resection of the affected, aganglionic bowel and anastomosis of the normal bowel to the anus.

Nursing Care

- Monitor vital signs.
- Assess the wound.
- Provide thermoregulation.
- Administer antibiotics for prophylaxis.
- Provide gastric decompression.
- Administer parenteral fluids with appropriate electrolytes for maintenance and the correction of gastric losses.
- Take action to combat the fluid shifts that are common after contrast medium–enhanced studies with hyperosmolar media.
- Closely monitor rectal area after rectal biopsy.
- Control any bleeding with digital pressure (Chang, 1980b).
- Give preoperative colonic lavage or enema to evacuate and prepare the bowel for surgery. Only isotonic solutions such as normal saline should be used to avoid water intoxication and resulting hyponatremia (Kenner & Brueggemeyer, 1984; Leape, 1987).

Postoperative Care

- Assess for respiratory compromise.
- Assess for abdominal distention.
- Assess for hemorrhage.
- Watch for wound dehiscence.
- Monitor for infection.
- Assess stomal perfusion/appearance.
- Provide appropriate skin care.

- Continue intravenous fluids until oral feedings can be started (Sugar, 1981).
- Provide routine rectal irrigations with normal saline to reduce the incidence of postoperative enterocolitis (Marty et al., 1995b).

Small Left Colon Syndrome

PATHOPHYSIOLOGY

Neonatal small left colon syndrome is a condition of functional immaturity of the large bowel in which the left colon is uniformly narrowed from the anus to the splenic flexure. The proximal colon above the flexure is dilated and distended with meconium. A cone-shaped transition zone lies between the dilated and narrowed distal segments (Davis & Campbell, 1975). The etiology is unclear but is generally thought to involve the myenteric plexuses that innervate the gastrointestinal tract in a cephalocaudal direction between 5 and 12 weeks' gestation. Once the plexuses are in position, their maturation and function are largely determined by gestational age. The impression that this condition results from intramural immaturity is supported by histologic findings of increased numbers of small, immature neuronal elements in contrast to the larger, multipolar ganglion cells that normally predominate at term. The neuronal plexuses are present but immature, morphologically resembling the structure expected at approximately 32 weeks' gestation. The syndrome might therefore be best described as a disease of decreased intestinal motility (Davis, Allen, Favara, & Slovis, 1974; Philippart, Reed, & Georgeson, 1975).

INCIDENCE

Small left colon syndrome occurs in 1 in 855 deliveries.

RISK FACTORS

Approximately 40 percent of those with small left colon syndrome are the infants of diabetic mothers (Davis et al., 1974; Philippart, Reed, & Georgeson, 1975).

CLINICAL MANIFESTATIONS

Presenting signs and symptoms are those associated with low intestinal obstruction. These manifestations include the following:

- Bile-stained vomitus
- Abdominal distention
- Failure to spontaneously pass meconium
- Rectal examination followed by the passage of very small amounts of meconium in approximately a third of patients

DIFFERENTIAL DIAGNOSIS

On clinical presentation and with plain radiographic studies, this condition is indistinguishable from Hirschsprung's disease and meconium plug syndrome.

Multiple gas-filled loops of bowel are seen proximally, with decreased air noted distally (Davis & Campbell, 1975).

Barium enema will show the uniformly small left colon with a zone of transition at the splenic flexure. Although a zone of transition may also be noted with Hirschsprung's disease, the margins of the distal colon generally appear smooth with small left colon syndrome rather than jagged or serrated as described in Hirschsprung's disease (Davis et al., 1974; Davis & Campbell, 1975). Perhaps more distinguishing from Hirschsprung's disease is the incidental finding that after contrast medium–enhanced studies the majority (71 percent) of infants with small left colon syndrome will promptly evacuate the barium and begin passing stools spontaneously. As a consequence, the signs and symptoms of low intestinal obstruction disappear. The meconium rarely (5 percent) contains a significant rubbery plug (Davis et al., 1974; Philippart, Reed, & Georgeson, 1975).

Rectal biopsy for the presence of ganglion cells, although they may appear atypically immature in small left colon syndrome, may ultimately be required to differentiate this syndrome from Hirschsprung's disease (Ricketts, 1984). If the possibility of meconium plug persists, a follow-up contrast examination should be performed. Despite the passage of meconium, the transition zone persists in infants suffering from small left colon syndrome (Philippart, Reed, & Georgeson, 1975).

PROGNOSIS

Although the initial presentation may be dramatic, many cases are apparently asymptomatic and go undiagnosed. In either case, the condition spontaneously resolves within the neonatal period with no subsequent stooling problems encountered (Cowett & Schwartz, 1987; Davis et al., 1974; Davis & Campbell, 1975). Late intermittent obstruction with or without cecal perforation is reported rarely (Philippart, Reed, & Georgeson, 1975).

COLLABORATIVE MANAGEMENT

Management is of a conservative nature. The diagnostic barium enema is generally curative. Only in the rare cases of significant intermittent obstruction or cecal perforation is a colostomy required. If the diagnosis of small left colon syndrome is made in the presence of a negative maternal history, the suggestion of maternal diabetes may be made to the obstetric team (Davis et al., 1974; Philippart, Reed, & Georgeson, 1975).

As with all intestinal obstructions, initial management involves decompression, intravenous fluids for hydration, and the treatment of electrolyte imbalance. Symptoms generally resolve after barium enema, and oral feeding may be gradually instituted. The nurse must be diligent, however, for evidence of persistent or recurrent obstruction and report abnormal findings accordingly (Philippart, Reed, & Georgeson, 1975).

Meconium Ileus
PATHOPHYSIOLOGY

Meconium ileus is an obstruction of the distal ileum due to an accumulation of abnormally thick, tarry meconium. The condition is a result of pancreatic insufficiency. Pancreatic hydrolytic enzymes are normally responsible for the metabolism of fat and protein. Consequently, if these enzymes are absent, the meconium has an unusually high protein content and abnormal mucous glycoprotein, making it more viscid than usual. The resultant thick, tenacious material literally becomes impacted with the ileal lumen, producing a functional obstruction (Avery & Taeusch, 1984; Chang, 1980b; Cohn & Roth, 1983; Leape, 1987).

RISK FACTORS AND INCIDENCE

Virtually all children (95 percent) with meconium ileus have cystic fibrosis, although only a small proportion (10 to 15 percent) of infants with cystic fibrosis present with meconium ileus. Cystic fibrosis, also known as mucoviscidosis, is a genetic disorder with an autosomal recessive inheritance pattern that occurs in 1 of every 2000 live births. All exocrine glands are affected, producing tenacious mucus that causes not only gastrointestinal dysfunction but also ultimately respiratory malfunction (American Association of Pediatrics Committee on Genetics, 1989; Chawls, Lally, & Mahour, 1988; Leape, 1987; Wells & Meghdadpour, 1988).

Rarely (5 percent) meconium ileus occurs in the absence of cystic fibrosis, but generally pancreatic duct stenosis or partial pancreatic aplasia can be demonstrated. The cause of these isolated findings is not known (Leape, 1987; Lebenthal, Wynn, & Lebenthal, 1983).

Additional findings associated with meconium ileus include maternal polyhydramnios (5 to 10 percent) and prematurity (10 to 33 percent) (Chawls, Lally, & Mahour, 1988; Leape, 1987).

CLINICAL MANIFESTATIONS

Meconium ileus generally presents first with progressive abdominal distention (within 12 to 24 hours of birth), followed by bilious vomiting and a failure to pass meconium. On physical examination the meconium mass may be palpated as a movable, doughy or putty-like ball; smaller pellet-like concretions of inspissated meconium may be felt distally. Rectal examination should produce no meconium, but normal sphincter tone should be felt (Avery & Taeusch, 1984; Chang, 1980b; Chawls, Lally, & Mahour, 1988; Ghory & Sheldon, 1985; Leape, 1987).

DIFFERENTIAL DIAGNOSIS

Plain abdominal films show distended loops proximal to the point of obstruction, but unlike the uniformly lucent areas seen in jejunoileal atresia, the dilated areas typical of meconium ileus are of varying sizes and have a "soap bubble" or "ground glass" appearance. This appearance reflects the mixture of trapped air and meconium. Calcifications may also be noted that are the result of antenatal intestinal perforation and consequent meconium peritonitis. Barium enema demonstrates a distally unused microcolon, thus differentiating this condition from Hirschsprung's disease. The smaller pellet-like masses of meconium may also be noted in the distal segment (Chang, 1980b; Chawls, Lally, & Mahour, 1988; Dirkes et al., 1995; Ghory & Sheldon, 1985;

Leape, 1987; Ricketts, 1984). A history of cystic fibrosis in siblings virtually ensures the diagnosis of meconium ileus. An immunoreactive trypsin test using a dry blood spot provides a screen for cystic fibrosis, with confirmation by sweat test (American Association of Pediatrics Committee on Genetics, 1989).

PROGNOSIS

Cystic fibrosis is a condition of delayed mortality, with a mean survival of 22 years. At this age, death comes as a result of obstructive pulmonary disease and infection. The intervening period is marked by poor growth and chronic respiratory and gastrointestinal dysfunction. The infant mortality rate in cystic fibrosis is 13 percent, with these early deaths attributed to malabsorption and malnutrition (American Association of Pediatrics Committee on Genetics, 1989).

COLLABORATIVE MANAGEMENT

In the case of uncomplicated meconium ileus, the bowel can generally be evacuated using a hyperosmolar contrast enema such as Gastrografin. Because of its hyperosmolarity, fluid is drawn from the interstitial and intravascular spaces into the intestinal lumen, softening the impacted meconium and allowing it to pull away from the intestinal wall. The mass can then be evacuated by normal peristalsis. This nonoperative treatment is generally successful in 15 to 20 percent of patients (Chang, 1980b; Chawls, Lally, & Mahour, 1988; Leape, 1987).

If repeated enemas are not productive, or if meconium ileus is complicated by bowel ischemia, sepsis, or hypovolemic shock, the obstructing meconium may be surgically removed. A temporary ileostomy may be established and, if present, is irrigated daily with dilute acetylcysteine until any residual meconium is softened and evacuated. Chest physiotherapy, Mucomyst aerosols, and extra humidity may be helpful in preventing postoperative pulmonary complications (such as atelectasis and pneumonia), to which infants with cystic fibrosis are particularly prone (Avery & Taeusch, 1984; Bishop, 1976; Chang, 1980b; Ghory & Sheldon, 1985; Leape, 1987).

Genetic counseling should clearly be provided to parents of affected children, with appropriate referral to a geneticist or genetic counselor. A social worker or other mental health professional may help parents explore their feelings concerning their child's prognosis and their future reproductive plans (Wells & Meghdadpour, 1988). Extensive parent teaching of pulmonary toilet and enzyme supplementation is needed. Respiratory therapy personnel and the nutritional support team should consequently be included in parent teaching. Many larger communities have special follow-up clinics for cystic fibrosis patients that may be utilized to ensure continuity and coordination of care after discharge.

Immediate stabilization of the child with meconium ileus requires decompression with gastric suction and the correction of fluid and electrolyte imbalances. Hydration is particularly important in those patients being medically treated with hyperosmolar enemas. Fluids drawn into the intestinal lumen to allow softening and evacuation of the meconium are by default removed from the effective circulation, placing the infant at risk for severe hypovolemia and vascular collapse. The extracted fluids should be replaced accordingly. Generally, 4 ml of 0.5 normal saline solution is given for every 1 ml of retained enema. Fluids and suction are continued until the meconium is evacuated and the clinical manifestations of obstruction resolve. When intestinal function is deemed adequate, Pregestimil feedings may be started, together with the pancreatic enzyme supplement Viokase (Chawls, Lally, & Mahour, 1988; Leape, 1987).

If the obstruction is not relieved, decompression, fluids, and electrolytes are continued until surgical treatment can be carried out. Postoperatively, ostomy care becomes a part of nursing management, along with assistance in providing pulmonary toilet. The infant's respiratory status should be closely monitored. If there are adhesions secondary to meconium peritonitis or surgical manipulation, or if the meconium is incompletely removed, the signs of obstruction may recur. These signs of persistent or recurrent obstruction must be immediately reported to allow for early intervention and reoperation as needed. Feedings are delayed until the obstruction is relieved, the ileostomy is functioning, and bowel activity has returned. Pregestimil with added Viokase is initially given. Many of these infants feed quite poorly, however, and total parenteral nutrition may be required for these special cases (Chang, 1980b; Leape, 1987).

Meconium Plug Syndrome

PATHOPHYSIOLOGY

Meconium plug syndrome is a condition in which intestinal obstruction (generally of the lower colon and rectum) occurs as the result of unusually thick meconium in the absence of demonstrable enzymatic deficiency. The syndrome is most likely the result of abnormal gut motility associated with immaturity or hypotonia; ganglion deficiency is not found. The plug is primarily formed from mucus and secretions and therefore appears yellowish white and gelatinous, lacking the usual flow properties of normal meconium (Gryboski & Walker, 1983).

RISK FACTORS

Premature infants are especially prone to meconium plug syndrome; however, the condition may also be found in hypotonic infants with central nervous system damage, and some infants of diabetic mothers are also affected. In the latter case, meconium plug syndrome is considered to be a variant of small left colon syndrome. Maternal therapy with magnesium sulfate is an additional risk factor that has been noted by some clinicians (Avery & Taeusch, 1984; Sunshine et al., 1983). Meconium plugs are found in about 1 of every 100 newborns. A fourth of these infants are unable to spontaneously evacuate the plug and thus develop intestinal obstruction (Gryboski & Walker, 1983).

CLINICAL MANIFESTATIONS

The signs are those of low intestinal obstruction with failure to stool, followed by abdominal distention and bilious vomiting. Hyperactive bowel sounds are often noted on auscultation, and normal sphincter tone is generally felt on rectal examination. Often after digital examination, the meconium plug and flatus are passed (Gryboski & Walker, 1983; Sunshine et al., 1983).

DIFFERENTIAL DIAGNOSIS

Plain radiographs indicate a low intestinal obstruction with multiple distended loops of proximal bowel, thus bringing to mind a number of possible conditions, including jejunoileal atresia, meconium ileus, Hirschsprung's disease, small left colon syndrome, or meconium plug syndrome. On barium enema the colon is generally described as being of normal caliber with no evidence of microcolon, thus eliminating the diagnosis of jejunoileal atresia or meconium ileus. The presence of normal ganglion cells on rectal biopsy removes Hirschsprung's disease from the differential diagnosis. In the absence of a history of maternal diabetes, meconium plug syndrome becomes the most logical cause for the symptoms presented (Ricketts, 1984; Sunshine et al., 1983).

PROGNOSIS

Once the meconium plug is expulsed, complete recovery should follow (Gryboski & Walker, 1983).

COLLABORATIVE MANAGEMENT

Small enemas of warm saline, Gastrografin, or acetylcysteine are usually all that is needed to dislodge the obstructing meconium plug if it has not already been expelled after rectal examination. Normal stooling patterns should follow. Surgical intervention is rarely needed (Avery & Taeusch, 1984; Gryboski & Walker, 1983; Sunshine et al., 1983).

Decompression, hydration, and electrolyte balance are the immediate concerns. The special care required after Gastrografin enema and rectal biopsy has already been discussed. Once the plug is evacuated, symptomatology has resolved, and normal intestinal function has returned, feedings can be begun.

Anorectal Agenesis

PATHOPHYSIOLOGY

Anorectal agenesis (imperforate anus) refers to a group of congenital malformations involving the anus, rectum, or the junction between the two. If the urorectal septum deviates during its growth, the cloaca will be abnormally or incompletely partitioned, resulting in rectal stenosis or atresia. Rectourethral and rectovaginal fistulas frequently occur in association with these defects. If the anal membrane fails to rupture, the result is a membranous anal atresia (Boles, 1978; Moore & Persaud, 1993; Sadler, 1985).

A whole spectrum of defects is possible, but they are generally classified into four major types (Fig. 12–3). The cause of deviated or arrested anorectal development is not known.

INCIDENCE

The incidence of anorectal agenesis is 1 in 1500 to 5000 live births.

RISK FACTORS

Twenty to 75 percent of all affected infants have an associated anomaly. Considering its common origin from the cloaca, it is not surprising that

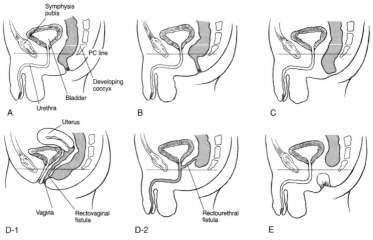

FIGURE 12–3. Anorectal agenesis. Shading represents areas of lucency typically found on radiograph. Percentages reflect relative occurrence. *A*, Normal anatomy. *B*, Type I or anal stenosis (5 to 6 percent): anus or lower rectum is narrowed but patent. *C*, Type II or anal membrane (5 to 7 percent): anal opening covered by a membranous diaphragm. *D*, Type III or anal agenesis (85 percent): anus is clearly imperforate; fistulas are present in three fourths of cases. *D-1*, Type IIIA or low agenesis: bowel ends as a blind pouch below the pubococcygeal (PC) line; most common in females. *D-2*, Type IIIB or high agenesis: bowel ends as a blind pouch above the pubococcygeal line; most common in males. *E*, Type IV or anal atresia (3 percent): rectum and anus are present as blind pouches but are separated by a variable distance. (Data from Avery, M. E., & Taeusch, H. W. [1984]. *Schaffer's diseases of the newborn* [5th ed.]. Philadelphia: W. B. Saunders; Chang, J. H. T. [1980b]. Neonatal surgical emergencies: V. Intestinal obstruction. *Perinatology/Neonatology*, 4([2], 34–40; deVries, P. A., & Cox, K. L. [1985]. Surgery of anorectal anomalies. *Surgical Clinics of North America*, 65, 1139–1169; Gryboski, J., & Walker, W. A. [1983]. *Gastrointestinal problems in the infant* [2nd ed.]. Philadelphia: W. B. Saunders; Moore, K. L., & Persaud, T. V. N. [1993]. *Before we are born: Basic embryology and birth defects* [4th ed.]. Philadelphia: W. B. Saunders; and Sadler, T. W. [1985]. *Langman's medical embryology* [5th ed.]. Baltimore: Williams & Wilkins.)

genitourinary tract abnormalities are most frequently found (25 to 50 percent); approximately 4 percent have the lethal defects of bilateral renal agenesis or dysplasia. Cryptorchidism is noted in 3 to 19 percent of affected males.

Congenital heart disease and esophageal atresia are also occasionally reported, and when the latter is found, the VATER and VACTERL associations should be considered.

Approximately half of these infants have spinal dysraphism, ranging from occult spina bifida (2.2 percent) to myelomeningocele (2.0 to 4.4 percent), including scoliosis (13.3 percent), hemivertebra (6.7 percent), extra segments (8.9 percent), tethered cord (4.0 to 13.3 percent), and fibrolipoma of the cord (8.9 to 38.0 percent).

CLINICAL MANIFESTATIONS

Presenting signs and symptoms vary slightly with the particular type of defect present. For the majority (those with type III agenesis), the anus is clearly imperforate. Owing to the high incidence of fistulas, meconium may be passed in the urine (in males) or its presence may be noted at the vaginal outlet (in females). With anal stenosis (type I), the anus and rectal vault are patent but narrowed, so that the pasty stools of the newborn may be passed. The stenosis is generally suspected by the microscopic appearance of the anus and confirmed on rectal examination. With the remaining two types, the anus may appear misleadingly normal on first inspection. In the membranous type (type II), the anal membrane may become visible within 24 to 48 hours as meconium bulges from beneath the thin epithelial covering, but by then the signs of low intestinal obstruction (distention, bilious vomiting, and failure to pass stool) are also becoming apparent. The atretic type (type IV), which fortunately is rare, generally first presents as the full-blown manifestations of obstruction (Avery & Taeusch, 1984; Boles, 1978; Chang, 1980b).

DIFFERENTIAL DIAGNOSIS

Visual and digital rectal examination is generally diagnostic. In the presence of a fistula, the urine may also be examined for meconium epithelial cells (Gryboski & Walker, 1983; Leape, 1987).

An inverted lateral radiograph (upside-down Wangensteen-Rice technique) may demonstrate air collected in the blind-ending upper rectal pouch but is generally unreliable for determining the level of obstruction, owing to the considerable time required for swallowed air to reach this portion of the gut. Even when sufficient time is given, air may be prevented by meconium from reaching the end of the pouch. Nevertheless, if a fistula is present, air may be seen in the bladder or vagina on the plain film (Boles, 1978; Gryboski & Walker, 1983; Leape, 1987).

Contrast medium–enhanced studies with barium injected into the blind rectum will confirm obstruction but provide no indication of the distance that separates the distal and proximal pouches. Barium injected through the urethra or vagina will confirm the presence of a fistula and through retrograde filling indicates the level of the rectal pouch (Boles, 1978; Leape,

1987; Flake & Ryckman, 1992). In those rare situations in which a fistula is not present and the level of the obstruction has still not been determined, a perineal puncture contrast rectogram or needle aspiration may be required. For the rectogram, a needle is inserted through the perineum and guided (by sonography) into the rectal pouch to inject the barium. The needle aspiration is a more conservative alternative and involves advancement of the needle while attempting to aspirate. If the needle has been advanced to a depth of 1.5 cm and no meconium has been obtained, the defect is assumed to be of a high type (Adkins & Kiesewetter, 1976; deVries & Cox, 1985; Leape, 1987).

PROGNOSIS

The outcome is largely dependent on the type of defect and the level of the upper rectal pouch in relation to the puborectal muscle, which is the main muscle of sphincter function and continence. This muscle is a central component of the levator ani muscle, which spans the pelvis much like a sling to support the lower end of the rectum. On radiograph, the position of this muscle can be estimated by drawing an imaginary line between the symphysis pubis and the developing coccyx. Based on the relation of the pouch to this pubococcygeal line, anorectal anomalies can be classified into three groups, indicating a low, high, or intermediate level defect. In low (translevator) types, the rectum descends through and is surrounded by the puborectalis and levator ani muscles, so the sensorimotor mechanisms are generally intact. With high (supralevator) defects, the rectal pouch ends above the puborectalis and levator ani muscles, so the neurologic and muscular mechanisms of continence may be impaired. In intermediate types (supralevator), the rectum again ends above the puborectalis, but the pouch is cradled in the muscular hammock formed by the levator ani so that neuromuscular function is variable and repair more complicated (Adkins & Kiesewetter, 1976; Chang, 1980b; deVries & Cox, 1985; Leape, 1987).

The overall mortality rate is approximately 20 percent, with death largely a reflection of the nature of the defect and the presence of associated anomalies. In general, the supralevator types of defects carry the highest mortality (31 percent), with intermediate supralevator lesions having the highest death rate of all (45 percent), followed by high supralevator lesions (29 percent) and low translevator defects (7 percent). As a group, the cause of death for most is due to the presence of associated anomalies (Adkins & Kiesewetter, 1976).

For survivors, the main criterion for outcome is fecal continence. When anorectal anomalies are reviewed as a whole, 74 percent of patients can be expected to have good results, with normal anal function and control of defecation; 14 percent will have fair results, with only occasional soiling or straining; and 12 percent will have poor results, being nearly or completely incontinent or requiring permanent colostomy. Here again, however, outcome will be largely determined by the level of the defect. Most low translevator (92 percent) and intermediate supralevator (83 percent) types will have a good outcome. Far fewer (51 percent) of the high supralevator types will have good postoperative results, and a large proportion (23 percent) will have frankly poor results (Adkins & Kiesewetter, 1976).

COLLABORATIVE MANAGEMENT

As might be expected, the treatment of anorectal anomalies varies with the nature of the defect. The higher the lesion, the more technically complicated its repair becomes.

The treatment of anal stenosis (type I defect) consists of repeated dilation using Hegar dilators. When the anus is sufficiently enlarged, and if the infant is otherwise stable, the patient is discharged, with daily digital dilation (using the little finger) to be performed by the parents (Adkins & Kiesewetter, 1976; Chang, 1980b; Leape, 1987).

Membranous defects (type II) require minimal surgical therapy. The membrane is simply punctured with a hemostat or excised using a scalpel. Repeated dilation is performed as needed (Adkins & Kiesewetter, 1976; Chang, 1980b).

Low agenesis (translevator, type III lesion) is corrected by perineal anoplasty. After locating the position of the superficial external sphincter using a nerve stimulator, the rectal pouch is brought down through the sphincter to the opening on the anal skin. The fistulous connection, if present, is removed. Gentle irrigations help facilitate stooling and keep the anastomotic site clean until daily dilations can be started, generally between 10 and 14 postoperative days (Adkins & Kiesewetter, 1976; Chang, 1980b; Hendren & Kim, 1974; Leape, 1987).

High agenesis (intermediate or high supralevator, type III lesions) and atresia (supralevator, type IV lesions) generally are treated in two phases. The first step is immediate placement of a colostomy for decompression and diversion of fecal contents. If present, the urethrorectal fistula is generally closed or excised so as to avoid "spill-over" fecal contamination with resultant urinary tract infection. The definitive repair is generally delayed 3 to 12 months to allow for growth and pelvic enlargement. At that time, an abdominal-perineal pull-through procedure is performed in which the rectal pouch is literally pulled through the levator sling and anchored to the skin. The colostomy is left intact until healing is complete (Boles, 1978; Chang, 1980b; deVries & Cox, 1985; Leape, 1987).

Nonemergent cases (typically stenosis) usually require little in the way of stabilization, other than replacement and correction of fluid and electrolyte imbalance. If a fistula is present, these infants are at risk of developing hyperchloremic acidosis owing to the absorption of urine from the colon (Leape, 1987). Gastric suction for decompression is instituted prophylactically (in the case of agenesis when the defect is obvious on inspection) or therapeutically (when membranous and atretic types begin to display symptoms of obstruction).

Postoperatively, wound care and monitoring for postoperative complications are added to the regimen. If anoplasty is performed, the site should be inspected (as allowed by the surgical team) for mucosal prolapse, which may occur if there is inadequate sphincter preservation. A colostomy placed for higher defects should receive the standard care and monitoring. Dilatory procedures are initially carried out by the surgeon, but when digital dilation becomes possible, the nurse may assume this task, making sure to provide bedside parent teaching. Throughout recuperation the urine (or vaginal outlet) should be closely observed for the presence of meconium, which would indicate a recurrent fistula. If such a fistula is suspected, electrolyte and acid–base status should also be monitored for hyperchloremic acidosis. Otherwise, feeding may begin when the colostomy or anoplasty is sufficiently healed and intestinal function resumes. Stool-softening agents may be required (Leape, 1987).

Malrotation With Volvulus

PATHOPHYSIOLOGY

Malrotation is an anomaly of intestinal rotation and fixation. Although alternative theories have been offered (Kluth, Kaestner, Tibboel, & Lambrecht, 1995) the abnormality most likely arises as the intestine rotates around the axis of the superior mesenteric artery during its entry into and movement from the umbilical cord. Once returned to the abdominal cavity, the intestinal mesentery lies along and eventually adheres to the posterior abdominal wall, thus fixing the intestine in place (Chang, 1980a; Moore & Persaud, 1993; Sadler, 1985). The normal 270-degree counterclockwise rotation can be interrupted or deviated at any time, and consequently a variety of rotation and fixation anomalies are possible.

The major danger with malrotation is that the intestinal loops may become kinked, knotted, or otherwise obstructed. This knotting and twisting of the bowel is called a volvulus. The resultant occlusion of the intestinal tract or its blood supply can lead to widespread ischemia and necrosis. Nearly two thirds of all cases of malrotation are complicated by volvulus, with incidence varying with age at onset of symptoms. Eighty-five percent of patients younger than 1 month of age have volvulus, compared with 43 percent of older children (Gryboski & Walker, 1983; Messineo, MacMillan, Palder, & Filler, 1992; Seashore & Touloukian, 1994).

RISK FACTORS

Owing to the rarity of rotational anomalies, their incidence is not known. However, the busiest surgical referral services typically see only two to four cases a year (Ducharme & Ghosn, 1987; Messineo, MacMillan, Palder, & Filler, 1992; Reyes, Meller, & Loeff, 1989; Seashore & Touloukian, 1994). The anomaly does appear to predominate in males; however, no specific etiology has been identified (Chang, 1980a).

Because of the nature of these defects, almost all cases of omphalocele, gastroschisis, and diaphragmatic hernia entail some component of malrotation. The frequency is, in fact, so high that many clinicians do not consider malrotation an anomaly associated with these conditions but rather an expected component of them. In addition to these defects, associated anomalies such as intestinal atresias, annular pancreas, Meckel's diverticulum, urinary tract malformation, and congenital heart disease are found in 8 to 24 percent of patients (Chang, 1980a; Messineo, MacMillan, Palder, & Filler, 1992; Reyes, Meller, & Loeff, 1989; Seashore & Touloukian, 1994).

CLINICAL MANIFESTATIONS

Only about half of patients present with symptoms in the first week of life, which are generally intermittent or recurrent, indicating that most of these obstructions are partial rather than complete. Sudden, progressive, bilious vomiting (Chang, 1980a) in a well infant suggests a malrotation with volvulus. Abdominal distention and bloody stools may be noted. Bleeding occurs when twisting is severe enough to interfere with venous return from the bowel, causing the vessels to become engorged and leak blood into the gut (Hendren & Kim, 1974).

DIFFERENTIAL DIAGNOSIS

The differential diagnosis generally includes pyloric stenosis, duodenal atresia, and jejunoileal atresia. On plain radiograph, the stomach and upper small intestine are generally distended with air and may mimic the characteristic "double bubble" of duodenal atresia. However, the presence of small amounts of gas in the distal positions of the gut is more reflective of a partial obstruction by malrotation than of an atresia in the jejunum or ileum. In adults, the gas-filled loops may appear to converge to a point (convergency sign). A spoke-wheel sign of mucosal folds radiating from the center has also been described. However, these radiographic signs have not been reported in neonates (Lee et al., 1995). If doubt persists, a barium enema can be given to locate the position of the cecum under fluoroscopy. If a misplaced colon is seen, the diagnosis of malrotation is confirmed. However, some malrotations (notably reverse rotation) may not be demonstrated. An upper gastrointestinal series is diagnostic in all cases, allowing the exact position of the duodenum to be seen. When volvulus is present, the barium column is noted to end with a peculiar "beaking" effect. This beaking appearance is pathognomonic of a volvulus and is caused by the twisting of the bowel into a sharp point resembling the beak of a bird (Chang, 1980a; Leape, 1987). Suspected malrotation is the only situation that warrants an upper gastrointestinal series; otherwise the procedure should not be carried out in infants (Ricketts, 1984).

PROGNOSIS

When the condition is uncomplicated by infarction or associated anomalies, the survival rate is excellent and may be as high as 99 percent. However, in the presence of necrosis, survival falls to 35 percent. An increased risk of dying is also noted with younger age (< 3 months) at the time of surgery (Chang, 1980a; Ducharme & Ghosn, 1987; Messineo, MacMillan, Palder, & Filler, 1992).

COLLABORATIVE MANAGEMENT

The goals for surgical management are the release of obstruction and counterclockwise rotational reduction of the bowel (Chang, 1980a). Viability of the bowel is determined with necrotic sections removed. If the necrosis is extensive, rather than perform massive bowel resection, the abdomen is closed. A return "second look" surgery is performed in 24 to 48 hours, at which time it becomes mandatory to remove any unrecovered, infarcted bowel. If the bowel appears viable, the Ladd bands (if present) are divided and the entrapped duodenum is freed. The entire length of the bowel is then inspected for patency and associated defects and returned to the abdominal cavity; the small intestine is placed on the right and the colon is placed on the left side of the abdominal cavity. Suture fixation of the replaced bowel is generally not necessary. Appendectomy and gastrostomy are generally done as well (Ducharme & Ghosn, 1987d; Ghory & Sheldon, 1985; Leape, 1987; Sunshine et al., 1983).

The major postoperative complication is short-bowel syndrome, resulting from the excision of major portions of the gut (Leape, 1987). (See previous discussion on short-bowel syndrome in this chapter.) Wound problems and prolonged ileus may also be noted (Seashore & Touloukian, 1994).

Preoperative Stabilization

- Gastric decompression and correction of fluid and electrolyte deficits are done.
- Hypovolemia and metabolic acidosis are prevented.

Postoperative Management

- Abdominal decompression is performed.
- Fluid and electrolyte resuscitation is instituted.
- Total parenteral nutrition is started and continued, often for months in the case of short-bowel syndrome, until the intestine has had an opportunity to recover and grow.
- When feedings are begun, very dilute formula (one-fourth strength Pregestimil or Nutramigen) is initially given; the volume and then the concentration are gradually increased until a normal amount of full-strength formula can be tolerated.

Intussusception

PATHOPHYSIOLOGY

Intussusception is an acquired obstruction in which a part of the intestine prolapses into the lumen of an adjoining, distal intestinal segment. This luminal prolapse may occur at any site in the gastrointestinal tract, but typically there are four varieties:

- Enteric intussusception, in which the small intestine prolapses into itself
- Colic intussusception, in which the large intestine prolapses into itself
- Ileocecal intussusception, in which the ileocecal valve is inverted and pushed into the cecum, pulling a segment of ileum with it
- Ileocolic intussusception, in which the ileocecal valve remains in place but the ileum prolapses through it into the colon (Taylor, 1988).

Rarely, a retrograde intussusception may occur in which a distal intestinal segment prolapses upward into a proximal part. In the neonate, the majority of cases are of the enteric (most often involving the terminal ileum) or ileocecal type (Avery & Taeusch, 1984).

INCIDENCE

Intussusception is extremely rare in the newborn period; consequently, an overall incidence rate is not known. It generally appears at 3 to 24 months.

RISK FACTORS

Intussusception is an acquired condition and therefore not easily explained by any one etiologic factor. Five to 13 percent have a "lead point," a demonstrable anatomic lesion or defect that may have been the cause of intussusception. Such lead points may include Meckel's diverticula, duplication defects, polyps, hematomas, lymphomas, or viscid stool, which is common in cystic fibrosis.

In most situations the etiology is not known (idiopathic intussusception). Often there is a history of preceding upper respiratory tract infection or gastroenteritis. Nearly half of all patients demonstrate infection with adenovirus on stool culture.

CLINICAL MANIFESTATIONS

Regardless of the site, the intussusception gives rise to two problems:

- It causes a simple mechanical obstruction as the result of the blockage of the distal intestinal lumen by the prolapsed proximal segment.
- As the intestinal walls are telescoped into one another, the mucosal blood vessels become compressed, congested, and prone to ischemia or infarction (Avery & Taeusch, 1984).

Thus, the symptoms of intussusception typically include vomiting, colicky pain, and bloody stools or red currant-jelly stools (Gryboski & Walker, 1983; Shanbhogue et al., 1994).

DIFFERENTIAL DIAGNOSIS

Plain radiographs may not be very helpful in diagnosis, with 20 to 30 percent showing only a general picture of intestinal obstruction with dilated proximal loops and an airless distal bowel. On ultrasound, the affected area often appears as a doughnut sign on cross section.

Definitive diagnosis is by barium enema with the contrast media outlining the gut and ending proximally in a characteristic "coiled spring" pattern. This pattern is caused by barium trickling into the transverse folds of the luminal mucosa between the intussusceptum and the intussuscipiens.

PROGNOSIS

The prognosis for intussusception in newborns is accompanied by a 41 percent mortality rate (Avery & Taeusch, 1984), because newborns present with so few of the signs that classically appear in infants and older children. Consequently, intussusception is rarely considered in the differential diagnosis of intestinal obstruction.

COLLABORATIVE MANAGEMENT

Medical Intervention

In older children and adults, an attempt is first made to reduce the intussusception using the hydrostatic pressure produced by a barium enema. Barium is injected into the rectum and allowed to flow distally until the "coiled spring" pattern appears. A balloon-tipped catheter is then inserted into the rectum. The balloon is inflated with air, and gentle traction is applied until the balloon is pulled back against the muscular sling of the levators, thus preventing any outflow of barium. The administration of barium is restarted, causing the intraluminal pressure to slowly rise as more and more contrast medium is added without an avenue for escape. The pressure is maintained until the intussusception is pushed distally and freed. The procedure can be likened to taking a surgical glove in which one fingertip has been pulled inward, closing the cuff around the mouth, and slowly exhaling until the fingertip of the glove is blown outward. If the intussusception is fully reduced, the barium is seen to suddenly flow freely into the proximal bowel and the clinical status of the patient should immediately improve. Unfortunately, in infants, full reduction is generally not accomplished and surgical reduction is required (Avery & Taeusch, 1984; Gryboski & Walker, 1983; Leape, 1987).

An alternate approach by rectal insufflation of air has been reported. Pneumatic reduction, however, is generally not performed in infants younger than 3 months of age owing to the risk of bowel perforation and rapid tension pneumoperitoneum (Lipschitz, Patel, & Kazlow, 1995; Shiels, 1995; Zheng, Frush, & Guo, 1994).

Surgical Intervention

Surgical intervention involves a manual reduction of the intussusception using a "milking" motion on the proximal bowel. The pressure and squeezing are continued until the loop is freed; traction and pulling should never be applied. The bowel is carefully inspected, any necrotic tissue is removed, and lead points are resected (Avery & Taeusch, 1984; Leape, 1987).

Associated Management

- Sepsis should be suspected, and blood samples for cultures drawn, owing to the strong association with adenovirus and the frequent history of gastroenteritis or respiratory tract infection.
- Antibiotic therapy is initiated pending cultures.
- Shock from fluid loss into the wall of the trapped intestine and/or blood lost from congested vessels into the lumen of the intestine should be watched for and managed with fluid resuscitation and volume expansion. Decompression by gastric suction is also recommended (Leape, 1987).
- Fluid and electrolyte support is required.
- Intussusception may recur and such clinical signs as increasing gastric drainage should be sought. The recurrence risk is 2 to 20 percent, being more common after hydrostatic reduction (8 to 13 percent) than

after surgical reduction (0 to 4 percent) (Champous, DelBeccaro, & Nazar-Stewart, 1994; Leape, 1987).

Necrotizing Enterocolitis

PATHOPHYSIOLOGY

Necrotizing enterocolitis (NEC) is an acquired disorder characterized by necrosis of the mucosal and submucosal layers of the gastrointestinal tract. Any portion of the bowel can be affected, but the ileocecal area predominates (66 percent), with the antimesenteric side being most typically involved (Lemelle et al., 1994). To the naked eye, the affected intestine appears irregularly dilated with patchy areas of discoloration ranging from pale to dark purple. The pale color indicates areas of ischemic necrosis where the tissues have been deprived of their blood supply; the purple color indicates areas of hemorrhagic necrosis where blood has leaked into the tissues from capillary hemorrhage. Gas-containing cysts (pneumatosis) may be seen in the wall of the intestine as the result of gas dissecting beneath the serosa or submucosa. If perforation has occurred, it is usually found in the ileocecal area.

On microscopic examination, the mucosa appears edematous, and the necrotic areas may extend beyond the mucosa and submucosa into the muscular layers. Microthrombi may also be noted in the tiny arterioles and venules of the mesentery, but frank thrombosis of the larger arteries or veins rarely occurs. Contrary to what the name NEC implies, there is really little inflammation in the acute stages of the disease (Kosloske & Musemeche, 1989).

The etiology and pathogenesis of NEC have been the focus of extensive debate and research for the past 30 years. At present the sum of knowledge indicates there are three major pathologic mechanisms occurring in combination that lead to the development of NEC. These three mechanisms involve selective ischemia of the bowel, establishment of bacterial flora, and the effect of feeding (Kosloske & Musemeche, 1989; Santulli et al., 1975).

- The selective bowel ischemia is really an asphyxial defense mechanism, serving to protect the brain and heart from hypoxia by shunting blood away from the mesenteric, renal, and peripheral vascular bed.
- Establishment of bacterial flora within the lumen of the bowel is a postnatal process that occurs by 10 days in healthy infants. Intestines are sterile at birth, becoming seeded with a wide variety of aerobic and anaerobic bacteria, which multiply and spread with enteral feedings. The organisms typically isolated are *Enterobacter, Escherichia coli, Klebsiella,* and clostridial species. These enteric bacilli do not usually invade normal tissue but are opportunistic pathogens (Blakey et al., 1985; Chan et al., 1994; Kosloske, 1994a; Kosloske & Musemeche, 1989; Santulli et al., 1975).
- Formula feedings have also been cited as an important factor in making the gut susceptible to NEC. Ninety-eight percent of all infants who develop NEC have been fed formula or dextrose solution (Kliegman & Fanaroff, 1981; Santulli et al., 1975), which provides a substance on which bacteria can feed and flourish. In comparison, infants who re-

ceive fresh breast milk are rarely affected with NEC, being presumably protected by the secretory immunoglobulin (IgA) and anti-inflammatory components it provides (Barlow et al., 1974; Buescher, 1994; Kosloske, 1994a; Kosloske & Musemeche, 1989).

- Hyperosmolar loads of formula or medications may further compound the situation.

The development of NEC apparently occurs as a result of the three pathologic mechanisms—ischemia, bacteria, and feeding (particularly hyperosmolar feeding)—operating in concert. Injured by ischemia, the mucosal cells lining the gut stop secreting protective enzymes. The unprotected luminal cells are destroyed by the digestive enzymes present (autodigestion). Enteric bacteria proliferate in the substrate-rich but immunologically deficient environment and invade the intestinal wall, where they release toxins and produce hydrogen gas. The gas is formed as a result of the catalytic activity of bacterial enzymes acting on formula as a substrate (Engel, Virnig, Hunt, & Levitt, 1973). The gas initially dissects beneath the serosal and submucosal layers of the intestine (pneumatosis intestinalis); but if this gas ruptures into the mesenteric vascular bed, it can be distributed through the systemic vessels into the venous system of the liver (portal venous gas). The bacterial toxins together with ischemia result in necrosis. If the full thickness of the intestinal wall is damaged, perforation can result, with the release of free air into the peritoneal cavity (pneumoperitoneum), and a true surgical emergency exists (Avery & Tausch, 1984; Leape, 1987; Santulli et al., 1975).

RISK FACTORS

The most common gastrointestinal disorder seen in the intensive care nursery, NEC affects approximately 5 percent of all admissions, although wide center-to-center differences are reported (from a low of 1 to a high of 8 percent).

- Any condition or situation leading to ischemia and bacterial overgrowth in the presence of formula feedings is a risk factor.
- Sixty-two to 94 percent of infants are premature, with the highest rates in those with lowest birth weight and gestational age. No consistent associations between NEC and sex, race, socioeconomic status, or season of the year have been found (Kliegman & Fanaroff, 1981; Kosloske, 1994a; Kosloske & Musemeche, 1989; Stoll, 1994).

CLINICAL MANIFESTATIONS

Symptoms generally present on an overall average (mean) at 12 days of age, with the most common age at onset (mode) of 3 days and a range up to 90 days (Kliegman & Fanaroff, 1981). Early signs include nonspecific signs of gastrointestinal compromise (abdominal distention, gastric residuals, vomiting that may or may not be bilious, and bloody stools) or nonspecific signs of infection (lethargy, temperature instability, apnea, and bradycardia), or both.

Laboratory findings include abnormal blood gases, abnormal blood cell counts, thrombocytopenia, and reducing substances. Hypovolemia occurs as a result of the third spacing of fluids in the interstitial compartments of the damaged intestine. Blood pressure falls, urinary output decreases, and the poorly perfused, often septic infant appears gray, pale, or mottled. Peritonitis is evident by erythema, edema, and tenderness of the abdominal wall. If clotting factors continue to be consumed, disseminated intravascular coagulation may even occur (Gupta, Burke, & Herson, 1994; Kanto, Hunter, & Stoll, 1994; Kliegman & Fanaroff, 1981; Kosloske & Musemeche, 1989; Leape, 1987; Santulli et al., 1975; Schober & Nassiri, 1994).

DIFFERENTIAL DIAGNOSIS

Radiographs taken very early in the course of the disease generally exhibit little more than fixed, dilated bowel loops with thickened walls, all due to local edema. The invasion of gas-forming bacteria into the intestinal wall produces the diagnostic picture of pneumatosis intestinalis. This intraluminal air, found in 85 percent of affected infants, generally appears as very tiny, lucent bubbles that may come so close together in some places that they coalesce to form curvilinear or crescent-shaped streaks. If extensive disease is present, air may enter the venous system and outline the hepatic veins. Portal venous gas, found in 15 to 30 percent of patients, is also diagnostic of NEC. Ultimately, perforation may occur, presenting the characteristic appearance of pneumoperitoneum with a layer of free air lying immediately inferior to the abdominal wall. This free air is best seen by a lateral view, but on anteroposterior view it may be noted by the characteristic "football sign" due to air outlining the falciform ligament (Fotter & Sorantin, 1994; Kosloske & Musemeche, 1989; Leape, 1987; Morrison & Jacobson, 1994; Rabinowitz & Siegle, 1976; Santulli et al., 1975).

PROGNOSIS

Mortality rates have dramatically reduced from a rate of 24 to 65 percent in the 1960s and 1970s to a rate of 9 to 28 percent in the 1990s. There is a lower mortality among infants who respond to medical management as compared with those requiring surgical intervention. Persistent acidosis, severe pneumatosis, and the presence of portal venous air are poor prognostic indicators (Buras, Guzzetta, Avery, & Naulty, 1986; Kosloske, 1994b; Stoll, 1994).

Of those who survive, approximately 31 percent develop strictures (mostly colonic) as the result of structural changes in nonperforated, healed ischemic sites.

- Nine to 23 percent suffer from short-bowel syndrome.
- Nine percent become septic.
- Recurrent NEC has been reported in 4 to 6 percent of patients with average onset of symptoms approximately 5 weeks after the original episode.

COLLABORATIVE MANAGEMENT

Aggressive medical management may be successful in approximately half of all affected neonates (Ricketts, 1994). Such management is based on three traditional principles:

- Bowel rest
- Prevention of progressive injury
- Normalization of systemic responses

Enteral nutrition is discontinued, the stomach is decompressed by low intermittent suction through a large-bore orogastric tube, and fluids and electrolytes are closely monitored and adjusted. Antibiotic therapy (after blood samples for cultures are drawn), early intubation and ventilation, management of acid–base derangements, and efforts to support blood pressure and blood flow to the gut are undertaken to both prevent continuing injury and correct systemic responses. Serial abdominal films are made at 6- to 8-hour intervals during acute illness to monitor progression of the disease and to detect perforation (Kanto, Hunter, & Stoll, 1994; Kosloske & Musemeche, 1989; Leape, 1987).

Criteria for surgery are somewhat controversial. Expedient laparotomy is ideally performed after the advent of intestinal gangrene but before perforation. Absolute indications are pneumoperitoneum or confirmation of intestinal gangrene by positive paracentesis (peritoneal tap producing ≥ 0.5 ml of fluid that is yellowish brown or brown and/or contains bacteria that are demonstrated on Gram's stain). Nonspecific but supportive findings include clinical deterioration in spite of vigorous clinical management (metabolic acidosis, ventilatory failure, thrombocytopenia, leukopenia or leukocytosis with shift to the left, oliguria, etc.), portal venous air, erythema of the abdominal wall, or persistently dilated and fixed bowel loop (Kosloske, 1994b; Kosloske & Musemeche, 1989; Parigi, Bragheri, Minniti, & Verga, 1994; Ricketts, 1994).

The principles of surgical management are as follows:

- The bowel is examined carefully, with resection of all grossly necrotic intestine or perforated sites.
- If the viability of extensive portions of the gut is in question, resection is deferred, with a follow-up second-look operation carried out in 24 to 48 hours.
- Bowel ends are brought to the surface to create an ostomy (Kosloske & Musemeche, 1989; Ricketts, 1994).

Extensive respiratory therapy may be required throughout hospitalization, especially when marked abdominal distention may interfere with ventilation. Long-term parenteral nutrition can be anticipated, making collaboration with the nutritional support team essential.

Because of the high incidence of NEC in the intensive care nursery, a premature infant who develops any of the early signs of obstruction (vomiting, distention, increased gastric aspirates), who demonstrates increased episodes of apnea and bradycardia, or who passes bloody stools should be regarded with a high index of suspicion. Should two or more of the early signs appear together, one should presume NEC until other diagnostic studies can be performed. Feedings are immediately stopped and venous access obtained. A gastric tube is placed to intermittent suction for decompression. Vigorous hydration and antibiotic therapy are provided, and total parenteral nutrition is initiated as soon as possible. Circulatory status must be evaluated frequently by monitoring perfusion, vital signs including blood pressure, and urinary output. All stools are routinely checked for blood.

Hematologic studies are performed to look for anemia, thrombocytopenia, and disordered coagulation; and blood, platelets, or fresh frozen plasma is given as needed. Oxygenation and acid-base status are also monitored, with respiratory support provided accordingly. Careful, gentle re-examination of the abdomen should be carried out every 8 hours (Kosloske & Musemeche, 1989; Leape, 1987).

Ventilatory and circulatory support are maintained in the postoperative period, and antibiotic therapy is continued for 10 to 14 days past resolution of pneumatosis. Ostomy care is performed as previously described. When stabilized gastrointestinal function has resumed (generally in 7 to 14 days), feedings are cautiously and slowly begun with small amounts of dilute elemental formula. The amount and concentration of feedings are advanced as tolerated, but these attempts are frequently frustrated by malabsorption associated with short-bowel syndrome or the development of strictures. Recurrent distention, residuals, vomiting, intractable constipation, or bloody stools may be noted with partial or complete obstruction due to such strictures (Rushton, 1990).

REFERENCES

Adkins, J. C., & Kiesewetter, W. B. (1976). Imperforate anus. *Surgical Clinics of North America, 56,* 379–394.

American Association of Pediatrics Committee on Genetics. (1989). Newborn screening fact sheets. *Pediatrics, 83,* 449–464.

Ashcraft, K. W., & Holder, T. M. (1981). Esophageal atresia and tracheoesophageal fistula malformations. *Continuing Education, 15*(4), 51–60.

Avery, M. E., Fletcher, B. D., & Williams, R. G. (1981). *The lung and its disorders in the newborn infant* (4th ed.). Philadelphia: W. B. Saunders.

Avery, M. E., & Taeusch, H. W. (1984). *Schaffer's diseases of the newborn* (5th ed.). Philadelphia: W. B. Saunders.

Barlow, B., Santulli, T. V., Heird, W. C., et al. (1974). An experimental study of acute necrotizing enterocolitis: The importance of breast milk. *Journal of Pediatric Surgery, 9,* 587–595.

Berenberg, W., & Neuhauser, E. B. D. (1950). Cardioesophageal relaxation (chalasia) as a cause of vomiting in infants. *Pediatrics, 5,* 414–419.

Bergstrom, L. V. (1978). Congenital and acquired deafness in clefting and craniofacial syndromes. *Cleft Palate Journal, 15,* 254–261.

Bettex, M., & Oesch, I. (1983). The hiatus hernia saga. Ups and downs in gastroesophageal reflux: Past, present, and future perspectives. *Journal of Pediatric Surgery, 18,* 670–680.

Bishop, H. C. (1976). Small bowel obstructions in the newborn. *Surgical Clinics of North America, 56,* 329–348.

Blakey, J. L., Lubitz, L., Campbell, N. T., et al. (1985). Enteric colonization in sporadic neonatal necrotizing enterocolitis. *Journal of Pediatric Gastroenterology and Nutrition, 4,* 591–595.

Boles, E. T. (1978). Imperforate anus. *Clinics in Perinatology, 5,* 149–161.

Boley, S. J., Dinari, G., & Cohen, M. I. (1978). Hirschsprung's disease in the newborn. *Clinics in Perinatology, 5,* 45–60.

Bowers, D. G. (1970). Congenital lower lip sinuses with cleft palate. *Plastic and Reconstructive Surgery, 45,* 151–154.

Breaux, C. W., Georgeson, K. E., Royal, S. A., & Curnow, A. J. (1988). Changing patterns in the diagnosis of hypertrophic pyloric stenosis. *Pediatrics, 81,* 213–217.

Buescher, E. S. (1994). Host defense mechanisms of human milk and their relations to enteric infections and necrotizing enterocolitis. *Clinics in Perinatology, 21,* 247–262.

Buras, R., Guzzetta, P., Avery, G., & Naulty, C. (1986). Acidosis and hepatic portal venous gas: Indications for surgery in necrotizing enterocolitis. *Pediatrics, 78,* 273–277.

Cassani, V. L. (1984). Tracheoesophageal anomalies. *Neonatal Network, 3,* 20–27.

Chaet, M. S., Farrell, M. K., Ziegler, M. M., & Warner, B. W. (1994). Intensive nutritional support and remedial surgical intervention for extreme short bowel syndrome. *Journal of Pediatric Gastroenterology and Nutrition, 19,* 295–298.

Champous, A. N., DelBeccaro, M. A., & Nazar-Stewart, V. (1994). Recurrent intussusception. *Archives of Pediatric and Adolescent Medicine, 148,* 474–478.

Chan, K. L., Saing, H., Yung, R. W. H., et al. (1994). A study of pre-antibiotic bacteriology in 125 patients with necrotizing enterocolitis. *Acta Paediatrica, 83*(Suppl. 396), 45–48.

Chang, J. H. T. (1979). Neonatal surgical emergencies: II. Esophageal atresia and tracheoesophageal fistula. *Perinatology/Neonatology, 3*(2), 26–27, 78.

Chang, J. H. T. (1980a). Neonatal surgical emergencies: IV. Malrotation of the intestine. *Perinatology/Neonatology, 4*(1), 50–52.

Chang, J. H. T. (1980b). Neonatal surgical emergencies: V. Intestinal obstruction. *Perinatology/Neonatology, 4*(2), 34–40.

Chawls, W. J., Lally, K. P., & Mahour, G. H. (1988). Neonatal surgical casebook: Meconium ileus in premature twins. *Journal of Perinatology, 8,* 62–64.

Cohen, M. M. (1978). Syndromes with cleft lip and cleft palate. *Cleft Palate Journal, 15,* 306–328.

Cohn, R. M., & Roth, K. S. (1983). *Metabolic disease: A guide to early recognition.* Philadelphia: W. B. Saunders.

Conner, G. K. (1993). Abdomen assessment. In E. P. Tappero & M. E. Honeyfield (Eds.), *Physical assessment of the newborn: A comprehensive approach to the art of physical examination* (pp. 81–89). Petaluma, CA: NICU Ink.

Cowett, R. M., & Schwartz, R. (1987). Glucose metabolism and homeostasis. In L. Stern & P. Vert (Eds.), *Neonatal medicine* (pp. 809–830). New York: Masson Publishing.

Cusick, E. L., Batchelor, A. A. G., & Spicer, R. D. (1993). Development of a technique for jejunal interposition in long-gap esophageal atresia. *Journal of Pediatric Surgery, 28,* 990–994.

Davis, D. W. (1985). Congenital duodenal obstruction. *Neonatal Network, 3*(6), 9–13.

Davis, W. S., Allen, R. P., Favara, B. E., & Slovis, T. L. (1974). Neonatal small left colon syndrome. *American Journal of Roentgenology, 120,* 322–329.

Davis, W. S., & Campbell, J. B. (1975). Neonatal small left colon syndrome. *American Journal of Diseases of Children, 129,* 1024–1027.

Desmond, M. M., & Rudolph, A. J. (1965). Progressive evaluation of the newborn infant. *Postgraduate Medicine, 37,* 207–212.

deVries, P. A., & Cox, K. L. (1985). Surgery of anorectal anomalies. *Surgical Clinics of North America, 65,* 1139–1169.

Dienno, M. E. (1987). Esophageal atresia: Corrective procedures and nursing care. *AORN Journal, 45,* 1356–1367.

Dirkes, K., Crombleholme, T. M., Craigo, S. D., et al. (1995). The natural history of meconium peritonitis diagnosed in utero. *Journal of Pediatric Surgery, 30,* 979–982.

Dorney, S. F. A., Ament, M. E., Berquist, W. E., et al. (1985). Improved survival in very short small bowel of infancy with use of long-term parenteral nutrition. *Journal of Pediatrics, 107,* 521–525.

Ducharme, J. C., & Ghosn, P. B. (1987). Intestinal malrotation. In L. Stern & P. Vert (Eds.), *Neonatal medicine* (pp. 1065–1068). New York: Masson Publishing.

Engel, R. R., Virnig, N. L., Hunt, C. E., & Levitt, M. D. (1973). Origin of mural gas in necrotizing enterocolitis. *Pediatric Research, 7,* 292.

Flake, A. W., & Ryckman, F. C. (1992). Selected anomalies and intestinal obstruction. In A. A. Fanaroff & R. J. Martin (Eds.), *Neonatal-perinatal medicine: Diseases of the fetus and infant* (5th ed., pp. 1038–1065). St. Louis: C. V. Mosby.

Fotter, R., & Sorantin, E. (1994). Diagnostic imaging in necrotizing enterocolitis. [Review]. *Acta Paediatrica, 83*(Suppl. 396), 41–44.

Fraser, F. C. (1970). The genetics of cleft lip and cleft palate. *American Journal of Human Genetics, 22,* 336–352.

Frentner, S. (1987). Abdominal wall defects: Omphalocele and gastroschisis. *Neonatal Network, 6*(3), 29–41.

Gantt, L., & Thompson, C. (1985). Short gut syndrome in the infant. *American Journal of Nursing, 85,* 1263–1266.

Ghory, M. J., & Sheldon, C. A. (1985). Newborn surgical emergencies of the gastrointestinal tract. *Surgical Clinics of North America, 65,* 1083–1098.

Gryboski, J., & Walker, W. A. (1983). *Gastrointestinal problems in the infant* (2nd ed.). Philadelphia: W. B. Saunders.

Gupta, S. K., Burke, G., & Herson, V. C. (1994). Necrotizing enterocolitis: Laboratory indicators of surgical disease. *Journal of Pediatric Surgery, 29,* 1472–1475.

Guyton, A. C. (1996). *Textbook of medical physiology* (9th ed.). Philadelphia: W. B. Saunders.

Guzzetta, P. C., Anderson, K. D., Eichelberger, M. R., et al. (1994). Surgery of the neonate. In G. B. Avery (Ed.), *Neonatology: Pathophysiology and management of the newborn* (4th ed., pp. 914–984). Philadelphia: J. B. Lippincott.

Haber, B. A., & Lake, A. M. (1990). Cholestatic jaundice in the newborn. *Clinics in Perinatology, 17,* 483–506.

Habib, Z. (1978a). Factors determining occurrence of cleft lip and cleft palate. *Surgery, Gynecology and Obstetrics, 146,* 105–110.

Habib, Z. (1978b). Genetic counseling and genetics of cleft lip and cleft palate. *Obstetrical and Gynecological Survey, 33,* 441–447.

Harrell-Bean, H. A., & Klell, C. A. (1983). Neonatal ostomies. *Journal of Obstetric, Gynecologic, and Neonatal Nursing* (supplement), *12,* 69s–73s.

Hendren, W. H., & Kim, S. H. (1974). Abdominal surgical emergencies of the newborn. *Surgical Clinics of North America, 54,* 489–527.

Herbst, J. J. (1983). Diagnosis and treatment of gastroesophageal reflux in children. *Pediatrics in Review, 5,* 75–79.

Hlusko, D. L., & McMurray, J. (1991). Gastroesophageal reflux: Treatment and nursing care. *Neonatal Network, 9*(5), 33–35.

Holder, T. M., & Ashcraft, K. W. (1981). Developments in the care of patients with esophageal atresia and tracheoesophageal fistula. *Surgical Clinics of North America, 61,* 1051–1061.

James, L. S. (1987). Emergencies in the delivery room. In A. A. Fanaroff & R. J. Martin (Eds.), *Neonatal-perinatal medicine: Diseases of the fetus and infant* (4th ed., pp. 360–378). St. Louis: C. V. Mosby.

Jedd, M. B., Melton, L. J., Griffin, M. R., et al. (1988). Factors associated with infantile hypertrophic pyloric stenosis. *American Journal of Diseases of Children, 142,* 334–337.

Johnson, C. B. (1993). Head, eyes, ears, nose, throat (HEENT) assessment. In E. P. Tappero & M. E. Honeyfield (Eds.), *Physical assessment of the newborn: A comprehensive approach to the art of physical examination* (pp. 41–54). Petaluma, CA: NICU Ink.

Jones, K. L. (1988). *Smith's recognizable patterns of human malformation: Genetic, embryologic and clinical aspects* (4th ed.). Philadelphia: W. B. Saunders.

Kanto, W. P., Hunter, J. E., & Stoll, B. J. (1994). Recognition and medical management of necrotizing enterocolitis. *Clinics in Perinatology, 21,* 335–346.

Kemmotsu, H., Joe, K., Nakamura, H., & Yamashita, M. (1995). Cervical approach for the repair of esophageal atresia. *Journal of Pediatric Surgery, 30,* 549–552.

Kenner, C., & Brueggemeyer, A. (1984). Hirschsprung's disease: Current trends and practices. *Neonatal Network, 3*(1), 7–16.

Kenner, C., Harjo, J., & Brueggemeyer, A. (Eds.) (1988). *Neonatal surgery: A nursing perspective.* Orlando, FL: Grune & Stratton.

Kiernan, B. S., & Scoloveno, M. A. (1986). Assessment of the neonate. *Topics in Clinical Nursing, 8*(1), 1–10.

Kim, S. H. (1976). Omphalocele. *Surgical Clinics of North America, 56,* 361–371.

Kimura, K., & Soper, R. T. (1994). Multistaged extrathoracic esophageal elongation for long gap esophageal atresia. *Journal of Pediatric Surgery, 29,* 566–568.

Kliegman, R. M., & Fanaroff, A. A. (1981). Neonatal necrotizing enterocolitis: A nine-year experience. I. Epidemiology and uncommon observations. *American Journal of Diseases of Children, 135,* 603–607.

Kluth, D. (1976). Atlas of esophageal atresia. *Journal of Pediatric Surgery, 11,* 901–919.

Kluth, D., Kaestner, M., Tibboel, D., & Lambrecht, W. (1995). Rotation of the gut: Fact or fantasy? *Journal of Pediatric Surgery 30,* 448–453.

Kosloske, A. M. (1994a). Epidemiology of necrotizing enterocolitis. *Acta Paediatrica, 83*(Suppl. 396), 2–7.

Kosloske, A. M. (1994b). Indications for operation in necrotizing enterocolitis revisited. *Journal of Pediatric Surgery, 29,* 663–666.

Kosloske, A. M., & Musemeche, C. A. (1989). Necrotizing enterocolitis of the neonate. *Clinics in Perinatology, 16,* 97–111.

Krogman, W. M. (1979). Craniofacial growth: Prenatal and postnatal. In H. K. Cooper, R. L. Harding, W. M. Krogman, et al. (Eds.), *Cleft palate and cleft lip: A team approach to clinical management and rehabilitation of the patient* (pp. 22–107). Philadelphia: W. B. Saunders.

Lambrecht, W., & Kluth, D. (1994). Esophageal atresia: A new anatomic variant with gasless abdomen. *Journal of Pediatric Surgery, 29,* 564–565.

Leape, L. L. (1987). *Patient care in pediatric surgery.* Boston: Little, Brown.

Lebenthal, E., Wynn, R., & Lebenthal, H. (1983). Digestive disorders in neonates: II. Congenital and acquired disease. *Perinatology/Neonatology, 7*(4), 53–59.

Lee, T. Y., Ko, S. F., Wan, Y. L., et al. (1995). Spoke wheel sign of small intestinal volvulus. *American Journal of Emergency Medicine, 13,* 477–478.

Lemelle, J. L., Schmitt, M., deMiscault, G., et al. (1994). Neonatal necrotizing enterocolitis: A retrospective and multicenter review of 331 cases. *Acta Paediatrica, 83*(Suppl. 396), 70–73.

Lepley, C. J. (1980). *Assessment of risk in the newborn: Evaluation during the transitional period.* White Plains, NY: March of Dimes Birth Defects Foundation.

Lipschitz, B., Patel, Y. T., & Kazlow, P. (1995). Endoscopic pneumatic reduction of an intussusception with simultaneous polypectomy in a child. *Journal of Pediatric Gastroenterology and Nutrition, 21,* 91–94.

Lynn, M. R. (1986). Use of infant seats for gastroesophageal reflux. *Journal of Pediatric Nursing, 1,* 127–129.

Martin, L. W., & Alexander, F. (1985). Esophageal atresia. *Surgical Clinics of North America, 65,* 1099–1113.

Martin, L. W., & Torres, A. M. (1985). Hirschsprung's disease. *Surgical Clinics of North America, 65,* 1171–1180.

Marty, T. L., Seo, T., Matlak, M. E., et al. (1995a). Gastrointestinal function after surgical correction of Hirschsprung's disease: Long-term follow-up in 135 patients. *Journal of Pediatric Surgery, 30,* 655–658.

Marty, T. L., Seo, T., Sullivan, J. J., et al. (1995b). Rectal irrigations for the prevention of postoperative enterocolitis in Hirschsprung's disease. *Journal of Pediatric Surgery, 30,* 652–654.

McCormack, M. K. (1979). Medical genetics and family practice. *American Family Physician, 20,* 142–154.

Meire, F., Standaert, L., deLaey, J. J., & Zeng, L. H. (1987). Waardenburg syndrome, Hirschsprung megacolon, and Marcus Gunn ptosis. *American Journal of Medical Genetics, 27,* 683–686.

Meller, J. L., Reyes, H. M., & Loeff, D. S. (1989). Gastroschisis and omphalocele. *Clinics in Perinatology, 16,* 113–122.

Merenstein, G. B. (1970). Rectal perforation by thermometer. *Lancet, 1,* 1007.

Merenstein, G. B., & Gardner, S. L. (1989). *Handbook of neonatal intensive care.* St. Louis: C. V. Mosby.

Messineo, A., MacMillan, J. H., Palder, S. B., & Filler, R. M. (1992). Clinical factors affecting mortality in children with malrotation of the intestine. *Journal of Pediatric Surgery, 27,* 1343–1345.

Methany, N. M. (1987). *Fluid and electrolyte balance: Nursing considerations.* Philadelphia: J. B. Lippincott.

Meyers, W. F., & Herbst, J. J. (1982). Effectiveness of positioning therapy for gastroesophageal reflux. *Pediatrics, 69,* 768–772.

Mitchell, L. E., & Risch, N. (1993). The genetics of infantile hypertrophic pyloric stenosis: A reanalysis. *American Journal of Diseases of Children, 147,* 1203–1211.

Moore, K. L., & Persaud, T. V. N. (1993). *Before we are born: Basic embryology and birth defects* (4rd ed.). Philadelphia: W. B. Saunders.

Morrison, S. C., & Jacobson, J. M. (1994). The radiology of necrotizing enterocolitis. *Clinics in Perinatology, 21,* 347–363.

Nagaya, M., Akatsuka, H., & Kato, J. (1994). Gastroesophageal reflux occurring after repair of congenital diaphragmatic hernia. *Journal of Pediatric Surgery, 29,* 1447–1451.

Oellrich, R. G., & Cusumano, M. M. (1987). Biliary atresia. *Neonatal Network, 5,* 25–32.

Oka, S. W. (1979). Epidemiology and genetics of clefting: With implications for etiology. In H. K. Cooper, R. L. Harding, W. M. Krogman, et al. (Eds.), *Cleft palate and cleft lip: A team approach to clinical management and rehabilitation of the patient* (pp. 108–143). Philadelphia: W. B. Saunders.

Orenstein, S. R. (1992). Controversies in pediatric gastroesophageal reflux. *Journal of Pediatric Gastroenterology and Nutrition, 14,* 338–348.

Orenstein, S. R., Magill, H. L., & Brooks, P. (1987). Thickening of infant feedings for therapy of gastroesophageal reflux. *Journal of Pediatrics, 110,* 181–186.

Parigi, G. B., Bragheri, R., Minniti, S., & Verga, G. (1994). Surgical treatment of necrotizing enterocolitis: When? How? *Acta Paediatrica, 83*(Suppl. 296), 58–61.

Pate, C. M. H. (1987). Care of the family following the birth of a child with a cleft lip and/or palate. *Neonatal Network, 5,* 30–37.

Pereira, G. R., & Ziegler, M. M. (1989). Nutritional care of the surgical neonate. *Clinics in Perinatology, 16,* 233–253.

Philippart, A. I., Reed, J. O., & Georgeson, K. E. (1975). Neonatal small left colon syndrome: Intramural not intraluminal obstruction. *Journal of Pediatric Surgery, 10,* 733–740.

Pickering, L. K., & Adcock, E. W. (1980). Gastrointestinal disorders in infants. *Family Practice Annual, 2,* 57–76.

Poland, R. L., & Ostrea, E. M. (1993). Neonatal hyperbilirubinemia. In M. H. Klaus & A. A. Fanaroff (Eds.), *Care of the high-risk neonate* (4th ed., pp. 302–322). Philadelphia: W. B. Saunders.

Quinn, D., & Shannon, L. (1996). Congenital anomalies of the gastrointestinal tract: III. The colon and rectum. *Neonatal Network, 15*(2), 63–67.

Rabinowitz, J. G., & Siegle, R. L. (1976). Changing clinical and roentgenographic patterns of necrotizing enterocolitis. *American Journal of Roentgenology, 126,* 560–566.

Reyes, H. M., Meller, J. L., & Loeff, D. (1989). Neonatal intestinal obstruction. *Clinics in Perinatology, 16,* 85–96.

Reyna, T. M. (1994). Familial Hirschsprung's disease: Study of a Texas cohort. *Pediatrics, 94,* 347–349.

Richey, D. A. (1990). Transporting the infant with an abdominal wall defect. *Neonatal Network, 9,* 53–56.

Richman, R. A., Sheehe, P. R., McCanty, T., et al. (1988). Olfactory deficits in boys with cleft palate. *Pediatrics, 82,* 840–844.

Ricketts, R. R. (1984). Workup of neonatal intestinal obstruction. *American Surgeon, 50,* 517–521.

Ricketts, R. R. (1994). Surgical treatment of necrotizing enterocolitis and the short bowel syndrome. *Clinics in Perinatology, 21,* 365–387.

Roberts, F. B. (1977). *Perinatal nursing: Care of newborns and their families.* New York: McGraw-Hill.

Rushton, C. H. (1990). Necrotizing enterocolitis: Part II. Treatment and nursing care. *MCN American Journal of Maternal Child Nursing, 15*(5), 309–313.

Ryckman, F. C., Flake, A. W., & Balistreri, W. F. (1992). Upper gastrointestinal disorders. In A. A. Fanaroff & R. J. Martin (Eds.), *Neonatal-perinatal medicine: Diseases of the fetus and infant* (5th ed., pp. 1024–1029). St. Louis: C. V. Mosby.

Sadler, T. W. (1985). *Langman's medical embryology* (5th ed.). Baltimore: Williams & Wilkins.

Santulli, T. V., Schullinger, J. N., Heird, W. C., et al. (1975). Acute necrotizing enterocolitis in infancy: A review of 64 cases. *Pediatrics, 55,* 376–387.

Scanlon, J. W., Nelson, T., Grylack, L. J., & Smith, Y. F. (1979). *A system of newborn physical examination.* Baltimore: University Park Press.

Schneider, E. L. (1973). Lip pits and congenital absence of second premolars: Varied expression of the lip pits syndrome. *Journal of Medical Genetics, 10,* 346–349.

Schober, P. H., & Nassiri, J. (1994). Risk factors and severity indices in necrotizing enterocolitis. *Acta Paediatrica, 83*(Suppl. 396), 49–52.

Seashore, J. H. (1978). Congenital abdominal wall defects. *Clinics in Perinatology, 5,* 61–77.

Seashore, J. H., Collins, F. S., Markowitz, R. I., & Seashore, M. R. (1987). Familial apple peel jejunal atresia: Surgical, genetic, and radiographic aspects. *Pediatrics, 80,* 540–544.

Seashore, J. H., & Touloukian, R. J. (1994). Midgut volvulus: An ever-present threat. *Archives Pediatrics and Adolescent Medicine, 148,* 43–46.

Shah, C. P., & Wong D. (1980). Management of children with cleft lip and palate. *Canadian Medical Association Journal, 122,* 19–24.

Shanbhogne, R. L. K., Hussain, S. M., Meradji, M., et al. (1994). Ultrasonography is accurate enough for the diagnosis of intussusception. *Journal of Pediatric Surgery, 29*(2), 324–328.

Shiels, W. E. (1995). Childhood intussusception: Management perspectives in 1995. *Journal of Pediatric Gastroenterology and Nutrition, 21,* 15–17.

Sigalet, D. L., Nguyen, L. T., Adolph, V., et al. (1994). Gastroesophageal reflux associated with large diaphragmatic hernias. *Journal of Pediatric Surgery, 29,* 1262–1265.

Sinatra, F. R., & Rosenthal, P. (1987). Cholestasis in the neonate. In G. B. Avery (Ed.), *Neonatology: Pathophysiology and management of the newborn* (3rd ed., pp. 630–637). Philadelphia: J. B. Lippincott.

Sinkin, R. A., Phillips, B. L., & Adelman, R. D. (1985). Elevation in systemic blood pressure in the neonate during abdominal examination. *Pediatrics, 76,* 970–972.

Spitz, L., Kiely, E. M., Morecroft, J. A., & Drake, D. P. (1994). Oesophageal atresia: At-risk groups for the 1990s. *Journal of Pediatric Surgery, 29,* 723–725.

Stoll, B. J. (1994). Epidemiology of necrotizing enterocolitis. *Clinics in Perinatology, 21*, 205–218.

Stringer, M. D., Brereton, R. J., Drake, D. P., et al. (1994). Meconium ileus due to extensive intestinal aganglionosis. *Journal of Pediatric Surgery, 29*, 501–503.

Styer, G. W., & Freeh, K. (1981). Feeding infants with cleft lip and/or palate. *Journal of Obstetric, Gynecologic, and Neonatal Nursing, 10*, 329–332.

Sugar, E. C. (1981). Hirschsprung's disease. *American Journal of Nursing, 81*, 2065–2067.

Sunshine, P., Sinatra, F. R., Mitchell, C. H., & Santulli, T. V. (1983). The gastrointestinal system. In A. A. Fanaroff & R. J. Martin (Eds.), *Behrman's neonatal-perinatal medicine: Diseases of the fetus and infant* (3rd ed., pp. 477–535). St. Louis: C. V. Mosby.

Surana, R., Quinn, F. M. J., & Puri, P. (1994). Short-gut syndrome: Intestinal adaptation in a patient with 12 cm of jejunum. *Journal of Pediatric Gastroenterology and Nutrition, 19*, 246–249.

Swaniker, F., Guo, W., Fonkalsrud, E. W., et al. (1995). Adaptation of rabbit small intestinal brush-border membrane enzymes after extensive bowel resection. *Journal of Pediatric Surgery, 30*, 1000–1003.

Taylor, E. J. (Ed.). (1988). *Dorland's illustrated medical dictionary* (27th ed.). Philadelphia: W. B. Saunders.

Touloukian, R. J. (1978). Intestinal atresia. *Clinics in Perinatology, 5*, 3–18.

Tsakayannis, D. E., & Shamberger, R. C. (1995). Association of imperforate anus with occult spinal dysraphism. *Journal of Pediatric Surgery, 30*, 1010–1012.

Warner, B. W., & Ziegler, M. M. (1993). Management of the short bowel syndrome in the pediatric population. *Pediatric Clinics of North America, 40*, 1335–1350.

Wells, P. W., & Meghdadpour, S. (1988). Research yields new clues to cystic fibrosis. *MCN, American Journal of Maternal Child Nursing, 13*, 187–190.

Yazbeck, S., & Bensoussan, A. L. (1987). Omphalocele and gastroschisis. In L. Stern & P. Vert (Eds.), *Neonatal medicine* (pp. 1078–1081). New York: Masson Publishing.

Young, T. E., & Mangum, O. B. (1997). *Neofax 97: A manual of drugs used in neonatal care* (10th ed.). Columbus, OH: Ross Products Division, Abbott Laboratories.

Zheng, J. Y., Frush, D. P., & Guo, J. Z. (1994). Review of pneumatic reduction of intussusception: Evolution not revolution. *Journal of Pediatric Surgery, 29*, 93–97.

Zink, M. (1985). Biliary atresia: Nursing diagnoses and management. *Journal of Enterostomal Therapy, 12*, 128–139.

CHAPTER 13

Assessment and Management of Metabolic Dysfunction

ROUTINE NEONATAL SCREENING TESTS

The purpose of routine neonatal screening for metabolic disease is to search for the population of subjects with a certain genotype, or change of the gene structure, either already associated with the disease or predisposed to the disease. There are reliable tests to screen infants on a large scale, and these disorders should receive priority in detection:

- Phenylketonuria
- Congenital hypothyroidism
- Galactosemia
- Maple syrup urine disease
- Congenital adrenal hyperplasia

Newborn screening, the purpose of which is to diagnose shortly after birth those infants with genetic diseases for which early treatment will prevent or minimize serious, irreversible complications or even death, is not mandated by the federal government.

PRENATAL AND NEONATAL DIAGNOSIS OF INHERITED METABOLIC DISORDERS

The prenatal diagnosis of inherited metabolic disorders is not often indicated. In the analysis and investigation of metabolic disorders, a positive screening test must be followed by complementary determinations of compounds. For example, a positive screening test for phenylketonuria (PKU) must be followed by determining the levels of phenylalanine, tyrosine, orthohydroxy-phenylacetic acid, phenylpyruvic acid, and urinary biopterins to confirm the diagnosis and specify the exact type of hyperphenylalaninemia (Blaskovics, Schaeffler, & Hack, 1974; Qu, Miller, Slocum, & Shapira, 1991; Scriver, Kaufman, Eisensmith, & Woo, 1995). This confirmational stage is critical.

History and Clinical Manifestations

When an infant is being evaluated for an inherited metabolic disorder, the history and clinical manifestations may include the following:

- History of recurrent spontaneous abortions
- Unexplained neonatal deaths or psychomotor deficiencies in the family
- Evidence of consanguinity for autosomal recessive disorders
- Previous children with a history of hypoglycemia, acute encephalopathy,

ataxia, metabolic acidosis, hepatomegaly, or acute episodes of "intoxication" or vomiting
- Circumstances leading to the onset of symptoms
  - Interval of variable duration—intermittent or cyclic
- Neurologic manifestations:
  - Hypotonia
  - Hypertonia
  - Lethargy
  - Alternating hyperexcitability
  - Somnolence
  - Myoclonia
  - Abnormal eye movements
  - Alteration in levels of consciousness
- Vomiting
- Diarrhea
- Poor feeding
- Weight loss
- Dehydration
- Failure to thrive
- Hepatomegaly with hyperbilirubinemia
- Hemorrhagic syndrome and splenomegaly
- Unusual odor of the infant's breath or sweat
- Unusual odor or color of the urine

Laboratory Tests

Laboratory tests to be ordered may include the following:

- Serum glucose determination
- Acid–base determination
- Ammonia level
- Complete blood cell count
- Coagulation studies

The following should be evaluated to rule out other causes:

- Serum electrolytes
- Calcium
- Magnesium
- Blood urea nitrogen
- Creatinine
- Urine ketones (Acetest)
- Urine reducing sugars (Clinitest)
- Urine glucose (Clinistix)
- Urine phenylpyruvic acid (Phenistix)
- Urine toxicology

CARBOHYDRATE METABOLISM

Glucose occupies a unique position in intermediary metabolism for two reasons: (1) the substrate of glycolysis is the sole pathway that produces adenosine triphosphate (ATP) in anaerobic life, and (2) glucose is the major substrate of brain metabolism.

The main dietary carbohydrates are starch, sucrose, and lactose, which are hydrolytically degraded into the free sugars glucose, fructose, and galactose.

Glucose is utilized by all tissues of the body, and its penetration into muscle and adipose tissue is controlled by insulin. As the primary regulator of blood glucose, the liver takes up glucose during times of abundance after meals and converts it mostly to glycogen. The liver uses very little of this glucose for its own energy needs but instead consumes mostly fatty acids. By the breakdown of glycogen and gluconeogenesis during times of fasting, the liver delivers a large amount of glucose to the blood for utilization by the brain, erythrocytes, and other tissues. The concentration of glucose in the blood is the primary stimulus that elicits glucose uptake or glucose output by the liver. The hepatic threshold of glucose is the glucose concentration at which the liver is converted from an organ of glucose output to an organ of glucose uptake (Burman, Holton, & Pennock, 1978; Cornblath & Schwartz, 1966; Cornblath, Wybregt, & Bacens 1963).

Disorders of Carbohydrate Metabolism

Defects in hydrolysis or absorption result in retention of residues in the intestinal tract and gastrointestinal symptoms. Carbohydrate intolerance is a common clinical problem and may have serious consequences, particularly when it occurs in early life.

The predominant symptoms of carbohydrate intolerance are intestinal. The osmotic pressure of the unabsorbed carbohydrate in the small intestine leads to a secretion of water and electrolytes into the lumen until osmotic equilibrium is reached. A proportion of the carbohydrate may be excreted unchanged in the stool, but the majority is hydrolyzed (reduced) by ideal and colonic bacteria to small carbohydrate molecules, short-chain organic acids, hydrogen, carbon dioxide, and other fermentative products. The organic acids lower the stool pH, inhibit water absorption from the colon, and contribute to the increased mobility (Burman, Holton, & Pennock, 1978; Wapnir, 1985; Winick, 1979).

Watery acid diarrhea with excoriated buttocks is the *hallmark of carbohydrate intolerance,* and fluid losses may be profound and life threatening. Dehydration may be complicated by metabolic acidosis. Large amounts of bicarbonate are secreted into the intestinal lumen to neutralize the contents and hydrogen ions produced by bacterial fermentation of the carbohydrate (Burman, Holton, & Pennock, 1978). Untreated lactose intolerance in infancy can lead to a more generalized malabsorption of other sugars, nitrogen compounds, and fats, with further impairment of nutrition.

The most important information is obtained from a detailed dietary history, linking the symptoms to carbohydrate ingestion. This linkage requires full knowledge of the composition of infant formulas and weaning foods.

An empirical diagnosis based on the history, clinical manifestations, and stool examination results in the prescription of lactose-free, disaccharide-free, or even carbohydrate-free diets (Winick, 1979). The diagnosis is confirmed later after stabilization and recovery.

The examination of stools includes the measurement of reducing substances, glucose, carbohydrate chromatography, pH, and organic acid content (Burman, Holton, & Pennock, 1978; Cornblath & Schwartz, 1966; Schmidt, 1989; Wapnir, 1985; Winick, 1979). The indices are listed below:

- Concentrations of the reducing substances of more than 0.25 percent, 1+ glucose
- Stool pH of less than 6.0

All tests must be performed on the liquid portion of fresh stool specimens, preferably collected on nonabsorbent material. The tests must be performed immediately, because fecal bacteria hydrolyze sugars very rapidly at room temperature and pH decreases and lactic acid content increases quickly (Burman, Holton, & Pennock, 1978; Wapnir, 1985). All stools must be tested, because some specimens may be carbohydrate free even in infants with severe intolerance (Burman, Holton, & Pennock, 1978).

Tests for reducing substances of stool are very useful but can result in false-positive and false-negative results. Antibiotic therapy and type of sugar in the diet must be considered in interpreting the results of the measurements of pH and sugar in stools. Carbohydrate chromatography may be necessary to test the significance of the stool-reducing substances.

The shape of the blood sugar curve after ingestion of an oral sugar load is a measure of absorption, whereas the symptoms after ingestion (coupled with stool examination) indicate clinical intolerance (Burman, Holton, & Pennock, 1978; Scriver, Beaudet, Sly, Valle, 1995; Wapnir, 1985).

Breath tests have also been used diagnostically. If $^{14}CO_2$ is recovered in the breath after oral ingestion of ^{14}C radioactive-labeled compound, at least a portion of the compound has been absorbed and metabolized (Burman, Holton, & Pennock, 1978).

Hydrogen breath tests do not require the use of radioactive-labeled compounds. The amount of hydrogen excreted in the breath correlates well with the amount produced in the intestine by fermentation of carbohydrates. Breath hydrogen measurement is the most accurate, sensitive, and specific indirect test for detecting lactose deficiency.

Disorders of Galactose Metabolism

Three inherited abnormalities of galactose metabolism are known. They are transmitted by autosomal recessive inheritance. Metabolic disorders result from a deficiency of galactokinase, galactose 1-phosphate uridyltransferase, or uridine diphosphate (UDP) galactose 4-epimerase, the enzymes of the pathway converting galactose to glucose.

Clinical features of these disorders are listed here:

- Galactokinase deficiency: mild clinical symptoms; cataracts
- Galactose 1-phosphate uridyltransferase deficiency: failure to thrive, vomiting, liver disease, cataracts, and developmental delay
- Long-term complications, despite a lactose-free diet:
  - Poor growth
  - Speech abnormality
  - Mental deficiency
  - Neurologic syndromes
  - Ovarian failure in females

- Uridine diphosphate galactose 4-epimerase deficiency (two forms): one is benign and one is clinically similar to transferase deficiency and responds to a restriction of dietary galactose.

Most galactose in the diet is in the form of the disaccharide lactose, which is synthesized in the mammary gland from glucose. Lactose is the primary carbohydrate source for nursing mammals and provides approximately 40 percent of the energy in human milk (Winick, 1979).

Lactose digestion is initiated by the hydrolysis of the disaccharide into absorbable monosaccharides glucose and galactose. Hydrolysis of lactose by the galactosidase lactase occurs in the brush border of the small intestine.

The main pathway of galactose metabolism is the conversion of galactose to glucose. In the normal pathway of galactose metabolism, galactose is phosphorylated with ATP to form galactose-1-phosphate. The galactose-1-phosphate reacts with uridine diphosphate glucose (UDP-glucose) catalyzed by galactose-1-phosphate uridyltransferase to produce two products, glucose-1-phosphate and UDP-galactose. Classic galactosemia occurs as a result of a block in this step. The UDP-galactose formed is converted to UDP-glucose by UDP-galactose 4-epimerase. The UDP-glucose formed can then serve as a substrate for the transferase reaction. These reactions function in a cyclic fashion until all of the galactose-1-phosphate entering the pathway from galactose is converted to glucose-1-phosphate and subsequently to glucose (Scriver, Beaudet, Sly, & Valle, 1995).

When no galactose is introduced to the pathway from an external source, protective processes do exist to produce galactose and its metabolites, which are critical to the formation of complex lipids and glycoprotein. If galactose is unable to be metabolized owing to a deficiency or inefficiency of galactokinase, transferase, or epimerase, two alternate pathways are available. Galactose can be reduced to galactitol by aldolase reductase or oxidized to galactonate by an oxidase or dehydrogenase (Scriver, Beaudet, Sly, & Valle, 1995).

HEREDITARY GALACTOKINASE DEFICIENCY

This autosomal recessive disorder of galactose metabolism is caused by a deficiency in the enzyme galactokinase.

Incidence

The incidence varies from 1 in 40,000 to 1 in 155,000 across European populations.

Clinical Manifestations and Diagnosis

Because galactokinase-deficient newborns are asymptomatic, or develop cataracts as their first and only abnormality, the diagnosis in early infancy depends on the routine screening of blood and urine for galactose.

The diagnosis can be made by the finding of normal amounts of galactose-1-phosphate uridyltransferase and an absence of galactokinase in the red blood cells (Gitzelmann, 1967; Scriver, Beaudet, Sly, & Valle, 1995). High blood galactose levels are best detected after milk feedings. The presence of reducing substances in the urine may be identified as galactose. The urine of any newborn with cataracts should be examined for sugar with a method that does not use glucose oxidase.

The nuclear cataracts develop from an accumulation of galactitol in the lens. The trapped galactitol causes swelling and disruption of lens fibers. The formation of cataracts is caused by a complex sequence of events, including disturbances in the balance of water, electrolytes, amino acids, proteins, energy-rich phosphates, and reduced glutathione (Crawford, Gibbs, & Watts, 1982; Scriver, Beaudet, Sly, & Valle, 1995).

Collaborative Management

Treatment with a galactose exclusion diet must be continued throughout life (Levy & Hammersen, 1978; Winick, 1979).

HEREDITARY GALACTOSE-1-PHOSPHATE URIDYLTRANSFERASE DEFICIENCY

This autosomal recessive disorder results from a deficiency of galactose-1-phosphate uridyltransferase, which catalyzes the metabolism of galactose-1-phosphate to galactose to UDP (Ampola, 1982; Burman, Holton, & Pennock, 1978; Galjaard, 1980; Levy & Hammersen, 1978; Wapnir, 1985; Winick, 1979).

Incidence

The incidence of this deficiency is 1 in 155,000 live births.

Diagnosis

The absence of transferase activity of erythrocytes is the basis for diagnosing galactosemia (Levy & Hammersen, 1978; Scriver, Beaudet, Sly, & Valle, 1995). The presumptive diagnosis may be made by the identification of galactose in urine and blood. Although this is a useful, noninvasive screening test, normal newborns may excrete up to 60 mg/dl of galactose in the first 5 days of life, and this level may be detected for up to 2 weeks in premature infants (Dahlqvist & Svenningsen, 1969).

Clinical Manifestations

Infants with galactosemia have normal birth weights but fail to gain weight after they start ingesting milk. Usually symptoms appear in the second half of the first week of life and include jaundice, vomiting, and diarrhea (Ampola, 1982; Burman, Holton, & Pennock, 1978; Levy & Hammersen, 1978; Wapnir, 1985; Winick, 1979). Many of the affected newborns receive exchange transfusions before diagnosis. Nuclear cataracts appear within days or weeks and become irreversible within weeks (Ampola, 1982; Burman, Holton, & Pennock, 1978; Levy & Hammersen, 1978; Scriver, Beaudet, Sly, & Valle, 1995). If milk feedings continue, the disease usually progresses, resulting in abnormal results of liver function tests, hepatomegaly, cirrhosis, and death. There also appears to be a high frequency of *Escherichia coli* sepsis and neonatal death in infants with transferase deficiency galactosemia (Levy et al., 1977), probably owing to inhibition of leukocyte bactericidal activity (Litchfield & Wells, 1978).

In general, the clinical manifestations of the disorder are reversed a few weeks after initiation of appropriate treatment, but the long-term outcome and intellectual development are uncertain. Follow-up of galactosemic individuals has shown that many have developed very well, whereas others have had more severe problems involving growth, development, brain function, and, in females, ovarian dysfunction (Ampola, 1982; Burman, Holton, & Pennock, 1978; Komrower, 1980; Levy & Hammersen, 1978; Lloyd & Scriver, 1985; Scriver, Beaudet, Sly, & Valle, 1995; Winick, 1979).

HEREDITARY URIDINE DIPHOSPHATE GALACTOSE 4-EPIMERASE DEFICIENCY

This disorder, inherited as a recessive trait, is due to the absence of UDP galactose 4-epimerase in the blood.

Incidence

The incidence is 1 in 23,000 in Japan, where there are screening programs.

Clinical Manifestations

Two forms of UDP galactose 4-epimerase deficiency exist. The benign condition, which is more common, is due to the absence of UDP galactose 4-epimerase in the blood. The only metabolic consequence of galactose ingestion is the elevation of galactose 1-phosphate in red cells, without any further red cell abnormality (Scriver, Beaudet, Sly, & Valle, 1995).

In contrast, a severe form exists in which UDP galactose 4-epimerase activity is absent in liver and other tissues as well as in red blood cells. The clinical presentation is similar to transferase deficiency with jaundice, vomiting, weight loss, hepatomegaly, aminoaciduria, and galactosuria (Henderson, Holton, & MacFaul, 1983; Scriver, Beaudet, Sly, & Valle, 1995).

Collaborative Management

Treatment includes providing small amounts of dietary galactose that will not produce toxicity but will be adequate for galactoprotein and galactolipid synthesis (Scriver, Beaudet, Sly, & Valle, 1995).

Disorders of Fructose Metabolism

Fructose is metabolized predominantly in the liver, kidney, and small intestine and, to a lesser extent, in adipose tissue. Three inherited abnormalities are known, and all are autosomal recessive traits:

- Essential fructosuria is a benign, asymptomatic disorder caused by the absence of fructokinase, resulting in hyperfructosemia and fructosuria.
- Hereditary fructose intolerance is characterized by hypoglycemia and vomiting after the ingestion of fructose. In infants, prolonged fructose ingestion leads to poor feeding, vomiting, jaundice, hepatomegaly, hem-

orrhage, and potentially hepatic failure and death. The disorder results from a deficiency of fructose 1-phosphate aldolase in the liver, kidney cortex, and small intestine. Hypoglycemia after fructose ingestion is caused by fructose l-phosphate inhibiting glycogenolysis and gluconeogenesis. Patients remain healthy on a diet free of fructose and sucrose.

- Hereditary fructose 1,6-diphosphatase deficiency is characterized by episodes of hyperventilation, apnea, hypoglycemia, ketosis, and lactic acidosis. Gluconeogenesis is severely impaired owing to the enzyme defect and leading to accumulation of amino acids, lactate, and ketones (gluconeogenic precursors) as liver glycogen stores are depleted.

Glycogen Storage Diseases

All proteins involved in the synthesis or degradation of glycogen or its regulation have been discovered to cause some type of glycogen storage disease. In these disorders the quantity or the quality of glycogen is abnormal. The different types of glycogen storage diseases have been categorized by numerical type in the chronological order of the identification of the disorder.

Most seriously affected tissues are liver and muscle—the tissues with the most abundant quantities of glycogen. The liver is responsible for maintaining plasma glucose through its regulation of carbohydrate metabolism. Thus, glycogen storage diseases have hepatomegaly and hypoglycemia as the most common presenting features. The role of glycogen in muscle is to provide substrates that enable the ATP generation necessary for muscle contraction. The predominant features of glycogen storage diseases that primarily affect the muscle include the following:

- Muscle cramps
- Exercise intolerance
- Susceptibility to fatigue
- Progressive weakness

TYPE I GLYCOGEN STORAGE DISEASE

Type Ia glycogen storage disease (von Gierke disease) results from a deficiency of glucose-6-phosphatase activity in the liver, kidney, and intestinal mucosa. Excessive accumulation of glycogen occurs in these tissues. The clinical manifestations of this disorder include growth retardation, hepatomegaly, hypoglycemia, lacticacidemia, hyperuricemia, and hyperlipidemia. A variant caused by the transport of glucose-6-phosphate (type 'Ib) has the additional findings of neutropenia and impaired neutrophil function, resulting in recurrent bacterial infections and gastrointestinal ulceration. Defects in microsomal phosphate or pyrophosphate transport (type Ic) and in microsomal glucose transport (type Id) have been identified.

In the past, the prognosis for type I glycogen storage disease was associated with a high mortality. The morbidity in the survivors included gout, hepatic adenomas, osteoporosis, renal disease, and short stature. Continuous nocturnal feedings of glucose or of uncooked cornstarch are effective for sustaining the metabolic indices of adequate therapy. With early diagnosis and initiation of therapy, the prognosis for type I glycogen storage disease has markedly improved. Normal growth and pubertal development can now be achieved, and many patients who have survived to adulthood have no evidence of hepatic adenomas or symptoms of gout.

TYPE II GLYCOGEN STORAGE DISEASE

Type II glycogen storage disease (Pompe disease) is caused by a deficiency of lysosomal acid α-glucosidase. It is the prototype of a lysosomal storage disease that results from inherited inborn errors of metabolism.

TYPE III GLYCOGEN STORAGE DISEASE

Type III glycogen storage disease results from a defect in the glycogen debranching enzyme activity. A deficiency in this enzyme impairs the release of glucose from glycogen but not from gluconeogenesis. The glycogen that accumulates resembles dextrin. Patients with type II glycogen storage disease have both liver and muscle involvement (type IIIa). A small percentage of patients have only liver involvement (type IIIb), without apparent muscle disease. During infancy, both forms of type III disease resemble type I disease with hepatomegaly, hypoglycemia, hyperlipidemia, and growth retardation as clinical manifestations. However, in type III disease, the blood lactate and uric acid levels are normal and increases in hepatic transaminases are prominent. The hepatic symptoms actually improve with age. Overt liver cirrhosis is rare. In those patients with muscle involvement (type IIIa), muscle weakness increases with age, manifested by progressive weakness and distal muscle wasting. There may be ventricular hypertrophy and electrocardiographic abnormalities.

Treatment is symptomatic. Frequent meals high in carbohydrates, cornstarch supplements, or nocturnal continuous gastric feedings are effective in treating hypoglycemia. There is no effective treatment for the progressive myopathy or cardiomyopathy.

TYPE IV GLYCOGEN STORAGE DISEASE

Type IV glycogen storage disease results from a deficiency of branching enzyme activity that causes the accumulation of glycogen with unbranched, long, outer chains in the tissues. This form appears frequently in the first year of life with hepatomegaly and failure to thrive. Hypoglycemia is rare. Progressive liver cirrhosis with portal hypertension, ascites, esophageal varices, and death occurs before age 5 years. Liver transplantation may be an effective treatment for the hepatic manifestations. However, because type IV disease affects other tissues, the long-term success of liver transplantation is not yet known.

TYPE V GLYCOGEN STORAGE DISEASE

Type V glycogen storage disease (McArdle disease) results from a deficiency of muscle phosphorylase activity. Symptoms usually appear in adulthood and present as exercise intolerance, muscle cramps, and myoglobinuria. Avoidance of exercise prevents the symptoms, and there is no need for specific therapy.

TYPE VI GLYCOGEN STORAGE DISEASE

Type VI glycogen storage disease is a heterogeneous group of disorders caused by a deficiency of the liver phosphorylase system. Clinical manifestations occur in early childhood with hepatomegaly and growth retardation. Mild hypoglycemia and hyperlipidemia are found occasionally. Lactic acid and uric acid levels are normal. Treatment is symptomatic and includes frequent feedings and a high carbohydrate diet. These disorders are considered benign forms of glycogen storage disease, and most patients do not require any therapy. Prognosis is good; adult patients have normal stature and minimal hepatomegaly. Type VI is inherited as an X-linked pattern, in contrast to the other glycogen storage diseases, which are transmitted in an autosomal recessive manner.

TYPE VII GLYCOGEN STORAGE DISEASE

Type VII glycogen storage disease is caused by a deficiency of muscle phosphofructokinase activity. The clinical manifestations include exercise intolerance, muscle cramps, and myoglobinuria similar to type V glycogen storage disease. However, in type VII glycogen storage disease there is usually a compensated hemolytic anemia, early-onset myogenic hyperuricemia, and a glucose-induced exertional fatigue.

AMINO ACID METABOLISM

Amino acids play a major role as constituents of intracellular and extracellular proteins. Essential amino acids have to be derived from exogenous sources such as dietary protein and nonprotein nitrogen. Estimates of the daily requirements of these essential amino acids (isoleucine, leucine, lysine, methionine, phenylalanine, threonine, tryptophan, and valine) have been made. Although histidine is not an essential amino acid, its presence is essential for the normal growth of the infant (Nyhan, 1984).

Alanine, arginine, asparagine, aspartic acid, cysteine, glutamic acid, glutamine, glycine, histidine, proline, serine, and tyrosine can be synthesized from a reduced form of nitrogen and a carbon skeleton. Major sources of the carbon chain are α-ketoglutarate, pyruvate, and oxaloacetate, and the reduced form of nitrogen becomes available from recycling of other compounds (Nyhan, 1984).

Synthesis of any protein is a complex multistep process that results in macromolecule formation from the 20 individual amino acids in a specific sequence that is under genetic control. There are two basic steps of all protein synthesis: (1) DNA that has the genetic code for the protein makes RNA; and (2) RNA makes the protein from cytosolic amino acids.

Gastrointestinal digestion and absorption of released amino acids are well developed in neonates. This is evidenced even in small preterm infants by the total stool nitrogen content, which does not exceed 15 percent of intake (Nyhan, 1984; Stave, 1978).

Disorders of Amino Acid Metabolism

AMINO ACID DISORDERS THAT INVOLVE A SPECIFIC ENZYME DEFICIENCY

The Hyperphenylalaninemias

The hyperphenylalaninemias are disorders of phenylalanine hydroxylation. Hyperphenylalaninemia (plasma phenylalanine levels above 2 mg/dl [120 μmol]) is a heterogeneous disease caused by mutations at the genetic sites that encode components of the hydroxylation reaction. The known and putative forms involve the following:

- Primary deficiency in phenylalanine hydroxylase activity (phenylketonuria [PKU] and nonphenylketonuria [non-PKU])
- Impaired synthesis of tetrahydrobiopterin (BH4) due to enzyme deficiency
- Impaired recycling of BH4 due to deficient activity of dihydropterin reductase (DPHR) or other putative enzyme systems

Overall incidence is approximately 100 cases per 1 million live births among whites and Asians. Non-PKU is less prevalent than PKU and it shows less variation in the incidence (15 to 75 cases per 1 million live births).

Associated diseases are autosomal recessive. Two conditions are necessary to cause clinical manifestations—the genetic mutation and exposure to L-phenylalanine. In the BH4-deficient forms, mutation alone is the principal cause of the disease. Infants with PKU have plasma values >1000 μmol; infants with non-PKU hyperphenylalaninemia have plasma values < those of PKU-affected infants. PKU is a disease of impaired cognitive and neurophysiologic consequences; non-PKU hyperphenylalaninemia signifies less clinical harm and may be a benign condition. The BH4-deficient forms of the hyperphenylalaninemias have no categorical degree of hyperphenylalanine; they impair two other hydroxylation reactions involving tyrosine and tryptophan and the synthesis of the corresponding neurotransmitter derivatives (L-dopa and 5-hydroxytryptophan). Pathogenesis of the brain disorder in the different hyperphenylalaninemias involves the effects of phenylalanine on essential cellular processes in the brain, notably myelination, protein synthesis, and the consequences of deficient neurotransmitter supply.

Genes that encode the components of the hydroxylation reaction are at various stages of analysis in normal and mutant genomes. Loci on chromosomes 4, 12, and 14 have been identified as having a role in the hydroxylation reactions associated with hyperphenylalaninemia.

Newborn screening is the best method of screening for hyperphenylalaninemia.

Maternal hyperphenylalaninemia compromises fetal growth and causes congenital malformations, including microcephaly and mental retardation.

Treatment requires restoration of blood phenylalanine levels to values as near normal as possible for as long as possible throughout life. The BH4-deficient forms of hyperphenylalaninemias require adjunct therapy, including supplements of L-dopa and 5-hydroxytryptophan, and of BH4 in disorders of the cofactor synthesis and of folinic acid in DHPR deficiency.

The Hypertyrosinemias

Tyrosine is obtained from two sources in humans: dietary intake and hydroxylation of phenylalanine. Degradation of tyrosine occurs primarily in the liver and is both glucogenic and ketogenic. The rate of tyrosine degradation is determined by the activity of tyrosine aminotransferase.

Most inborn errors of tyrosine catabolism produce hypertyrosinemia. Hypertyrosinemia may also occur in various acquired conditions, including severe hepatocellular disease.

Hepatorenal hypertyrosinemia, or type I tyrosinemia, is an autosomal recessive disease caused by a deficiency of fumarylacetoacetate hydrolase. Symptoms are highly variable and include the following:

- Acute liver failure
- Cirrhosis
- Hepatocellular carcinoma
- Renal Fanconi's syndrome
- Glomerulosclerosis
- Crises of peripheral neuropathy

In untreated patients, the tyrosine levels are elevated. The presence of increased levels of succinylacetone in plasma or urine is diagnostic of this condition. There may be a partial response to dietary restriction of tyrosine and phenylalalnine in many patients. Hepatic transplantation cures the liver manifestations and prevents further neurologic crises. Treatment with 2-(2-nitro-4-trifluoromethylbenzoyl)-1,3-cyclohexanedione (NTBC), an inhibitor of 4-hydroxyphenylpyruvate dioxygenase (pHPPD), has been reported to cause a marked improvement in hepatic and renal function.

Type II tyrosinemia is a deficiency of the enzyme tyrosine aminotransferase, which results in oculocutaneous tyrosinemia. The ocular and cutaneous symptoms are characterized by palmoplantar keratosis and painful corneal erosions associated with photophobia. Half of the reported patients have mental retardation. The ocular and cutaneous symptoms respond to dietary restriction of tyrosine and phenylalanine.

Type III tyrosinemia results in three different conditions associated with dysfunction of the enzyme pHPPD:

- Primary pHPPD deficiency
- Hawkinsinuria
- Transient tyrosinemia of the newborn

Primary pHPPD deficiency has been in two case reports of neurologically abnormal individuals. Biochemically, the patients demonstrated hypertyrosinemia and elevated urinary excretion of 4-hydroxyphenyl derivatives.

Hawkinsinuria is an autosomal dominant condition putatively caused by dysfunction of pHPPD. It results in acidosis and failure to thrive in infancy. Hypertyrosinemia is minimal or absent. The urinary excretion of hawkinsin, an amino acid thought to be an intermediate of the pHPPD reaction, is diagnostic for this condition. Symptoms may respond to dietary protein restriction and to the administration of ascorbate.

Transient tyrosinemia of the newborn results from a combination of pHPPD immaturity, elevated tyrosine and phenylalanine intake, and a relative ascorbate deficiency. Improvement is spontaneous but can be accelerated by the administration of ascorbate and by dietary protein restriction, especially of tyrosine and phenylalanine. The vast majority of children with transient tyrosinemia are asymptomatic and recover without adverse effects on development.

DISORDERS OF HISTIDINE METABOLISM

The two known disorders of histidine metabolism are histidinemia and urocanicaciduria. *Histidinemia* is an autosomal recessive trait and is due to a defect in histidase, which catalyzes the conversion of histidine to urocanic acid. This enzyme is most readily identified in the stratum corneum of the skin. As a result of the metabolic block, there is an increased concentration of histidine in the blood, urine, and cerebrospinal fluid (CSF) and a decreased concentration of urocanic acid in the blood and the skin. Histidine metabolites are increased in the urine. Histidinemia seems to be benign in most individuals, although some reports exist of neurologic dysfunction.

Urocanicaciduria is an autosomal recessive disorder. The enzyme urocanase is defective and cannot catalyze the conversion of urocanic acid to imidazolonepropionic acid. In this apparently benign disorder, an increase in urinary urocanic acid is the only known metabolic aberration.

Initially discovered in 1961, histidinemia has been found to be the most frequent and well-known disorder of histidine metabolism. In various world locations where neonatal screening is routinely performed, the incidence is 1 in 11,500 in over 20 million screened infants. The incidence is particularly high in Japan, with incidences reported as high as 1 in 8000.

Deficiency of urocanic acid in histidinemia may have implications for the putative functions of urocanic acid as a natural sunscreen against ultraviolet light and as a mediator of ultraviolet light–induced immunosuppression.

Atypical histidinemia is a biochemically milder form. Maternal histidinemia is most likely benign. Histidinuria without histidinemia has been reported.

NONKETOTIC HYPERGLYCINEMIA

Nonketotic hyperglycinemia is an inborn error of glycine degradation in which large amounts of glycine accumulate in all tissues, including the central nervous system. The diagnosis is established by calculating the CSF:plasma ratio of glycine. A value greater than 0.08 is diagnostic. The diagnosis is confirmed by measuring the activity of the glycine cleavage enzyme system in liver tissue.

The neonatal form is the most common presentation, occurring within the first few days of life. There is lethargy, pronounced hypotonia, and myoclonic jerking progressing to apnea and often death. Those infants who do regain spontaneous respirations develop intractable seizures and profound mental retardation.

A transient form of hyperglycinemia has been described in newborns with symptoms indistinguishable from those of the neonatal form. The elevated glycine levels are identical to those found in the neonatal form but return to normal by 8 weeks of age.

Glycine is a neurotransmitter. It functions to inhibit the neurotransmission in the spinal cord, and it is excitatory in the cortex. Excessive stimulation of the cortical brain is thought to be responsible for the seizures and brain damage.

The primary metabolic defect is in the glycine enzyme cleavage system found within the mitochondria. The glycine cleavage enzyme system consists of four components: a pyridoxal-phosphate-dependent glycine decarboxylase (P protein); a lipoic-acid-containing hydrogen carrier protein (H protein); a tetrahydrofolate-dependent protein (T protein); and lipoamide dehydrogenase (L protein). In the neonatal form of the disease, the P protein is defective. Metabolic variations in this disease may reflect defects in the T, H, or L proteins.

The gene for the P protein has been mapped to chromosome 9. Nonketotic hyperglycinemia is inherited as an autosomal recessive trait.

No effective treatment exists.

Neonatal Nonketotic Hyperglycinemia

This is the most common form of the disease, and patients present in a strikingly similar manner. The infants typically are products of normal, uncomplicated pregnancies with appropriate growth in all parameters at birth. No external congenital anomalies are present. The symptom-free interval ranges from 6 hours to 8 days, with 66 percent of the patients becoming symptomatic by 48 hours (Dalla Benardina, Aicardi, Goutieres, & Plouin, 1979). There is a progressive development of hypotonia, lethargy, and refusal to feed. Wandering eye movements and increased deep tendon reflexes are present. As the encephalopathy progresses to coma, the infant develops frequent segmental myoclonic jerks, apneic episodes, and hiccoughs. Most infants require assisted ventilation in the first weeks of life (Scriver, Beaudet, Sly, & Valle, 1995).

The diagnosis is established by determining the CSF:plasma ratio of glycine (Perry et al., 1975; Scriver, Beaudet, Sly, & Valle, 1995). Plasma concentrations of glycine in this disorder range from high normal to values eight times the normal mean and four times the upper normal limit. Urinary glycine levels are usually increased but may be difficult to interpret owing to the physiologic hyperglycinuria seen in the newborn period. Thus, screening urine for glycine is not useful in the diagnosis. The CSF concentration of glycine is elevated (15 to 30 times normal) to a much greater extent than the plasma levels. A CSF:plasma ratio of more than 0.08 is considered diagnostic of nonketotic hyperglycinemia. The normal CSF:plasma ratio of glycine is consistently less than 0.02. Patients with atypical nonketotic hyperglycinemia have ratios around 0.09, whereas neonatal patients have ratios ranging from 0.2 to 0.3 (Scriver, 1995). Definitive diagnosis can be established by measuring the glycine cleavage enzyme system activity of liver tissue. This procedure requires a liver biopsy and is not feasible in critically ill neonates.

Despite neonatal intensive care, approximately 30 percent of these patients die in the neonatal period. Those who survive usually regain spontaneous respirations by 3 weeks of age, and survival is reported to range from several months to 22 years. Most patients regain the ability to suck, but many must be gavage fed. If untreated, infants develop intractable seizures by age 12 months but rarely before 3 months. The seizure pattern evolves with the initial development of myoclonic jerks, progressing to infantile spasms, partial motor seizures, and/or tonic extension. Severe psychomotor retardation and little adaptive or social behavior is the usual outcome. Spastic quadriplegia replaces the initial hypotonia (Scriver, Beaudet, Sly, & Valle, 1995).

The electroencephalogram (EEG) progresses from an early initial burst-suppression pattern to a hypsarrhythmia pattern. It usually does not correlate to the clinical findings. After 1 year of age, the sleep and awake EEG patterns differ. During sleep, the hypsarrhythmia pattern is routine but the awake tracing reveals a slow background with lack of normal wake and sleep components and frequent independent multifocal spike discharges (Scriver, Beaudet Sly, & Valle, 1995). All patients have prolonged latencies on the auditory evoked responses, suggesting a slowing of the conduction system along the brain stem auditory pathway (Markland, Garg, & Brandt, 1982).

DISORDERS OF TRANSSULFURATION OF AMINO ACIDS

The transsulfuration pathway converts the sulfur atom of methionine into the sulfur atom of cysteine. This pathway is the chief route of disposal of methionine and explains why cysteine is not an essential amino acid in humans. Two additional metabolic sequences are also involved: the transmethylation reaction, by which the methyl group of methionine is ultimately transferred to form any of a host of methylated compounds, and the reformation of methionine by methylation of homocysteine (Nyhan, 1984). At least nine specific genetic disorders have been recognized that affect this metabolic pathway. Only three disorders are discussed here: methionine adenosyltransferase (MAT) deficiency, cystathionine beta-synthase (CBS) deficiency, and gamma-cystathionase deficiency.

A deficiency of MAT has been found in newborns screened for hypermethioninemia. All were clinically well at ages ranging to 38 years. Residual hepatic MAT activity was present in varying amounts, and the MAT activity of tissues other than the liver was normal.

CBS deficiency is the most frequently encountered cause of homocystinuria. Homocystine, methionine, and homocystine metabolites accumulate in the body or are excreted in the urine. Dislocation of the optic lens, osteoporosis, thinning and lengthening of the long bones, mental retardation, and thromboembolism are the most common clinical features. It is an autosomal recessive trait with considerable genetic heterogeneity.

CBS activity may range from none to a small percentage of residual activity. A small amount of residual activity may be required for clinical responsiveness to pyridoxine administration. Pyridoxine-responsive individuals have more slowly developing or milder manifestations of the disease.

Frequency of CBS deficiency detected by newborn screening for hypermethioninemia is 1 in 344,000 live births.

Management of CBS-deficient individuals involves the amelioration of the characteristic biochemical abnormalities with the use of low-methionine, cystine-supplemented diets. If the patient is pyridoxine responsive, then treatment with pyridoxine should be ordered. Dietary restriction in the newborn period has been shown to prevent mental retardation and possibly decrease the incidence of seizures. Pyridoxine treatment has been shown to decrease the incidence of initial thromboembolic events.

Gamma-cystathionase deficiency leads to persistent excretion of large amounts of cystathionine in the urine and accumulation of cystathionine in body tissues and fluids. There are no clinical abnormalities characteristically associated with this disorder. The deficiency is inherited as an autosomal recessive trait and likely has considerable genetic heterogeneity.

AMINO ACID DISORDERS THAT INVOLVE DEFECTS IN MEMBRANE TRANSPORT SYSTEMS

Cystinuria

Cystinuria is a defect of the amino acid transport affecting the epithelial cells of the renal tubule and the gastrointestinal tract. The defective transport of cystine, lysine, arginine, and ornithine is transmitted as an autosomal recessive trait. The heterozygous state may reflect true recessive or incompletely recessive inheritance. In the latter, the affected amino acids are excreted in urine in quantities greater than normal but less than in the homozygous state.

The intestinal defect is demonstrated by oral loading tests and by intestinal perfusion studies. The dibasic amino acids can be absorbed by cystinuric subjects in a normal fashion as dipeptides.

Renal lesions of all four amino acids and the mixed disulfide of cysteine-homocysteine are demonstrated by clearance studies. The clearance of cystine in adults with cystinuria is frequently greater than the glomerular filtration rate, suggesting active secretion. Affected kidneys have demonstrated a defect in the transport system for the dibasic amino acids but not for cystine. Cystine and the dibasic amino acids appear to share the low-saturation, high-affinity renal cortical transport system that is probably defective in the cystinuric kidney. There is probably an interaction of cystine and the dibasic amino acids at the luminal membrane of the renal tubule cells, which may play an important role in the regulation of cystine transport into renal cortical cells.

Cystinuria is expressed clinically as urinary tract calculus disease. Cystine stones are formed and cystine crystals appear in the urine. Diagnosis may be pursued by testing urine with nitroprusside, electrophoresis, or column amino acid analysis. Stones generally form when cystine is excreted at rates greater than 300 mg cystine per gram of creatinine in acid urine. Cystinuric patients are susceptible to all complications of stone disease. Treatment is aimed at reducing the concentration of cystine in urine by increasing urine volume, increasing cystine solubility by alkalinizing urine, and reducing cystine excretion by the use of drugs.

Hartnup Disorder

Hartnup disorder is an autosomal recessive impairment of neutral amino acid transport limited to the kidneys and small intestine. It is postulated that the disorder results from a genetic defect in the specific carrier for neutral amino acid transport across the brush border membrane of renal and intestinal epithelium. The diagnostic feature is the marked neutral aminoaciduria. Most affected individuals also have an increased excretion of indolic compounds. These indolic compounds arise from the intestine from bacterial degradation of unabsorbed tryptophan. Reduced intestinal absorption of tryptophan and increased tryptophan loss in the urine lead to reduced availability of tryptophan for the synthesis of niacin.

Pellagra-like clinical features have been described in patients with this disorder. Some affected individuals have also been mentally retarded to some degree. Treatment with nicotinamide has been associated with clearing of the rash and, on occasion, disappearance of ataxia. This has led researchers to suggest that the clinical manifestations are due to niacin deficiency. Renal and intestinal defects are not always expressed concordantly. Maternal Hartnup disorder is probably benign.

Most infants identified by newborn screening, as well as affected sibs of probands, have remained clinically well without treatment. Clinical expression of the disorder depends on the genetic defect, the predisposition to low amino acid levels, and environmental influences, such as poor diet or diarrhea.

DISORDERS OF BRANCHED-CHAIN AMINO AND KETO ACIDS: MAPLE SYRUP URINE DISEASE

Maple syrup urine disease (MSUD), or branched-chain ketoaciduria, is caused by a deficiency in the activity of the branched-chain alpha-keto acid dehydrogenase (BCKAD) complex. This metabolic block results in the accumulation of branched-chain amino acids (BCAAs) leucine, isoleucine, and valine and the corresponding branched-chain alpha-keto acids (BCKAs).

MSUD is divided into five phenotypic classes (classic, intermediate, intermittent, thiamine-responsive, and dihydrolipoyl dehydrogenase deficient) based on the clinical presentation and biochemical responses to thiamine administration. Classic MSUD has a neonatal onset of encephalopathy and is the most severe and common form. Persons with variant forms of MSUD generally have the initial symptoms by 2 years of age. The levels of BCAAs, especially leucine, are greatly increased in plasma and urine. Activity of BCKAD complex in skin fibroblasts or lymphoblast cultures is reduced and ranges from less than 2 percent of normal in the classic form to 30 percent of normal in the variant forms. The E3-deficient MSUD presents a combined deficiency of BCKAD, pyruvate dehydrogenase, and α-ketoglutarate dehydrogenase complexes.

MSUD is an autosomal recessive disorder of panethnic distribution. The worldwide incidence is 1 per 185,000 based on routine screening of 26.8 million newborns. In the inbred Old Order Mennonite population of Lancaster and Lebanon counties in Pennsylvania, MSUD occurs in approximately 1 in 176 newborns.

The BCAAs constitute about 35 percent of the indispensable amino acids in muscle and 40 percent of the preformed amino acids required by humans. The catabolic pathways for BCAAs begin with the transport of these amino acids into cells where they undergo reversible transamination by isoforms of the branched-chain aminotransferase to produce BCKA. Leucine is catabolized to α-ketoisocaproate, isoleucine is catabolized into α-keto-β-methylvalerate, and valine is catabolized into α-ketoisovalerate. Oxidative decarboxylation of the BCKA is catalyzed by the single BCKAD multienzyme complex generating the respective branched-chain acyl coenzymes A (CoA) that are further metabolized into separate pathways. The end products of leucine catabolism are acetyl CoA and acetoacetate. Valine yields succinyl CoA, and isoleucine produces acetyl CoA and succinyl CoA. BCAAs are the precursors for fatty acids and cholesterol synthesis through acetyl CoA. These amino acids are also substrates for energy production by means of succinyl CoA and acetoacetate.

The oxidation of BCAA occurs primarily in the liver, kidney, heart, and adipose tissue. There is evidence that transamination is the rate-limiting step in the catabolism of BCAA in the liver where aminotransferase activity is low. In extrahepatic tissues, oxidative decarboxylation of the alpha-keto acids is the rate-limiting step. A significant portion of BCKA appears to originate from the skeletal muscle and circulates to the liver, where it is oxidized.

The human BCKAD genes have been located on different chromosomes, including chromosomes 19, 6, 1, and 7. The genomic structure including the regulatory and promoter regions of the genes of the BCKAD complex have been characterized.

The majority of infants with untreated classic MSUD die within the early months of life of recurrent metabolic crisis and neurologic deterioration. Treatment involves both long-term dietary management and aggressive intervention during acute metabolic decompensation. Advances in both aspects of treatment have considerably decreased the morbidity, mortality, and length of individual hospitalization for patients during the 1990s. The age at diagnosis and the subsequent metabolic control are the most important determinants of long-term outcome. Patients in whom treatment is initiated after 10 days of age rarely achieve normal intellect.

There has been a successful pregnancy in a patient with classic MSUD. The major concerns are the stress of pregnancy on the metabolic homeostasis and the rapidly changing nutritional requirements during the course of pregnancy. These parameters require intensive monitoring.

Organic Acidemias: Disorders of Propionate and Methylmalonate Metabolism

Propionyl CoA is formed by the catabolism of several essential amino acids, odd-chain fatty acids, and cholesterol. It is metabolized primarily by enzymatic conversion to methylmalonyl CoA, which is subsequently converted into succinyl CoA. This metabolic sequence is dependent on the activity of several enzymes: propionyl CoA carboxylase, methylmalonic CoA racemase, and methylmalonic CoA mutase. Propionyl CoA requires biotin as a cofactor, whereas methylmalonyl CoA mutase requires a cobalamin (vitamin B_{12}) coenzyme—adenosylcobalamin.

Propionyl CoA carboxylase is composed of nonidentical subunits (alpha and beta) with biotin binding occurring only on the alpha subunit. The alpha subunit is regulated by a gene found on chromosome 13, whereas the beta subunit is regulated by a gene located on chromosome 3. Methylmalonyl CoA mutase has two identical subunits regulated by a gene on chromosome 6.

Isolated deficiency of propionyl CoA carboxylase is a major cause of ketotic hyperglycinemia syndrome. It results from the accumulation of propionate in the blood and of 3-hydroxypropionate, methylcitrate, triglycine, and unusual ketone bodies in urine. Clinically, the disorder is characterized by severe metabolic ketoacidosis, which often appears in the neonatal period and requires vigorous alkali therapy and protein restriction to reverse. Oral antibiotic therapy to reduce gut propionate production may also be useful.

Inherited deficiency of methylmalonic CoA mutase activity is caused by gene mutations at many different loci. Neonatal or infantile metabolic ketoacidosis is the clinical hallmark of isolated methylmalonic CoA mutase deficiency. Cells may have zero mutase activity, or the mutase may be structurally altered when it was synthesized and has a decreased affinity and reduced stability for adenosylcobalamin. These infants exhibit methylmalonicacidemia and methylmalonicaciduria that does not respond to cobalamin supplementation but can be treated with dietary protein restriction. Oral antibiotic therapy may also be useful.

Abnormalities of adenosylcobalamin synthesis lead to impaired methylmalonyl CoA mutase activity and the clinical manifestations identical to those seen in methylmalonic CoA mutase deficiency. In most of these infants, large pharmacologic doses of cyanocobalamin produce a distinct reduction in methylmalonate accumulation and offer a valuable adjunct to dietary protein restriction.

All of the disorders of propionate and methylmalonate metabolism for which there are adequate data are inherited as autosomal recessive traits. There is considerable genetic heterogeneity of the phenotype even among siblings.

Prenatal diagnosis of fetuses with propionyl CoA carboxylase deficiency, methylmalonyl CoA mutase deficiency, and defective synthesis of adenosylcobalamin has been accomplished by assays of cells from chorionic villus sampling or cultured amniotic fluid cells and by chemical determinations on amniotic fluid or maternal urine.

METHYLMALONICACIDEMIAS

The methylmalonicacidemias include two distinct defects in the mutase enzyme, two distinct defects of adenosylcobalamin synthesis, and three distinct defects of both adenosylcobalamin and methylcobalamin synthesis (Fenton & Rosenberg, 1995).

Clinical presentation includes lethargy, failure to thrive, recurrent vomiting, dehydration, respiratory distress, and muscular hypotonia (Fenton & Rosenberg, 1995; Matsui, Mahoney, & Rosenberg, 1983). Less commonly, the disorder presents as developmental retardation, hepatomegaly, or coma. Patients with the least enzymatic activity present earlier, usually within the first week of life, than those with some residual activity, who present later in the neonatal period.

The laboratory findings include normal serum cobalamin levels and metabolic acidosis, with blood pH values as low as 6.9 and serum bicarbonate levels as low as 5 mEq/L. Ketonemia or ketonuria is present in 80 percent of the cases, and hyperammonemia is only slightly less common. Leukopenia and thrombocytopenia are present in more than half of the patients (Matsui, Mahoney, & Rosenberg, 1983).

Diagnosis of methylmalonicacidemia must be considered in any infant in whom acidosis and ketosis develop after birth. After other sources of neonatal acidosis and infantile ketosis have been eliminated, blood and urine assays for methylmalonate must be obtained. If excessive amounts of methylmalonate are found in the urine, cobalamin deficiency can be determined by direct measurement of serum cobalamin.

Two treatment protocols exist and should be employed in tandem. A protein-restricted diet or a diet restricted in amino acid precursors of methylmalonate should be instituted as soon as life-threatening problems such as ketoacidosis, hypoglycemia, and hyperammonemia have been addressed. Supplementary cobalamin should be instituted as soon as the diagnosis of methylmalonicacidemia is seriously considered (Fenton & Rosenberg, 1995). Such measures have been shown to decrease the levels of methylmalonic and propionic acid. As is the case with propionicacidemia, the administration of L-carnitine has been shown to improve the clinical symptoms. Oral antibiotic therapy has been shown to improve appetite, decrease vomiting, increase growth, improve behavior, and decrease the number and severity of acidotic episodes (Scriver, Beaudet, Sly, & Valle, 1995).

Response to supplementary cobalamin and long-term outcome in affected patients depend on the nature of the biochemical abnormality causing the methylmalonicacidemia. The long-term outcome for affected patients with complete absence of enzyme activity is poorest, with the greatest mortality and degree of neurologic impairment. The affected patients who respond to cobalamin administration have the best long-term outcome (Shevell, Matiaszuk, Ledley, & Rosenblatt, 1993).

Lacticacidemia: Disorders of Pyruvate Carboxylase and Pyruvate Dehydrogenase

Lactic acid that circulates in the body is the product of the anaerobic metabolism of glucose that takes place primarily in red cells, skin, kidney medulla, and white skeletal muscle. Some of it is oxidized by red muscle and kidney cortex, but the bulk is taken up by the liver and made into glucose. Lactate is always produced by the reduction of pyruvate through lactate dehydrogenase and is always removed by a reversal of this process. The oxidation of pyruvate proceeds through pyruvate dehydrogenase, the tricarboxylic acid (Krebs) cycle, and the respiratory chain. Anaerobic utilization proceeds primarily through pyruvate carboxylase. A defect in any of these pathways may lead to inadequate removal of pyruvate and lactate from the circulation and lacticacidemia results.

Deficiency of pyruvate dehydrogenase complex is the most common of the disorders leading to lacticacidemia. It may be caused by a defect in the E1, E2, E3, X-lipoate, or pyruvate dehydrogenase phosphatase component of the complex. The most common of these is the defect in the E1 component. The clinical presentation of this disorder has a graded spectrum from most severe to least severe.

In its most severe form, it presents with overwhelming lactic acidosis at birth, with death in the neonatal period. In the second form of the disorder, the lacticacidemia is moderate but there is quite profound psychomotor retardation with increasing age, and in many patients concomitant damage to the basal ganglia and brain stem, leading to death in infancy. In the third form of the disorder, found only in males, there is carbohydrate-induced ataxic episodes coupled with mild developmental delay.

The E1 defects are caused by mutations in the E1 alpha gene, which is X linked. Males and females are equally affected, even though only one X chromosome in females carries the mutation. Thus, this disorder is classified as X-linked dominant. The E2 and protein X-lipoate defects are rare and result in severe psychomotor retardation. The E3 lipoamide dehydrogenase defect leads to deficient activity not only in the pyruvate dehydrogenase complex but also in the α-ketoglutarate and BCKAD complexes. Pyruvate dehydrogenase phosphatase deficiency has been documented in four cases. The most common pathologic feature of deficiency of pyruvate dehydrogenase complex is the development of cystic lesions in the cerebral cortex, basal ganglia, and brain stem.

Pyruvate carboxylase deficiency has three clinical presentations. In the simple form of the disease, the patient presents in the first few months of life with a mild to moderate lacticacidemia and delayed development. Survivors have severe mental retardation. These patients are believed to have some residual enzyme activity. In the more complex form of the disease, the patient presents soon after birth with a severe lacticacidemia accompanied by hyperammonemia, citrullinemia, and hyperlysinemia. These patients are believed to have no residual enzyme activity and rarely survive beyond 3 months of age. In a single case, a patient presented with only episodic attacks of lactic acidosis and with no psychomotor retardation.

Pyruvate Kinase Deficiency

Pyruvate kinase (PK) deficiency is the most common enzyme defect of anaerobic glycolysis. It results in a hereditary hemolytic anemia, has been documented to occur worldwide, and is characterized by lifelong chronic hemolysis of variable severity. Splenectomy often results in amelioration of the hemolytic process in more severely affected patients. The defective PK enzyme in affected erythrocytes results in increased concentrations of 2,3-diphosphoglycerate (2,3-DPG) and decreased ATP, relative to cells of comparable age.

PK deficiency is inherited as an autosomal recessive trait. Heterozygous carriers usually have 40 to 60 percent of the normal red cell PK activity, and they do not have any significant hematologic or clinical abnormalities. In the absence of consanguinity, clinically affected patients are usually compound heterozygotes with two mutant alleles. Thus, they have two intracellular mixtures of defective PK enzymes, which complicates the interpretation of the biochemical data. Genes encoding the principal natural PK enzymes have been identified, resulting in hemolytic anemia.

Glucose-6-Phosphate Dehydrogenase Deficiency

Glucose-6-phosphate dehydrogenase (G6PD) is an enzyme found in all cells that catalyzes the first step in the hexose monophosphate pathway. It produces the reduced form of nicotinamide-adenine dinucleotide phosphate (NADPH), which is required for reactions of various biosynthetic pathways as well as the preservation and regeneration of the reduced form of glutathione. Because catalase and glutathione are essential for detoxification of hydrogen peroxide, the defense of cells against this compound depends ultimately and heavily on G6PD. This is especially true of red cells, which are exquisitely sensitive to oxidative damage and in which other NADPH-producing enzymes are lacking.

The gene that encodes the protein for G6PD has been mapped to the long arm of the X chromosome. Therefore, one of the two G6PD alleles is subject to inactivation in females.

G6PD is the most commonly known red blood cell enzyme deficit. It is estimated to affect over 400 million people worldwide. The highest incidences are found in tropical Africa, in the Middle East, in tropical and subtropical Asia, in some areas of the Mediterranean, and in Papua New Guinea. The prevalence rates vary in these geographic regions from 5 to 25 percent.

The most common clinical manifestations are neonatal jaundice and acute hemolytic anemia. In some cases the hyperbilirubinemia is severe enough to cause permanent neurologic sequelae or death. The active hemolytic anemia is triggered by a number of drugs, by infections, or by the ingestion of fava beans. In a proportion of cases, the hemolysis can be life threatening. The mechanism of hemolysis is thought to occur as a result of the inability of red cells to withstand the oxidative damage produced, directly or indirectly, by the triggering agent. Red cell destruction is largely intravascular; therefore, there is hemoglobinuria. In between episodes of hemolytic anemia, most G6PD-deficient individuals are asymptomatic. A very small proportion of G6PD-deficient individuals have a chronic hemolytic disorder, which might be quite severe.

G6PD is genetically heterogeneous. Numerous different variants have been reported on the basis of diverse biochemical characteristics. This diversity suggests that these variants result from many allelic mutations in the G6PD gene seen in different parts of the world where this abnormality is prevalent. Genetic heterogeneity also explains the diversity of clinical manifestations.

LIPID METABOLISM

Lipids are a heterogeneous group of substances that can be extracted from tissues. Three main classes of lipids—fatty acids, triglycerides, and phospholipids—function as insulation and an energy source and provide structure to cell membranes. Fat insulation consists mainly of triglycerides packed densely into adipocytes. Triglycerides are hydrolyzed into fatty acids and glycerol, which serve as an energy source. Phospholipids provide an important component of all cellular membranes.

Classes of Lipids

FATTY ACIDS

The sources of fatty acids in the blood are the supply of fat in the diet and the release of fatty acids from adipose tissue. In suckling infants, there is a high level of fatty acids in the blood and there is greater fatty acid utilization at this time than at any time before birth or after weaning (Ampola, 1982; Stave, 1978; Wapnir, 1985). Fatty acids are synthesized in two metabolic pathways: malonyl-CoA and reversal of β-oxidation. The rate of fatty acid synthesis is greater in the fetus than in the adult. This rate of fatty acid synthesis decreases rapidly after birth, possibly linked to the accumulation of some metabolite (glycerol, fatty acids, and acyl-CoA) and the rise in the rate of gluconeogenesis, which decreases the availability of citrate (Stave, 1978; Wapnir, 1985). Fatty acid oxidation occurs in the mitochondria. As opposed to the passive, gradient-dependent transport across cell membranes, fatty acids must be converted from acyl-CoA to acylcarnitine to be transported across the mitochondrial membrane. Once inside the mitochondrion, the acylcarnitine is reassembled into acyl-CoA and oxidized (Scriver, Beaudet, Sly, & Valle, 1995; Stave, 1978).

Oxidation of fatty acids requires more oxygen than does oxidation of carbohydrates. After birth, fatty acid oxidation is greatly enhanced. In brown fat, fatty acid oxidation is completely dependent on the presence of carnitine and ATP. Carnitine is also important for acetate oxidation and for optimum ketone production by liver mitochondria. Lysine is the precursor of carnitine, and when protein ingestion is severely limited, there may also be a carnitine deficiency (Scriver, Beaudet, Sly, & Valle, 1995; Stave, 1978).

The liver lacks the enzyme needed for the transfer of CoA from succinyl-CoA to acetoacetate. Thus, the final products of fatty acid oxidation in the liver are the ketone bodies—acetoacetic acid, β-hydroxybutyric acid, and acetone. The rate of ketone body production depends on the supply of fatty acids to the liver. Fatty acids from the blood enter the liver in large amounts after birth. In the liver, the fatty acids are broken down into ketone bodies, which are then transported to other tissues and organs where they serve as a source of energy (Stave, 1978).

TRIGLYCERIDES

The triglyceride blood level is dependent on fat absorption from the intestines, the release of triglycerides from the liver, and the removal of triglycerides from the blood. Triglycerides cannot serve as an immediate energy source, because they must first be hydrolyzed into fatty acids and glycerol. In the blood, triglycerides are transported as lipoproteins and are removed from the blood by many tissues. After birth, chylomicrons appear in the blood 1 to 3 days after feedings have been initiated (Stave, 1978). The major storage site of triglycerides is adipose tissue.

Lipogenesis is the process in which fatty acids combine with CoA to form acyl-CoA. Three molecules of acyl-CoA and glycerol-3-phosphate combine to form a triglyceride molecule. Lipolysis is not a reversal of the synthetic process. The rate of fatty acid synthesis requires a sufficient supply of glycerol-3-phosphate. If fatty acid levels accumulate, the excess acyl-CoA inhibits further fatty acid synthesis and glycolytic reactions. In lipolysis, triglycerides are hydrolyzed by tissue lipases into fatty acids and glycerol. Glycerol-3-phosphate arises by phosphorylation of glycerol by glycerol kinase. The glycerol released from adipose tissue during lipolysis can be used for energy only after being phosphorylated (Stave, 1978).

PHOSPHOLIPIDS

Phospholipids are any lipid molecules that contain a radical derived from phosphoric acid. Phospholipids are an important part of cell walls and cell particle membranes, myelin sheaths, and lung secretions. The composition of fatty acids in phospholipids changes considerably with age and in various organs. Fatty acid composition of phospholipids is less dependent on dietary changes than is that of triglycerides.

Relationships Between Glucose and Fatty Acid Metabolism

The metabolism of fatty acids cannot be discussed without discussing the relationships between glucose and fatty acid metabolism. Several control points exist at which it is determined whether glucose or fatty acids will be predominantly synthesized or oxidized. For example, glucose synthesis is promoted by fatty acid oxidation. A high-fat diet enhances gluconeogenesis and fatty acid oxidation and results in a decrease in lipid synthesis. The elevated level of fatty acids supplied to the newborn after birth is responsible for the decreased rate of glycolysis in the liver and the brain, the increased rate of acetoacetate formation, the decreased rate of fatty acid synthesis in the liver, and the postnatal increase in the rate of gluconeogenesis (Ampola, 1982; Wapnir, 1985). After birth, the rate of fatty acid oxidation and ketone body formation increases dramatically, owing to sympathetic stimulation of lipolysis in adipose tissue and the resulting increased fatty acid delivery to the liver.

Disorders of Lipid Metabolism

Disorders of lipid metabolism may affect any component of fatty acid, triglyceride, or phospholipid synthesis or degradation. Disorders of lipid metabolism may also affect β-oxidation of fatty acids in the mitochondria. General clinical manifestations of a lipid metabolic disorder include vomiting, changes in level of consciousness, metabolic acidosis, sweaty feet odor, severe hypoglycemia without ketosis, hyperammonemia, and hepatic and/or muscular lipid accumulation. This clinical presentation may occur acutely after birth or intermittently. The fulminant neonatal course is rapidly fatal.

LIPOPROTEIN DISORDERS

Very low density lipoproteins (VLDL) and chylomicrons, which transport triglycerides to the peripheral tissues in the blood, are major lipoprotein secretory products of the liver and intestine. Each class of these lipoproteins contains a protein of high molecular weight (a β-lipoprotein) that is essential for the secretion of the lipoprotein particle and that has a high affinity for lipids, remaining with the lipoprotein complex throughout its metabolic processing in plasma or lymph. Familial β-lipoprotein deficiencies represent one of several classes of lipoproteins that are absent or are present in abnormally low concentrations in the plasma. Three most common types of disorders are abetalipoproteinemia, hypobetalipoproteinemia, and Tangier disease.

A single structural gene for β-lipoproteins is responsible for the synthesis of the two types of lipoproteins found in humans. The predominant β-lipoprotein of VLDL and low density lipoproteins (LDL) is apolipoprotein B-100. The predominant types of apolipoprotein B in chylomicrons is apolipoprotein B-48. Several disorders result from the abnormal secretion of apolipoprotein B–containing lipoproteins.

Abetalipoproteinemia is an autosomal recessive disorder characterized by the virtual absence of VLDL and LDL from plasma. Fat malabsorption is severe, and triglyceride accumulation occurs in erythrocytes and in the liver. Acanthocytosis of erythrocytes is common. Spinocerebellar ataxia, peripheral neuropathy, degenerative pigmentary retinopathy, and ceroid myopathy all appear to be secondary to defects of transport of tocopherol in blood. Intracellular accumulation of B protein results from an impairment in the assembly or secretion of triglyceride-rich proteins. The absence of activity of microsomal triglyceride transfer protein, a factor critical to the lipidation of B proteins, was the first recognized defect of lipoprotein deficiencies. Treatment involves the restriction of dietary fat to prevent steatorrhea and supplementation with tocopherol to prevent progression of the neuromuscular and retinal degenerative disease.

Clinical manifestations are indistinguishable from abetalipoproteinemia in the homozygous state: acanthocytosis, neuromuscular disability, and malabsorption. Clinically, this disorder is distinguished from recessive abetalipoproteinemia by the appearance of hypolipidemia in heterozygotes. The defects that underlie this disorder involve the gene for apolipoprotein B. A number of mutations have been identified that involve secretion of a truncated form of apolipoprotein B, abnormal rate of apolipoprotein B synthesis, or removal from the blood.

Chylomicron retention disease is characterized by fat malabsorption and the absence of chylomicrons in plasma after fat ingestion. Acanthocytosis and neurologic manifestations occur in some patients. Large numbers of nascent chylomicrons crowd the enterocyte, which results from a specific defect in the secretion of chylomicrons. High levels of apolipoprotein B-100 have been found in the cytoplasm and the endoplasmic reticulum of the enterocyte.

Familial combined hyperlipidemia is probably the most prevalent genetically determined disorder of lipoproteins. It carries a significantly increased risk of coronary atherosclerosis. It is recognized as an autosomal dominant trait with high penetrance that leads to high levels of apolipoprotein B-100 and elevated levels of VLDL, LDL, or both in plasma.

Abetalipoproteinemia

This autosomal disorder occurs as a result of the absence of apolipoprotein B and is characterized by very low plasma cholesterol and triglyceride levels. It has a higher incidence in Ashkenazic Jews, who constitute 25 percent of those affected (Ampola, 1982; Bickel, 1980; Scriver, 1995). It affects males more frequently than females, and there is good health of obligate heterozygotes. The clinical manifestations develop shortly after birth, with fat malabsorption, acanthocytosis, pigmented retinitis, and ataxia (Kane & Havel, 1995).

Malabsorption of fat is a central pathologic feature of abetalipoproteinemia. Steatorrhea occurs after birth and is associated with malabsorption of the fat-soluble vitamins A, D, E, and K. These infants are poor feeders and have frequent vomiting and voluminous steatorrheic stools, which results in somatic underdevelopment and failure to thrive. Hepatic steatosis occurs with severe disturbances in plasma lipid levels, which are less than 50 percent of normal. Triglyceride levels are often undetectable, phospholipid levels are lowered by 75 percent, and the cholesterol level is often less than 0.025 g/L. Unlike vitamins A and K, in which modest supplementation will achieve normal plasma levels, the transport of tocopherol is severely limited in this disorder. The abnormal lipoproteins of abetalipoproteinemia appear incapable of incorporating normal amounts of vitamin E even in the presence of relatively large supplements. Massive supplementation, however, somehow increases the flux into the body, eventually increasing the vitamin E levels in adipose tissue appreciably (Kane & Havel, 1995). The intestinal villi are normal but have a yellow discoloration of the mucosa that results from a greatly increased lipid content. Electron microscopy has demonstrated an increase in lipid droplets in the cells, even if no fat has been ingested for days (Kane & Havel, 1995). Despite the inability of the liver to secrete VLDL, abnormalities of liver function are uncommon.

Severe anemia develops secondary to abnormally shaped erythrocytes. Red cell survival is frequently shortened, and hyperbilirubinemia has been described. Reticulocytosis and erythroid hyperplasia occurs in many patients, suggesting that erythropoiesis is not notably impaired. Acanthocytosis is not found in the bone marrow, which suggests that the membrane changes leading to the malformation are acquired by contact with the plasma (Kane & Havel, 1995).

Ocular involvement presents as retinitis pigmentosa, decreased visual acuity, nystagmus, and ophthalmoplegia. The more severe cases of retinopathy occur in those patients with the more severe neurologic impairment, suggesting a common mechanism. Major pathologic features are the loss of photoreceptors, loss of pigmented epithelium, and relative preservation of submacular pigmented epithelium (Kane & Havel, 1995). These retinal changes closely resemble the retinopathy of vitamin E deficiency. Deficiency of vitamin A may also contribute to the retinopathy, and some patients benefit from additional supplementation. The onset of symptoms is variable. Compromise of visual acuity may occur during the first decade, although many cases have been asymptomatic until adulthood. Loss of night or color vision is often a presenting sign. Patients are frequently unaware of the slow progression of the ophthalmologic disease. Nystagmus and complete loss of vision can occur. Neuropathy affects the oculomotor nerve and results in ophthalmoplegia (Kane & Havel, 1995).

The most characteristic degenerative sites in the nervous system are the large sensory neurons of the spinal ganglia and their heavily myelinated axons. There is a progressive neuropathy and extensive demyelination of these areas. The first neurologic signs are diminution in the intensity of the deep tendon reflexes, which may occur in the first few years of life. Vibratory sense and proprioception tend to be lost progressively, and an ataxic gait develops. Neurologic problems are evident in 35 percent of the children by 10 years of age. By 20 years of age, there is mild to severe ataxia and intellectual deficits (Ampola, 1982; Bickel, 1980; Kane & Havel, 1995; Wapnir, 1985). Untreated patients are unable to stand by the third decade. Muscle contractions are common, leading to pes cavus, pes equinovarus, and kyphoscoliosis. Muscle weakness is a frequent feature of this disorder. The clinical determination that myopathy is present tends to be obscured by the frequent presence of degenerative peripheral neuropathy. Cardiomyopathy may lead to death early in the second decade of life (Kane & Havel, 1995). Slow neuromuscular development has been recorded in a number of cases. Attributing the developmental delay to this disorder is difficult because specific neuropathologic cerebral disease is lacking. In addition, slow neurologic development is common in infants who have steatorrhea and fail to thrive and may reflect nutritional deficiencies. Furthermore, because many patients with this disorder are products of consanguineous matings, other rare inborn errors may be responsible for the mental retardation.

The diagnosis of this disorder is suggested by the absence of apolipoprotein B, low serum cholesterol levels, low triglyceride levels, and plasma that has no chylomicrons (LeGrys, 1984). In addition, there are low levels of vitamins A, E, and K, of folic acid, and of iron (Ampola, 1982; Bickel, 1980; Kane & Havel, 1995).

Treatment includes early dietary restriction of long-chain triglycerides to control the gastrointestinal symptoms. Fatty acids derived from medium-chain triglycerides do not require the formation of chylomicrons for absorption. They are transported mainly by albumin as free fatty acids through the hepatic portal system and serve as energy substrate for the liver but are not necessary nutrients. Hepatic function should be followed in these patients receiving medium-chain triglyceride supplements. Infant formula should contain medium-chain triglycerides (Winick, 1979). Prolonged observation of vitamin E supplementation has shown that such supplementation does inhibit the progression of the neurologic disease and probably leads to the regression of symptoms even if it is started in adulthood (Kane & Havel, 1995).

The retinopathy may be prevented if therapy is started early, or it may be stabilized if disease is already present when therapy is started. The myopathy is also reversed with vitamin E therapy (Kane & Havel, 1995).

Treatment will require large doses (1000 to 10,000 mg/day) of oral vitamin E until the reliability and safety of parenteral preparations are established. Initiation of vitamin E therapy before the appearance of neurologic symptoms will prevent them. If vitamin A and carotene levels are low, additional supplementation may be of benefit. Because vitamin D has its own transport mechanism and because the symptoms of vitamin D deficiency are lacking in this disorder, no specific supplementation is necessary. Supplementation with vitamin K should be given if bruising, bleeding, or hypoprothrombinemia is present (Kane & Havel, 1995).

Familial Combined Hyperlipidemia

Familial combined hyperlipidemia was identified as a disease in studies of the survivors of myocardial infarction and their relatives. Three patterns of lipoprotein distribution were recognized: elevated plasma levels of VLDL or LDL or a combination of both. The pattern may change over time in an affected individual or within a family. Family pedigrees are compatible with an autosomal dominant pattern. Although evident in childhood, the manifestations are limited until about the third decade of life. Plasma triglyceride levels tend to distribute between 200 and 400 mg/dl but may be much higher. LDL levels are usually greater than 100 mg/dl. Most affected family members have apolipoprotein B levels greater than 85 mg/dl. Xanthoma formation is less common than in heterozygous familial hypercholesterolemia at similar LDL levels. The prevalence of familial combined hyperlipidemia is estimated at 1 to 2 percent of the population in North America and Europe. Treatment goals include the achievement of ideal body weight in addition to the restriction of cholesterol and saturated fats. Hypercholesterolemia appears to respond well to treatment with HMG-CoA reductase inhibitors. Triglyceride levels respond to a lesser extent. The addition of nicotinic acid often reduces the VLDL levels dramatically and appears to have a synergistic effect on LDL levels. The use of bile acid binding resins alone frequently increases the triglyceride level. The combined regimen of bile acid binding resins and nicotinic acid is often very effective.

Tangier Disease

Tangier disease is characterized by a severe deficiency or absence of normal high-density lipoproteins (HDL) in plasma and results in the accumulation of cholesterol esters in many tissues throughout the body, such as tonsils, liver, spleen, thymus, lymph nodes, intestinal mucosa, peripheral nerves, and the cornea.

Clinical manifestations include hyperplastic, orange tonsils, splenomegaly, and relapsing neuropathy. HDL deficiency and low plasma cholesterol concentration accompanied by normal or elevated triglyceride levels in combination with hyperplastic adenoidal tissue is pathognomonic. Despite the HDL deficiency, there is only a minimal risk of myocardial infarction.

Plasma apolipoprotein I concentration is less than 3 percent of controls, and the small amount of HDL in Tangier plasma differs from normal HDL. Chylomicron remnants and VLDL are very abnormal. Heterozygotes are asymptomatic and have half-normal concentrations of HDL, apolipoprotein I, and apolipoprotein II.

The molecular basis for the disease is still unknown but is likely related to a defect in the pathway in intracellular lipid transfer processes. There is no specific treatment for Tangier disease.

FAMILIAL HYPERLIPOPROTEINEMIA: FAMILIAL LIPOPROTEIN LIPASE DEFICIENCY

Familial lipoprotein lipase deficiency is one of three disorders in which chylomicrons accumulate in the plasma. Chylomicronemia can also occur in individuals with common familial forms of hypertriglyceridemia who also have an acquired cause of hypertriglyceridemia, such as untreated diabetes mellitus, estrogen or antihypertensive drug therapy, or alcohol use.

This rare autosomal recessive disorder is characterized by massive accumulation of chylomicrons in plasma and by a corresponding increase in the plasma triglyceride concentration. The concentration of VLDL may be normal.

The disorder is usually detected in childhood on the basis of repeated episodes of abdominal pain, recurrent attacks of pancreatitis, eruptive cutaneous xanthomatosis, and hepatosplenomegaly. The severity of the symptoms is directly related to the degree of hyperchylomicronemia, which, in turn, is related to dietary fat intake.

Over 30 structural defects in the lipoprotein lipase gene are associated with lipoprotein lipase defects. This lipolytic enzyme is present on the vascular endothelial cells of extrahepatic tissues and is essential for hydrolysis of chylomicron and VLDL triglycerides to provide free fatty acids to tissues for energy.

Diagnosis is based on low or absent enzyme activity and confirmed by demonstrating the defect in the structure of the lipoprotein lipase gene. The disorder is not associated with atherosclerotic vascular disease, but recurrent pancreatitis may threaten the patient's life.

Restriction of dietary fat to less than 20 g/day is usually sufficient to reduce plasma triglyceride levels and to keep the patient free from symptoms. Available lipid-lowering drugs are not effective.

Heterozygotes exhibit a 50 percent decrease in lipoprotein lipase but have normal or only slightly abnormal plasma lipid levels.

FAMILIAL CHOLESTEROLEMIA

Familial hypercholesterolemia is characterized by an elevated concentration of LDL, deposition of LDL-derived cholesterol in tendons and skin, and autosomal dominant inheritance.

Heterozygotes number approximately 1 in 500 persons, making familial hypercholesterolemia among the most common inborn errors of metabolism. Heterozygotes have twofold elevations in plasma cholesterol (350–550 mg/dl) from birth. Tendon xanthomas and coronary atherosclerosis develop after ages 20 and 30, respectively.

Homozygotes are more severely affected and number about 1 in 1 million persons. They have severe hypercholesterolemia (650–1000 mg/dl). Cutaneous xanthomas appear in the first 4 years of life. Coronary heart disease begins in childhood and frequently causes death from myocardial infarction before age 20.

The primary defect is an inability of the LDL receptors to bind with circulating LDL. When LDL receptors are deficient, the rate of removal of LDL from plasma declines and the level of LDL rises in inverse proportion to the receiver number. The excess plasma LDL is deposited in scavenger cells and other cell types, producing xanthomas and atheromas.

The LDL receptor gene has been mapped to chromosome 19. Five classes of mutations at the LDL receptor locus have been identified. Each class has been subdivided into multiple alleles and over 150 different mutant alleles have been described.

Heterozygotes have one normal and one mutant allele; thus, their cells are able to take up LDL at approximately one half the normal rate. Homozygotes show a total or near-total absence of LDL binding.

Treatment is directed at lowering plasma LDL. In heterozygotes, the most effective therapy is the administration of drugs that stimulate the single normal gene to produce additional messenger RNA for the LDL receptor, such as through the combined administration of a bile acid binding resin and an inhibitor of 3-hydroxy-3-methylglutaryl CoA reductase. These drugs enhance LDL receptor activity in the liver, which in turn increases LDL catabolism and decreases LDL production. Homozygotes with two nonfunctional genes are resistant to drugs that work by stimulating LDL receptors. Effective treatment can lead to a reduced rate of progression of coronary artery disease.

Disorders of Lysosomal Enzymes

GANGLIOSIDOSES

G_{M1} Gangliosidoses

This autosomal recessive disorder results from a deficiency of hydrolase ganglioside G_{M1} β-galactosidase (acid β-galactosidase), which normally uses ganglioside G_{M1} and galactose-containing glycoproteins as substrates (Scriver, 1995). As a result of this enzyme deficiency, ganglioside G_{M1} that is normal in composition accumulates in the gray matter of the brain and in lesser amounts in the liver (Ampola, 1982; Cohn & Roth, 1983; Scriver, 1995; Wapnir, 1985). Galactose-containing glycoprotein also accumulates in the liver (Ampola, 1982; Wapnir, 1985). The clinical manifestations are often evident at birth, with edema affecting the face and extremities and occasionally ascites. There is a poor appetite, weak sucking, ineffective swallowing, and subnormal weight gain. After several months, facial dysmorphism is apparent, with enlarged skull, large forehead, coarse facial features, flattened nose, low-set ears, macroglossia, and hypertelorism. There is progressive psychomotor deterioration. The infant has a dull expression, is hypoactive and hypotonic, and never learns to sit independently. Tonic-clonic seizures may develop. There is hepatomegaly (Ampola, 1982; Benson, 1983; Cohn & Roth, 1983; Scriver, Beaudet, Sly, & Valle, 1995; Wapnir, 1985). On ophthalmologic examination there is a cherry-red macular spot in 50 percent of these patients (Ampola, 1982; Scriver, Beaudet, Sly, & Valle, 1995; Wapnir, 1985). Survivors beyond the first year manifest decerebrate rigidity, blindness, deafness, spastic quadriplegia, and poor level of responsiveness. Death usually ensues by 3 years. Diagnosis of this disorder can be made by examination of bone marrow, liver, or spleen for the presence of foamy histiocytes (LeGrys, 1984; Scriver, Beaudet, Sly, & Valle, 1995). Prenatal diagnosis is possible. There is no treatment.

G$_{M2}$ Gangliosidoses

The G$_{M2}$ gangliosidoses are a group of inherited disorders caused by excessive intralysosomal accumulation of ganglioside G$_{M2}$, particularly in neuronal cells. Enzymatic hydrolysis of ganglioside G$_{M2}$ requires a substrate-specific cofactor. There are two isoenzymes of β-hexosaminidase. Defects in any of the three genes that regulate the synthesis of these proteins result in the accumulation of gangliosides in the cell. Only Tay-Sachs disease is discussed.

Clinical phenotypes in the G$_{M2}$ gangliosidoses vary widely, ranging from infantile onset, rapidly progressive neurodegenerative disease that culminates in death before age 4 years (Tay-Sachs) to later onset, subacute or chronic forms with more slowly progressive neurologic conditions compatible with survival into childhood or adolescence or with long-term survival. Chronic forms include several different presentations, including progressive dystonia, spinocellular degeneration, motor neuron disease, and psychosis.

At least 54 genetic mutations have been described. Most mutations are associated with the severe, infantile-onset disease. The subacute and chronic forms of the disease are associated with variable low levels of residual enzyme activity, with the level of activity correlating to severity.

All G$_{M2}$ gangliosidoses exhibit an autosomal recessive inheritance pattern. The defective genes have been mapped to chromosome 15 (HEX A) and chromosome 5 (HEX B and G$_{M2}$ activator/cofactor). Heterozygotes for any of the defects are completely asymptomatic.

Availability of rapid and inexpensive methods for identifying heterozygotes for HEX A defects has made large scale screening programs for family and population carriers possible. When combined with DNA-based diagnostics, the type of mutation (acute, subacute, or chronic) can be identified.

In the non-Jewish, general population, the incidence is approximately 6 in 1000 for HEX A and 36 in 10,000 for HEX B mutations. Of these mutations, about 35 percent are characterized by the acute, infantile type of disease and 5 percent are characterized by the chronic form.

Among the Ashkenazic Jews of North America and in Israel, a heterozygote frequency of 33 in 1000 was found for HEX A mutations, 95 percent of which were characterized as the infantile or acute form of the disease. Extensive genetic counseling and monitoring of at-risk pregnancies has reduced the incidence of Tay-Sachs disease in the Ashkenazic population by 90 percent.

Specific therapy for G$_{M2}$ gangliosidoses is not available. All HEX A deficiency disorders can be diagnosed prenatally from amniotic fluid, cultured amniotic fluid cells, or chorionic villus biopsies.

SPHINGOMYELIN LIPIDOSES: NIEMANN-PICK DISEASE (TYPES A AND B)

Types A and B Niemann-Pick disease (NPD) are lysosomal storage disorders that result from the deficient activity of acid sphingomyelinase. Type A NPD is a fatal disorder of infancy characterized by failure to thrive, hepatomegaly, and a rapidly progressive neurodegenerative course that leads to death in 2 to 3 years. In contrast, type B NPD is a variable disorder usually diagnosed in childhood by the presence of hepatomegaly. Most patients with type B have little to no neurologic impairment and survive into adulthood. In severely affected patients with type B NPD, progressive pulmonary infiltration causes insufficiency and lifestyle changes.

The hallmark of types A and B NPD is the lipid-laden foam cell, often referred to as the Niemann-Pick cell. These cells result from the accumulation of sphingomyelin and other lipids in the monocyte-macrophage system, which is the primary pathologic site of the disease.

Patients with type A NPD have less than 5 percent of normal acid sphingomyelinase activity in their cells and tissues. Patients with type B NPD, who have milder disease, may have residual enzyme activity that ranges from 5 to 10 percent of normal.

Both types A and B NPD are inherited as autosomal recessive traits. Type A NPD has a high incidence among Ashkenazic Jews as compared with the general population. The frequency of disease among this population is approximately 1 in 120, with a carrier frequency of 1 in 60.

The acid sphingomyelinase gene has been mapped to chromosome 11. Twelve mutations have been identified. Diagnosis of types A and B can be made by enzymatic determination of acid sphingomyelinase activity in cell or tissue extracts. Heterozygote detection requires molecular studies. Prenatal diagnosis by enzymatic and/or molecular analysis has been accomplished using chorionic villus sampling and cultured amniocytes.

There is no specific therapy for type A and B NPD.

CELLULAR CHOLESTEROL LIPIDOSES: NIEMANN-PICK DISEASE (TYPE C)

Type C NPD is an autosomal recessive lipidosis that results from an error in cellular trafficking of exogenous cholesterol that is associated with the lysosomal accumulation of unesterified cholesterol. Biochemically it is distinct from NPD types A and B. Most patients with NPD type C have progressive neurologic disease and hepatic damage.

Clinical manifestations in type C NPD are varied. Most patients present in late childhood with variable degrees of hepatosplenomegaly, ophthalmoplegia, progressive ataxia, dystonia, and dementia. Death occurs in the second decade. This disorder may also present in the neonatal period with fatal liver disease or in the infant period with hypotonia and developmental delay.

The distribution of type C NPD is panethnic. Genetic isolates have been described in Nova Scotia (formerly NPD type D) and southern Colorado. Despite the variable clinical manifestations, studies have not shown genetic heterogeneity.

Type C NPD is as least as frequent as types A and B combined. The true prevalence of the disease is underestimated owing to the lack of a definitive diagnostic test before the discovery of the abnormalities of cellular cholesterol processing.

Foams cells are present in many tissues and are not specific for type C NPD. Foam cells may be absent in patients lacking visceromegaly.

Primary molecular defect in NPD type C is unknown. Unesterified cholesterol, sphingomyelin, phospholipids, and glycolipids are stored in excess in the liver and spleen. Glycolipid levels are elevated in the brain.

The diagnosis of NPD type C requires both measurement of cellular cholesterol esterification and documentation of filipin-cholesterol staining in cultured fibroblasts during LDL uptake.

Symptomatic treatment of seizures, dystonia, and cataplexy is effective in many patients with NPD type C. Various drug protocols have been used to lower hepatic cholesterol levels, but it is not known if this therapy influences the neurologic progression of the disease.

Hypoxanthine-Guanine Phosphoribosyltransferase Deficiency: Lesch-Nyhan Syndrome

Lesch-Nyhan syndrome is caused by a complete deficiency of the purine salvage enzyme hypoxanthine-guanine phosphoribosyltransferase (HPRT). The disease is characterized by hyperuricemia, choreoathetosis, spasticity, mental retardation, and compulsive self-mutilation. Individuals with a partial deficiency of HPRT have hyperuricemia and gouty arthritis but are generally spared the neurologic consequences of Lesch-Nyhan syndrome.

Patients are clinically normal at birth. By 6 months of age, developmental delay is evident. Choreoathetoid movements begin within the first year. Self-mutilation is present in most patients and may begin as early as 6 months or as late as 16 years. Gouty arthritis in individuals with partial HPRT deficiency develops during adulthood.

HPRT enzyme is expressed in all tissues at low levels except in the basal ganglia, where the levels are higher, presumably because the rate of de novo purine synthesis is low.

Human HPRT gene lies on the X chromosome. Genetic lesions that lead to HPRT deficiency are heterogeneous. DNA mutation techniques are used in the diagnosis of affected males and for the determination of carrier status of asymptomatic females. Tissues can be analyzed for the presence or absence of HPRT activity.

Treatment with allopurinol, an inhibitor of xanthine oxidase, reduces serum uric acid levels and prevents most of the symptoms associated with hyperuricemia. There is no effective therapy for the neurologic complications of Lesch-Nyhan syndrome.

Hereditary Xanthinuria

Deficiency of the enzyme xanthine dehydrogenase results in the inability to degrade purine bases hypoxanthine and xanthine to uric acid, the normal end product of purine metabolism in humans. Xanthine and hypoxanthine accumulate in place of uric acid in plasma and urine. Xanthine is excreted; hypoxanthine is recycled by a salvage pathway. Excess xanthine in the defect is derived from guanine nucleotide catabolism, with guanine being converted to xanthine by way of the enzyme guanase.

Classic xanthinuria relates to the extreme insolubility of the purine base xanthine and its high renal clearance. It may present in the newborn period as renal damage due to xanthine calculi. The renal damage may be severe, resulting in renal failure and death.

Whereas classic xanthinuria results from a deficiency of xanthine dehydrogenase, a second type of xanthinuria results from a deficiency of three enzymes—xanthine dehydrogenase, sulfite oxidase, and aldehyde oxidase—which have a common (and, in this case, deficient) molybdenum cofactor.

Xanthine dehydrogenase is predominantly concentrated in the liver and intestinal mucosa. This mutant enzyme has not yet been studied on the molecular level; however, complementary DNA for the human enzyme has been cloned. The gene locus for xanthine dehydrogenase has been linked to chromosome 2.

The genetic defect in classic xanthinuria and the cofactor deficiency is inherited as an autosomal recessive trait. Heterozygotes for the classic defect have 50 percent of the normal enzyme activity and normal uric acid levels.

No specific treatment has proven successful for these patients, but a high fluid intake and avoidance of purine-rich foods may be of benefit.

Adenosine Deaminase Deficiency and Purine Nucleoside Phosphorylase Deficiency

Deficiencies of adenosine deaminase (ADA) and purine nucleoside phosphorylase (PNP) each cause abnormalities of purine metabolism that interfere with normal immune function. Patients with ADA deficiency are severely lymphopenic and lack both T cells and B cells, resulting in severe combined immunodeficiency (SCID). PNP-deficient patients have a lack of T cells but may have normal, hyperactive, or reduced B-cell activity. Most patients with these disorders are severely affected and present during infancy and early childhood with recurrent infections.

Diagnosis is made by finding absent or low ADA or PNP activity in erythrocytes. Heterozygotes have 50 percent of enzyme activity but normal immune function. Amniotic fluid cells or chorionic villi can establish a prenatal diagnosis.

ADA and PNP deficiencies are inherited in an autosomal recessive manner. Genes have been mapped to chromosomes 20 (ADA) and 14 (PNP). Several gene mutations for both ADA and PNP have been identified.

Primary lymphotoxic substrates of ADA and PNP are deoxyadenosine and deoxyguanosine. These substrates are derived from the dissolution in macrophages of the DNA of cells undergoing programmed cell death. The biochemical effects of deoxyadenosine in ADA deficiency impair lymphocyte differentiation, viability, and function by blocking DNA replication and division in thymocytes, selective depletion of cellular ATP, breakage of DNA strands, and depletion of cellular nicotinamide-adenine dinucleotide. In PNP deficiency, the cellular immunodeficiency that develops is believed to be a result of the accumulation of deoxyguanine triphosphate in T cells that inhibits DNA replication.

Complete or partial immune system restoration can be accomplished though a bone marrow transplant from an HLA-identical donor. Transplantation of T cell–depleted bone marrow has also been of benefit in the treatment of ADA deficiency but is associated with greater morbidity and mortality and is not as effective at restoring humoral immunity. Partial red cell exchange transfusion has been replaced by intramuscular injection of bovine ADA. The once- to twice-weekly injections have served to improve the specific immune function and have improved clinical status. Several of these patients have received gene therapy to transfer the ADA gene, and initial studies of stem cell–targeted gene therapy are in process. For patients with PNP deficiency, limited success has been made with the use of bone marrow.

Hereditary Oroticaciduria

Pyrimidines, along with purines, are the building blocks of DNA and RNA. Like purines, pyrimidines have two routes of nucleotide formation: the de novo pathway, which begins with ribose phosphate, amino acids, carbon dioxide, and ammonia; and the salvage pathway, which scavenges free bases and nucleosides back to nucleotides. The de novo and salvage pathways are balanced and connected through the enzymes that degrade the nucleotides.

Four defects of pyrimidine metabolism exist: hereditary oroticaciduria, pyrimidine 5'-nucleotase deficiency, dihydropyrimidine dehydrogenase deficiency, and dihydropyrimidinuria. Only hereditary oroticaciduria is discussed here.

The end product of purine metabolism is uric acid, which is easily recognized and quantified. There is no equivalent end product in pyrimidine metabolism.

Hereditary oroticaciduria results from a defect in the de novo pathway. It is an autosomal recessive disorder that results from a severe deficiency of the last two enzyme activities of the pathway. Although two enzymes are affected in this disorder, they are regulated by a single polypeptide encoded by a single gene localized to chromosome 3.

Only 15 reported cases of hereditary oroticaciduria have been reported in the literature. All of the patients have macrocytic hypochromic megaloblastic anemia and orotic acid crystalluria. Treatment with uridine has resulted in clinical improvement in most patients. Other clinical manifestations of the disorder include crystal lithiasis, cardiac malformations, and strabismus. Infections are a problem in some patients with various alterations of immune function. Mild intellectual impairment has not been a constant feature before treatment.

REFERENCES

Ampola, M. G. (1982). *Metabolic diseases in pediatric practice*. Boston: Little, Brown.

Benson, P. F. (1983). *Screening and management of potentially treatable genetic metabolic disorders*. Boston: MTP Press.

Bickel, H. (1980). Rationale of neonatal screening for inborn errors of metabolism. In H. Bickel, R. Guthrie, & G. Hammersen (Eds.), *Neonatal screening for inborn errors of metabolism* (pp. 1–6). New York: Springer-Verlag.

Blaskovics, M. E., Schaeffler, G. E., & Hack, S. (1974). Phenylalaninemia: Differential diagnosis. *Archives of Disease in Childhood, 49*, 835–843.

Burman, D., Holton, J. B., & Pennock, C. A. (Eds.). (1978). *Inherited disorders of carbohydrate metabolism*. Baltimore: University Park Press.

Cohn, R., & Roth, K. (1983). *Metabolic disease: A guide to early recognition.* Philadelphia: W. B. Saunders.

Cornblath, M., & Schwartz, R. (1966). *Disorders of carbohydrate metabolism in infancy.* Philadelphia: W. B. Saunders.

Cornblath, M., Wybregt, S. H., & Bacens, G. S. (1963). Studies of carbohydrate metabolism in the newborn infant. *Pediatrics, 32,* 1007.

Crawford, M. d'A., Gibbs, D. A., & Watts, R. W. E. (Eds.). (1982). *Advances in the treatment of inborn errors of metabolism.* New York: John Wiley & Sons.

Dahlqvist, A., & Svenningsen, N. W. (1969). Galactose in the urine of newborn infants. *Journal of Pediatrics, 75,* 454–462.

Fenton, W. A., & Rosenberg, L. E. (1995). Disorders of propionate and methylmalonate metabolism. In C. R. Scriver, A. L. Beaudet, W. S. Sly, & D. Valle (Eds.), *The metabolic and molecular bases of inherited metabolic disease* (7th ed.). New York: McGraw-Hill.

Galjaard, H. (1980). *Genetic metabolic diseases.* New York: Elsevier/North Holland Biomedical Press.

Gitzelmann, R. (1967). Hereditary galactokinase deficiency, a newly recognized cause of juvenile cataracts. *Pediatric Research, 1,* 14.

Kane, J. P., & Havel, R. J. (1995). Disorders of the biogenesis and secretion of lipoproteins containing the B apoproteins. In C. R. Scriver, A. L. Beaudet, W. S. Sly, & D. Valle (Eds.), *The metabolic basis of inherited disease* (7th ed.). New York: McGraw-Hill.

Komrower, G. M. (1980). Inborn errors of metabolism. *Pediatrics in Review, 2,* 175–181.

LeGrys, V. (1984). *The laboratory diagnosis of selected inborn errors of metabolism.* New York: Praeger Publishers.

Levy, H., & Hammersen, G. (1978). Newborn screening for galactosemia and other galactose metabolic defects. *Journal of Pediatrics, 92,* 871–877.

Levy, H. L., Sepe, S. J., Shih, V. E., et al. (1977). Sepsis due to *Escherichia coli* in neonates with galactosemia. *New England Journal of Medicine, 297,* 823–825.

Litchfield, W. J., & Wells, W. W. (1978). Effects of galactose on free radical reactions of polymorphonuclear leukocytes. *Archives Biochemistry and Biophysics, 188,* 26–30.

Lloyd, J. K., & Scriver, C. R. (Eds.). (1985). *Genetic and metabolic disease in pediatrics.* London: Butterworths.

Markland, O. N., Garg, B. P., & Brandt, I. K. (1982). Nonketotic hyperglycinemia: EEG and evoked potentials. *Abnormal Neurology, 32,* 151.

Matsui, S. M., Mahoney, M. J., & Rosenberg, L. E. (1983). The natural history of the methylmalonic acidemias. *New England Journal of Medicine, 308,* 857–861.

Nyhan, W. L. (1984). Hawkinsinuria. In W. L. Nyhan (Ed.), *Abnormalities in amino acid metabolism in clinical medicine* (p. 187). Norwalk, CT: Appleton-Century-Crofts.

Perry, T. L., Urquhart, N., Maclean, J., et al. (1975). Nonketotic hyperglycinemia. *New England Journal of Medicine, 292,* 1269–1273.

Qu, Y., Miller, J. B., Slocum, R. H., & Shapira, E. (1991). Rapid automated quantitation of isoleucine, leucine, tyrosine and phenylalanine from dried filter paper specimens. *Clinica Chimica Acta, 203,* 191–197.

Scriver, C. R., Beaudet, A. L., Sly, W. S., & Valle, D. (Eds.). (1995). *The metabolic basis of inherited disease* (7th ed.). New York: McGraw-Hill.

Scriver, C. R., Kaufman, S., Eisensmith, R. C., & Woo, S. L. C. (1995). The hyperphenylalaninemias. In C. R. Scriver, A. L. Beaudet, W. S. Sly, & D. Valle (Eds.). (1995). *The metabolic basis of inherited disease* (7th ed.). New York: McGraw-Hill.

Shevell, M. I., Matiaszuk, N., Ledley, F. D., & Rosenblatt, D. S. (1993). Varying neurologic phenotypes among muto and mut− patients with methylmalonyl CoA mutase deficiency. *American Journal of Medical Genetics 45,* 619–624.

Stave, U. (Ed.). (1978). *Perinatal physiology*. New York: Plenum Publishing.

Wapnir, R. A. (1985). *Congenital metabolic diseases: Diagnosis and treatment*. New York: Marcel Dekker.

Winick, M. (Ed.). (1979). *Nutritional management of genetic disorders*. New York: John Wiley & Sons.

••

CHAPTER 14

Assessment and Management of Endocrine Dysfunction

GROWTH HORMONE

Human growth hormone (GH, somatotropin) is a protein consisting of 191 amino acid residues. It is secreted from somatotroph cells in the anterior portion of the pituitary gland (Wallis, 1988).

Secretion of GH is under the control of two hypothalamic peptides: growth hormone–releasing factor (GHRF) and somatostatin (Gelato et al., 1987). GHRF stimulates the release of GH from the anterior pituitary gland.

Proliferation and differentiation of various cells are affected by GH. Uptake of GH by liver and skeletal muscle cells improves amino acid transport and protein synthesis. Liver cells increase glucose output and produce insulin-like growth factors (IGFs) called somatomedins. The IGFs, which are in synergy with GH, appear to stimulate skeletal growth. An anti-insulin effect occurs in muscle (Ganong, 1985; Wallis, 1988).

High levels of GH present in the cord blood of neonates have fetal origin because GH does not cross the placental barrier. Concentrations of GH in full-term and premature newborns have not been statistically different (Bona et al., 1994). Despite high levels, GH seems to have little effect on gestational size. Rather, somatomedins appear to play a bigger role in fetal tissue growth and differentiation (Bona et al., 1994). In all infants, a rapid decline of GH occurs 1 to 2 weeks postnatally; however, throughout the first 8 weeks of life, these levels are persistently higher than in adults (Lanes et al., 1989).

Growth Hormone Deficiency

PATHOPHYSIOLOGY

Growth hormone deficiency is not thought to be the root cause of the majority of short stature cases in humans. When GH and related hormones are involved, the etiology of deficiency is variable (Wallis, 1988).

Various defects produce low levels or absence of GH. For example, a defect of the hypothalamus limits stimulation of the pituitary to release GH. Developmental or degenerative lesions of the pituitary also prohibit GH secretion. The somatotrophs may be unable to produce GH if the gene response for its production is defective. Under such circumstances, target organs may be unable to respond to hormonal stimulation. Lastly, the hormone itself may be abnormal and rendered useless (Rimoin, 1990; Wallis, 1988).

295

CLINICAL MANIFESTATIONS

Signs and symptoms in neonates are as follows:

- Height and birth weight within normal range
- Persistent hypoglycemia, the mechanism of which is not clearly defined but which may be related to the production of IGFs (somatomedins)
- Micropenis in males (Herber & Milner, 1984)

Infants younger than 6 months of age often present with the following:

- Failure to thrive
- Poor feeding
- Subnormal height velocity
- Hypoglycemia (Herber & Milner, 1984)

A thorough history and physical examination includes assessment of other signs of GH deficiency:

- Pallor
- Lethargy
- Sweatiness

Any condition that disrupts GH production, stimulation, secretion, or tissue response can result in deficiency. For example, a neonate with congenital absence of the anterior pituitary gland manifests signs and symptoms like those of isolated GH deficiency. In addition, many other glands and hormones are affected because the pituitary is the master endocrine gland.

Additional clinical features in infants may include the following:

- Early lethargy
- Hyperbilirubinemia
- Micropenis in males
- Hypoplastic gonads
- Hypoplastic thyroid
- Hypoglycemia
- Cyanosis
- Convulsions
- Circulatory collapse

INCIDENCE

The incidence of GH deficiency is 1 in 4000 to 1 in 30,000; it is more prevalent in boys.

RISK FACTORS

Birth trauma has been implicated in some cases. It is postulated that perinatal trauma or difficulty compromises the blood supply to the pituitary gland, which can result in deficient GH secretion (Aetiology of growth hormone deficiency, 1988).

DIFFERENTIAL DIAGNOSIS

There are several ways to diagnose GH deficiency:

- Direct measurement of GH

- Measurement of GHRF, which evaluates anterior pituitary function
- Use of L-dopa, glucagon, or propranolol combined with GHRF evaluates ophthalmic function (Shimano et al., 1985)

COLLABORATIVE MANAGEMENT

- Closely monitor vital signs and laboratory values.
- If there is a suspected genetic cause of the deficiency, refer to a genetic center.
- Evaluate parents' support systems.
- Educate parents:
  - Explain how to give biosynthetic GH and other necessary medication.
  - Explain when to give medication.
  - Explain how to recognize adverse side effects and toxicity.
  - Give telephone numbers of the local poison control center and health care professionals.
  - Stress compliance to medication therapy. Hormone replacement is long term.
  - Treatment with biosynthetic human GH causes transient decreases in percentage of B lymphocytes and percentage of T lymphocytes. Instruct parents to notify their physician in charge of GH replacement therapy if there are recurring infections.

ANTIDIURETIC HORMONE

Syndrome of Inappropriate Secretion of Antidiuretic Hormone

PHYSIOLOGY

Antidiuretic hormone (ADH), or vasopressin (arginine vasopressin), is a hormone produced by the hypothalamus and stored in the anterior pituitary gland. It is normally secreted in physiologic states when there is an increase in serum osmolality. The primary function of ADH is to control fluid and electrolyte balance. It contributes to the adaptation to changes in intravascular (extracellular) volume by regulating renal clearance of free water (Weise & Zaritsky, 1987). ADH allows the renal distal tubules to absorb water from the collecting ducts and consequently decrease urine output. Specialized osmoreceptors in the anterior hypothalamus control the release of ADH in response to plasma osmolality. ADH also exerts a modest vasopressor effect on baroreceptors in the left atrium and carotid sinus, causing vasoconstriction in response to hypotension. Under normal conditions, the response of the kidney to plasma hypo-osmolality is to concentrate the urine maximally (Kinzie, 1987) (Fig. 14–1). Hence, disorders that affect the release and actions of ADH indicate ineffective maintenance and balance of fluid and electrolytes.

RISK FACTORS

The syndrome of inappropriate secretion of ADH (SIADH) has been reported in both term and preterm infants in association with the following:

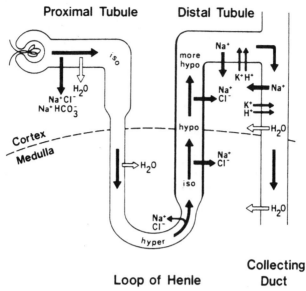

FIGURE 14–1. Tubular reabsorption and secretion: summary of changes in the osmolality of tubular fluid in various parts of the nephron. The thickened wall of the ascending limb of the loop of Henle indicates relative impermeability of the tubular epithelium to water. In the presence of vasopressin, the fluid in the collecting ducts becomes hypertonic, whereas in the absence of this hormone the fluid remains hypotonic throughout the collecting duct. Aldosterone promotes reabsorption of Na^+ and secretion of H^+ and K^+ in the distal convoluted tubule. (From Cannon, P. J. [1977]. The kidney in heart failure. *New England Journal of Medicine, 296,* 26–32. Reprinted with permission.)

- Asphyxia
- Meningitis
- Pneumonia
- Hypoplasia of the anterior pituitary and idiopathic ADH secretion
- Surgical repair of a patent ductus arteriosus
- Pneumothorax
- Pain
- Positive-pressure ventilation
- Periventricular/intraventricular hemorrhage

CLINICAL MANIFESTATIONS

Clinical features of SIADH include the following:

- Increased secretion or amount of ADH
- Water retention, edema
- Low serum osmolar state or relative fluid overload
- Plasma hypo-osmolality
- Hyponatremia

- Increased glomerular filtration rate
- Increased fractional excretion of sodium, further decreasing the sodium concentration (Kinzie, 1987)
- Low serum potassium level
- Low serum chloride level
- Low serum calcium level
- High urinary sodium level
- Decreased free water clearance
- Elevated urine specific gravity

The signs° of SIADH include the following:

- Hyponatremia (serum Na < 135 mEq)
- Serum hypo-osmolality (serum osmolality < 275 mOsm)
- Urine hyperosmolarity (urine osmolarity > 1000 mOsm)
- High urine sodium (urine Na > 220 mEq/24 hr)

DIAGNOSIS

The diagnosis of SIADH assumes that there is normal cardiac output as well as normal renal, adrenal, and thyroid function. Therefore, these systems must first be evaluated for normal function before the SIADH diagnosis can be made. It is based on laboratory findings and the previously listed clinical manifestations.

COLLABORATIVE MANAGEMENT

The treatment of choice is fluid restriction, which decreases the availability of free water. Exceptions are if the serum sodium level is less than approximately 120 mEq/L or if neurologic signs such as seizures are present. Treatment measures are listed below:

- More rapid elevation of serum tonicity may be achieved with furosemide (Lasix), 1 mg/kg intravenously every 6 hours.
- Urinary sodium is replaced milliequivalent for milliequivalent with hypertonic saline (3 percent solution). This therapy results in accelerated loss of free water with no net change in total body sodium.
- Fluid restriction alone should be relied on only once the serum sodium level exceeds 120 mEq/L (Cloherty & Stark, 1991).
- Interventions are related to finely tuned assessment skills, with close attention to perinatal history, physical examination, and evaluation of laboratory and clinical data.
- Overall responsibility involves a high degree of sensitivity to infants at risk.

The following lists appropriate collaborative actions or interventions:

- Monitor urine output.
- Check specific gravity and/or dipsticks with every void or every 4 hours.
- Maintain intravenous fluids.

. . . .

°Values vary according to institution.

- Monitor laboratory data.
- Document renal group serum, urine osmolarity, and urine electrolytes.
- Notify the physician or nurse practitioner of urine volumes exceeding the fluid intake. Adjust the intravenous fluids accordingly.
- Monitor for water intoxication:
  - Irritability
  - Lethargy
  - Seizure activity
  - Change in the neurologic examination or reflex activity

THYROID HORMONES

Thyroid Hormone Levels in Newborns

Neonatal serum thyroid-stimulating hormone (TSH) increases from mean cord serum values of 9 μU/ml to a mean peak of 85 μU/ml within 30 minutes after delivery. The placenta is impermeable to the passage of thyroid hormones from mother to fetus. Thus, the fetal hypothalamic pituitary–thyroid system appears to be independent of the maternal system. However, thyroid-releasing hormone (TRH) is capable of crossing the placental barrier, thus producing some effects on the fetus. One of these effects is suppression of the fetal thyroid hormone production.

Thyroid Screening

Triiodothyronine (T_3) levels have been found to be increased in amniotic fluid early in pregnancy and to decrease gradually to cord serum concentrations that are still higher than maternal values at term.

Premature infants frequently have low levels of thyroxine (T_4) when compared with the normal range for full-term infants (transient hypothyroidism). Cord blood levels of T_4 range from 6 to 15 μg/dl (Goetzman & Wennberg, 1991).

Thyroid Function Tests

Total T_4 ranges from 7.1 to 22.7 μg/dl during the first few months of life.

Congenital Hypothyroidism

PATHOPHYSIOLOGY

Abnormal embryologic development of the thyroid gland is most frequently the cause of congenital hypothyroidism, which includes the absence of the thyroid gland or the lack of development of the thyroid (ectopic) (Malvaux, 1981).

CLINICAL MANIFESTATIONS

Signs and symptoms of congenital hypothyroidism are as follows:

- Usually greater than or equal to 42 weeks' gestation

- Birth weight more than 4000 g
- Posterior fontanelle may be enlarged with delayed ossification
- Respiratory difficulty from goiter compression
- Hypothermia
- Lethargy
- Hypotony
- Feeding difficulties
- Delayed meconium
- Abdominal distention
- Elongated nasal bridge
- Enlarged tongue
- Hoarse cry

The latter findings are directly related to the function of the thyroid and its effect, along with GH, on bone maturation, calcium regulation, temperature regulation, and metabolic rate. A general slowdown of bodily functions occurs, including a shutdown or slowdown in terms of temperature.

DIFFERENTIAL DIAGNOSIS

Serum T_3, T_4, and TSH levels are measured. Approximately one third of all measurements are low and need follow-up blood sampling for TSH evaluation to confirm an abnormal level.

Long-bone radiographs are used to determine if the characteristic pattern of scattered bone growth centers are visible; if so, this indicates hypothyroidism.

COLLABORATIVE MANAGEMENT

The goal of treatment is to establish a euthyroid state as soon as possible. Two types of thyroid hormones are available; those from the extracts of pork and beef are not used as frequently as synthetic thyroid hormones. Thyroid extracts contain 0.21 iodide. Synthetic hormones are available as a sodium salt of L-thyroxine (L-T_4) and L-triiodothyronine (L-T_3). L-T_3 is more potent than L-T_4, and its intestinal absorption is more complete. The metabolic effects appear and disappear rapidly. In the long run, it is preferable to use L-T_4 because the effects are longer lasting (blood TSH levels remain constant), and thus it need be given orally only twice a day. The dose of thyroid hormone prescribed should be adequate to regulate metabolic functions. The T_4 level should increase rapidly to ensure a euthyroid level of this hormone. The dose of T_4 during the newborn period is 8 to 10 µg/kg/day for most full-term infants (Goetzman & Wennberg, 1991). Delay in instituting hormone replacement therapy or noncompliance with its administration leads to mental retardation.

Over the first few days after initiation of replacement therapy, observations must be made for cardiac problems. Cardiac failure or arrhythmias are possible. The infant becomes more active, and body temperature normalizes as therapeutic levels are reached. Observation of growth is crucial because it can be the only indicator that treatment is truly successful.

Before medication is deemed effective, metabolic demand is decreased.

Thus, the activity of the infant may be reduced because of fatigue and weakness. Constipation may result from decreased peristaltic action. The infant may become edematous secondary to infiltration of fluid into interstitial tissues. Cold intolerance may also develop, causing discomfort.

Congenital Hyperthyroidism

Neonatal hyperthyroidism is serious and potentially life-threatening. The infant may be born with a very small goiter or even a small thyroid gland. Serum T_4 levels may be low, normal, or even high at birth, depending on the degree of in utero thyroid suppression. Most often, this neonatal thyrotoxicosis is due to maternal Graves' disease. The condition may be temporary in the neonatal period (Becks & Burrow, 1990).

Infant of a Hyperthyroid Mother

Maternal hyperthyroidism is present in 1 in 500 pregnancies (Becks & Burrow, 1990). This creates a great threat to the unborn fetus, with an increase in spontaneous abortions as well as premature births (Parks, 1981). After the first trimester, the maternal–fetal pituitary–thyroid axes are independent. T_3, T_4, and TSH do not cross the placenta, but antibodies in the form of immunoglobulin G do cross the placental barrier. These antibodies act on the thyroid gland of the fetus, causing thyroid function and growth hormone to be increased. The hyperthyroid state occurs as the passage of these antibodies increases during the second and third trimesters of pregnancy. Maternal antithyroid medications and stable iodine can also affect the fetus and neonate (Becks & Burrow, 1990). These substances, although effective therapy for both mother and fetus because they cross the placenta, can also adversely affect the fetus. Use of stable iodine in pregnant mothers is contraindicated because of the blockage of fetal thyroid hormone release, which, in turn, leads to hypothyroidism and goiter. Excess dosage of maternal antithyroid medications is also likely to cause fetal and neonatal hypothyroidism.

DIFFERENTIAL DIAGNOSIS

The diagnosis is determined by the presence of maternal thyroid-stimulating antibodies and clinical manifestations (Becks & Burrow, 1990).

CLINICAL MANIFESTATIONS

Effects on the fetus of maternal hyperthyroidism include the following:

- Heart rates greater than or equal to 160 beats per minute
- Goiter
- Intrauterine growth retardation
- Mature bone growth greater than expected for gestational age
- Craniosynostosis (Becks & Burrow, 1990)

COLLABORATIVE MANAGEMENT

The overall objective of therapy is to restore and maintain a euthyroid state.

- Use medications, such as methimazole and carbimazole, that will interfere with thyroid hormone synthesis. These agents decrease the active transport of iodine into the thyroid gland. Propranolol is given to the severely hyperthyroid infant to reduce heart rate and to lessen tremors. This drug is generally used in the first week of replacement therapy.
- If medical treatment is not chosen, surgical removal of part or all of the thyroid gland is possible.

In radioiodine treatment a dose is given that is dependent on the individual mass and geometry of the thyroid gland. Reservations about the use of radioiodine therapy in children relate to concerns about the development of thyroid carcinoma or leukemia during adulthood. Damage to the thymus gland, a major immune organ in the neonate, is possible, which leaves the neonate vulnerable to infections.

The disease process of hyperthyroidism results in increased metabolic demands (Avery, Fletcher, & MacDonald, 1994).

- A higher caloric intake is needed, often more than 180 kcal/kg/day (up from about 100 to 120 kcal/kg/day) to maintain positive growth.
- Propranolol is used to decrease the heart rate and to combat the occurrence of heart failure (Avery, Fletcher, & MacDonald, 1994).
- Fatigue and exhaustion occur, owing to the hypermetabolic state and use of energy stores (Parks, 1981). Energy conservation with minimal stimulation may be necessary.
- Diarrhea may result because of increased peristalsis, thus leading to even more loss of nutrients as well as fluids.
  - Monitor weight daily.
  - Monitor intake and output values every 4 to 8 hours.
- Heat intolerance and profound diaphoresis are side effects of the increased basal metabolic rate.
  - Observe for signs of heat increases.
  - Closely monitor temperature.
- If exophthalmos occurs, provide lubricating drops or ointment to protect the eye from damage.
- Perform weekly head circumference and growth curve determinations.
- Teach parents that therapy is a lifelong commitment.

DIABETES

Infant of a Diabetic Mother

MATERNAL CONSIDERATIONS

During pregnancy, a woman experiences increasing levels of estrogen and progesterone. This hormonal increase stimulates pancreatic beta cell hyperplasia and increases the secretion of insulin. This pancreatic beta cell hyperplasia continues as the pregnancy progresses. Pregnant women with diabetes also experience these hormonal changes, making it more difficult to manage their glucose levels (Hoskins, 1990).

Gestational diabetes occurs during pregnancy and is usually self limiting to the pregnancy.

INCIDENCE

The incidence of gestational diabetes is 2 to 3 percent of pregnancies.

RISK FACTORS

Risk factors for delivery of an infant with a diabetic mother are as follows:
- Previous pregnancy with gestational diabetes
- Maternal obesity
- Previous infant macrosomatia shown by ultrasonography
- Maternal glycosuria
- Uterine size larger than normal for gestational date

The severity of maternal diabetes can be determined by using the White classification system (White, 1974) (see Chapter 4, High-Risk Pregnancy).

FETAL AND NEONATAL RISKS

No matter what the maternal class is, the fetus is at risk for the following:
- Spontaneous abortion
- Stillbirth
- Cephalopelvic disproportion
- Asphyxia
- Respiratory distress
- Hypoglycemia
- Macrosomatia
- Congenital anomalies
- Hypocalcemia
- Hypomagnesemia
- Hyperbilirubinemia
- Polycythemia
- Major problem: labile glucose level

Hypoglycemia

Hypoglycemia is signified by a blood sugar level below 40 mg/dl for the term infant and below 20 mg/dl for the preterm infant. Insulin is a larger molecule than glucose, and it does not cross the placenta easily, so maternal glucose levels are mirrored with the neonatal system and amniotic fluid.

This maternal hyperglycemia leads to fetal hyperglycemia. Because maternal insulin does not cross the placenta, elevated glucose levels stimulate the fetal pancreas to secrete insulin. This stimulation also leads to hyperplasia of the beta cells and increased productions of insulin, which continues after delivery. Insulin is the main growth hormone for the fetus so this hyperinsulinemia leads to fat accumulation and macrosomatia (Hoskins, 1990).

Because of this hyperinsulinism, and then the loss of maternal glucose at

delivery, the infant can become hypoglycemic within a few hours after delivery and needs to be monitored closely.

Common signs of hypoglycemia are listed below:

- Jitteriness
- Cyanosis
- Irritability
- Seizures
- Apnea

Macrosomia

The infant of a diabetic mother has a characteristic appearance:

- Large for gestational age with increased adipose tissue
- Full face liberally covered with vernix
- Plethoric
- Large placenta and umbilical cord
- Growth acceleration
- Smaller head circumference:weight ratio
- Larger weight:length ratio

These infants can experience cephalopelvic disproportion, leading to difficult deliveries secondary to their size. Birth trauma may include the following:

- Brachial plexus trauma
- Fractured clavicle
- Facial palsy
- Shoulder dystocia
- Asphyxia
- Subdural hemorrhage

According to Neufeld (1987), hyperinsulinemia influences the fetal lung maturity in infants of diabetic mothers by inhibiting the fetal lung synthesis of surfactant.

Hypocalcemia and Hypomagnesemia

Hypocalcemia and hypomagnesemia are major metabolic problems exhibited by infants of diabetic mothers. The incidence is related to the severity of the maternal diabetes; both problems need to be followed closely. The symptoms are similar to those seen with hypoglycemia (Perelman, 1983).

Hypocalcemia develops within the first 3 days of life and is seen primarily in the infant of the insulin-dependent diabetic mother. It is thought that hypocalcemia may be secondary to decreased hypoparathyroid functioning resulting from hypomagnesemia. The infant should be observed for hypocalcemia and hypomagnesemia and treated as needed (Cowett & Schwartz, 1982).

Hyperbilirubinemia and Polycythemia

Hyperbilirubinemia is a common occurrence in an infant of a diabetic mother. Most infants of diabetic mothers have the unconjugated form of bilirubin circulating in their system. This finding suggests an impairment of

the glucuronidation system (Neufeld, 1987). Hyperbilirubinemia may also be related to decreased albumin levels, leaving less albumin available for binding bilirubin.

Polycythemia is also frequently observed in infants of diabetic mothers. The infant with polycythemia may exhibit signs and symptoms such as jitteriness, tachypnea, cyanosis, priapism, and oliguria.

A complication of polycythemia that occurs frequently in an infant of a diabetic mother is renal vein thrombosis. Signs include hematuria and a palpable renal mass.

Congenital Anomalies

Preconceptual glucose control is essential because anomalies may occur before the woman knows she is pregnant. Many of these defects occur before the seventh week of gestation as a result of maternal hyperglycemia. Hyperglycemia inhibits cellular mitosis, resulting in anomalies (Hitti, Glasberg, Huggins-Jones, & Sabet, 1994; Hoskins, 1990; Novak & Robinson, 1994).

The occurrence of congenital heart disease in the infant of a diabetic mother can be as high as five times that of normal infants and can include the following:

- Atrial or ventricular septal defects
- Transposition of the great vessels
- Coarctation of the aorta

Skeletal malformations including the following may occur:

- Delayed ossification
- Osseous defects
- Caudal regression syndrome
- Femur agenesis or hypoplasia

Central nervous system anomalies may include any of the following:

- Hydrocephalus
- Meningomyelocele
- Anencephaly

A gastrointestinal anomaly is small left colon syndrome.

COLLABORATIVE MANAGEMENT

Signs and symptoms of hypoglycemia must be sought to prevent adverse effects on the central nervous system:

- Jitteriness
- Extreme hunger (sucking vigorously on hands and fingers)
- Diaphoresis
- Cyanosis
- Tachypnea
- Lethargy
- Seizures
- Apnea

Serum glucose levels need to be monitored frequently until stable at 80

to 120 mg/dl. After delivery, the infant's glucose level must be monitored at least every hour until it has stabilized. Perelman (1983) identifies hypoglycemia as less than 30 mg/dl for the term infant, 20 mg/dl for the preterm infant, and 40 mg/dl for any infant who is showing signs and symptoms of hypoglycemia. If the infant's condition is stable, early feedings should be given. Intravenous fluids of 10 percent dextrose in water ($D_{10}W$) at 6 to 8 mg/kg/min should be started for the infant unable to take oral feedings. If the glucose level remains low, administering an intravenous bolus of dextrose may be necessary with a concentration no greater than $D_{10}W$. Administration of more concentrated dextrose solutions may cause rebound hypoglycemia.

Signs of birth trauma such as brachial plexus damage or a fractured clavicle should be watched for. If decreased movement is noted in an arm or the infant cries when an extremity is moved, a radiograph should be obtained to assess for a fracture. If a fracture is present, the affected extremity should be stabilized and an orthopedic consultation obtained.

Bottle feeding may be difficult for the macrosomic infant. These infants have weaker reflex functioning and poor motor behavior during the first 2 days of life (Pressler, 1991).

The infant of a diabetic mother with poor glucose control during her pregnancy may have respiratory distress. If this is the case, treatment should be the same as for other infants with respiratory distress syndrome.

Monitoring is necessary for hypocalcemia and hypomagnesemia. The signs, such as jitteriness or lethargy, usually appear within the first 3 days of life and are similar to those seen in hypoglycemia.

A spun hematocrit should be obtained to assess for polycythemia. A partial exchange transfusion may need to be done for a central hematocrit over 65 percent. Phototherapy may need to be started for treatment of hyperbilirubinemia.

Many of the problems that occur are transient and resolve within a few days.

ABNORMAL SEXUAL DIFFERENTIATION

When the sperm fertilizes the ovum at conception, the genetic sex of the embryo is determined. However, during the first 7 weeks of gestation, the primitive gonads contain both ovarian (cortical) and testicular (medullary) components (Avery, Fletcher, & MacDonald, 1994), creating a "bipotential environment" in which either gender's characteristics may emerge. This initial stage of "sexual indifference" lasts until the seventh week of gestation, when the gonads, which are the future testes or ovaries, begin to acquire sexual characteristics (Moore & Persaud, 1993).

Although most conditions resulting in ambiguous genitalia are not life threatening (with the exception of the salt-wasting form of congenital adrenal hyperplasia), it is vitally important that early diagnosis be made and treatment instituted to minimize any negative sequelae and maximize outcome.

The more common disorders of sexual differentiation can be categorized into two generalized groups: congenital adrenal hyperplasia (CAH) and disorders of gonadal differentiation. The most common cause of ambiguous genitalia in the newborn is CAH, but not all patients with the disorder show sexual ambiguity. The same is true for disorders of gonadal differentiation.

Congenital Adrenal Hyperplasia

Congenital adrenal hyperplasia is an autosomal recessive inborn error of metabolism that equally affects male and female fetuses.

INCIDENCE

One in 5000 to 15,000 births results in CAH. Affected females often present with some degree of virilization of the external genitalia, but the internal female structures remain normal. Conversely, few male infants show any genital anomalies and they may go unrecognized until later infancy or childhood (Griffin & Wilson, 1986; Shapiro, Santiago, & Crane, 1989).

PATHOPHYSIOLOGY

The adrenal cortex consists of three regions: the outer zona glomerulosa, the middle fasciculata, and the inner zona reticularis, which adjoins the adrenal medulla. The reticularis, however, does not complete differentiation until about 3 years of age. There are three classes of hormones produced by the adrenal gland: mineralocorticoids, glucocorticoids, and sex steroids. Specific enzymes are necessary for the biosynthesis of these hormones. Adrenocorticotropic hormone (ACTH) stimulates the adrenal gland to produce the steroids. When sufficient quantities are released into the blood stream, ACTH is turned off by a negative feedback mechanism (Mininberg, Levine, & New, 1982; New et al., 1990).

Many forms of CAH exist. Abnormally high ACTH with low plasma cortisol levels is pathognomonic of all forms of CAH. Each type is the result of a separate enzyme deficiency necessary for production of a particular steroid. No matter which form of CAH is operating, a deficiency in cortisol results. This deficiency, in turn, prohibits the natural negative feedback loop necessary to turn off pituitary secretion of ACTH. Thus, ACTH continues to stimulate the adrenal gland to synthesize and secrete deficient steroids, and adrenal hyperplasia ensues (Kelnar, 1993; Miller & Levine, 1987; Mininberg, Levine, & New, 1982).

The types and symptoms of CAH depend on which steroids are deficient and which are produced in excess (Miller & Levine, 1987).

CAH may be separated into three categories: rare enzyme defects, nonclassic forms, and classic forms. The rare enzyme defects may be incompatible with life and are thus rarely seen clinically. The nonclassic forms are usually hidden at birth, with no major developmental abnormalities noted. If signs of the disorder appear at all, they are typically seen later in life. One of the classic forms of CAH, 21-hydroxylase deficiency, is the most common autosomal recessive disorder in humans (New et al., 1990). Although the nonclassic forms are more prevalent in the general population, the classic forms of CAH are expressed most commonly in the neonatal population.

CONGENITAL ADRENAL HYPERPLASIA DUE TO 21-HYDROXYLASE DEFICIENCY

CAH due to 21-hydroxylase deficiency accounts for 90 to 95 percent of all CAH cases (Mininberg, Levine, & New, 1982; New, 1988).

Incidence

The severe form occurs in 1 in 5000 to 14,000 births. A milder form is present in 0.3 percent of whites and in 1 to 3 percent of European Jews (Kalaitzoglou & New, 1993; White, New, & Dupont, 1986).

Pathophysiology

Congenital adrenal hyperplasia due to 21-hydroxylase deficiency results in a build-up of 17-hydroxyprogesterone that is not converted to 11-deoxycortisol. Without sufficient circulating cortisol, the negative feedback loop to the hypothalamus and pituitary does not operate. Increasing amounts of ACTH continue to be secreted, resulting in high levels of circulating androgens. Excess circulating androgens lead to progressive virilism, which begins during prenatal development. Female neonates can present with mild clitoral enlargement with or without labioscrotal folds or, in severe cases, with a penile urethra (Kalaitzoglou & New, 1993). Premature female neonates are at risk for delayed diagnosis because prominent clitoris and electrolyte imbalance caused by renal immaturity are not uncommon (Cruz, MacMillan, Browning, & Stewart, 1995). The increased testosterone does not, however, interfere with normal development of internal genitalia, uterus, or fallopian tubes. Consequently, virilized females have the potential for a normal female reproductive life, complete with childbearing. Androgen excess also contributes to initial rapid skeletal growth with early closure of the epiphyses and consequent short adult stature.

Males with 21-hydroxylase deficiency often appear normal at birth. An enlarged penis with small testes may be present. The disorder may go unrecognized until the male develops precocious puberty during later infancy or early childhood. This may be shown in the development of early pubic hair, advanced muscular development, and rapid growth. Infertility may result without treatment intervention (New & Josso, 1988).

Clinical Manifestations

The classic form of 21-hydroxylase deficiency is the most common presenting CAH disorder. Twenty-five percent of affected newborns have a simple virilizing form. Seventy-five percent of patients with classic 21-hydroxylase deficiency are unable to synthesize adequate aldosterone. Aldosterone is a necessary component for the transport of sodium ions across cell membranes (New et al., 1990). A defect in aldosterone biosynthesis results in the inability of the distal and collecting tubules of the kidney to reabsorb sodium. Salt wasting occurs and creates high urinary sodium. Serum sodium levels drop while serum potassium levels rise. In an effort to increase levels of aldosterone, large amounts of renin are released into the plasma. As a result, circulating angiotensin II is also increased. Despite high levels of the natural vasoconstrictor, blood pressure falls, presumably owing to downregulation of angiotensin receptors in vascular smooth muscle. Patients with this form of CAH may die in the neonatal period as a result of hyponatremic shock (Ganong, 1985; New, 1988). Rapid diagnosis with accurate treatment is clearly an important goal for these newborns.

Diagnosis

Blood spots routinely collected for newborn screening can be used to detect 17-hydroxyprogesterone concentration.

Treatment

Treatment involves replacing deficient cortisol with hydrocortisone or a similar synthetic substitute, such as dexamethasone. In addition, mineralocorticoid replacement is necessary in the salt-wasting form (New & Josso, 1988). The goal of hormone replacement therapy is to prevent adrenal crisis, achieve normal growth and development, and suppress excessive androgen production (Einaudi et al., 1993). Supplemental medication is taken lifelong (DiGrande, 1984). Surgical repair of ambiguous genitalia may also be indicated.

CONGENITAL ADRENAL HYPERPLASIA DUE TO 3β-HYDROXYSTEROID DEHYDROGENASE DEFICIENCY

Congenital adrenal hyperplasia due to 3β-hydroxysteroid dehydrogenase deficiency is also due to recessive genes that have been mapped to the short arm of chromosome 1. Testosterone, aldosterone, and cortisol values are all reduced. Males have incomplete prenatal genital development from decreased androgen synthesis in the testes as well as in the adrenal gland. Females can experience mild masculinization because of the increased production of a weak androgen that is produced before the deficient enzyme in the hormone biosynthesis pathway of the adrenal gland. The majority of patients with 3β-hydroxysteroid dehydrogenase deficiency have varying degrees of salt wasting due to insufficient aldosterone (Kalaitzoglou & New, 1993; Miller & Levine, 1987; New et al., 1990).

CONGENITAL ADRENAL HYPERPLASIA DUE TO 11β-HYDROXYLASE DEFICIENCY

The second most common form of CAH is 11β-hydroxylase deficiency. The recessive genes involved in this disorder are located on the long arm of chromosome 8. Unlike the other two described forms of CAH, 11β-hydroxylase deficiency is distinguished by hypertension, hypokalemia, and sodium retention in the majority of patients. 11-Deoxycortisol is not converted to cortisol, and deoxycorticosterone is usually not converted to corticosterone. Again, because there is deficient cortisol, which acts as a negative feedback to turn off adrenal production of steroids, excess prenatal androgen secretion results in female virilization with normal internal female reproductive organs (Kalaitzoglou & New, 1993; New, 1988; New et al., 1990).

CONGENITAL ADRENAL HYPERPLASIA DUE TO 17α-HYDROXYLASE/17,20-LYASE DEFICIENCY

A defect in the microsomal enzyme $P450_{c17}$, which catalyzes both 17α-hydroxylase and 17,20-lyase, is present in both the adrenals and gonads. Consequently, a reduction in all androgens and estrogens results. Males present with pseudohermaphroditism and gynecomastia. Females express infantile genitalia. Neither male nor female adolescents experience pubertal changes. Owing to elevated concentrations of deoxycorticosterone, hypertension and hypokalemia may develop. The recessive gene for the $P450_{c17}$ enzyme has been mapped to chromosome 10 (Kalaitzoglou & New, 1993).

COLLABORATIVE MANAGEMENT

Newborns

- Evaluation is done by an endocrinologist and geneticist.
- Serum hormone concentrations are monitored and blood is drawn for chromosome analysis.
- Signs of acute adrenal insufficiency are sought.
- Replacement hormone therapy may be started when CAH is suggested.
- Eventually, virilized females can undergo surgical correction (Miller & Levine, 1987; New, 1988).

Emphasis has been placed on prenatal diagnosis and treatment of CAH due to 21-hydroxylase deficiency (Kuller, Chescheir, & Cefalo, 1996). The goal is to avoid corrective genital surgery after birth by preventing virilization of females.

- Oral dexamethasone or hydrocortisone is administered to the mother as early as possible during the first trimester.
- Chorionic villus sampling is done between 8 and 12 weeks' gestation.
- Amniocentesis, done between 14 to 18 weeks' gestation, can be performed for DNA analysis and gender determination. If the fetus is male or an unaffected female, the mother can discontinue treatment. Therapy is continued to term if the fetus is an affected female.

Parents

Parents of a newborn with CAH-induced ambiguous genitalia require immediate information about questionable sex assignment. Naming their child is postponed until sex can be genetically determined. Health care providers should refer to the neonate as the "baby," "infant," or "child." It must be emphasized that virilized females possess normal internal reproductive organs and that external genitalia can be surgically corrected.

Medication administration and schedules must be taught to the parents. Compliance must be stressed and the need for lifelong hormone replacement therapy emphasized.

Parents also need to be educated about the signs and symptoms of dehydration.

Frequent and regular evaluation of affected infants is necessary to monitor and adjust the dosage of cortisone when ACTH suppression may be inadequate.

Certain stressors, such as illness, trauma, and surgery, may trigger an adrenal crisis requiring medication adjustment (DiGrande, 1984).

Disorders of Gonadal Differentiation

Disorders of gonadal differentiation involve abnormal combinations of the sex chromosomes X and Y. Basic descriptions of these disorders can be classified into three separate categories based on phenotypic expression or the observable characteristics of the individual.

The first general category involves phenotypic females with abnormal gonadal differentiation. Two specific types include Turner's syndrome and Swyer's syndrome. The second general category consists of phenotypic males with abnormal gonadal differentiation. Included are Klinefelter's syndrome and XX male phenotypes. A third general category comprises sexually ambiguous individuals with gonadal dysgenesis. Identifiable types include (1) male pseudohermaphroditism, (2) true hermaphroditism, (3) Leydig cell hypoplasia, and (4) testicular regression syndrome.

TURNER'S SYNDROME

Individuals with Turner's syndrome have a 45,X genotype with characteristic congenital anomalies that include skeletal defects, webbing of the neck, lymphedema of the hands and feet at birth, and shortened stature in adulthood. The gonads are eventually reduced to fibrous streaks, which leads to primary amenorrhea, sexual infantilism, and infertility (New & Josso, 1988). Recognition of the syndrome before puberty may be done by obtaining a karyotype of the chromosomal set.

Incidence

The incidence of Turner's syndrome is 1 in 2200 female births.

Treatment

Sex hormone (estrogen) replacement therapy is begun at puberty, followed by low-dose maintenance estrogen administration (New & Josso, 1988; Ross et al., 1983).

SWYER'S SYNDROME

Swyer's syndrome, like Turner's syndrome, often presents at puberty with primary amenorrhea. Streak gonads are seen, but without the congenital anomalies that accompany Turner's syndrome. The karyotype may reveal a 46,XX or 46,XY genotype. Treatment involves hormone replacement therapy and exploratory surgery to remove streak gonads.

KLINEFELTER'S SYNDROME

The karyotype of individuals with Klinefelter's syndrome shows one additional X chromosome. Mosaic combinations (usually 46,XY, 47,XXY) may also be possible. Adult XXY males present with small testes, sterile seminiferous tubules, and gynecomastia owing to lowered testosterone levels. Mental retardation may also be seen. Diagnosis is made through Barr screening to determine the sex chromosomal arrangement.

Treatment includes testosterone replacement therapy in individuals with postpubertal hypogonadism (New & Josso, 1988).

GONADAL DYSGENESIS

Infants with XX male phenotypes have testicular development in the absence of a Y chromosome. These individuals usually present with infertility problems.

Individuals with pseudohermaphroditism with mixed gonadal dysgenesis have impaired testicular function, which leads to early fetal testicular dysgenesis. Sexual ambiguity occurs with the presence of one or two testes, hypospadias, cryptorchidism, and an intact uterus. There is an increased risk of gonadal tumors. In addition, Turner's syndrome–like characteristics may be seen. The sex of rearing is preferably female if the infant is diagnosed and treated at an early age, usually under 2 years. If the child is older, sex reassignment may psychologically impair the individual. Thus, it is better to correct the hypospadias and cryptorchidism surgically, remove gonadal streaks, and monitor for tumor development. Testosterone hormone replacement should be provided at puberty, and the individual should retain his male gender (New & Josso, 1988).

True hermaphrodites possess both testicular and ovarian tissue, often combined in the same gonad, called an ovotestis. The newborn presents with ambiguous genitalia and abnormal internal anatomic structures. Whereas internal testicular tissue usually degenerates, the ovarian tissue remains functional, and thus fertility may be possible in the female sex. For this reason, the female sex is the desired sex of rearing.

Treatment involves surgical removal of internal organs contradictory to desired sex.

Leydig cell hypoplasia and embryonic testicular regression syndrome are both rare occurrences. Sexual ambiguity is often seen, and these disorders may be genetically transmitted.

Additional Causes of Ambiguous Genitalia

Other causes of ambiguous genitalia are maternal exposure to androgens, 5α-reductase deficiency, and end-organ androgen insensitivity (Hamblin, Assimos, & Kroovand, 1989). Maternal exposure to androgens may be either exogenous (through the use of certain prescribed oral contraceptives) or endogenous (by increased circulating androgens due to a maternal tumor).

Strategies in Assessment

Assessment of the newborn with ambiguous genitalia includes a complete family history and physical examination, followed by a thorough diagnostic evaluation.

CLINICAL MANIFESTATIONS

The features of ambiguous genitalia include the following:

- Structure that resembles an enlarged clitoris or micropenis with hypospadias
- Partial fusion of labioscrotal folds
- Absence of gonads or one palpable gonad in the incomplete scrotum of a term infant (Mazur, 1983)
- Downward bowing of the penile-clitoral structure, called chordee

DIAGNOSTIC EVALUATION

The goals of diagnostic evaluation are to determine the cause of the abnormality and to develop an appropriate plan of care. It should be explained to the parents that although their infant was born with sexual organs that appear underdeveloped or unfinished, a thorough evaluation will help define the extent of the condition and determine the most effective strategy to complete the unfinished sex organs (Mazur, 1983).

A comprehensive diagnostic evaluation involves three areas of testing: (1) measurement of the circulating hormones, (2) analysis of the chromosomes, and (3) visualization of the internal organs.

First, measurement of the circulating hormones will identify the presence of abnormal levels. Evaluating specific hormone levels can be accomplished through measurement of urinary 17-ketosteroids and blood pregnanetriol. Elevation of these hormonal levels may indicate CAH. These levels may also be assessed prenatally by sampling amniotic fluid to identify an affected fetus (Frasier, Weiss, & Horton, 1974; Pang et al., 1977).

Infants with ambiguous genitalia in which CAH has been ruled out may be further evaluated with serum testosterone measurement and a human chorionic gonadotropin stimulation test. When performed when the newborn is between 2 and 9 weeks of age, these tests can help to determine the integrity of the hypothalamic–pituitary axis in male infants and can identify the presence of testicular tissue in infants with ambiguous genitalia (Ismail, Walker, Macfaul, & Gindal, 1989).

Second, analysis of the chromosomes determines the chromosomal or genetic sex of the infant. Complete chromosomal analysis can be done through the establishment of a karyotype.

Advances in genetics (Erickson, Verga, & Dasouki, 1990) have provided information about the sex-determining gene, zinc finger Y, which can be identified on part of the Y chromosome with the use of a probe. The probe can determine the integrity of the gene and can be useful in the diagnosis of an infant with ambiguous genitalia.

Third, visualization of the internal organs provides a comprehensive picture of the anatomic structures involved in an infant with abnormal sexual differentiation. Pelvic ultrasonography is an important diagnostic tool for determining the presence of a uterus or urogenital sinus or both. Contrast studies (genitography) may further clarify the presence of a urogenital sinus. Magnetic resonance imaging can be useful in identifying undescended testes. Endoscopy of the urogenital sinus may determine if there is a small or abnormal vagina. Laparotomy or laparoscopy and gonadal biopsy in the infant is controversial, owing to limited availability of smaller-sized instruments. These procedures should be done only in infants who will require removal of the gonads, such as true hermaphrodites and infants with mixed gonadal dysgenesis (Hamblin, Assimos, & Kroovand, 1989).

COLLABORATIVE MANAGEMENT

Medical Management

Medical management involves assessment and diagnosis of the disorder, as well as physical stabilization of the neonate experiencing a salt-wasting adrenal crisis from CAH.

Through an extensive diagnostic process, a determination as to the desired sex of rearing should be made. Gender assignment is based on the infant's anatomy (Hamblin, Assimos, & Kroovand, 1989), with less emphasis on the chromosomal sex or the prospect for future fertility except in females with CAH. It is usually more difficult to masculinize than to feminize an affected individual. Therefore, only those infants with a satisfactory phallic structure typically greater than 2.0 cm in length from the symphysis pubis to the tip should be considered a candidate for male sex assignment. Adequate phallic structure will respond to testosterone replacement therapy, whereas an inadequate phallic structure will not (Penny, 1990). Infants with a micropenis assigned the female gender will require surgical correction of the external genitalia, gonadectomy, estrogen supplementation therapy at puberty as well as maintenance therapy in adulthood, and possible additional surgery for the construction of a neovagina (Castiglia, 1989; Rock & Jones, 1989).

Nursing Management

Three levels of concern include immediate, midrange, and long-term needs and goals. The immediate needs and goals involve the potential for a life-threatening adrenal crisis, as may be seen in the neonate with salt-wasting CAH. The primary goal is directed toward achieving elevation of circulating cortisol and replacement of sodium and water deficits. Fluid and electrolyte status and circulating cortisol levels should be carefully monitored.

The midrange needs and goals of the sexually ambiguous infant relate to the assessment and diagnosis of the disorder that led to the ambiguous genitalia. The needs and goals of the infant at the long-term level pertain to the therapeutic intervention developed to manage the disorder and correct the ambiguous genitalia.

Parents often wonder about the risk of recurrence, which, in fact, depends on the actual diagnosis of their affected child. In the more common classic 21-hydroxylase deficiency of CAH, there is a 25 percent risk of a subsequent affected sibling (Shapiro, Santiago, & Crane, 1989). The parents should undergo genetic counseling to determine their risk for subsequent childbearing.

Families may benefit from a referral to social services to assist them with available community resources. Support groups may be established so that families and affected individuals can gain confidence in knowing that they are not alone in dealing with the disorder.

CYSTIC FIBROSIS

Cystic fibrosis (CF), formerly known as mucoviscidosis or CF of the pancreas, is an inherited, chronic, progressive, metabolic disorder affecting the exocrine (mucus-secreting) glands. Classic CF is characterized by chronic pulmonary infection, pancreatic insufficiency, and increased salt loss through the sweat glands.

PATHOPHYSIOLOGY

Pulmonary disease probably begins with the development of mucus plugging or obstruction of small airways. Eventually, the patient experiences chronic inflammation and obstruction of larger airways. As the patient is colonized with bacteria, infection sets in. Repeated infection and inflammation lead to structural changes in the airway, consisting of damage to respiratory epithelium, supporting structures, airway, wall, and pulmonary vasculature. Repeated exacerbations can result in bronchiectasis and pulmonary fibrosis. Pulmonary parenchymal changes cause an increase in pulmonary vascular resistance, leading to pulmonary hypertension, cor pulmonale, and cardiorespiratory failure (Hilman, 1989).

The course of CF is chronic and progressive, characterized by frequent respiratory infections with *Haemophilus influenzae, Staphylococcus aureus,* and *Pseudomonas aeruginosa. Burkholderia cepacia* (formerly *Pseudomonas cepacia)* is seen less commonly but may be associated with greater morbidity and mortality than *P. aeruginosa* colonization.

Early radiographic findings include (1) hyperinflation or emphysema due to partial airway obstruction and (2) patchy areas of atelectasis due to complete airway obstruction. Characteristically, patients develop generalized nodulocystic shadowing and increased bronchial markings. Destructive changes within the airways eventually lead to severe bronchiectasis with a "honeycomb" appearance of the lung on the radiograph (Hilman, 1989).

INCIDENCE

Cystic fibrosis occurs in 1 in 2000 people of European ancestry. Incidence in the African-American population is 1 in 17,000 (Kulczycki & Schauf, 1974); the disorder is estimated to be much less common in Asians and Native Americans (Wood, Boat, & Doershuk, 1976). It is the most common fatal genetic disorder affecting the white population. The trait is recessive with a carrier frequency of 1 in 20.

CLINICAL MANIFESTATIONS

There may be a combination of the following findings:

- Recurrent respiratory tract infections
- Abnormal stools
- Failure to thrive

Less common presentations are listed below:

- Intestinal obstruction (e.g., meconium ileus), rectal prolapse

- Nasal polyps
- Prolonged neonatal jaundice
- Hyponatremic/hypochloremic dehydration
- Hypoproteinemia

Pulmonary disease is usually a major clinical problem for the patient with CF later in life, but it can also present in the neonatal period.

The following are additional signs:

- Cough that is initially dry and that later becomes productive and increased at night
- Decreased exercise tolerance
- Tachypnea
- Retractions
- Flaring
- Increased anteroposterior diameter of the chest
- Crackles
- Wheezes
- Digital clubbing
- Pneumonia

Once generalized bronchiectasis is evident, the clinical course steadily progresses with the following (Wood, Boat, & Doershuk, 1976):

- Frequent exacerbations
- Eventual respiratory failure
- Cor pulmonale
- Death

In CF, the pancreatic duct becomes obstructed with thick mucus, which does not allow for the passage of enzymes. This obstruction leads to fibrosis and destruction of the pancreas. Consequently, food (predominantly proteins and fats) cannot be digested and absorbed normally, leading to signs and symptoms of malnutrition. Absorption of the fat-soluble vitamins A, D, E, and K is therefore impaired, resulting in frequent, bulky, loose, greasy stools (steatorrhea) and poor growth.

Ten to 20 percent of newborns with CF present with meconium ileus, which is a functional bowel obstruction presenting between 24 and 48 hours of age caused by large quantities of thick meconium in the small and large intestine. There may be abdominal distention, vomiting, failure to pass meconium, and, rarely, meconium peritonitis (Orenstein, 1989).

DIFFERENTIAL DIAGNOSIS

The diagnosis of CF is based on a combination of typical clinical signs and symptoms as well as a positive sweat test. The accepted method to confirm the diagnosis of CF is the Gibson-Cooke sweat test. A sweat chloride concentration of greater than 60 mEq/L is diagnostic in children; 70 mg of sweat is needed to obtain an accurate result. Sweat testing in the newborn period is difficult, because infants may not produce sufficient quantities of sweat. If a sufficient quantity is collected, the results are as valid as in older individuals (Gibson & Cooke, 1959; Orenstein, 1989).

The most common cause of a false-positive sweat test is laboratory error.

False-positive results can also be found in malnutrition, adrenal insufficiency, ectodermal dysplasia, nephrogenic diabetes insipidus, hypothyroidism, and mucopolysaccharidosis. False-negative results can occur in the presence of edema and hypoproteinemia (Wood, Boat, & Doershuk, 1976).

DNA analysis can be performed on buccal smears (cheek cell smears) of infants weighing less than 8 pounds or when sufficient sweat is unobtainable. This test is 90 percent sensitive for the white North American population (Richards et al., 1992).

Prenatal testing for CF includes DNA analysis of chorionic villus samples during the first trimester (8 to 10 weeks) or of amniotic fluid samples collected after 14 weeks. If a positive family history of CF exists, the risk can usually be assessed in the fetus by testing through mutation analysis or restriction fragment length polymorphism markers to determine haplotype.

Another screening test is the immunoreactive trypsin assay, which is performed on a dried blood spot. A newborn with CF can have extremely high levels of plasma trypsinogen compared with normal infants. This elevation is presumed to occur because of pancreatic duct obstruction.

COLLABORATIVE MANAGEMENT

There is still no cure for CF. Care revolves around preventing the progression of the disease and treating the symptoms.

The first goal of therapy is to minimize pulmonary infections and prevent the progression of disease. This goal is accomplished by using mucus clearance techniques such as chest physiotherapy and postural drainage. Occasionally, aerosols of bronchodilators and mucolytic agents are used in combination with chest physiotherapy.

Oral or intravenous antibiotics are used during respiratory exacerbations to help decrease bacterial colonization and minimize inflammation. Supplemental oxygen becomes necessary when hypoxemia occurs.

A second goal of therapy is to ensure adequate nutrition. The aim of nutritional therapy is to foster normal growth and development while contributing to the general health of the individual.

Pancreatic enzyme replacement therapy is used to replace the enzymes that normally reach the intestine via the pancreatic duct. A diet high in calories (120 to 150 percent recommended daily allowance) and protein (200 percent recommended daily allowance) is needed, along with vitamin supplementation, with emphasis on the fat-soluble vitamins (A, D, E, and K) in a water-soluble form. Infants are often prescribed an elemental or predigested formula such as Pregestimil or Portagen, especially if the infant is nutritionally deprived at the time of diagnosis. To meet an individual's nutritional goals, an increased calorie per ounce formula may be given (e.g., 24 or 27 cal/oz). Individuals may also receive feedings by nasogastric, gastrostomy, or jejunostomy tubes if oral intake is poor.

A third goal of treatment is to facilitate family coping skills and adaptation to a condition that will be lifelong. Families are confronted by enormous psychological stresses, financial obligations, and time burdens. The nurse can assist in the adjustment process, and referral to the social worker or psychologist may be indicated. Families can be referred to a genetic specialist for genetic counseling and future planning.

Nursing Management

If an infant is suspected of having CF, the nurse may provide help to the family, as follows:

- Makes a referral to the CF clinic and collaborates with the nurse on the CF team to help coordinate efforts and avoid confusing the family with conflicting information.
- Provides clarification regarding the following:
  - Diagnosis
  - Genetic issues
  - Therapy
  - Home management
  - Medications
  - Equipment
  - Normal growth and development
  - Follow-up routine
- Refers the family to their local Cystic Fibrosis Foundation and parent support group and assists them in locating community informational, service, and support resources as well as funding sources.

PROGNOSIS

Survival statistics are improving steadily, and the median age of survival is now approaching 30 years of age (Cystic Fibrosis Genotype-Phenotype Consortium, 1993; Cystic Fibrosis Foundation, 1994).

REFERENCES

Aetiology of growth hormone deficiency [Letter]. (1988). *Archives of Disease in Childhood, 63,* 219–220.

Avery, G. B., Fletcher, M. A., & MacDonald, M. G. (Eds.). (1994). *Neonatology: Pathophysiology and management of the newborn* (4th ed.). Philadelphia: J. B. Lippincott.

Becks, G. P., & Burrow, G. N. (1990). Thyrotoxicosis in pregnancy. In N. M. Nelson (Ed.), *Current therapy in neonatal–perinatal medicine 2* (pp. 108–111). Philadelphia: B. C. Decker.

Bona, G., Aquili, C., Ravanini, P., et al. (1994). Growth hormone, insulin-like growth factor-I and somatostatin in human fetus, newborn, mother plasma and amniotic fluid. *Panminerva Medica, 36*(1), 5–12.

Cannon, P. J. (1977). The kidney in heart failure. *New England Journal of Medicine, 296,* 26–32.

Castiglia, P. T. (1989). Ambiguous genitalia. *Journal of Pediatric Health Care, 3,* 319–321.

Cloherty, J. P., & Stark, A. R. (Eds.). (1991). *Manual of neonatal care* (3rd ed.). Boston: Little, Brown.

Cowett, R. M., & Schwartz, R. (1982). The infant of the diabetic mother. *Pediatric Clinics of North America, 29,* 1213–1231.

Cruz, T. V. D., MacMillan, D. R., Browning, R. M., & Stewart, D. L. (1995). Delayed diagnosis of congenital adrenal hyperplasia in a premature female infant. *Journal of Kentucky Medical Association, 93*(1), 19–21.

Cystic Fibrosis Foundation. (1994). Patient Registry 1993, Annual Data Report, Bethesda, Maryland.

Cystic Fibrosis Genotype Phenotype Consortium. (1993). Correlation between genotype and phenotype in patients with cystic fibrosis. *The New England Journal of Medicine, 329*, 1308–1313.

DiGrande, A. (1984). The child born with ambiguous genitalia: Family assessment and nursing intervention. *Issues in Comprehensive Pediatric Nursing, 7*, 307–318.

Einaudi, S., Lala, R., Corrias, A., et al. (1993). Auxological and biochemical parameters in assessing treatment of infants and toddlers with congenital adrenal hyperplasia due to 21-hydroxylase deficiency. *Journal of Pediatric Endocrinology, 6*, 173–178.

Erickson, R. P., Verga, V., & Dasouki, M. (1990). Use of a probe for the putative sex determining gene, zinc finger Y, in the study of patients with ambiguous genitalia and XY gonadal dysgenesis. *American Journal of Medical Genetics, 36*, 232–236.

Frasier, S. D., Weiss, B. A., & Horton, R. (1974). Amniotic fluid testosterone: Implications for the prenatal diagnosis of congenital adrenal hyperplasia. *Journal of Pediatrics, 8*, 738.

Ganong, W. F. (1985). *Review of medical physiology* (12th ed.). Los Altos, CA: Lange Medical Publications.

Gelato, M. C., Malozowski, S., Pescovitz, O. H., et al. (1987). Growth hormone–releasing hormone: Therapeutic perspectives. *Pediatrician, 14*, 162–167.

Gibson, L., & Cooke, R. (1959). A test for concentration of electrolytes in sweat in cystic fibrosis of the pancreas utilizing pilocarpine by iontophoresis. *Pediatrics, 23*, 545–549.

Goetzman, B. W., & Wennberg, R. P. (1991). *Neonatal intensive care handbook* (2nd ed.). St. Louis: Mosby–Year Book.

Griffin, J. E., & Wilson, J. D. (1986). Disorders of sexual differentiation. In P. C. Walsh, R. F. Gittes, A. D. Perlmutter, & T. A. Stamey (Eds.), *Campbell's urology* (5th ed.). Philadelphia: W. B. Saunders.

Hamblin, J. E., Assimos, D. G., & Kroovand, R. L. (1989). Pediatric urology. *Primary Care, 16*, 889–904.

Herber, S. M., & Kay, R. (1987). Aetiology of growth hormone deficiency. *Archives of Disease in Childhood, 62*, 735–736.

Herber, S. M., & Milner, D. G. (1984). Growth hormone deficiency presenting under age 2 years. *Archives of Disease in Childhood, 59*, 557–560.

Hilman, B. (1989). Cystic fibrosis—changing concepts. *Schumpert Medical Quarterly, 7*, 345–370.

Hitti, I. F., Glasberg, S. S., Huggins-Jones, D., & Sabet, R. (1994). Bilateral femoral hypoplasia and maternal diabetes mellitus. *Pediatric Pathology, 14*, 567–574.

Hoskins, S. K. (1990). Nursing care of the infant of a diabetic mother. *Neonatal Network, 9*, 39–46.

Ismail, A. A., Walker, P. L., Macfaul, R., & Gindal, B. (1989). Diagnostic value of serum testosterone measurement in infancy: Two case reports. *Annals of Clinical Biochemistry, 26*(Pt. 3), 259–261.

Kalaitzoglou, G., & New, M. I. (1993). Congenital adrenal hyperplasia: Molecular insights learned from patients. *Receptor, 3*, 211–222.

Kelnar, C. J. H. (1993). Congenital adrenal hyperplasia (CAH)—the place for prenatal treatment and neonatal screening. *Early Human Development, 35*, 81–90.

Kinzie, B. J. (1987). Management of the syndrome of inappropriate secretion of antidiuretic hormone. *Clinical Pharmacy, 6*, 625–633.

Kuller, J. A., Chescheir, N. C., & Cefalo, R. C. (1996). (Eds.). *Prenatal diagnosis & reproductive genetics.* Philadelphia: J. B. Lippincott.

Kulczycki, L., & Schauf, V. (1974). Cystic fibrosis in blacks in Washington, D.C.: Incidence and characteristics. *American Journal of Diseases of Children, 127*, 64.

Lanes, R., Nieto, C., Bruguera, C., et al. (1989). Growth hormone release in response to growth hormone–releasing hormone in term and preterm neonates. *Biology of the Neonate, 56*, 252–256.

Malvaux, P. (1981). Hypothyroidism. In C. Brook (Ed.), *Clinical paediatric endocrinology* (pp. 329–336). London: Blackwell Scientific Publications.

Mazur, T. (1983). Ambiguous genitalia: Detection and counseling. *Pediatric Nursing, 9,* 417–422, 431.

Miller, W. L., & Levine, L. S. (1987). Molecular and clinical advances in congenital adrenal hyperplasia. *Journal of Pediatrics, 111,* 1–17.

Mininberg, D. T., Levine, L. S., & New, M. I. (1982). Current concepts in congenital adrenal hyperplasia. In T. V. N. Persaud (Ed.), *Advances in the study of birth defects: Genetic disorders, syndromology and prenatal diagnosis* (Vol. 5, pp. 181–196). New York: Alan R. Liss.

Moore, K. L., & Persaud, T. V. N. (1993). *Before we are born: Basic embryology and birth defects* (4th ed.). Philadelphia: W. B. Saunders.

Neufeld, N. D. (1987). Infants of diabetic mothers: Prenatal care and outcomes for the infant. *Mount Sinai Journal of Medicine, 54,* 266–271.

New, M. (1988). Congenital adrenal hyperplasia. *Biochemical Society Transactions, 16,* 691–694.

New, M. I., & Josso, N. (1988). Disorders of gonadal differentiation and CAH. *Endocrinology and Metabolism Clinics of North America, 17,* 339–366.

New, M. I., White, P. C., Speiser, P. W., et al. (1990). Congenital adrenal hyperplasia. In A. E. H. Emery & D. L. Rimoin (Eds.), *Principles and practice of medical genetics* (Vol. 2., pp. 1559–1586). Edinburgh: Churchill Livingstone.

Novak, R. W., & Robinson, H. B. (1994). Coincident DiGeorge anomaly and renal agenesis and its relation to maternal diabetes. *American Journal of Medicine Genetics, 50,* 311–312.

Orenstein, D. (1989). *Cystic fibrosis: A guide for patient and family.* New York: Raven Press.

Pang, S., Hotchkiss, J., Drash, A. L., et al. (1977). Microfilter paper method for 17 alpha-progesterone radioimmunoassay: Its application for rapid screening for congenital adrenal hyperplasia. *Journal of Clinical Endocrinology and Metabolism, 4,* 1003.

Parks, J. S. (1981). Hyperthyroidism. In C. Brook (Ed.), *Clinical paediatric endocrinology* (pp. 340–361). London: Blackwell Scientific Publications.

Penny, R. (1990). Ambiguous genitalia [editorial]. *American Journal of Diseases of Children, 144,* 753.

Perelman, R. H. (1983). The infant of the diabetic mother. *Primary Care, 10,* 751–760.

Pressler, J. L. (1991). Strategies useful in caring for macrosomic newborns. *Journal of Pediatric Nursing, 6,* 149–153.

Richards, B., Skoletsky, J., Shuber, A., et al. (1992). Multiplex PCR amplification from the *CFTR* gene using DNA prepared from buccal brushes/swabs. *Human Molecular Genetics, 2,* 159–163.

Rimoin, D. L. (1990). Genetic disorders of the pituitary gland. In A. E. Emery & D. L. Rimoin (Eds.), *Principles and practice of medical genetics* (Vol. 2, pp. 1461–1488). Edinburgh: Churchill Livingstone.

Riordan, J., Rommens, J., Kerem, B., et al. (1989). Identification of the cystic fibrosis gene: Cloning and characterization of complementary DNA. *Science, 245,* 1066–1073.

Rock, J. A., & Jones, H. W., Jr. (1989). Construction of a neovagina for patients with a flat perineum. *American Journal of Obstetrics and Gynecology, 160,* 845–853.

Ross, J. L., Cassorla, F. G., Skerda, M. C., et al. (1983). A preliminary study of the effect of estrogen dose on growth in Turner's syndrome. *New England Journal of Medicine, 309,* 1104.

Shapiro, E., Santiago, J. V., & Crane, J. P. (1989). Prenatal fetal adrenal suppression following in utero diagnosis of CAH. *Journal of Urology, 142,* 663–666.

Shimano, S., Suzuki, S., Nagashima, K., et al. (1985). Growth hormone response to growth hormone releasing factor in neonates. *Biology of the Neonate, 47,* 367–370.

Wallis, M. (1988). The molecular basis of growth hormone deficiency. *Molecular Aspects of Medicine, 10,* 429–509.

Weise, K., & Zaritsky, A. (1987). Endocrine manifestations of critical illness in the child. *Pediatric Clinics of North America, 34,* 119–130.

White, P. (1974). Diabetes mellitus in pregnancy. *Clinics in Perinatology, 1,* 331–347.

White, P. C., New, M. I., & Dupont, B. (1986). Structure of human steroid 21-hydroxylase genes. *Proceedings from the National Academy of Science, 83,* 5111–5115.

Wood, R., Boat, T., & Doershuk, C. (1976). Cystic fibrosis. *American Review of Respiratory Disease, 113,* 833–878.

CHAPTER 15

Assessment and Management of Immunologic Dysfunction

MATERNAL–FETAL–NEONATAL RELATIONSHIPS

The predominant transfer of antibody occurs by way of passage of immunoglobulin (Ig) G from the maternal to the fetal circulation by an active transport process. Such immunity is transient but nevertheless may provide protection during a vulnerable time of life. Although this passive antibody may protect the newborn, this process may interfere with active antibody synthesis after immunization. Secretory IgA in breast milk may also interfere with successful immunization, particularly with live poliovirus, by neutralization of virus by antibody in the gastrointestinal tract. Maternal antibodies may have other harmful effects on the newborn.

Inherited Newborn Immunodeficiencies

PHAGOCYTIC DISORDERS

Neutropenia (low neutrophil count) is the most common sign of phagocytic dysfunction and is easily detected by a simple complete blood cell count with differential. Neutropenia can be further worked up by bone marrow examination, by blood smear examination, and by other specific tests such as the dye test for chronic granulomatous disease. Defects in neutrophil chemotaxis, described in patients with recurrent abscesses, can be evaluated by special tests.

DISORDERS OF ANTIBODY FORMATION

Evaluation of antibody-mediated immunity begins with quantitative immunoglobulins; however, because most of the neonate's immunoglobulin is maternal, this test is not particularly helpful during the first 3 months of life. IgM elevation in the cord blood may indicate intrauterine infection, and elevations of both IgM and IgA suggest maternal–fetal bleeding (Fanaroff & Martin, 1997). Studies of circulating B lymphocytes should be performed on infants with immunoglobulin deficiency. Some infants who cannot make immunoglobulins do have circulating B lymphocytes, but these cannot differentiate into plasma cells and secrete immunoglobulins or antibodies, as is common in patients with acquired agammaglobulinemia (now called common variable immunodeficiency) (Fanaroff & Martin, 1997).

T-LYMPHOCYTE IMMUNODEFICIENCY

Because T lymphocytes constitute the vast majority of the circulating peripheral lymphocyte population, lymphopenia is noted when the number of T

323

lymphocytes is decreased. Delayed hypersensitivity skin reactions are not elicited in patients with cell-mediated immunodeficiency.

SEVERE COMBINED IMMUNODEFICIENCY (SCID)

This group of disorders is characterized by the absence of both T-lymphocyte and B-lymphocyte immunity. The congenital absence of cell-mediated and antibody-mediated immunity causes a profound susceptibility to a broad range of bacterial, viral, protozoal, and fungal infections. Infants with SCID usually develop symptoms of life-threatening infection during the first 3 months of life and often die quickly without immunologic reconstitution. There is some speculation from work on the Human Genome Project that at least one form of SCID may be an inborn error of metabolism that can potentially be successfully treated in utero (Bellanti, Pung, & Zeligs, 1994).

COMPLEMENT DISORDER

Both persistent and transient deficiencies of components of serum complement have been reported in the literature. The usual serum screening for complement levels of serum proteins detects defects in the classical pathway but will not ascertain deficiencies in the alternative pathway.

ASSESSMENT OF THE IMMUNE SYSTEM

Subjective Data

Areas to be covered in the history include family history of immune diseases, previous stillbirths or newborn deaths in the family, infections during pregnancy, maternal medications, previous diseases in the mother, and prior isoimmunization of the mother.

Objective Data

A meticulous physical examination of the neonate, in conjunction with the history, should provide a solid basis for interpretation of further objective data, including laboratory data.

Diagnostic Work-Up

Initial screening tests should be performed, moving on to more definitive testing to establish a specific diagnosis. The definitive tests may be available only at a tertiary care center.

INFECTION IN THE NEONATE

Clinical Manifestations

Clinical manifestations of infection are as follows:

- Hypothermia, the inability of the neonate to maintain temperature in the neutral thermal zone (usually between 97.7°F and 99°F axillary)

- Lethargy, poor feeding, and perhaps a poor Moro reflex
- Abdominal distention
- Delayed gastric emptying time
- Diarrhea or loose green or brown stools
- Poor weight gain
- Hypoglycemia or hyperglycemia, as well as glycosuria
- Decreased vascular perfusion
- Gray, mottled, or ashen color
- Cyanosis with petechiae and, potentially, thrombocytopenia
- Sclerema and/or disseminated intravascular coagulation affecting the prothrombin time, partial thromboplastin time, and split fibrin product laboratory values of the newborn
- Hemolytic anemia, significantly decreasing oxygen-carrying capacity
- Apnea in a term infant
- Respiratory distress (may be an early sign of pneumonia)
- Unexplained bradycardia
- Jaundice
- Hepatosplenomegaly
- Irritability

A preterm infant who demonstrates apnea in the first 24 hours of life is likely to be infected with foreign organisms. Shock can be a sudden clinical sign of fulminant sepsis and demands immediate and aggressive intervention to restore adequate circulation (Cairo et al., 1987; Levy & O'Rourke, 1995).

The following are laboratory studies that should be done:

- Complete blood cell count
- Leukopenia, especially neutropenia with a cell count of polymorphonuclear leukocytes less than 5000/mm^3, or a large number of immature leukocytes, in particular bands, with the band:leukocyte ratio greater than 0:2.

Indications of bacterial infection include the following:

- Increased total neutrophils—neutrophilia
- Decreased total neutrophils—neutropenia
- Increased immature forms (bands, metamyelocytes, sometimes promyelocytes, and myeloblasts)
- Increased band:segmented neutrophil ratio equal to or greater than 0:3 or immature:total neutrophil ratio greater than or equal to 0:2
- Döhle's bodies (aggregates of reticuloendothelial system)
- Vacuoles in nucleus
- Toxic granules in cell

Risk Factors

There are a number of risk factors:

- Prematurity
- Prolonged rupture of membranes longer than 24 hours
- Increased maternal temperature. If maternal temperature of 101°F is noted at delivery, a sepsis work-up is indicated. Maternal cervical or amniotic fluid cultures may be helpful to determine the causative agent.

If the maternal illness suggests viral infection, neonatal blood samples should be drawn for viral cultures.

- Foul-smelling amniotic fluid. This is an indication for neonatal antimicrobial therapy in symptomatic infants. The placenta should be sent for pathologic evaluation.
- Antenatal or intrapartal asphyxia
- Iatrogenic complications of treatment modalities
- Postnatal invasive procedures
- Indomethacin therapy for patent ductus arteriosus
- Stress, which inhibits the newborn's ability to fight infection

Maternal risk factors associated with sepsis are as follows:

- Low socioeconomic status
- Malnutrition
- No prenatal care
- Substance abuse
- Premature rupture of membranes (before 37 weeks' gestation or at the start of labor)
- Presence of a urinary tract infection at delivery
- Peripartum infection
- Clinical amnionitis
- General bacterial colonization

Differential Diagnosis

Microorganisms commonly responsible for early-onset infection include streptococci, *Listeria monocytogenes,* and gram-negative enteric rods. Late-onset infections are most often caused by staphylococci, *Pseudomonas,* or *Bacteroides fragilis* (anaerobes). After 7 days of age, nosocomial microorganisms should be considered. These microorganisms include *Staphylococcus epidermidis,* particularly with invasive medical devices, such as endotracheal tubes and arterial lines; *Staphylococcus aureus* (common skin contaminant); and the spectrum of gram-negative bacilli, including *Klebsiella, Pseudomonas, Serratia,* and *Escherichia coli.*

The evaluation for infection generally includes a complete blood cell count with differential, platelet count, and blood, urine, and cerebrospinal fluid (CSF) cultures. Gram stain of the CSF can give an indication of the type of microorganism responsible for the infection. Cell count and protein and glucose levels of the CSF may also indicate the presence of infection. A chest radiograph is performed to detect pneumonia. Other tests that may be useful include latex agglutination or counterimmunoelectrophoresis of urine or CSF, erythrocyte sedimentation rate, and acute phase proteins. Other nonspecific findings, such as hypoglycemia, hypocalcemia, thrombocytopenia, hyponatremia, or metabolic acidosis, may also be present. Definitive diagnosis is based on recovery of a microorganism in blood, CSF, urine, or other body fluids.

Collaborative Management

Collaborative management for an infected infant focuses on ventilatory support, oxygen therapy, correction of acidosis, immune therapy, volume expanders, extracorporeal membrane oxygenation if persistent pulmonary hypertension is present, and antimicrobial agents.

ANTIMICROBIAL AGENTS

The selection of antimicrobial agent is based on the microorganism present and the infant's response to therapy. Infectious microorganisms fall into two broad classes: gram positive and gram negative. The shape of the microorganism categorizes it as either a coccus or a rod. Generally, the gram-positive organisms respond to broad-spectrum antibiotics such as penicillin analogues and first-generation cephalosporins (beta-lactamases) and the beta-lactamase penicillins. The gram-negative microorganisms are most often susceptible to aminoglycosides, cephalosporins, and chloramphenicol. Tests must be run to determine the specific sensitivity of a microorganism to the antimicrobial agent selected.

Most gram-positive cocci respond to penicillin, unless the microorganism produces beta-lactamase (or penicillinase). The beta-lactamase destroys the penicillin. *S. aureus* is a beta-lactamase–producing microorganism and is therefore not usually responsive to penicillin. A group of semisynthetic penicillins with added side chains are used for treatment of *S. aureus* sepsis. Of this group, nafcillin and oxacillin are most often used. Other, similar drugs are methicillin, dicloxacillin, and cloxacillin. First-generation cephalosporins, such as cefazolin, cephalexin, and cephalothin, are also resistant to beta-lactamase.

S. epidermidis and *S. aureus* strains may be resistant to penicillin, semisynthetic penicillins, and cephalosporins. Methicillin-resistant *S. aureus* is unresponsive to semisynthetic penicillins. In this case, vancomycin is the drug of choice. It may also be used for *S. epidermidis* and sepsis related to foreign bodies or invasive procedures.

Third-generation cephalosporins are used to treat gram-negative cocci that are penicillin and methicillin resistant. *L. monocytogenes*, a gram-positive rod, is most successfully treated with ampicillin. Aminoglycosides or third-generation cephalosporins are the drugs of choice for gram-negative enteric rods. Some gram-negative rods are classified according to their lactose fermentation ability. The lactose fermenters are *E. coli* and *Klebsiella*. They are sensitive to aminoglycosides and third-generation cephalosporins. *Shigella* and *Salmonella* are nonlactose fermenters, which respond well to ampicillin and third-generation cephalosporins.

Haemophilus influenzae is usually sensitive to ampicillin and third-generation cephalosporins, although some strains are ampicillin resistant. *Pseudomonas* requires a combination therapy: aminoglycoside and anti-*Pseudomonas* penicillin such as azlocillin, carbenicillin, imipenem, mezlocillin, piperacillin, and ticarcillin.

Anaerobes are a subset of gram-negative and gram-positive rods. Two anaerobes associated with sepsis are *Bacteroides* and *Clostridium*. *Bacteroides* is susceptible to metronidazole, clindamycin, chloramphenicol, or some of the newer beta-lactamases, such as imipenem and ampicillin/sulbactam. *Clostridium* is usually susceptible to penicillin.

A combination of ampicillin and gentamicin is useful for antibacterial action against streptococci, *L. monocytogenes*, and gram-negative enteric rods. This combination of antimicrobial agents has a synergistic effect, increasing the efficacy of either drug therapy used by itself. Additional therapy or selection of other agents is necessary if staphylococcal infection is suspected, if *Pseudomonas* or *Bacteroides* (most often iatrogenically acquired) is present, if there is an outbreak of resistant organisms, or if prolonged ampicillin and gentamicin therapy has been used. Antibacterial agents must be re-evaluated after completion of cultures and sensitivity testing (Lott & Kilb, 1992).

TYPES OF NEONATAL INFECTION

Congenital Infections

The microorganisms most often responsible for congenitally acquired infections have been grouped together as the TORCH infections. These include *t*oxoplasmosis, *o*thers, *r*ubella, *c*ytomegalovirus, and *h*erpes. The "others" category includes various microorganisms that have been responsible for congenital infections.

TOXOPLASMOSIS

The life cycle of *Toxoplasma gondii* is complicated. The predominant host is the ordinary house cat. Other animals can serve as hosts. Congenital toxoplasmosis is transmitted from undercooked meat or food or from fomites in cat feces (Carter & Frank, 1986).

Clinical Manifestations

Women sometimes report a mononucleosis-like syndrome that may have a febrile course, with malaise, headache, fatigue, sore throat, and sore muscles. These symptoms may persist up to 6 months (Daffos et al., 1988).

In an infant, toxoplasmosis can present with hydrocephalus, chorioretinitis, and intracranial calcification. There is an incredible variety of clinical signs in the scope of the disease. A normal picture at birth, or even severe erythroblastosis, hydrops fetalis, and other clinical signs, can occur (Remington, McLeod, & Desmonts, 1995).

Neurologic signs similar to encephalitis occur, including convulsions, bulging fontanelles, nystagmus, and abnormal increase in circumference of the head. If the infant is treated, signs and symptoms may disappear, allowing normal cerebral growth and development.

Mild cases of the disease go unrecognized in the newborn. Signs and symptoms of delayed onset of disease in premature infants include very severe central nervous system or eye lesions appearing at 3 months of age.

In term infants, delayed disease may occur in the first 2 months of life and is usually more mild. Clinical signs may be generalized sepsis, enlarged liver and spleen, late-onset jaundice, enlarged lymph nodes, or late-onset central nervous system problems, including hydrocephalus and eye lesions. Infants with congenital toxoplasmosis may have new lesions appearing until age 5 years (Koppe, Loewer-Sieger, & deRoever-Bonnet, 1986).

Collaborative Management

Treatment of congenital toxoplasmosis is pyrimethamine plus sulfon-amides. The suggested dose is 1 mg/kg/day orally, with a maximum dose of 25 mg/day. Duration of treatment is varied, depending on the presentation of the congenital disease. Sulfonamides (sulfadiazine or trisulfapyrimidine) are given in doses of 85 mg/kg/day (two divided oral doses). Spiramycin can be given, 100 mg/kg/day orally in two doses every other month, as an alternative treatment. These drugs are potentially toxic and need close monitoring (Remington, McLeod, & Desmonts, 1995).

Toxoplasmosis is one of the most common causes of deafness and may include microcephaly and low IQ (less than 70) (Remington, McLeod, & Desmonts, 1995).

RUBELLA

Clinical Manifestations

The features of rubella are listed below:

- Malaise
- Low-grade fever
- Headache
- Conjunctivitis
- Rash. In 1 to 5 days, a macular rash appears on the face and usually disappears after 3 to 4 days. Often rashes that resemble rubella may occur as a result of adenovirus, enterovirus, or other respiratory virus infections.

Congenital rubella syndrome (CRS) is described by the Centers for Disease Control and Prevention (CDC) as hearing loss, mental retardation, cardiac malformations, and eye defects. Myocarditis, pneumonitis, hepato-splenomegaly, and vascular stenosis can also be present because of these processes. Unfortunately, as seen with other severe congenital infections, signs and symptoms may continue to develop until 10 to 20 years of age. Late clinical signs of this disease include insulin-dependent diabetes, thyroid abnormalities, hypoadrenalism, hearing loss, and eye damage (Sever, Smith, & Shaver, 1985).

Differential Diagnosis

The possibility of subclinical infection with rubella highlights the need for laboratory confirmation. It takes 4 to 6 weeks to obtain clinical confirmation of rubella isolation. The detection of rubella antibody confirms the presence of the infection. Rubella-specific IgG persists for life and can be detected by enzyme immunoassay. With confirmed serologic studies, the risk of fetal damage after 16 weeks' gestation appears to be small (Munro et al., 1987).

Demonstration of rubella-specific IgM in fetal blood obtained by cordo-centesis has been used to establish diagnosis in utero. Chorionic villus sampling has also demonstrated recovery of the virus during the first trimester (Enders & Jonatha, 1987).

Collaborative Management

All infants should be vaccinated against rubella at 15 months of age. Also, women who do not have detectable IgG rubella antibody and are of childbearing age (and not pregnant) should be immunized (CDC, 1984a). After immunization, they should avoid pregnancy for at least 3 months to decrease the risk for development of rubella syndrome in the fetus.

Today, treatment in the nursery of the rubella-infected infant is fortunately a rare occurrence. Supportive therapy for identified problems, such as respiratory, cardiac, or neurologic deficits, is in order, because there is no specific recommended therapy. Rubella-specific IgM can usually accurately identify these infants. Persistent shedding of the virus may last until 1 year of life, and thus pregnant women should avoid contact with these patients. Follow-up care for surgical corrections of heart defects and cataracts as well as special schooling may be needed for these infants.

CYTOMEGALOVIRUS

Cytomegalovirus (CMV), a member of the herpes family, is a very common infection. By adulthood, most people have been exposed and have developed antibodies to CMV. In the United States, women of childbearing age from lower socioeconomic groups have an incidence of about 6 percent, whereas those from higher socioeconomic groups have an incidence of about 2 percent. CMV may lie dormant, with periods of exacerbation followed by remission. During remission, the patient is asymptomatic, but the virus is shed (Stagno, 1995). The virus is usually transmitted person to person through body fluids and secretions. Blood, urine, breast milk, cervical mucus, semen, and saliva harbor CMV. The virus can cause an infectious mononucleosis-like syndrome, with general malaise, liver complications, fever, and general fatigue.

Perinatal transmission can occur within 2 to 3 days of infection by transplacental crossing of the organism. The fetus can also contract the virus intrapartally from infected maternal cervical secretions while descending through the birth canal. CMV can also be transmitted through infected breast milk (Nelson & Grossman, 1986).

Clinical Manifestations

More damage occurs to the fetus when the exposure to and acquisition of CMV occur from a primary lesion. Congenital CMV occurs in 0.2 to 2.2 percent of all newborns.

Primary lesions result in the following:

- Intrauterine growth retardation
- Microcephaly
- Periventricular calcifications
- Deafness
- Blindness
- Congenital cataracts
- Profound mental retardation
- Hepatosplenomegaly

- Jaundice
- "Blueberry muffin" syndrome

The American Academy of Pediatrics (1994) reports the incidence of neonatal complications to be 5 to 10 percent for hearing loss; 2 percent for chorioretinitis; and less than 1 percent for mental retardation.

Diagnosis

Suspicious clinical findings or obstetric history warrant further investigation.

- Urine culture–the most rapid and sensitive indicator
- IgG and IgM antibody titers. Elevated neonatal IgG titers indicate perinatally acquired CMV infection. A negative maternal IgG titer and a positive neonatal IgG titer indicate postnatal transmission.

Prevention

Transmission of CMV by infected blood products has been significantly decreased through the use of CMV-negative donors and irradiation of blood products.

Collaborative Management

Treatment is symptomatic. Specific therapy for CMV is still in the experimental stage but includes immunoglobulin therapy, vaccines, and chemotherapy. Intravenous immunoglobulin therapy provides passive immunity to at-risk infants but not to those already infected. Chemotherapeutic agents under investigation include idoxuridine, 5-fluoro-2'-deoxyuridine, cytarabine, vidarabine, acyclovir, leukocyte interferon, interferon stimulators, and ganciclovir. Toxicity and immunosuppression associated with these agents raise concern about widespread neonatal use (Stagno, 1995).

SYPHILIS

Syphilis is on the rise because of an increase in substance abuse, sexual practices involving multiple partners, and human immunodeficiency virus (HIV)–positive immunocompromised individuals, who act as reservoirs for *Treponema pallidum.*

Antenatal screening involves the use of the Venereal Disease Research Laboratory (VDRL) test or rapid plasma reagin (RPR) test, each of which measures anticardiolipin antibody. These tests are reactive in almost 80 percent of all patients with secondary or early latent (less than 1 year's duration) primary syphilis. A definitive diagnosis can be made with a rising VDRL or RPR accompanied by a positive *T. pallidum* fluoroantibody test or a reactive serologic test for *T. pallidum* in the CSF. Condylomata lata, bony changes, or snuffles in the presence of a positive serologic test are diagnostic (Ingall, Sanchez, & Musher, 1995).

The microorganisms can cause preterm labor, premature rupture of membranes, stillbirth, congenital infection, or neonatal death. Current untreated secondary infection causes the greatest risk of damage to the fetus, particularly if it occurs during the period of organogenesis. Late untreated syphilis usually presents as an asymptomatic infection in an infant who needs treatment in the newborn nursery.

Clinical Manifestations

When newborns acquire syphilis from hematogenous spread across the placenta, the effects are on the major organ systems of the fetus, especially the central nervous system (Chawla, Pandit, & Nkrumah, 1988):

- Hepatosplenomegaly
- Jaundice
- Low birth weight
- Intrauterine growth retardation
- Anemia
- Osteochondritis
- Bilateral superficial peeling of the skin (desquamation) on the neonatal palms and soles
- Nonimmune hydrops

Differential Diagnosis

A lumbar puncture for CSF analysis and radiographs of the long bones facilitate the definitive diagnosis. Radiologic changes such as osteochondritis (a blurring of the epiphyseal borders) demonstrate recent fetal infection (within 5 weeks), and periostitis represents prolonged involvement, probably 16 weeks or second-trimester infection.

Stillborns should be examined by whole-body radiography and autopsy if possible. Spirochetes can be visualized by special staining techniques (Ingall, Sanchez, & Musher, 1995).

VDRL titers at least two dilutions higher than maternal VDRL titers indicate probable fetal infection.

Prognosis

Serologic specimens can be measured at follow-up visits at 1, 2, 3, 6, and 12 months of age. The infection can be effectively treated, but the physiologic and developmental prognosis depends on the degree of organ damage sustained during fetal development.

Collaborative Management

The recommended treatment is aqueous penicillin G. In many perinatal centers, the presence of a positive VDRL in a neonate dictates treatment as if positive for syphilis. If neonatal clinical manifestations are highly suggestive of syphilis and there is a positive VDRL test but the titer is not significantly higher than the maternal titer, syphilis treatment should be instituted. A newborn with an antibody titer four times or more higher than the maternal level should be treated as if a definitive diagnosis has been obtained.

To prevent neurosyphilis, the infant should be treated with aqueous penicillin G, 100,000 to 150,000 units/kg intravenously in two or three divided doses for at least 10 to 14 days, or 50,000 units/kg/day of procaine penicillin in a daily dose for 10 to 14 days.

Asymptomatic infants whose mothers were treated adequately during pregnancy do not need treatment unless follow-up cannot be ensured. Some clinicians recommend benzathine penicillin, 50,000 units/kg intramuscularly in a single dose, if the infant is not likely to be observed. If maternal treatment did not include penicillin and if neonatal follow-up is likely to be unreliable, the neonate is treated for a full 10-day course.

Isolation of an infant with suspicious symptoms may be necessary until appropriate treatment has been given. There is a definite role for nursing education and support in the treatment of an infant exposed to syphilis. The 10- to 14-day course of penicillin treatment may lead to the establishment of a trusting relationship between the nurse and family, and thus more information regarding sexual risk factors can be given.

HERPES SIMPLEX VIRUS

Herpes simplex virus (HSV) is a member of a family of large DNA viruses. The herpesvirus family also includes CMV, varicella zoster, and Epstein-Barr virus. A strand of the viral DNA persists in an infected individual for a lifetime, and thus the virus is able to maintain a foothold in its unsuspecting host. Clinical experiences demonstrate that after primary HSV infection, at the site of the infection (perhaps an oral or genital site), the microorganism invades the sensory nerve endings and sets up housekeeping.

Potential stimuli for HSV reactivation include periods of stress, emotional trauma, or prolonged exposure to the sun.

Maternal HSV is usually the source of neonatal infection. The risk of neonatal infection is estimated to be 5 percent if it is recurrent herpes and higher if it is a primary infection (Arvin, 1988).

Transmission of the infection to the fetus can be caused by passage through infected genital secretions in the intrapartum period or by ascending infection from the vaginal vault through ruptured (or not) membranes. Unfortunately, many women can be asymptomatic and can be shedding HSV. Although primary infection is less common, it causes the most severe neonatal disease, most likely including central nervous system problems, disseminated disease into other organ systems, and probable death. The incidence of intrapartum transmission with a primary infection is 40 to 50 percent. Many neonatal complications such as prematurity, intrauterine retardation, and respiratory distress syndrome can potentiate the neonate's illness, limiting the ability to fight off HSV (Prober et al., 1988). There is a broad range of severity of neonatal infection, from very severe to benign and asymptomatic, but the incidence of neonatal herpes is 1500 to 2000 cases per year (Overall, 1994).

Clinical Manifestations

Clinical manifestations of neonatal HSV infection include the following:

- Skin vesicles and/or scarring
- Hypopigmentation
- Chorioretinitis

- Microcephaly
- Hydranencephaly

Neonatal patients are divided into three categories. The first category includes those with localized infections of the skin, eyes, or mouth. The second category includes those who present with encephalitis. In this group, neurologic sequelae are very high (approximately 50 percent). About one third of these patients do not have skin vesicles, and they are identified by history alone. The CSF is positive for the virus in 25 to 40 percent of these patients. The presence of cells and increased protein are very common in the CSF of patients with encephalitis, and they will die if not treated. The third category of neonatal patients includes those with disseminated disease characterized by irritability, seizures, respiratory distress, jaundice, disseminated intravascular coagulation, shock, and other symptoms of viral and bacterial sepsis. All major neonatal organs may be involved. Liver and the adrenals are the most common reservoirs for the virus. The central nervous system is involved in 70 to 90 percent of affected neonates. Unfortunately, more than 20 percent of the newborns with disseminated disease do not develop skin vesicles, making identification of positive infants more difficult (Whitley & Arvin, 1995).

Differential Diagnosis

Routine cultures should include any vesicle on the skin, oropharyngeal or eye secretions, or stool. Viral typing is done for epidemiologic purposes only. HSV types 1 and 2 are the most common. Type 1 has been most closely associated with any herpes found outside the genital area; type 2 is commonly referred to as genital herpes. However, either type can occur almost anywhere in the body.

Risk Factors

Intrapartal transmission is more likely to occur in the presence of ruptured membranes. Other risk factors include intrauterine fetal monitoring and fetal scalp sampling. Transmission from mother to infant from an infected breast lesion has been reported. Transmission has also been documented from oral lesions.

Prevention

Presence of maternal active HSV genital lesions is a contraindication to vaginal delivery. If the membranes have been ruptured 4 hours or longer, cesarean section may or may not prevent transmission to the neonate. Postnatal nosocomial transmission is greatly reduced with good handwashing and universal precautions.

Collaborative Management

The most recent methods of treatment include the antiviral drugs acyclovir and vidarabine.

Vidarabine is usually given intravenously in dosages of 15 to 30 mg/kg/day over a 12-hour period for 10 to 14 days. It has been reported that newborns receiving the higher dosages of 30 mg/kg/day seem to progress to less serious forms of the disease. In some circumstances, longer periods of treatment may be necessary, because infants can have either a clinical recurrence or a clinical progression of the disease.

Acyclovir, a relatively new antiviral agent undergoing clinical study, has become the recommended mode of therapy. Acyclovir appears to be very helpful in decreasing the frequency of the reactivation of the virus, particularly in the treatment of herpes simplex encephalitis. It is a selective inhibitor of viral replication and thus has few side effects. The recommended dose is 30 mg/kg/day intravenously divided over 8 hours. Duration of therapy is 10 to 14 days.

Newborns with eye involvement should be treated with topical antiviral agents such as trifluridine, 1 drop every 2 hours, as well as intravenous therapy. Vidarabine and acyclovir are potent drugs with a potential for toxicity. Neonatal therapeutic ranges for these drugs have not been established. Monitoring of the infant's physiologic status is necessary to detect potential side effects. Isolation of the identified infected infant is essential, because viral shedding provides a reservoir for infecting other infants in the nursery.

Primary nursing responsibilities in the management of a family with HSV are education and support. Careful history taking and thorough questioning can often identify potentially infected patients early.

All family members with active lesions anywhere on the body should be taught careful handwashing before handling the newborn. All family members or friends with an oral HSV infection must wash well, wear a mask, and not kiss the infant anywhere until their lesions are completely crusted over and healed.

Breastfeeding is contraindicated if the mother has a lesion on her breast. Infants are not isolated unless they themselves are infected. Many nurseries have guidelines regarding a 24- to 48-hour observation period to check cultures on an infant who was delivered vaginally through an infected genital area. An uninfected child does not require prolonged hospitalization, and on discharge the family needs information and education. Families should be informed that immediate medical consultation should be obtained with the development of major findings, including malaise, irritability, fever, temperature instability, respiratory distress, apnea, large abdomen or liver, sudden changes in skin color, new skin vesicles, lesions on the mucous membranes, or conjunctivitis. Sudden onset of systemic disease in a small recovering preterm infant can include disseminated intravascular coagulation and shock. Skin lesions are often absent in these severe cases, which may delay diagnosis.

VARICELLA

Varicella is the member of the herpesvirus family that commonly causes chickenpox as well as varicella zoster. Most women of childbearing age in the United States have been exposed to or have contracted this virus; yet women from other parts of the world may not be seropositive. Incidence of this virus in pregnant women is very low, probably about 0.5 in 10,000 pregnancies (Gershon, 1995).

Symptoms of varicella are usually present 10 to 20 days after exposure and include fever, malaise, and an itchy rash. The maculopapular rash eventually forms vesicles and crusts over. Potential complications include pneumonia, encephalitis, arthritis, and bacterial cellulitis. If the virus is contracted early in pregnancy, the damage is likely to be cutaneous, musculoskeletal, neurologic, and ocular. Infants can have intrauterine growth retardation, microcephaly, cerebellar and cortical atrophy, cataracts, and chorioretinitis (Freij & Sever, 1988).

Viral infection in the last 3 weeks of pregnancy will infect one in four newborns. The severity of neonatal disease is determined by the timing of the exposure. Infections are generally severe if contracted within 4 days before and 2 days after delivery. Severe viral respiratory distress with significantly depleted maternal passive antibody transmission puts the infant at an even greater risk for other complications. When maternal varicella occurs 5 to 21 days before delivery, the newborn has a much milder course of the disease and appears more capable of defending itself. This milder course is probably due to passive immunity transmitted to the infant through maternally derived antibodies.

The diagnosis of varicella is isolation of HSV. Strict isolation of positive or highly suspicious infants is necessary. Vidarabine or acyclovir can be used for treatment of severe newborn disease. Varicella zoster immune globulin (VZIG) can be given to newborns in an attempt to decrease the severity of infection in those exposed (CDC, 1984b).

Prevention

Typically, if a mother has contracted this disease late in pregnancy, others, such as health care workers, family members, or other newborns, may have been exposed. Exposed susceptible persons should be protected with VZIG. A live attenuated varicella vaccine has been approved by the Food and Drug Administration and is produced by Merck & Company (Clark, 1995). There is skepticism among pediatricians as to the efficacy of use of the vaccine for a usually benign childhood illness. However, for childbearing women who have not contracted varicella, it may be advocated rather than risking the disease during pregnancy.

GONORRHEA

Neisseria gonorrhoeae is a species of small gram-negative diploid bacteria. This organism appears most frequently in young adults, ages 15 to 24 years. There are approximately 1 million new cases each year. In females, this organism presents in an asymptomatic fashion, which compromises the detection of the disease. The organism is easily transmitted by infected tissue and secretions from the cervix, pharynx, urethra, or rectum. The incubation period is 2 to 7 days. Pelvic inflammatory disease is often caused by the organism.

Clinical Manifestations

Infections with gonorrhea are often mild but may cause blockage of the fallopian tubes. Perhaps 50 percent of women are asymptomatic when their

cervix is infected. In a pregnant woman, colonization of the cervix with gonorrhea can cause inflammation and weakening of the fetal membranes and early rupture. Chorioamnionitis with gonorrhea as the causative organism can occur in the antepartum period and during labor and delivery and is related to increased risk of postpartum endometritis.

Disseminated gonococcal infection may present during pregnancy, causing arthritis, tendinitis, general aching, fever, and malaise. A previous history of gonorrhea presents a strong possibility that it may recur during pregnancy. Sexual partners should be screened and treated, because reinfection after treatment is common.

Gonococcal conjunctivitis in the newborn has historically been a risk from transmission through the birth canal. Prophylaxis has been mandated by law in the United States, with the use of silver nitrate 1 percent solution or erythromycin in both eyes at birth. Fetal scalp electrodes have been identified as a potential method of organism transmission to the fetus. Gonorrhea has been isolated from scalp abscesses, gastric and pharyngeal aspirates, conjunctival aspirates, and other blood and body fluids. Infected women have a higher incidence of premature labor, premature rupture of membranes, and infectious complications (Fletcher & Gordon, 1990).

Prevention

Use of silver nitrate solution or erythromycin for prevention of gonococcal ophthalmia neonatorum is one of the early achievements in preventive medicine. Use of erythromycin ointment in both eyes is now a more common practice because it covers both gonococcus and chlamydia (Hammerschlag et al., 1989).

Collaborative Management: Mother

The appropriate treatment for a pregnant woman includes ceftriaxone, 250 mg intramuscularly once, plus erythromycin, 500 mg orally four times a day for 7 days (CDC, 1987). If gastrointestinal side effects are too severe, amoxicillin can be used (Majeroini, 1994). Follow-up, per the CDC, requires cervical and rectal cultures for *N. gonorrhoeae* obtained 4 to 7 days after treatment. Ideally, pregnant women should also be treated for chlamydial infection. In the nonpregnant woman, treatment with doxycycline, ofloxacin, and azithromycin is very effective but their use in pregnancy is not advised. Azithromycin has not been tested on pregnant women but if proven safe would require one dose for effective treatment (Majeroini, 1994).

Collaborative Management: Neonate

Infants who are delivered of an infected untreated mother are usually given a complete sepsis work-up, including a lumbar puncture, and placed on ampicillin and gentamicin. If cultures confirm the microorganism and resistance is an issue, infants should be treated with ceftriaxone, 25 to 50 mg/kg/day intravenously or intramuscularly in single doses, or cefotaxime, 25 mg/kg intravenously or intramuscularly every 12 hours (CDC, 1989).

HEPATITIS B VIRUS

The hepatitis B virus (HBV) is fairly large, approximately 42 mm in diameter. Exposure to infected blood and body fluids, percutaneous introduction of blood, and administration of infected blood products are the principal ways the virus is transmitted. Contamination or infection of wounds can easily transmit the disease. The virus is fairly strong and able to live on inanimate objects or fomites. Deactivation requires at least 1 minute in boiling water and extended autoclaving time.

In the adult, this virus produces systemic illness with general malaise, jaundice, anorexia, and nausea. Early stages of the disease may present with fever, rash, and sore joints. A carrier state of HBV can precipitate chronic liver disease (Lott & Kenner, 1994a, 1994b).

Hepatitis B surface antigen (HB_sAg) is an important test in assessing a woman's risk of transmitting HBV to her unborn child. The presence of HB_sAg and hepatitis B e antigen (HB_eAg) are the best indicators of infectiousness. It is recommended that all pregnant women be screened at their first prenatal visit for HB_sAg and HB_eAg to prevent prenatal transmission (ACIP, 1990).

Infection early in pregnancy with HBV causes 50 percent risk of neonatal HBV. Ninety percent of infants born to women who are HB_sAg and HB_eAg positive are at risk for developing HBV by their first birthday if not treated. Infants born to women who are HB_sAg positive and HB_eAg negative have lower rates of perinatal infection (20 percent) (Lee et al., 1986). Untreated infants are likely to become carriers, which may eventually lead to primary hepatocellular carcinoma (Lott & Kenner, 1994a, 1994b).

Treatment for these infants should be HBV vaccine along with hepatitis B immunoglobulin. For neonates whose mothers are HB_sAg positive or exposed, HBV vaccine 0.5 ml (10 μg/ml) should be given intramuscularly in the anterolateral thigh at or within 24 hours of birth. Immunoglobulin (0.5 ml) should be given concurrently at a separate site. The vaccine is repeated at 1 and 6 months: 0.5-ml booster injections are suggested at 12 months and may need repeating at 5-year intervals (American Academy of Pediatrics, 1992). It can be used in infants who have been exposed to HIV. There is usually an immune response in these infants despite an altered CD4 count. The response does appear to be somewhat diminished (Rutstein, Rudy, Codispoti, & Watson, 1994).

Vertical transmission may occur during vaginal deliveries. The sharing of bodily secretions during sexual intercourse can result in disease transmission also. HBV has a long incubation period—50 to 190 days (average 90 days). Current recommendations are that all pregnant women be screened initially and again before delivery. Family clustering of HBV has been identified through spread by household contacts.

Clinical Manifestations

Prematurity and low birth weight as well as hyperbilirubinemia are clinical signs of HBV infection. Hepatosplenomegaly is also a common presenting symptom of an infant who is infected with a virus. An infant infected with HBV can be asymptomatic or present with a picture of fulminant sepsis.

Risk Factors

Pregnant women in high-risk categories (known to have sexual contact with persons having HBV) need to be screened so that appropriate follow-up can be provided. Certain ethnic groups, such as Asians (Taiwanese especially) and Australian aborigines, intravenous drug users, and health care professionals are at risk for the development of HBV. Individuals living in poor sanitary conditions are also at risk (Lott & Kenner, 1994a, 1994b).

Collaborative Management and Prevention

Vaccination is recommended for individuals who are at risk for exposure to HBV, including health care workers, family members of chronic carriers, people with large numbers of heterosexual partners, and intravenous drug users. Hb_sAg protein is administered to the deltoid muscle once, and then again 1 month and 6 months later.

If the mother's antigen status is unknown at delivery, titers are drawn and vaccination is done if the result is Hb_sAg positive. If the test results are unavailable or cannot be obtained, the neonate is treated as if the mother is positive. The infant of a mother with confirmed HBV should be bathed with soap and water immediately, with special attention to removing all blood and secretions present on the skin and hair. The infant may be breastfed (unless the mother's nipples are cracked) and cared for routinely.

HUMAN PAPILLOMAVIRUS

Genital warts, or condylomata acuminata, are caused by human papillomavirus (HPV). Two specific strains of HPV have been identified as causing venereal warts and thus are of concern as sexually transmitted viruses. The time lag between exposure and infection can be up to 6 months (Bennett, 1987).

Symptoms are warty growths on the vagina, cervix, vulva, perineum, buttocks, or inner thigh.

Intrapartal transmission is possible if genital warts are visible. Current maternal treatment includes carbon dioxide laser therapy and 85 percent trichloroacetic acid. The incidence of maternal-to-newborn transmission is approximately 2 percent with this treatment (Schwartz, Greenberg, Daould, & Reid, 1988). Newborns can contract a respiratory or laryngeal papillomatosis from this virus.

Prenatal treatment is associated with low complication and recurrence rate. The treatment alleviates the need for a cesarean delivery. Examination, treatment, and follow-up of sexual partners are important aspects of treatment, because 50 percent of partners are infected (Bourcier & Seidler, 1987).

Clinical Manifestations

Laryngeal papillomatosis causes newborns to have a "weak cry" or hoarseness. The expected incidence of laryngeal papilloma in an infant born to a woman with untreated HPV is about 78 percent (Arvin & Maldonado, 1995). The newborn may have stridor or other respiratory symptoms.

Collaborative Management

Education and counseling of mothers and their partners are the primary concerns in the treatment of this disease.

Early identification of newborns at risk for laryngeal papillomas is important to prevent respiratory complications. Newborns experiencing respiratory distress accompanying stridor require an evaluation for laryngeal papillomas. Supportive ventilatory therapy may be needed.

CHLAMYDIA

Chlamydia is a bacterium that grows between cells. Chlamydial infection is one of the most common sexually transmitted diseases. Probably 50 percent of infected women of childbearing age are asymptomatic. The infection can present as cervicitis, salpingitis, urethritis, or pelvic inflammatory disease.

C. trachomatis has been identified as causing a significant increase in the incidence of premature rupture of membranes, low birth weight infants, and infant mortality (Ryan et al., 1990). Thus, screening pregnant women for *Chlamydia* is important. Treatment with erythromycin or clindamycin may prevent transmission to the newborn.

Clinical Manifestations

Chlamydial conjunctivitis can present in the newborn with a very watery discharge that may progress to purulent exudate. Application of erythromycin ointment at birth for ocular prophylaxis will successfully treat both chlamydial and gonococcal conjunctivitis. Pneumonia can occur in newborns who have contracted chlamydial infection from their mother's genital tract. The incubation period is anywhere from 5 days to 3 to 4 months. Typical presentation is tachypnea, barrel chest, and an increased oxygen requirement. The infant may have interstitial infiltrations, hepatosplenomegaly, and increased eosinophils.

Diagnosis is based on examination, and, in the case of conjunctivitis, Giemsa-stained conjunctival scrapings provide a method of direct fluorescent antibody testing. The definitive diagnosis for chlamydial pneumonia is made by culture of the respiratory tract or high levels of IgM antibodies to *Chlamydia*.

Collaborative Management and Prevention

Once the organism is identified, treatment is with erythromycin for 10 to 14 days.

If chlamydial infection is confirmed in a pregnant woman and treated, her sexual partners require treatment. Rapid screening and diagnosis are now available with the use of monoclonal antibodies. Some laboratories offer a chlamydia test called Chlamydiazme. Positive tests indicate the need for treatment, but negative tests indicate that repeated screening is needed.

Without medical treatment, the severe complications for the woman include pelvic inflammatory disease, ectopic pregnancy, and endometritis. Neonatal pneumonia is a complication and may require supportive ventilation.

Bacterial Infections

GROUP B *STREPTOCOCCUS*

The number of newborn deaths associated with either early-onset (prior to the first week of life) or late-onset infection continues to be high, particularly in high-risk urban centers. Potential for permanent neurologic sequelae for infant survivors of meningeal infections is approximately 15 percent (Baker & Edwards, 1995). The mortality of infected newborns is also estimated to be 15 percent (Opal, Cross, Palmer, & Almazen, 1988).

Pathophysiology

Streptococcus is a gram-positive diplococcus with an ultrastructure similar to other gram-positive cocci. It was classified as hemolytic because of its double zone of hemolysis surrounding colonies on blood agar plates. Cultures of body fluids such as blood, urine, CSF, or other secretions are the most common methods of identifying group B streptococci. Counterelectrophoresis and latex agglutination are rapid assays that enable a presumptive diagnosis before the return of cultures. Rapid identification of the group B *Streptococcus* organism is important in treating colonized pregnant women and in the early diagnosis and treatment of the sick, unstable septic infant. To accurately predict maternal colonization with group B streptococci, both vaginal and rectal areas should be cultured on more than one occasion (Minkoff & Mead, 1986).

Clinical Manifestations

Group B *Streptococcus* has been identified as a relatively common cause of midgestational fetal loss in women who experience vaginal hemorrhage, premature rupture of membranes, fetal membrane infection, and spontaneous abortion. Stillborns are reported to be as high as 61 percent with these bacteria. Early-onset neonatal infections with group B *Streptococcus* can be asymptomatic or can present with severe symptoms of respiratory distress and shock, which can rapidly progress to death (Klein & Marcy, 1995).

Early-onset group B *Streptococcus* usually appears within the first 24 hours of life and is most common in premature infants. Infants who weigh 1000 g or less usually present with congenital pneumonia.

The following are the signs of streptococcal infection:

- Pneumonia
- Meningitis
- Respiratory distress
- Apnea
- Grunting
- Tachypnea
- Cyanosis
- Hypotension (found in 25 percent)
- Risk for cardiopulmonary collapse

Nonspecific signs of sepsis include the following:

- Lethargy

- Poor feeding
- Temperature instability
- Abdominal distention
- Pallor
- Tachycardia
- Jaundice

Overwhelming group B streptococcal septicemia is often compounded by meningitis. Lumbar puncture and examination of the CSF is the only way to exclude meningeal involvement. Seizures are a possible presenting sign in infants with group B streptococcal meningitis.

Late-Onset Infection. This problem usually occurs in term newborns 7 days to 12 weeks of age. The fatality rate is less than that with early-onset infection, but meningitis is a common complication. Other complications are listed below:

- Global or profound mental retardation
- Spastic quadriplegia
- Cortical blindness
- Deafness
- Uncontrolled seizures
- Hydrocephalus
- Diabetes insipidus

Screening tests, such as a complete blood cell count with differential, are often used to identify the need for further evaluation for sepsis. Abnormal results indicate the necessity for definitive testing and implementation of antimicrobial therapy.

Collaborative Management

Generally, ampicillin and gentamicin are selected until culture results and sensitivities are available. Group B *Streptococcus* is usually very sensitive to penicillin G, and in many institutions it is substituted for ampicillin once the diagnosis is made. See Table 15–1 for dosages.

Therapy is maintained for 7 to 10 days for sepsis and 14 to 21 days for meningitis. The lumbar puncture may be repeated midway or at the end of therapy to ensure that there are no microorganisms remaining in the CSF.

Fluid management, volume expansion, and appropriate antimicrobial therapy are the key components of nursing care. Infants with group B streptococcal infection are often very labile and do not tolerate frequent interventions. Minimal handling is sometimes required for their care.

STAPHYLOCOCCUS

Ill neonates and premature infants who are already immunocompromised are particularly vulnerable to infections. Any open skin lesions, surgical incisions, or puncture wounds secondary to diagnostic tests or procedures are good sites for bacterial growth, especially of *S. aureus* or *S. epidermidis* (Howells & Jones, 1988). Nosocomial infections may also be transmitted to the neonate by contaminated articles or from the hands of health care professionals. Overgrowth of *S. epidermidis* may occur in nurseries where

TABLE 15–1. Selected Antimicrobial Agents and Their Dosages

Antimicrobial Agent	Dosage
Penicillin G	Sepsis 　25,000–50,000 IU/kg/dose 　　q 12 hr <7 days 　　q 8 hr <7 days 　　q 6 hr >7 days Group B streptococcus 　Higher dose + aminoglycoside
Ampicillin	Sepsis 　100–200 mg/kg/dose 　　q 8–12 hr <7 days 　　q 6–8 hr >7 days Meningitis 　200–400 mg/kg/dose 　　q 8–12 hr <7 days 　　q 6–8 hr >7 days
Methicillin	25–50 mg/kg/dose IV 　q 8–12 hr <7 days 　q 6–8 hr >7 days
Gentamicin	<7 days postnatal age 　≤29 wk: 2.5 mg/kg/dose q 24 hr 　30–34 wk: 3 mg/kg/dose q 24 hr 　≥35 wk: 2.5 mg/kg/dose q 12 hr >7 days postnatal age 　≤29 wk: 3.0 mg/kg/dose q 24 hr 　30–34 wk: 2.5 mg/kg/dose q 12 hr 　≥35 wk: 2.5 mg/kg/dose q 8 hr
Vancomycin	≤29 wk: 18 mg/kg/dose q 24 hr 30–36 wk: 15 mg/kg/dose q 12 hr 37–44 wk: 10 mg/kg/dose q 8 hr ≥45 wk: 10 mg/kg/dose q 6 hr

Adapted with permission from Lott, J.W., & Kilb, J.R. (1992). The selection of antibacterial agents for treatment of neonatal sepsis. *Neonatal Pharmacology Quarterly, 1*(1), 19–29.

an attempt has been made to reduce colonization of *S. aureus.* Resistant organisms pose a threat to preterm infants who require extensive invasive treatments. They are particularly susceptible to colonization with coagulase-negative staphylococci or even methicillin-resistant *S. aureus* (Reboli, John, & Levkoff, 1989).

Staphylococci release endotoxins that have systemic effects. One of these effects is alteration of the skin's protective layer. Scalded staphylococcal skin syndrome is one of the most dramatic results of these endotoxins.

Collaborative Management

Antimicrobial therapy begins with ampicillin and gentamicin. Once definitive results of culture and sensitivity studies are available and if the organism is ampicillin resistant, the drug of choice is one of the synthetic penicillins: oxacillin, methicillin, cloxacillin, dicloxacillin, or nafcillin. If the organism is methicillin resistant, the best available drug is vancomycin (Lott, 1994).

ESCHERICHIA COLI

Escherichia coli is a gram-negative, non–spore-forming motile rod. It is a normal inhabitant of the gastrointestinal tract and the most common cause of gram-negative sepsis in the newborn. Colonization of the gastrointestinal tract with *E. coli* occurs postnatally through environmental exposure and enteral feedings.

LISTERIA MONOCYTOGENES

Listeria monocytogenes is found in unpasteurized milk, soil, and fecal material. Infection with this bacterial organism appears to be underdiagnosed and also an underreported cause of congenital sepsis. Antepartum factors such as high maternal leukocyte count, fetal tachycardia, decreased fetal heart rate variability, and absence of intrapartum fetal heart rate accelerations were identified in the history of the newborns diagnosed with congenital *Listeria* (Boucher & Yonekura, 1986).

The incidence of *Listeria* in the United States is unknown, and the route of transmission is unclear. It can be foodborne.

Clinical Manifestations

A mother infected with *Listeria* commonly has flu-like symptoms, including malaise, fever, chills, diarrhea, and back pain. It is also possible to contract the infection and remain asymptomatic or have only minor symptoms. This organism has been identified as a cause of spontaneous abortion (Lennon et al., 1984).

If infection is contracted between 17 and 28 weeks' gestation, *Listeria* can cause fetal death or premature birth of an acutely ill newborn who may die hours later. However, early maternal treatment with intravenous ampicillin and gentamicin has been associated with normal newborn outcome (Bortolussi & Schlechi, 1995). Late infection in pregnancy may cause the infant to be born with a congenital infection, usually pneumonia. Mortality rates are high but are usually related to the amount of prematurity. Late-onset listeriosis, which can occur up to 4 weeks after delivery, can easily result in meningitis. A *term* newborn who becomes sick has less chance of dying but often suffers complications of hydrocephalus and mental retardation (Visintine, Oleske, & Nahmias, 1977). However, neonates, either preterm or term, who develop meningitis have a 70 percent mortality rate if treatment is delayed (Bortolussi & Schlechi, 1995).

Neonatal signs of infection with *Listeria* include the following (Visintine, Oleske, & Nahmias, 1977):

- Prematurity
- Meconium staining
- Apnea
- Flaccidity

- Papular erythematous rash
- Hepatosplenomegaly
- Poor feeding

Preterm birth associated with meconium staining should always be considered suggestive of listeriosis.

Collaborative Management

Intrapartum administration of antibiotics may decrease fetal morbidity and mortality. Ampicillin in combination with an aminoglycoside is the most common treatment. Institutional policy may require that the infant be isolated for the first 24 hours, until the antibiotics are on board. The mother's urine, stool, and lochia should be cultured; and if results are positive, she should be treated with ampicillin.

NEONATAL MENINGITIS

Pathophysiology

Meningitis can be a sequela of newborn sepsis. The incidence of neonatal sepsis is reported to be 1 to 8.1 in 1000 live births (Klein & Marcy, 1995). The incidence of meningitis associated with newborn sepsis is thought to be about 25 percent of those presenting with sepsis. Meningitis is a more common complication of late-onset sepsis. Morbidity is higher for preterm infants than for term infants. Morbidity of survivors of gram-negative bacilli or group B streptococci approaches 20 to 50 percent.

Complications of neonatal meningitis are listed below (Wald et al., 1986):

- Mental and motor problems
- Seizure disorders
- Hydrocephalus
- Hearing loss
- Blindness
- Abnormal speech patterns

In most cases, meningitis results from bacteremia. Thus, an inoculation of organisms may pass the blood–brain barrier and infect the CSF. Cytologic tests on the CSF can identify an inflammatory response. A Gram stain of the CSF fluid should be prepared and other appropriate cultures taken. High CSF protein and low glucose levels are also indicators of meningitis.

Clinical Manifestations

The clinical signs and symptoms of meningitis are as follows (Klein & Marcy, 1995):

- Generalized sepsis
- Increased irritability
- Crying
- Increased intracranial pressure leading to bulging fontanelles
- Lethargy
- Tremors or twitching
- Seizure activity

- Vomiting
- Alterations in consciousness
- Diminished muscle tone
- Focal signs: hemiparesis, horizontal deviation of the eyes, and some cranial nerve involvement

Risk Factors

It appears that male infants are more vulnerable to sepsis and meningitis. There has been a suggestion regarding a sex-linked factor; that is, that a particular gene located on the X chromosome is involved with the function of the thymus or with synthesis of immunoglobulin to defend the newborn host (Schlegel & Bellante, 1969). Female infants have lower rates of respiratory distress syndrome and lower rates of most congenital infections compared with males (Portillo & Sullivan, 1979).

Geography and socioeconomic factors are influential in patterns of neonatal disease.

Prognosis

Brain abscess is associated with a poor prognosis; approximately 50 percent of those affected die. Destruction of brain tissues, hemorrhages, and infarcts causing necrosis to vital brain cells may cause extensive brain damage, leading to death or poor neurologic outcomes. Fortunately, with the introduction of ultrasonography and computed tomography, brain abscesses are being identified earlier (Renier, Flandin, Hirsch, & Hirsch, 1988).

Collaborative Management

Selection of antimicrobial therapy is based on the causative microorganism. Supportive therapy is necessary for the newborn with meningitis. Acute observation and monitoring of vital signs and activity level are crucial. Infants who become critically ill with meningitis may deteriorate quickly and need rapid, acute interventions. Infants often require long-term antibiotic therapy, and often venous access is a problem. Placement of a percutaneous line for parenteral nutrition may be necessary.

Viral Agents

RESPIRATORY SYNCYTIAL VIRUS

Respiratory syncytial virus (RSV) is an infection usually found in older infants. It is thought that maternal antibodies protect infants for the first few weeks of life, but as passive immunity diminishes, these infants become more vulnerable. Premature infants, already immunocompromised, are more susceptible to the virus during their long-term hospitalizations.

Clinical Manifestations

An infant who is infected before 4 weeks of age may be asymptomatic or may have an upper respiratory tract infection with fever, bronchiolitis, apnea, or pneumonia. There may be a definite need for assisted ventilation; deaths have occurred in rapidly fulminating disease, for which there is little available treatment. Nosocomial transmission is possible. The first clinical signs of transmission include a clear nasal discharge at 10 to 52 days, followed by cough and wheezing. Radiologic changes compatible with pneumonia may also be found.

Treatment and Prevention

Any RSV-infected secretions can remain viable for up to 6 hours on countertops, 45 minutes on cloth gowns and paper tissues, and 20 minutes on skin (Hall, Douglas, & German, 1980). Thus, all infected infants should be cared for in cohort. Caretakers should be consistently assigned to decrease transmission rates. Gown and glove precautions can significantly reduce nosocomial transmission of RSV (Leclair et al., 1987).

Any infant with a runny nose or nasal congestion or unexplained apnea should be considered to be isolated and investigated for RSV. Attention should be specific for those infants older than 4 weeks of corrected age. Cultures and screening tests should be performed because specific treatment is available if RSV is found.

Collaborative Management

Treatment of RSV infection is with ribavirin. Methods have been developed to administer ribavirin safely to infants receiving mechanical ventilation, as well as those in an oxygen hood. Specific safety precautions should be taken to protect the caregiver, because this drug has been identified as being potentially teratogenic (Prows, 1989). These measures include gown, glove, and mask protection when in direct contact with the particles or mist containing ribavirin. Ideally, no pregnant woman should take care of an infant with RSV who is receiving ribavirin. Close monitoring of the pulmonary status, including the use of oxygen and mechanical ventilation, may be necessary. Isolation from other infants who could potentially be infected is important.

ADENOVIRUS AND ROTAVIRUS

Adenoviruses can be enteric and are very small; rotaviruses are approximately 70 nm. Both these categories of organisms can cause significant viral gastroenteritis and are considered medically important because of their ability to cause neonatal diarrhea. Breastfeeding, with the transmission of secretory IgA, is thought to be one of the best protections against illness caused by adenovirus or rotavirus (Welsh & May, 1979).

Rotavirus is a double-stranded RNA virus that has a wheel-like appearance on electron microscopy. Rotavirus infection, like other acute diarrhea diseases in general, is uncommon in neonates. Infants are usually at greater risk at 3 or 4 months of age.

Some of the ways a newborn could acquire infection include the following:

- Ingestion of viral particles at or shortly before the time of delivery
- Transfer from infants or toddlers excreting the virus by hands of nursery personnel or parents

- Transmission by direct contact with adults or older children excreting the virus
- Airborne or droplet infection
- Fomites
- Contaminated foods or formula

Transfer of particles from infant to infant on the hands of nursery and medical staff is probably the most common means of viral spread (Duffy et al., 1986).

CLINICAL MANIFESTATIONS

An infected newborn can be asymptomatic or may have severe gastrointestinal problems. Early signs are listed below:

- Lethargy
- Irritability
- Poor feeding
- Passage of watery yellow or green stools free of blood but containing mucus
- Vomiting
- Slight fever

Rotavirus has been identified as a potential cause of necrotizing enterocolitis (Rotbart et al., 1988).

Several specific methods of virus detection are available, including radioimmunoassay, immunofluorescence, latex agglutination, and enzyme-linked immunosorbent assay. Some nurseries use the commercially available product Rotozyme II, which is quick and effective.

Collaborative Management

The primary goal is minimizing fluid and electrolyte losses due to diarrhea. Persistent or recurrent diarrhea with the use of milk-based formulas or breast milk demands further investigation of carbohydrate intolerance or cow's milk intolerance. Some critically ill infants who may have reduced gastrointestinal absorptive surface (short bowel syndrome) or severe mucosal damage may require an elemental diet or parenteral nutrition.

Handwashing after each contact with the affected infant remains the single most important method of preventing the spread of the infection. These viruses are often excreted in infants' stools 2 or 3 days before the illness is recognized.

The isolation of an infant with diarrhea is often too late to prevent cross-contamination. Infants who develop gastroenteritis should be moved out of the nursery area if there are adequate facilities. The use of an incubator is helpful, because it may serve as a reminder that appropriate gowning and gloving are necessary before handling the infant. Encouraging the rooming in of infants with their mothers can be helpful in containing nursery epidemics.

Several live orally administered rotavirus vaccines are being tested for their effectiveness in young infants (Losonsky et al., 1988). Also, milk containing concentrates of immunoglobulin prepared from rotavirus-hyperimmunized cows has been fed to infants hospitalized for acute rotavirus gastroenteritis. This practice appears to reduce excretion of the virus significantly and has prevented rotavirus diarrhea outbreaks in nurseries (Hilpert et al., 1987).

Fungal Agents

CANDIDA ALBICANS

Candida albicans produces endotoxins, hemolysis, pyrogens, and proteolytic enzymes that are damaging to tissues (Kotloff et al., 1989). Early recognition and treatment of fungal sepsis is imperative to prevent severe central nervous system complications and death.

Prolonged broad-spectrum antibiotic treatment for small premature infants may predispose infants to *Candida* overgrowth in the gastrointestinal tract. This overgrowth may predispose the infant to disseminated fungemia. Administration of hyperalimentation, frequent use of indwelling venous lines, and invasive procedures may also predispose the infant to *C. albicans* infection.

Clinical Manifestations

The features of infection with *Candida* include the following (Miller, 1995):

- Sepsis, often worsening with no presence of positive cultures
- Age typically of 20 to 30 days
- Oral feeding difficulties
- Need for hyperalimentation
- Has been treated with multiple courses of antibiotics
- May have respiratory distress syndrome
- Abdominal distention
- Guaiac-positive stools
- Carbohydrate intolerance
- Candiduria
- Temperature instability
- Hypotension

Differential Diagnosis

A positive *Candida* culture should never be considered a contaminated specimen. Intermittently positive cultures may reflect transient candidemia, and usually removal of any indwelling catheters and lines and changing of antibiotic therapy may be indicated.

Collaborative Management

In symptomatic low birth weight infants with positive systemic cultures, treatment should begin pending cultures. The most effective drug is amphotericin B. This is a very toxic and potent antifungal agent and must be used very cautiously. The initial dose is 0.1 to 0.3 mg/kg given intravenously over a period of 2 to 6 hours. The maintenance dose is 0.5 to 1.0 mg/kg daily over 2 to 6 hours. Lower doses are started until higher doses can be tolerated. Increments of 0.1 mg/kg/day are used to increase the daily dose slowly.

Many infants will tolerate a total dose of 20 mg/kg if it is titrated over about 1 month's time. If minimal organ involvement is present, infants can often be successfully treated on lower doses. If meningitis is suspected, flucytosine may be used. This antifungal agent acts to inhibit DNA synthesis so that *Candida* replication cannot occur.

Kidney toxicity is a major side effect, because amphotericin B causes renal vasoconstriction and decreases both renal blood flow and glomerular filtration rate. This damage can result in hyponatremia, hypokalemia, increased blood urea nitrogen, and increased creatinine, as well as acidosis. If the medication makes the patient oliguric, most physicians recommend stopping the drug until the next day. Thrombocytopenia, granulocytopenia, fever, nausea, and vomiting are the common side effects associated with amphotericin B. One major side effect of flucytosine is bone marrow depression, resulting in a decreased platelet count.

Because of the insidious onset of this disease, the septic infant who is not responding to traditional antibiotic treatment may be infected with *Candida*. Changing of intravenous sites and percutaneous lines should be considered with a culture of the catheter tip. Urine can easily be cultured for the presence of *Candida*. Thrush and candidal rashes indicate candidiasis. These can easily be treated with oral and local antifungal agents.

Monitoring of infants receiving amphotericin B is challenging, because infants may have reactions to this medication. Blood pressure should be monitored every half hour, and urine output should be followed very closely. Vital signs and laboratory work, including liver enzymes, should be followed daily to detect early signs of neonatal toxicity.

HUMAN IMMUNODEFICIENCY VIRUS

Human immunodeficiency virus-1 is part of the lentivirus subfamily of human retroviruses and requires a cell-surface receptor for attachment and penetration into the cell.

Neonates and infants younger than 15 months of age will most likely contract HIV infection by way of vertical or transplacental transmission, although some cases may be contracted through contact with maternal blood or vaginal secretions or from breastfeeding.

Prevention

Clinical trials are exploring the possibility of ways to stop or minimize vertical HIV transmission from the mother to the infant during pregnancy or before delivery (Minkoff, 1990). These trials may include the use of zidovudine (azidothymidine, AZT), soluble CD4-positive (rs CD4+), CD4-positive immunoadhesion, dideoxyinosine (ddI), and HIV immunoglobulin (Viscarello, 1990). Newer techniques include the prenatal/intrapartal use of zidovudine (Research Project AIDS Clinical Trial Group or ACTG 076) (Baker & Edwards, 1995).

Clinical Manifestations

There are usually no characteristic symptoms. Factors that may be associated with the acceleration and development of AIDS in both the adult and infant populations include the following:

- Decreased number of CD4-positive cells
- Increased number of CD8-positive cells
- Reduced level of HIV antibodies
- Increased level of cytomegalovirus antibody

The progression of HIV may also be linked to (1) age, (2) physiologic stress, and (3) poor nutritional status.

CARE OF THE NEONATE IN THE DELIVERY ROOM

Recommendations for the management of the exposed neonate are the same as those that apply for all neonates.

Collaborative Management

Routine care involves use of universal precautions. Isolation is not necessary specifically for the HIV infection. Physicians in the United States do not recommend breastfeeding.

Follow-up Care

Immunizations should be given on time as long as the immune system can mount a response. Monthly follow-up is done for 6 months, unless the infant was drug exposed. These infants should be seen on a biweekly basis. After 6 months, the visits should occur every 2 to 3 months until 1 year of age.

Early signs of development of HIV positive status are listed below:

- Recurrent bacterial infections with sepsis
- Herpetic lesions
- Failure to thrive
- Anemia
- Candidiasis (thrush)
- Encephalopathy
- Lymphoid interstitial pneumonia
- Lymphopenia (specifically with a positive HIV culture)
- Normal or increased immunoglobulin levels
- Laboratory and physical findings consistent with specific opportunistic infections and neurologic alterations

Later manifestations include the following:

- Lymphadenopathy
- Hepatosplenomegaly
- Chronic or recurrent diarrhea
- Enlarged salivary glands
- Failure to thrive
- Developmental delays

- Neurologic disease
- Thrombocytopenia

Once symptoms appear, management includes monitoring the hemoglobin, hematocrit, prothrombin time, partial thromboplastin time, platelet counts, gammaglobulin levels, CD4-positive cell counts, and other serologic studies. The hemoglobin and hematocrit should be carefully evaluated for anemia. The frequency of serologic testing should be every 6 months to correspond with other laboratory studies. Bruising and bleeding problems have also been noted in the HIV-infected infant. Occult bleeding in gastric secretions, stool, and urine should be assessed. If the laboratory evidence indicates that an infant is experiencing bleeding problems, then replacement transfusion may be necessary.

Diagnosis

For the infant, the enzyme-linked immunosorbent assay and Western blot test may not be useful in detecting the presence of HIV because maternal antibodies for HIV (IgG) cross the placenta. Other tests being used are the p24 core antigen, which may be positive after 1 month of age, and the HIV IgA Immunoblot test.

Treatment

Opportunistic infections can be treated with appropriate therapy. Specific HIV therapy is gammaglobulin therapy and zidovudine. Zidovudine works by blocking the virus from reproducing in the newly infected cells.

Another drug that has been considered for the critically ill adult is dideoxyinosine (ddI).

Other forms of treatment are specific to the clinical problems presented and not to the HIV.

Nosocomial Infections

The incidence of nosocomial infections in neonatal intensive care units is 5 to 25 percent (Donowitz, 1989). Infants who are critically ill and remain in a pathogen-filled environment are often in jeopardy because of their prolonged length of stay in the hospital. Mortality associated with these infections is anywhere from 5 to 20 percent, depending on the geographic area and specific birth weight groups (Kotloff et al., 1989).

Coagulase-negative *Staphylococcus* has been identified as a major cause of nosocomial infections.

Nursery epidemics can be caused by gram-negative and gram-positive or viral organisms because they have (1) the ability to colonize or infect human skin or the gastrointestinal tract; (2) the ability to be carried from person to person by hand contact; and (3) characteristics that allow existence on hands of personnel or in fluids or on inanimate objects, including intravenous fluids, respiratory support equipment, solutions used for medications, disinfectants, and banked breast milk (Bishop, 1996).

Resistance to antibiotics is a very serious problem. Aminoglycoside resistance is a problem in many urban nurseries, as well as colonization and infection with methicillin-resistant *S. aureus*. Respiratory infections, including RSV, influenza virus, parainfluenza virus, rhinovirus, and echovirus, have occurred in many nurseries.

CMV infection has been reported as a transfusion-related problem in low birth weight infants and thus has prompted the current policy of using CMV-screened donors (Lamberson et al., 1988). Hepatitis A has also been reported as a transfusion-related problem that may develop in infants and staff in neonatal intensive care units (Azimi et al., 1986). Hepatitis C has been linked to use of immunoglobulins such as Gammagard by Baxter (Burton, 1995). Thus, almost any organism given the right environment and support can become a nosocomially transmitted infection.

REFERENCES

ACIP. (1990). Protection against viral hepatitis. *Morbidity and Mortality Weekly Report, 39*(RR-2).

American Academy of Pediatrics. (1992). Universal hepatitis B immunization. Policy statement. *AAP News, 8*(2), 13–15, 22.

American Academy of Pediatrics. (1994). *Report of the Committee on Infectious Diseases: The red book.* Elk Grove Village, IL: Author.

Arvin, A. (1988). Antiviral treatment of herpes simplex infection in neonates and pregnant women. *Journal of the American Academy of Dermatology, 18*, 200–203.

Arvin, A. M., & Maldonado, Y. A. (1995). Other viral infections of the fetus and newborn. In J. S. Remington & J. O. Klein (Eds.), *Infectious diseases of the fetus and newborn infant* (4th ed., pp. 745–756). Philadelphia: W. B. Saunders.

Azimi, P. H., Roberto, R. R., Guralnik, J., et al. (1986). Transfusion acquired hepatitis A in a premature infant with secondary nosocomial spread in an intensive care nursery. *American Journal of Diseases of Children, 140*, 23–27.

Baker, C. J., & Edwards, M. S. (1995). Group B streptococcal infection. In J. S. Remington & J. O. Klein (Eds.), *Infectious diseases of the fetus and newborn infant* (4th ed., pp. 980–1054). Philadelphia: W. B. Saunders.

Bellanti, J. A., Pung, Y-H., & Zeligs, B. J. (1994). Immunology. In G. B. Avery, M. A. Fletcher, & M. G. MacDonald. (Eds.), *Neonatology: Pathophysiology and management of the newborn* (4th ed., pp. 1000–1029). Philadelphia: J. B. Lippincott.

Bennett, E. C. (1987). Sexually transmitted diseases. *NAACOG Newsletter, 14*(8).

Bishop, B. E. (1996). It's time to talk about infections, again. *MCN, American Journal of Maternal Child Nursing, 21*, 63.

Bortolussi, R., & Schlechi, W. F. (1995). Listeriosis. In J. S. Remington & J. O. Klein (Eds.), *Infectious diseases of the fetus and newborn infant* (4th ed., pp. 1055–1073). Philadelphia: W. B. Saunders.

Boucher, M., & Yonekura, M. L. (1986). Perinatal listeriosis (early onset), correlation of antenatal manifestations and neonatal outcome. *Obstetrics and Gynecology, 68*, 593–597.

Bourcier, K. M., & Seidler, A. J. (1987). *Chlamydia* and condylomata acuminata: An update for the nurse practitioner. *Journal of Obstetric, Gynecologic, and Neonatal Nursing, 16*, 17–22.

Burton, T. M. (1995). A drug from Baxter is said to have posed a risk of hepatitis. *The Wall Street Journal, LXXVI*(194), July, 20, A1, A7.

Cairo, M. S., Worcester, C., Rucker, R., et al. (1987). Role of circulating complement and polymorphonuclear leukocyte transfusion in treatment and outcome in critically ill neonates with sepsis. *Journal of Pediatrics, 110*, 935–941.

Carter, A. O., & Frank, J. W. (1986). Congenital toxoplasmosis, epidemiology, features and control. *Canadian Medical Association, 135*, 618–623.

Centers for Disease Control. (1984a). Rubella prevention. *Morbidity and Mortality Weekly Report 33*(84), 301.

Centers for Disease Control. (1984b). Varicella zoster immune globulin for the prevention of chicken pox. *Morbidity and Mortality Weekly Report 33*(84), 301.

Centers for Disease Control. (1987). Progress towards achieving the national 1988 objectives for sexually transmitted disease. *Morbidity and Mortality Weekly Report 36*(12).

Centers for Disease Control. (1989). Sexually transmitted disease treatment guidelines. *Morbidity and Mortality Weekly Report 38*(58).

Chawla, V., Pandit, P. B., & Nkrumah, F. K. (1988). Congenital syphilis in the newborn. *Archives of Disease in Childhood, 63,* 1393–1394.

Clark, G. (1995). Varicella vaccine approved. *AAP News, 11*(4), 1, 10.

Daffos, F., Forestier, F., Capella-Pavlovsky, M., et al. (1988). Prenatal management of 746 pregnancies at risk for congenital toxoplasmosis. *New England Journal of Medicine, 318,* 271–275.

Donowitz, L. G. (1989). Nosocomial infection in neonatal intensive care units. *American Journal of Infection Control, 17,* 250–257.

Duffy, L. C., Riepenoff-Talty, M., Byers, T. E., et al. (1986). Modulation of rotavirus enteritis during breast feeding. *American Journal of Diseases of Children, 140,* 1164.

Enders, G., & Jonatha, W. (1987). Prenatal diagnosis of intrauterine rubella. *Infection, 15,* 162–164.

Fanaroff, A. A., & Martin, R. J. (Eds.). (1997). Neonatal-perinatal medicine (6th ed.). St. Louis: C. V. Mosby.

Fletcher, J. E., Jr., & Gordon, R. C. (1990). Perinatal transmission of bacterially sexually transmitted disease: Part I. Syphilis and gonorrhea. *Journal of Family Practice, 30,* 448–456.

Freij, B. J., & Sever, J. L. (1988). Herpesvirus infections in pregnancy: Risks to embryo, fetus and neonate. *Clinics in Perinatology, 15,* 203–231.

Gershon, A. A. (1995). Chickenpox, measles, and mumps. In J. S. Remington & J. O. Klein (Eds.), *Infectious diseases of the fetus and newborn infant* (4th ed., pp. 565–618). Philadelphia: W. B. Saunders.

Hall, C. B., Douglas, R. G., Jr., & German, J. M. (1980). Possible transmission by families for respiratory syncytial virus. *Journal of Infectious Diseases, 141,* 98–102.

Hammerschlag, M. R., Cummings, L., Roblin, P. M., et al. (1989). Efficacy of neonatal ocular prophylaxis for the prevention of chlamydial and gonococcal conjunctivitis. *New England Journal of Medicine, 320,* 769–772.

Hilpert, H., Brüssow, H., Mietens, L., et al. (1987). Use of bovine milk concentrate containing antibody to rotavirus to treat rotavirus gastroenteritis in infants. *Journal of Infectious Diseases, 156,* 158–166.

Howells, C. H., & Jones, H. E. (1988). Neonatalogy—then and now. Neonatal sepsis (1960). Two outbreaks of neonatal skin sepsis caused by *Staphylococcus aureus,* phage type 71. *Archives of Disease in Childhood, 63,* 1506.

Ingall, E., Sanchez, P. J., & Musher, D. (1995). Syphilis. In J. S. Remington & J. O. Klein (Eds.), *Infectious diseases of the fetus and newborn infant* (4th ed., pp. 529–564). Philadelphia: W. B. Saunders.

Klein, R. O., & Marcy, S. M. (1995). Bacterial sepsis and meningitis. In J. S. Remington & J. O. Klein (Eds.), *Infectious diseases of the fetus and newborn infant* (4th ed., pp. 835–890). Philadelphia: W. B. Saunders.

Koppe, J. G., Loewer-Sieger, D. H., & de Roever-Bonnet, H. (1986). Results of 20 year following of congenital toxoplasmosis. *Lancet, 1,* 2594–2596.

Kotloff, K. L., Blackmon, L. R., Tenney, J. H., et al. (1989). Nosocomial sepsis in the neonatal intensive care unit. *Southern Medical Journal, 82,* 699–704.

Lamberson, H. V., Jr., McMillian, J. A., Weiner, L. B., et al. (1988). Prevention of transfusion-associated cytomegalovirus infection in neonates by screening blood donors for IgM to CMV. *Journal of Infectious Diseases, 157,* 820–823.

Leclair, J. M., Freeman, J., Sullivan, B. F., et al. (1987). Prevention of nosocomial respiratory syncytial virus infections through compliance with glove and gown precautions. *New England Journal of Medicine, 317,* 329–334.

Lee, S. D., Lo, K. J., Wu, J. C., et al. (1986). Prevention of maternal–infant hepatitis B virus transmission by immunization: The role of serum hepatitis B virus DNA. *Hepatology, 6,* 369–373.

Lennon, D., Lewis, B., Mantall, C., et al. (1984). Epidemic perinatal listeriosis. *Pediatric Infectious Disease Journal, 3,* 30–34.

Levy, F. H., & O'Rourke, P. P. (1995). Topics in pediatric critical care. In S. L. Barnhart & M. P. Czervinske (Eds.), *Perinatal and pediatric respiratory care* (pp. 548–570). Philadelphia: W. B. Saunders.

Losonsky, G. A., Rennels, M. B., Lim, Y., et al. (1988). Systemic and mucosal immune response to rhesus rotavirus vaccine MMU 18006. *Pediatric Infectious Disease Journal, 7,* 388–393.

Lott, J. W. (1994). *Neonatal infection: Assessment, diagnosis, and management.* Petaluma, CA: NICU Ink.

Lott, J. W., & Kenner, C. (1994a). Keeping up with neonatal infections: Designer bugs: I. *MCN, American Journal of Maternal Child Nursing, 19,* 207–213.

Lott, J. W., & Kenner, C. (1994b). Keeping up with neonatal infection: Designer bugs: II. *MCN, American Journal of Maternal Child Nursing, 19,* 264–271.

Lott, J. W., & Kilb, J. R. (1992). The selection of antibacterial agents for treatment of neonatal sepsis or Which drug kills which bug? *Neonatal Pharmacology Quarterly, 1,* 19–29.

Majeroini, B. A. (1994). Chlamydial cervicitis: Complications and new treatment options. *American Family Physician, 49,* 1825–1829, 1832.

Miller, M. J. (1995). Fungal infections. In J. S. Remington & J. O. Klein (Eds.), *Infectious diseases of the fetus and newborn infant* (4th ed., pp. 703–744). Philadelphia: W. B. Saunders.

Minkoff, H., & Mead, P. (1986). An obstetric approach to prevention of early onset group B beta-hemolytic streptococcal sepsis. *American Journal of Obstetrics and Gynecology, 154,* 973–977.

Munro, N. D., Sheppard, S., Smithells, R. W., et al. (1987). Temporal relations between maternal rubella and congenital defects. *Lancet, 2,* 201–204.

Nelson, B. I., & Grossman, J., II. (1986). Perinatal infections. In S. E. Gabbe, J. R. Neible, & J. L. Simpson (Eds.), *Obstetrics: Normal and problem pregnancies.* New York: Churchill Livingstone.

Opal, S. M., Cross, A., Palmer, M., & Almazen, R. (1988). Group B streptococcal sepsis in adults and infants: Contrasts and comparisons. *Archives of Internal Medicine, 148,* 641–645.

Overall, J. C., Jr. (1994). Herpes simplex virus infection of the fetus and newborn. *Pediatric Annals, 23,* 131–136.

Portillo, D. T., & Sullivan, J. L. (1979). Immunological basis for superior survival of females. *American Journal of Diseases of Children, 133,* 1251–1253.

Prober, C. G., Hensleigh, P. A., Boucher, F. D., et al. (1988). Use of routine viral cultures at delivery to identify neonates exposed to herpes simplex virus. *New England Journal of Medicine, 318,* 887–891.

Prows, C. A. (1989). Ribavirin risks in reproduction—how great are they? *MCN, American Journal of Maternal Child Nursing, 14,* 400–404.

Reboli, A. C., John, J. R., Jr., & Levkoff, A. H. (1989). Epidemic methicillin-gentamicin resistant *Staphylococcus aureus* in a neonatal intensive care unit. *American Journal of Diseases of Children, 143,* 34–39.

Renier, D., Flandin, C., Hirsch, E. E., & Hirsch, J. F. (1988). Brain abscesses in neonates: A study of 30 cases. *Journal of Neurosurgery, 69,* 877–882.

Remington, J. S., McLeod, R., & Desmonts, G. (1995). Toxoplasmosis. In J. S. Remington & J. O. Klein (Eds.), *Infectious diseases of the fetus and newborn infant* (4th ed., pp. 140–267). Philadelphia: W. B. Saunders.

Rotbart, H. A., Nelson, W. L., Glode, M. P., et al. (1988). Neonatal rotavirus-associated necrotizing enterocolitis: Case control study and prospective surveillance during an outbreak. *Journal of Pediatrics, 112,* 87–93.

Rutstein, R. M., Rudy, B., Codispoti, C., & Watson, B. (1994). Response to hepatitis B immunization by infants exposed to HIV. *AIDS, 8,* 1281–1284.

Ryan, G. M., Jr., Adbella, T. N., McNeeley, S. G., et al. (1990). *Chlamydia trachomatis* infection in pregnancy and effect of treatment on outcome. *American Journal of Obstetrics and Gynecology, 162,* 34–39.

Schlegel, R. J., & Bellante, J. A. (1969). Increased susceptibility of males to infection. *Lancet, 2,* 826–827.

Schwartz, D. B., Greenberg, M. D., Daould, Y., & Reid, R. (1988). Genital condylomas in pregnancy: Use of trichloroacetic acid and laser therapy. *American Journal of Obstetrics and Gynecology, 158*(6 Pt 1), 1407–1416.

Sever, J. L., Smith, M. A., & Shaver, K. A. (1985). Delayed manifestations of congenital rubella. *Reviews of Infectious Diseases, 7*(Suppl 1), S164–S169.

Stagno, S. (1995). Cytomegalovirus. In J. S. Remington & J. O. Klein (Eds.), *Infectious diseases of the fetus and newborn infant* (4th ed., pp. 312–353). Philadelphia: W. B. Saunders.

Visintine, A. M., Oleske, J. M., & Nahmias, A. J. (1977). Infection in infants and children. *American Journal of Diseases of Children, 131,* 393–397.

Wald, E. R., Bergman, I., Taylor, H. G., et al. (1986). Long-term outcome of group B streptococcal meningitis. *Pediatrics, 77,* 217–221.

Welsh, J. K., & May, J. T. (1979). Anti-infective properties of breast milk. *Journal of Pediatrics, 94,* 1–9.

Whitley, R. J., & Arvin, A. M. (1995). Herpes simplex virus infections. In J. S. Remington & J. O. Klein (Eds.), *Infectious diseases of the fetus and newborn infant* (4th ed., pp. 354–376). Philadelphia: W. B. Saunders.

CHAPTER 16

Assessment and Management of Hematologic Dysfunction

NORMAL HEMATOLOGIC VALUES IN THE NEWBORN

Factors Affecting Laboratory Values

Blood values at birth depend on (1) the timing of cord clamping, (2) the infant's gestational age, (3) the blood sampling site, and (4) the technique used to obtain adequate blood flow. Blood volume in the newborn can be significantly influenced by the timing of cord clamping and the positional differences between the infant and the level of the placenta at the time of clamping. Complete emptying of placental vessels before clamping can increase blood volume by 61 percent (Oski & Naiman, 1982c).

Average blood volume in the term infant is approximately 85 ml/kg of body weight, whereas in the preterm infant it can average 90 to 105 ml/kg. The younger the gestational age of the infant, the greater the blood volume per kilogram (Usher et al., 1975). The average hemoglobin concentration at 32 to 33 weeks' gestation is 18.5 g/dl, with an average hematocrit of 60 percent (Zaizov & Matoth, 1976). In the term infant, hemoglobin values range between 17.1 and 21.5 g/dl, with hematocrit values between 53.6 and 67.8 percent. The mean hemoglobin values in postmature infants as early as 40 weeks' gestation are higher than in the term infant, possibly secondary to progressive lack of oxygen that stimulates erythropoietin release and subsequent red blood cell (RBC) production.

Fetal and Neonatal Blood Components

The life span of the RBC in the fetus and newborn is much shorter than the 120 days of the adult RBC. The term newborn's RBC can last 50 to 90 days, with that of the preterm infant lasting several days less (Oski & Naiman, 1982c; Stockman, 1988).

The total RBC count in the term newborn is in the range of 4.6 to 5.2 million/ml, with an elevated reticulocyte count of 4.2 to 7.2 percent during the first 24 to 48 hours of life. RBC counts in the premature infant range from 3.5 to 4.6 million/ml, with a greater number of circulating immature RBCs reflected in a higher reticulocyte count. The reticulocyte count falls abruptly to about 1 percent by the first week of life, and erythropoietin levels reach low, often undetectable levels in both groups of infants.

During the first 12 hours of life, the white blood cell (WBC) count rises, reaches a plateau, and then slowly declines. The normal WBC range in both term and preterm infants is 5000 to 26,000/mm^3 at birth and 5000 to

357

31,000/mm³ at 12 hours of age. The neutrophils average about 12,000/mm³ at this time, remaining constant from day 3 to the end of the first month of life. In infants younger than 37 weeks' gestation, the neutrophil count averages about 8000/mm³; and in infants younger than 32 weeks' gestation, it is about 6000/mm³. By 4 days of age, no difference is noted between different gestational age groups. In well newborns, the average number of bands (a form of immature neutrophil) is 10 percent of the total WBC count. Neutrophil counts can be lowered by conditions such as maternal hypertension, intraventricular hemorrhage, hemolytic disease, and infection. As the newborn increases in age, WBC composition changes. At birth, only a 72 percent correlation exists between the number of WBCs counted in a capillary sample and a simultaneous umbilical sample, with the umbilical sample having the lower count. When comparing peripheral venous and arterial samples with capillary samples, venous counts average 82 percent and arterial samples average 77 percent of the values obtained by capillary sampling (Christensen & Rothstein, 1979).

Because immature RBCs still maintain their nuclei and are relatively high in number for the first 4 days of life, they can be incorrectly counted in the total WBC count. Therefore, the WBC count needs to be corrected to adjust for any nucleated RBCs (NRBCs). This is usually done automatically by the hematology laboratory when the blood slide is read. If the count is not automatically adjusted, this can easily be done by multiplying the total WBC count by the percentage of NRBCs observed and subtracting this sum from the total WBC count.

Adjusted WBC count = total WBC count − (total WBC count × NRBCs)

Platelet counts in the newborn do not vary much in relation to gestational age (Sell & Corrigan, 1973). At 27 to 40 weeks' gestation, counts are quite similar, with the range of normal being 215,000 to 378,000/mm³. Platelet counts less than 150,000/mm³ are considered thrombocytopenic (Hathaway & Bonnar, 1978).

Assessment of Hematologic Function

Many clinical findings such as hypoglycemia, hypocalcemia, hypothermia, apnea, bradycardia, cyanosis, lethargy, and poor feeding warrant at least a complete blood cell count (CBC). In the presence of active bleeding, platelet counts, clotting studies, and levels of fibrinogen and fibrin split products or fibrinogen degradation products can shed light on the type of blood dyscrasia present and the most therapeutic approach to the problem. The presence of cutaneous abnormalities such as hematomas, abrasions, petechiae, and bleeding should alert one to the possibility of a hematologic abnormality. Hepatosplenomegaly can also herald the presence of abnormal breakdown of RBCs. Hepatosplenomegaly concurrent with hyperbilirubinemia and hemolysis can denote alloimmune problems (e.g., Rh and ABO incompatibilities) or acquired congenital and postnatal infections (e.g., cytomegalovirus, toxoplasmosis, herpes simplex, and hepatitis).

HEMATOLOGIC DYSFUNCTION IN THE NEONATE

Blood Group Incompatibilities

Before the use of RhIG or RhoGAM in 1964, Rh incompatibility accounted for one third of all blood group incompatibilities, with ABO being responsible for the remainder. Since the use of RhIG, ABO has become the main blood group incompatibility, occurring in 3 percent of all infants, and the incidence of Rh incompatibility has dropped. Both incompatibilities involve maternal antibody response to fetal antigen, leading to RBC destruction by means of hemolysis. Rh antibody response is elicited on exposure to antigen and does not exist spontaneously, whereas anti-A and anti-B antibodies occur naturally. These entities also differ in the severity with which they affect the fetus and newborn, as well as in the method of treatment.

ABO INCOMPATIBILITY

Antigens or agglutinogens, present on the RBC surface of each blood type, react with antibodies or agglutinins found in the plasma of opposing blood types. Of the 30 common antigens involved in antigen–antibody reactions, the ABO antigens are one of two groups most likely to be problematic, the other being the Rh group (Guyton, 1996a, 1996b). The four major blood types are A, B, O, and AB, with antigens A and B occurring on the surface of the RBCs in the large majority of the population, making A and B the most common blood types. Type A blood has A antigens on the cell surface but has circulating anti-B antibodies in the plasma. Type B blood has just the opposite: B antigens on the cell surface and anti-A antibodies in the plasma. Type AB blood has A and B antigens on the cell surface and neither antibody in the plasma, whereas type O has neither antigen on the cell surface and both anti-A and anti-B antibodies in the plasma. Unlike antigens, which are either glycoproteins or glycolipids, antibodies are gamma globulins, mostly IgG and IgM.

With antigen and antibody in harmony, no RBC destruction occurs. However, when a conflicting antibody is introduced into the circulation, RBC destruction may occur. An antibody is capable of simultaneously attaching to several RBCs, resulting in a clump of cells (agglutination). Hemolysis can occur without preliminary agglutination, but it is a more delayed process because the body must first activate its complement system. High antibody titers (hemolysins) are required, however, to stimulate this response, which causes the release of proteolytic enzymes that rupture the cell membrane.

In a transfusion reaction, the plasma portion of donor blood, which contains antibodies, becomes diluted by the recipient's blood volume, which decreases the available titer of donor antibodies in the recipient's circulation. However, recipient antibody titers are adequate to destroy the donor RBCs by means of agglutination and hemolysis or by hemolysis alone. This situation is what occurs in the case of ABO incompatibility. In this entity, the maternal blood type is usually O, containing anti-A and anti-B antibodies in the serum, whereas the fetus or newborn is type A or B. Although incompatibility can occur between A and B types, it does not occur as frequently as AO or BO because of the globulin composition of the antibodies. In the type O mother, the antibodies are usually IgG and can cross the placenta, whereas the antibodies of the type A or B mother frequently are IgM, which are too large to cross the placenta.

When transplacental hemorrhage occurs, fetal blood entering the maternal circulation undergoes agglutination and hemolysis by maternal antibodies. This rapid response prevents the development of antibodies to other antigens present on fetal red cells, because a necessary time lapse is required for activation of the immune system. Consequently, fetal RBCs that are Rh positive in addition to being type A or B are destroyed by naturally occurring anti-A or anti-B antibodies before any other maternal antibodies to Rh factor (anti-D) can be produced. This naturally occurring phenomenon provides the basis for the use of RhIG, in which extrinsic anti-D destroys fetal cells before the maternal antibody system can be activated.

In spite of this destruction of fetal RBCs, maternal anti-A or anti-B antibodies of the IgG form can freely cross the placenta and adhere to RBCs in the fetal circulation. For this reason, ABO incompatibility can occur in the first pregnancy (40 to 50 percent of total occurrence involves primigravidas) because transplacental hemorrhage and inoculation of the mother by foreign fetal blood are not necessary for the development of these naturally occurring antibodies (Oski & Naiman, 1982b). The A and B antigens on the fetal and neonatal RBCs are not well developed, so only a small amount of antibodies actually attaches to the antigen. Other body tissues also have antigen sites to which some of the circulating antibodies can adhere, thereby decreasing the potential for RBC destruction. The resulting small amounts of IgG in the plasma do not stimulate activation of the complement system, so hemolysis is minimal. This may explain why 15 to 20 percent of infants are ABO incompatible with their mothers (Bowman, 1988) but only 3 percent become symptomatic (Mollison, 1984).

Erythrocyte antibodies are not usually present in the circulating blood until 2 to 8 months of postnatal age. Antibody production then increases, reaching a maximum titer at 8 to 10 years of age (Guyton, 1996a, 1996b). The newborn becomes inoculated with A and B antigens after birth through the ingestion of food and bacterial colonization. This inoculation initiates the generation of anti-A or anti-B antibodies that will circulate in the plasma, depending on the antigens present on the RBCs.

Clinical Manifestations

The chief symptom is jaundice within the first 24 hours of life (Maisels, 1990), with 90 percent of all affected infants being female.

Additional laboratory findings include a positive result in the direct Coombs test in only 3 percent of the cases (Glader & Naiman, 1991) and positive results in both direct and indirect Coombs tests in 80 percent of the cases when microtechniques are used. The direct Coombs test is a measurement of the presence of antibody on the RBC surface; the indirect Coombs test is a measurement of antibody in the serum. ABO incompatibility can also be identified by the performance of an eluate test, which involves washing the RBCs of the newborn and testing the wash for the presence of anti-A or anti-B antibodies. Anemia tends not to be a problem, owing to the limited amount of hemolysis present.

Hepatosplenomegaly can be observed.

Treatment

Because the antibodies involved in ABO incompatibility occur naturally, the elimination of this type of incompatibility is virtually impossible. However, its effects on the fetus and newborn are much less dramatic and life threatening than those of Rh incompatibility. Consequently, amniocentesis and monitoring of amniotic fluid bilirubin levels, intrauterine transfusions, and early delivery are usually not necessary. However, the problems associated with postnatal bilirubin clearance can exist, with phototherapy and possibly exchange transfusion becoming part of the repertoire of care.

Rh INCOMPATIBILITY

There are three Rh gene loci with six recognized antigens in the Rh complex: C, D, E, and c, d, e. Each individual has a paired set of these factors, having inherited a single set of either C or c, D or d, and E or e from each parent. A predilection exists toward three particular combinations, two Rh-positive (CDe, cDE) and one Rh-negative (cde). Of these six factors, the two involved in Rh determination are D and d. The D antigen is most prevalent; its presence on the RBC indicates an Rh-positive cell, whereas its absence indicates an Rh-negative cell. Because of single-set inheritance from each parent, the potential for three different combinations of paired antigens exists, one pair being both d (Rh-negative, homozygous), another pair being both D (Rh-positive, homozygous), and the third pair being a combination of d and D (Rh-positive, heterozygous).

The Rh antigen can be detected as early as 38 days of gestation on the fetal RBC and is completely developed during fetal life. These antigens are necessary for normal function of red cell membranes and, unlike A and B antigens, are confined exclusively to the RBC. Antibodies never occur naturally in the Rh system; exposure to the antigen is necessary to produce antibodies. Such exposure is thought to occur through maternal inoculation with fetal RBCs through transplacental hemorrhage or undetectable hemorrhage during labor, abortion, ectopic pregnancy, or amniocentesis.

Spontaneous transplacental hemorrhage occurs during 50 to 75 percent of all pregnancies (Bowman, 1988), with the greatest and most severe occurrence at the time of delivery. At this time, fetal RBCs are passed into maternal circulation, where antibodies develop in response to any RBC antigen the mother does not possess. The risk of immunization depends on the ABO status of both mother and fetus and the size of the hemorrhage. Based on blood type, the risk of maternal Rh immunization in an ABO-compatible Rh-negative mother with a Rh-positive fetus is 16 percent, whereas an ABO-incompatible pregnancy with an Rh-negative mother and Rh-positive fetus runs a 1.5 to 2 percent risk with each pregnancy (Woodrow, 1970). If the hemorrhage is less than 0.1 ml RBCs, the risk of immunization is 3 percent. If the hemorrhage is greater than 5 ml, the risk increases to 50 to 65 percent (Bowman, 1988).

The maternal Rh antibody is very slow to develop and, at first, may consist exclusively of IgM that cannot cross the placenta because of its molecular size. This is followed by the production of IgG that can cross the placenta into fetal circulation. The maximum concentration of the IgG form of antibody occurs within 2 to 4 months after termination of the first sensitizing pregnancy (Guyton, 1996a, 1996b). If initial immunization occurs shortly before or at time of delivery, the first Rh-positive infant born to such a mother may trigger the initial antibody response but will not be affected by it. However, subsequent exposure to RBCs of Rh-positive fetuses produces a rapid antibody response that consists mostly of IgG. This response does affect these fetuses, by antibody attachment to antigen sites on the fetal RBCs. This antibody coating of the RBCs forms the basis for a positive result in the direct Coombs test. The affected RBCs undergo agglutination and phagocytosis and eventually extravascular hemolysis in the spleen. The rate of destruction of fetal RBCs depends on the amount of anti-D antibodies present on the cells, the effectiveness of anti-D antibodies in promoting phagocytosis, and the capability of the reticuloendothelial system of the spleen to remove antibody-coated cells (Oski & Naiman, 1982b).

Erythroblastosis Fetalis

Hemolysis in the fetus due to Rh incompatibility results in the disease known as erythroblastosis fetalis (EBF), with the major consequences being anemia and hyperbilirubinemia. EBF derives its name from the presence of immature circulating RBCs (erythroblasts) found in the blood of affected infants. Rapid destruction of fetal blood cells forces immature erythroblasts into the circulation. The severity of the disease depends on the degree of hemolysis and the ability of the fetus' erythropoietic system to compensate for the amount of cell destruction. The severely affected fetus must produce 10 times more RBCs than are normally needed. In the attempt to compensate for rapid destruction, the fetus continues to utilize extramedullary organs, especially the liver and spleen, that would normally have ceased RBC production after the seventh month of gestation (Tuchmann-Duplessis, David, & Haegel, 1975).

Clinical Manifestations

The clinical manifestations of EPF include the following:

- Jaundice
- Hepatosplenomegaly
- Petechiae
- Varying degrees of hydrops

Altered hepatic synthesis can cause impaired production of vitamin K and vitamin K–dependent clotting factors, which can lead to hemorrhage in these infants. The presence of petechiae and prolonged bleeding from cord and blood sampling sites may be initial signs of clotting abnormalities.

Hypoglycemia, secondary to hyperplasia of the pancreatic islet cells, has also been identified as a problem. Low blood glucose levels and elevated plasma insulin levels are present in approximately one third of surviving erythroblastotic infants.

Antenatal Therapy
RhIG Therapy

With the use of RhIG after delivery, the incidence of Rh immunization has been dramatically decreased to 1 to 1.8 percent. Antenatal administration has further decreased the incidence to as low as 0.1 percent (Sacher & Queenan, 1987). However, there will always be pregnancies in which the RhIG fails to suppress the formation of antibodies, administration is not feasible, sensitization has already occurred, or massive fetal-maternal hemorrhage has occurred. Because of these reasons, it is estimated that the incidence cannot be reduced beyond 4 in 10,000 pregnancies, despite the use of RhIG (Bowman, 1988).

RhIG has a half-life of 25 to 27 days, so the timing of its administration is very important. It is effective for as long as 2 weeks after antigen exposure. The anti-D from RhIG does enter the fetal circulation, but it does not seem to cause significant hemolysis.

The postdelivery dosage allows for a maximum estimated fetal transfusion of 30 ml, which will leave 0.2 to 0.6 percent of postpartum mothers without full coverage. RhIG should be administered within 72 hours of delivery. One caution should be noted, because it is common practice to give RhIG and rubella vaccine together. When a mother receives RhIG or blood products along with rubella vaccine, the rubella vaccine may be inactivated (Edgar & Hamblin, 1977; Govoni & Hayes, 1988; McEvoy, 1990). This caution is contained in the manufacturer's package insert for the rubella vaccine. The rationale is that RhIG and blood products may come from donors whose sera contain circulating antibodies for rubella. These antibodies block the stimulation of the mother's own immune system. So as with any passive immunity, protection is only transient in most cases. Thus, a mother may still remain vulnerable to rubella. Titers should be repeated 6 to 8 weeks after the combination of RhIG and rubella has been given.

Antenatal Screening

The mother should initially have a test for blood type and Rh factor. If she is Rh negative, the father's blood type should also be ascertained. If the father is Rh positive, it becomes essential to determine the presence of Rh immunization by Coombs testing, specifically the indirect Coombs test. Because antibody titers can change, serial antibody titers should be done at least at 28 weeks, 34 weeks, and then every 1 to 2 weeks until pregnancy is terminated. In addition to blood typing, a concise obstetric history in any Rh-negative mother regarding any previous spontaneous or therapeutic abortions is also exceedingly important.

Several obstetric conditions present at the time of delivery can increase the risk of sensitization:

- Therapeutic or spontaneous abortion beyond 7 to 8 weeks' gestation
- Amniocentesis, which has a 10 percent chance of causing transplacental hemorrhage
- Ectopic pregnancies or hydatidiform moles
- Abdominal trauma

Amniocentesis

Amniocentesis becomes a consideration as early as 18 to 20 weeks of gestation in a previously immunized mother, or at any time that prenatal maternal blood titers indicate sensitization has occurred. Maternal serum of 1:16 or more is considered a critical level. Amniocentesis is done to extract amniotic fluid samples for evaluation of bilirubin levels. Results are expressed as levels, which are then divided into three zones of severity. Zone I (0.04 mg/dl) is considered normal; zone II (more than 0.1 mg/dl) indicates Rh hemolytic disease; and zone III (levels in excess of 0.8 mg) indicates imminent fetal death (within 7 to 10 days). If zone III is reached in an advanced pregnancy (i.e., 31 to 33 weeks), and a reasonable lecithin-sphingomyelin ratio is present, preterm delivery may be indicated after an attempt to enhance lung maturation with maternal steroid therapy. If zone III is reached between 23 and 31 weeks' gestation, intrauterine transfusion or plasmapheresis may be necessary to maintain the fetus (Bowman, 1978; Bowman & Pollock, 1965).

Intrauterine Transfusions

Intrauterine transfusion involves the instillation of packed O-negative red blood cells with a hematocrit of approximately 90 percent into the fetal peritoneal cavity (intraperitoneal transfusion [IPT]) or into the umbilical vein or artery (intrauterine intravascular transfusion [IUIVT]). Eighty percent of the cells infused into the peritoneal cavity are absorbed through the right lymphatic duct into venous circulation, but IVIUT infuses blood directly into fetal circulation. Both procedures are repeated in 10 to 14 days, and then every 3 to 4 weeks until delivery. The volume of blood infused is dependent on gestational age, and the dosage can be calculated in the following manner:

$$\text{(Gestational age in weeks} - 20) \times 10 = \text{ml of blood}$$

Instillation of RBCs into the fetal peritoneal cavity consists of the following steps done while constantly monitoring fetal heart tones:

1. Ultrasonographic localization of placenta and fetal peritoneal cavity
2. Insertion of needle, usually 16-gauge, into the fetal peritoneal cavity, through which an epidural catheter is threaded
3. Insertion of contrast medium through the catheter, and radiographic verification of placement in the peritoneal cavity
4. Infusion of O-negative RBCs that have been crossmatched against the mother's blood into the peritoneal cavity

Direct intravascular fetal transfusions employing the umbilical vein and artery have been done, initially using fetoscopy, then ultrasonography.

Plasmapheresis

By using a continuous-flow cell separator to filter maternal blood, plasmapheresis can decrease levels of anti-D antibodies in maternal serum by as much as 80 percent (Graham-Pole, Barr, & Willoughby, 1977). This technique is most effective when the Rh antibody is present in the intravascular compartment, lending itself to easier removal. Presence of Rh antibody in the intravascular space occurs when antibody production is low. However, when production is elevated, the antibody is found in both the extravascular and the intravascular spaces, making plasmapheresis less effective. Uncontrollable rebound in anti-D antibody levels often occurs after discontinuation of plasmapheresis and during therapy in pregnancies of 24 to 26 weeks' duration, despite continued intense plasmapheresis (Bowman, 1978). This phenomenon necessitates the use of intrauterine transfusion to prolong fetal life until delivery.

Prenatal Pharmacologic Agents to Control Hemolysis

Attempts to either suppress antibody action on fetal RBCs or improve bilirubin conjugation and elimination are the reasons behind the antenatal use of medications in the Rh-sensitized mother. Some of the more commonly used medications are listed below:

- *Promethazine.* This immunosuppressive drug has had controversial results. It reportedly reduces the severity of hemolysis by two methods: decreasing antibody coating of fetal RBCs and interfering with phagocytosis to enhance bilirubin conjugation and excretion. Its potential to interfere with T-lymphocyte function can reduce antibody response to an antigen challenge but can also intensify any graft-versus-host response if intrauterine transfusions are deemed necessary.

- *Oral antigen.* Oral administration of a specific antigen composed of Rh-positive erythrocyte membrane in an enteric-coated capsule is used in Rh-negative mothers to establish a tolerance to the antigen. T-suppressor (CD8) cells resulting from the use of O-positive erythrocyte membrane (EMOT) are theorized to produce a reduction in antibody response to a subsequent antigen challenge. However, investigational results are not in agreement (Gold et al., 1983).

- *Immune serum globulin.* This is given intravenously in a dosage of 400 mg/kg/day over 5 days (Berlin, Selbing, & Ryden, 1985). It is thought to interfere with fetal receptor sites in the trophoblast (primitive embryonic structure giving rise to fetal membranes and the placenta), thereby preventing passage of maternal Rh antibodies across the placenta into the fetus. It is also theorized to interfere with antibody receptor sites in fetal organs that normally destroy antibody-coated RBCs. Also by raising the amount of circulating IgG in the mother through the administration of immune serum globulin, a concurrent reduction in her overall IgG, and specifically anti-D IgG, is considered feasible.

- *Phenobarbital.* This agent is administered as 30 mg three times a day to the mother 48 to 72 hours before delivery. Peak bilirubin levels are noted to be decreased in the neonate. There is a latent period of 2 to 3 days from initiation of this therapy to stimulation of the hepatic enzyme system.

Phenobarbital has multiple effects on the conjugation and excretion of bilirubin by the liver: (1) it increases the synthesis of Y protein, one of the two proteins required to transport bilirubin from the plasma into the liver; (2) it increases the production of glucuronyl transferase, an enzyme necessary to the conjugation of bilirubin; and (3) it enhances excretion of bilirubin into bile and its elimination through the intestine.

Postnatal Care and Management of the Erythroblastotic Infant

On delivery of an infant with EBF, assessment of the cardiorespiratory status is of utmost importance. As the result of ascites, pleural effusions, and circulatory collapse, these infants often require stabilization of the airway with intubation and mechanical ventilation. When peritoneal or pleural fluid prevents adequate chest excursion, it may be necessary to perform a paracentesis to remove fluid from the abdominal cavity and a thoracentesis, or chest tube insertion, to drain excess pleural fluid.

Delivery of an infant shortly after intrauterine transfusion may not allow adequate time for absorption of blood from the peritoneal cavity. The unabsorbed portion could lead to decreased lung expansion, resulting in respiratory failure or restricted mechanical ventilation. Such infants may require paracentesis for the removal of blood from the peritoneal cavity.

After the initiation of respiratory support, the infant needs to be assessed for adequate circulating blood volume. If the infant is severely hydropic, the inevitable anemia needs to be corrected by transfusions of packed RBCs before any exchange transfusions can be attempted. The severely affected infant will likely be unable to tolerate an exchange until the intravascular and circulating RBC volume is replenished. Transfusion is accomplished using O-negative or type-specific Rh-negative blood crossmatched against maternal blood. After cardiovascular stabilization, utilization of a single-volume or partial exchange may offer a cushion of safety before a double-volume exchange is attempted. Congestive heart failure, not present at the time of intravascular volume depletion, may become apparent as the infant is transfused. Often, the severely affected infant may benefit from digitalization and diuretic therapy.

Damage to the liver during gestation can also adversely affect the coagulation factors in such infants. It can intensify any hyperbilirubinemia present, because the hepatic substances required for conjugation may also be impaired.

Laboratory evaluation of the infant affected by EBF should consist of liver function studies, hematocrits, and evaluation of coagulation status.

All of these infants require careful monitoring of vital signs and blood volume status. Vital signs are usually done every hour until the infant's condition has stabilized. Hematocrits and bilirubin levels should be checked frequently during the first few hours and days of life. If the cord bilirubin levels are significantly elevated, exchange transfusion may be necessary shortly after birth. If bilirubin levels do not require immediate exchange, blood levels should be checked every 4 to 8 hours, depending on the initial cord blood levels and subsequent rate of rise. In Rh incompatibility, exchange is imminent if the rate of rise exceeds 1 mg/hr for the first 6 hours of life. The interval of blood sampling for bilirubin may be increased to 6 to 12 hours after the first 48 hours of life.

Analysis of Laboratory Data

The following laboratory data can be helpful in the diagnosis and treatment of EBF:

- Maternal and infant's blood and Rh types
- Coombs reactivity. The infant's RBCs will be coated with anti-D antibodies, causing a positive result in a direct Coombs test. On occasion, the heavy coating of neonatal RBCs with antibody can lead to a false

Rh typing (Rh negative). If the result of a direct Coombs test is positive, the infant should be considered Rh positive.

- Infant's hematocrit, reticulocyte count, and RBC morphology. The presence of immature cells or spherocytes assists in distinguishing Rh from ABO incompatibility.
- Plasma bilirubin levels. The initial cord blood bilirubin level and the rate of rise determine the appropriate timing of any exchange transfusions needed to control bilirubin levels. Cord bilirubin levels are closely associated with the severity of disease and mortality rate. There are three forms of circulating bilirubin: (1) direct or conjugated, (2) indirect, and (3) free. Measurement of direct bilirubin identifies the amount of conjugated bilirubin that will react directly with van den Bergh reagent. The unconjugated portion of bilirubin is found in albumin and is lipid soluble. It does not react with van den Bergh reagent until it is combined with alcohol, thus the term *indirect bilirubin*. Free bilirubin, the other form of unconjugated bilirubin, is not attached to albumin and can easily cross over the blood–brain barrier, causing the damage experienced in kernicterus. All three measurements become important in the evaluation of the hyperbilirubinemic infant.

Bilirubin Metabolism and Hyperbilirubinemia

Bilirubin is produced after completion of the natural life span of the RBC, but ineffective erythropoiesis or premature destruction of blood cells can increase its production. In RBC destruction, the aging or hemolyzed RBC membrane ruptures, releasing hemoglobin that is phagocytized by macrophages. The hemoglobin molecule then splits into a heme portion and a globulin portion. Bilirubin is derived from the breakdown of the heme ring in the heme portion.

Although bilirubin is found in stool and amniotic fluid, the major route of elimination in the fetus is through the placenta.

All bilirubin found in the cord blood is of the unconjugated variety, owing to the effective handling of bilirubin metabolism, conjugation, and excretion by the maternal liver and gallbladder. The mean cord blood bilirubin concentration in the infant unaffected by hemolytic disease is 1.8 mg/dl, regardless of the gestational age or weight of the infant. Jaundice becomes noticeable when the serum concentration reaches three times the normal amount present in the serum. The conjunctivae become visibly jaundiced at serum levels of more than 2.5 mg/dl. In the full-term infant, jaundice usually becomes apparent within 2 to 4 days after birth and lasts until the sixth day, reaching a peak concentration of 6 to 7 mg/dl. The preterm infant has cord blood levels similar to those of the term infant, but peak levels are higher, jaundice lasts longer, and levels peak later, at 5 to 7 days. Sixty-three percent of preterm infants achieve levels of 10 to 19 mg/dl, and 22 percent will reach levels greater than 15 mg/dl.

Initially, bilirubin is transported in the plasma, bound to albumin at two sites: (1) a primary binding site that has a strong bond and (2) a secondary site that has a weak bond. When available albumin-binding sites are saturated, bilirubin then circulates freely in the plasma. It is this portion of unconjugated bilirubin that can migrate into brain cells, causing damage known as kernicterus. The occurrence of kernicterus is related to the amount of diffusible, loosely bound bilirubin and availability of albumin-binding sites.

When bilirubin reaches the liver, it is transferred from plasma albumin, across the cell membrane of the liver, and into the liver cell. Two proteins, Y and Z, also called ligandins, affect bilirubin transfer from plasma to liver. Here it is either stored in the cell cytoplasm or removed from the ligandins and conjugated in the hepatic endoplasmic reticulum. Conjugation is essential for the excretion of bilirubin into bile. Eighty percent of the bilirubin is conjugated with glucuronic acid, becoming bilirubin glucuronide. Glucuronyl transferase is the important hepatic enzyme required for the production of bilirubin glucuronide. Ninety-five percent of bilirubin glucuronide is excreted into bile and subsequently into the intestine (Oski & Naiman, 1982b).

The effective excretion of bilirubin from the intestine is dependent on the length of time needed for the passage of stool and on the presence of substances that break down conjugated bilirubin.

KERNICTERUS

When albumin-binding sites are filled, increased amounts of free bilirubin are available for passage into the central nervous system (CNS). Free bilirubin easily crosses the blood–brain barrier and is transferred into the brain cells, causing obvious yellow staining of the brain tissue, similar to its effect on the skin. The areas of the brain usually affected by the staining are the hypothalamus, dentate nucleus, and cerebellum. Kernicterus is associated with varying degrees of neurologic damage, but a direct correlation between serum bilirubin levels and the severity of involvement cannot be drawn.

Many factors can influence the bilirubin-binding capacity and increase the risk of kernicterus at lower bilirubin levels. Some of these factors are listed here:

- The total amount of available serum albumin. Premature infants normally experience a relative hypoproteinemia and have fewer albumin-binding sites available for free bilirubin.
- Presence of other substances competing for available binding sites. Certain drugs, such as sulfisoxazole and salicylates, compete with bilirubin for binding sites or replace bilirubin loosely attached to binding sites.
- Acidosis and hypoxia. Increased production of hydrogen ions and implementation of anaerobic metabolism can impede bilirubin binding. Albumin's ability to bind bilirubin drops to one half of its potential at a serum pH of 7.1, with free fatty acids, produced during anaerobic metabolism, competing for albumin-binding sites (Bowman, 1988). When acidosis and hypoxia, which can open the blood–brain barrier, are concurrently present in a sick infant, such an infant can be exposed to kernicterus at much lower serum bilirubin levels. Evidence also suggests that subsequent CNS abnormalities are better correlated with tests evaluating bilirubin-binding capacity rather than serum bilirubin concentrations (Oski & Naiman, 1982b).

Clinical Manifestations

The signs and symptoms of kernicterus are as follows:

- Lethargy
- Irritability
- Hypotonia
- Paralysis of upward gaze
- High-pitched cry
- Poor eating
- Opisthotonic posturing
- Spasticity
- Deafness
- Cerebral palsy
- Tooth enamel abnormalities

The risk of kernicterus is 50 percent if serum bilirubin levels are 30 mg/dl or greater and 10 percent if levels are between 20 and 25 mg/dl.

Common Nonimmune Causes of Hyperbilirubinemia

Elevated bilirubin levels within the first 24 hours of life or levels that exceed 12 mg/dl are not considered normal physiologic jaundice and deserve investigation. Many conditions other than blood group incompatibilities can cause jaundice. These pathologic conditions can be classified as (1) problems causing increased RBC breakdown, such as sepsis, drug reactions, and extravascular blood; (2) problems that interfere with bilirubin conjugation, such as breast milk jaundice, drug interactions, hypothyroidism, hypoxia, and asphyxia; or (3) problems causing abnormal bilirubin excretion, such as bowel obstruction. However, the single factor most responsible for hyperbilirubinemia is prematurity.

Increased Red Blood Cell Breakdown

Neonatal bacterial and viral infections and intrauterine viral infections, especially those of the TORCH complex (*t*oxoplasmosis, *o*ther diseases, *r*ubella, *c*ytomegalovirus, and *h*erpes), have been implicated in the hemolytic destruction of the RBC. Certain medications, such as the synthetic analogues of vitamin K or large doses of natural vitamin K, also induce RBC destruction. Other conditions prevalent in the premature and term newborn can result in the extravasation of large quantities of blood (e.g., cephalhematoma and pulmonary or intracerebral hemorrhages). These extravascular collections of blood cells must undergo hemolysis to be resorbed by the body.

Interference with Bilirubin Conjugation

Breast Milk Jaundice. Breast milk jaundice affects 2 to 4 percent of all breastfed babies, with symptoms becoming apparent at 3 to 5 days of life. Bilirubin levels can reach 12 to 20 mg/dl between 8 and 15 days and may remain elevated for as long as 2 months (Maisels, 1990).

Two substances found in breast milk, pregnanediol and fatty acids, inhibit glucuronyl transferase, the enzyme necessary for bilirubin conjugation in the liver. Another substance present in breast milk, β-glucuronidase, enhances the breakdown of conjugated bilirubin deposited in the intestine as bile before it has the opportunity to be eliminated in the stool. This conjugated bilirubin is then broken down to the unconjugated form and subsequently resorbed by the small and large bowel. Unconjugated bilirubin present in the intestine diffuses easily into the blood supply of the bowel, where it is redistributed into the circulation.

When breastfeeding is discontinued, the bilirubin level falls within 24 to 48 hours, decreasing to one half of its previous peak level by 48 hours. With resumption of breastfeeding, the bilirubin level will again start to rise, but at a much slower pace (Maisels, 1990).

Drugs Interfering With Bilirubin Conjugation. Certain medications ingested by the mother and transplacentally passed to the fetus, such as salicylates and sulfa preparations, can interfere with the ability of albumin to bind bilirubin. Administration of these drugs to the newborn can produce the same effect. Other medications, such as sodium benzoate, which is commonly used as a preservative, compete with bilirubin for albumin-binding sites.

Hypothyroidism. Twenty percent of all infants with hypothyroidism have elevated bilirubin levels lasting 3 to 4 weeks, with normalization of levels requiring up to 4 months. The suspected mechanisms for jaundice are theorized to be a delay in glucuronyl transferase development or impaired hepatic proteins that bind bilirubin and remove it from the plasma. The plasma membrane of the liver may also be altered, resulting in decreased bilirubin influx into the hepatic cells.

Acidosis and Hypoxia. A drop in serum pH alters albumin's ability to bind bilirubin. The accompanying increase in free fatty acid production promotes competition between fatty acids and bilirubin for binding sites.

Abnormal Bilirubin Excretion

Any disease state resulting in decreased bowel motility or hepatocellular damage that causes abnormal bilirubin excretion can raise serum bilirubin levels significantly.

TREATMENT OF HYPERBILIRUBINEMIA

Phototherapy

Photo-oxidation and photoisomerization are the two mechanisms theorized to change bilirubin into water-soluble and excretable forms. Photo-oxidation involves the oxidation of bilirubin pigment deposited in the skin and its conversion into colorless products that can be excreted into the urine. Of the total body bilirubin concentration, 15 percent can undergo photodegradation through oxidation.

Phototherapy is also thought to enhance the hepatic excretion of unconjugated bilirubin and to increase bowel transit time. With the initiation of early phototherapy, a 20 to 35 percent reduction in serum bilirubin concentrations is noted by day 2 of life, with a reduction of 41 to 55 percent by day 4. This reduction is more significant than the naturally occurring drop in the untreated infant.

Adverse effects include the following:

- Dermal rash
- Lethargy
- Abdominal distention
- Possible eye damage
- Dehydration
- Thrombocytopenia
- Hypocalcemia
- Secretory diarrhea
- "Bronze baby" syndrome

The administration of albumin to an infant who is undergoing phototherapy may reduce the amount of bilirubin available in the skin for photoisomerization.

Collaborative Management

Infants requiring phototherapy benefit most from blue light in the wavelength range at which photoisomerization occurs most efficiently (i.e., 420 to 460 nm). In addition to appropriate wavelength, effective illumination must also be maintained. Spectroradiometer readings of 4 to 6 μW/cm^2/nm are considered in the effective therapeutic range.

Because the effects of prolonged exposure to phototherapy lights can potentially cause retinal damage, infants undergoing phototherapy require eye protection. Phototherapy units and eye protection should be periodically removed throughout the day to provide the infant with visual stimulation and interaction with parents and caregivers.

Infants undergoing phototherapy require temperature stabilization appropriate for their size and overall condition. Adequate fluid intake and compensatory fluid adjustments for increased insensible water loss may be required to prevent dehydration in these infants. Whereas the infant is under phototherapy, bilirubin levels must be monitored frequently to assess the need for exchange transfusion and the effectiveness of therapy. Because phototherapy lights can alter blood bilirubin results, the lights should be turned off during blood drawing for serum bilirubin determinations.

Many hyperbilirubinemic infants who are healthy and not in need of thermoregulation or exchange transfusion can easily be cared for at home. Their parents must have access to home phototherapy equipment and a medical supply company to service the equipment, as well as the support of their medical caregiver. If the infant can remain normothermic in an open crib without clothing, home phototherapy should be considered as a cost-effective alternative to hospitalization. The same precautions regarding protective eye covering and adequate fluid intake must be observed in these infants. Blood for the required frequent bilirubin levels can be drawn on a daily basis at the physician's office or neighborhood hospital laboratory or by a home health care worker.

Exchange Transfusion

If bilirubin levels start to approach those associated with kernicterus in spite of phototherapy, exchange transfusion may be necessary to protect the

CNS status of the jaundiced infant. The object of this procedure is to remove bilirubin and the antibody-coated RBCs from the newborn's circulation. After a single-volume exchange, 75 percent of the newborn's RBC mass is removed; a double-volume exchange removes 85 to 90 percent of the cells (Valaes, 1963). However, bilirubin removal is much less effective, with only 25 percent of the infant's total body bilirubin being removed during a double-volume exchange. This probably occurs because the major portion of bilirubin is in the extravascular compartment, an area not affected by the exchange of blood volume. Rebound in bilirubin levels occurs within 1 hour of the exchange, and they reach as much as 55 percent of the pre-exchange values (Valaes, 1963).

The following criteria are used to determine the need and timing of exchange transfusions, particularly in infants with erythroblastosis fetalis (Bowman, 1988):

- Cord blood indirect bilirubin level of more than 4 mg/dl
- Hemoglobin of less than 8 g/dl and bilirubin level of more than 6 mg/dl within 1 hour of delivery in a term infant
- Hemoglobin of less than 11.5 g/dl and bilirubin level of more than 3.5 mg/dl within 1 hour of delivery in a preterm infant
- Increase in bilirubin levels by 0.5 mg/dl despite phototherapy
- Bilirubin level of more than 20 mg/dl by 24 to 48 hours in an uncompromised term infant and 17 to 18 mg/dl in the high-risk term newborn
- Bilirubin level of more than 15 mg/dl in the stable preterm infant and of 10 to 12 mg/dl if hypoxia and acidosis are present

Identical criteria pertaining to rate of rise and elevation of bilirubin level are used to determine the need for repeat exchange transfusion.

Preparation of an Infant for an Exchange Transfusion

A double-volume exchange is usually done as soon as the need arises. The most common methods use umbilical artery catheters (UACs) and umbilical vein catheters (UVCs), although central venous and peripheral arterial lines can also be used. One procedure uses the intermittent push-pull method in which an aliquot of infant's blood is withdrawn and replaced with an aliquot of donor blood. This can be done using one or two indwelling lines. Another method is the constant infusion of donor blood through the umbilical vein and the constant withdrawal of the infant's blood through an umbilical artery. This method provides for more consistent arterial blood pressure. When peripheral arterial lines are used, blood can be withdrawn from them but should be returned through a central or peripheral venous line to prevent arterial spasm and clotting of the line.

Before and during an exchange, albumin can be administered to infants considered to have low reserves of albumin-binding sites (Bowman, 1988). Its administration is thought to provide more available binding sites for circulating free bilirubin and bilirubin deposited in the extravascular compartment. Theoretically, albumin should implement movement of bilirubin into the intravascular space, where it can be removed during an exchange. The recommended dosage is 1 g/kg administered 1 to 2 hours before the exchange. However, because intravascular albumin rapidly equilibrates with the extravascular compartment, its administration could potentially increase the amount of bilirubin pulled out of the plasma and into the tissue. For this reason, albumin administration before or during an exchange remains controversial. In the presence of severe anemia, hydrops, or congestive heart failure, use of albumin is contraindicated.

Selection of Blood Products

Selection and preparation of blood products are aimed at: (1) decreasing antigen–antibody reaction, thus preventing hemolysis and additional bilirubin production; (2) removal of toxic substances or endotoxins; (3) substitution of a higher, more efficient circulating RBC volume for a low RBC mass; and (4) prevention of biochemical imbalances caused by blood products during the exchange transfusion.

When exchange is imperative shortly after birth, O-negative blood cross-matched against the mother is usually used. The cells may need to be partially packed if anemia is significant and congestive heart failure is present. If exchange is not urgent, the blood used in Rh incompatibility can be type specific and Rh negative. If the exchange is done for ABO incompatibility, O-type Rh-specific or low-titered (low anti-A and anti-B) O-type cells suspended in AB plasma can be used.

Blood used for exchange should be as fresh as possible, preferably less than 48 hours old, to prevent problems associated with elevated potassium levels. If blood less than 48 hours old is not available, reconstituting RBC concentrates less than 7 days old with fresh-frozen plasma is suggested. This preparation not only ensures adequate oxygen-carrying capacity of the red cell but also provides a greater measure of safety in regard to potassium levels, in comparison with whole blood older than 48 hours. It is also recommended that RBC concentrates more than 4 days old be washed to further remove excess potassium.

Because of the unpredictable nature of potassium levels in banked blood, it may be advisable to measure the level in any blood before its use. In one study measuring citrate-phosphate-dextrose (CPD)–preserved banked blood, 21 percent of 28 units less than 4 days old had potassium levels of 11 mEq/L or higher (Scanlon & Krakaur, 1980). In a similar study, 14 percent of units less than 4 days old had potassium levels in this range, but 8 units less than 24 hours old had levels as high as 8.8 mEq/L. However, the serum potassium levels of infants receiving blood having an elevated potassium content may not significantly increase from pretransfusion levels (Barnard, 1980).

Physiologic Effects of Exchange Transfusion

Exchange transfusion has a marked effect on the cardiovascular status and the intravascular compartment, which is reflected in pressure changes, volume fluctuations, and biochemical balance.

Intravascular Pressure and Volume Changes. With slow blood exchange, 3 minutes for one exchange cycle (withdrawal and replacement of an aliquot), the blood pressure drops but returns to baseline during the infusion cycle. However, in a rapid exchange cycle lasting 45 to 60 seconds, the pressure drops, then rises, but does not return to baseline. At aliquots of 5 ml/kg every 3 minutes, an average exchange should take 100 to 110 minutes.

Because both cardiac return and output drop during hypotension, the potential risk of decreased ileocolonic blood flow due to sustained arterial hypotension exists during an exchange transfusion. In an exchange using an umbilical vein catheter, a rise in portal vein pressure during the injection phase can also result in diminished colonic blood flow at the end of injection. Regardless of the cause of gut hypoperfusion, ischemic damage of the intestinal mucosa can occur, resulting in necrotizing enterocolitis and perforation (Aranda & Sweet, 1977). Difficult or traumatic insertion or prolonged placement of the umbilical vein catheter can also lead to thrombosis of the portal vein and infection.

When arterial pressure decreases in response to blood withdrawal and increases in response to infusion, intracranial pressure changes accordingly, a reflection of the immature autoregulatory mechanisms of neonatal cerebral blood flow. Marked fluctuations in intracranial pressure, especially in the preterm infant, can predispose these infants to the risk of intraventricular and intracerebral hemorrhage.

Electrocardiographic Changes. During exchange transfusion, cardiac conduction abnormalities can occur. The precise reasons for these electrocardiographic changes are unclear, because several causative factors are present concurrently. The most common changes include P wave elevation, tachycardia, bradycardia, ST segment changes, and abnormal QRS complex.

Metabolic Disturbances. The common anticoagulants used to preserve banked blood are acid-citrate-dextrose (ACD), CPD, CPD-adenosine, and heparin. Heparin is not widely used because it offers only a limited shelf life and predisposes its receiver to a state of hypocoagulability. However, it does not cause rebound hypoglycemia, acidosis, and hypocalcemia, which occur with use of the other three preparations. The citrate found in ACD and CPD blood binds calcium, and if not metabolized quickly, as is the case in the preterm or seriously ill infant, it can lead to acidosis and hypocalcemia. CPD and CPD-adenosine blood are actually used more frequently because they contain one half of the acid load of ACD blood. CPD-adenosine blood has the longest shelf life.

Controversy regarding the use of calcium supplementation and correction of acidosis during an exchange still exists (Baumgart & Kim, 1988; Oski & Naiman, 1982b). Although total serum calcium level may be lowered, the ionized calcium level does not change during an exchange transfusion (Baumgart & Kim, 1988). However, if the initial ionized calcium level is low or drops during the exchange, or if symptoms of hypocalcemia occur, administration of 100 mg of calcium gluconate for 100 ml of blood is recommended. Blood calcium levels are only transiently raised by the administration of calcium supplements.

Excess heating of blood during an exchange produces hemolysis, resulting in elevated serum potassium levels. Levels should be monitored closely before, during, and after exchange. In the infant who is already hyperkalemic, it may be beneficial to screen the donor blood for its potassium level before starting the transfusion.

Because the dextrose concentration used in blood preservation is equivalent to 300 mg of glucose per liter of blood, rebound hypoglycemia can occur shortly after completion of an exchange transfusion. The compensatory insulin release requires adequate supplemental glucose if hypoglycemia is to be avoided. Blood glucose levels should be monitored during and after the exchange.

Alteration of Pharmacokinetics. Exchange transfusion alters blood levels of certain medications. The determining factors are the timing of doses in relation to the start of the exchange and the rate of metabolism of the medication. Table 16–1 lists medications that were evaluated for the percentage of decrease after single- and double-volume exchanges (Lackner, 1982).

Medications known to have significant decreases in blood levels owing to an exchange should be scheduled for administration after completion of the exchange.

Hematologic Changes. During the early phase of exchange transfusion in the term newborn, the neutrophil count drops but rises rapidly within hours after completion of the procedure (Phibbs, 1970). This phenomenon also occurs in the preterm infant but more gradually.

Collaborative Management

Management of an infant undergoing an exchange transfusion is as follows:

- The infant should be in the most stable cardiorespiratory status possible.
- The infant should be placed in an open warmer with continuous monitoring of temperature to ensure adequate thermoregulation during the procedure.
- Pre-exchange laboratory data should include blood type and cross-match; direct and indirect Coombs tests; electrolytes, bilirubin, calcium, and glucose levels; and hematocrit. All blood work except type, cross-match, and Coombs test should be repeated midway through and at the completion of the exchange.
- Necessary catheters and lines should be placed and kept patent with appropriate intravenous fluids until the procedure begins. Most central venous, UAC, and UVC lines can be kept open with 5 or 10 percent dextrose solutions. Normal saline or 0.45 percent saline solutions can be infused through peripheral arterial lines. The addition of calcium and electrolytes should be dictated by the infant's metabolic status.
- Blood administration sets should be assembled and placed on a blood

TABLE 16–1. Percentages of Decrease in Blood Levels after Transfusion

Drug	Single-Volume (% loss)	Double-Volume (% loss)
Ampicillin	7.7	14.2
Gentamicin	5.2	10.1
Digoxin	1.2	2.4
Phenobarbital	6.4	12.3
Vancomycin	5.7	11.0

warmer that is set at the manufacturer's recommended temperature. If a blood warmer is not used, donor blood should be allowed to reach room temperature before use. Parental consent for blood transfusion and exchange transfusion should be obtained beforehand.

- Vital signs should be taken before the procedure begins and at 15-minute intervals thereafter. Cardiorespiratory and blood pressure monitoring should be continuous throughout the procedure. If the infant is on a ventilator or oxygen, transcutaneous CO_2 and saturation monitors should be utilized, with blood gas sampling before, during, and after the procedure.
- Accurate tally of blood withdrawal and infusion and medication administration during the procedure should be kept. Blood is usually exchanged in aliquots of 10 to 20 ml for a term infant and 5 to 10 ml for a severely anemic, hydropic, or preterm infant.
- Readjustment of medication schedules, based on completion time of the exchange, may be required. Drug levels are needed to evaluate this.
- The infant will require the resumption of phototherapy and observation of postprocedural vital signs every 15 minutes for approximately 2 hours or until stable.

Anemia

PATHOPHYSIOLOGY

The presence of anemia, defined in RBC volume rather than hematocrit, is associated with increased mortality rates in both term and preterm infants. RBC volume is determined by multiplying the blood volume per kilogram times the hematocrit. The average blood volume of the term newborn is estimated at 82 to 85 ml/kg, with blood volume in the preterm approaching 100 ml/kg as gestational age decreases (Brown, 1988). For example, for an 800-g infant with 100 ml/kg blood volume and hematocrit of 25, the RBC volume would be calculated by the following:

$$100 \times 25 = 25 \text{ ml/kg}$$

CLINICAL MANIFESTATIONS

Acute Anemia

An infant experiencing an acute anemic episode, with hemorrhage being the most common cause, exhibits symptoms reflecting compromise of the cardiorespiratory system (Oski & Naiman, 1982a):

- Shock
- Poor peripheral perfusion
- Poor respiratory effort
- Respiratory distress
- Tachycardia
- Pallor
- Lethargy
- Hypotension
- Hemoglobin level less than 12 g/dl

Acute blood loss results in a recognizable sequence of symptoms based on the amount of volume loss (Oski & Naiman, 1982a):

- *7.5 to 15 percent volume loss.* Little change is noticed in heart rate and blood pressure, but the stroke volume and subsequent cardiac output are decreased. Peripheral vasoconstriction occurs, resulting in decreased blood flow to skeletal muscles, gut, and general body.
- *20 to 25 percent volume loss.* Hypotension and shock become apparent. Cardiac output is decreased, and peripheral vasoconstriction is present. Low tissue oxygen levels and acidosis become apparent.

Chronic Anemia

Prolonged or chronic anemia may not require rapid intravascular volume expansion, but it is by no means completely benign. Because these infants have had considerable time to adjust to chronic blood loss or hemolysis, the changes in vital signs may reflect poor oxygen-carrying capacity rather than hypovolemia. The blood smear may also reflect the long-standing nature of the problem, with RBCs appearing hypochromic and small and with an increased number of immature forms of RBCs.

Hemorrhage

Fetal-Maternal Transfusion due to Transplacental Hemorrhage. This phenomenon occurs in 50 percent to 75 percent of all pregnancies and can be an acute or a chronic process (Bowman, 1988; Jones, 1969). In an estimated 8 percent of pregnancies fetal-maternal transfusion is in the range of 0.5 ml to 40 ml of blood, whereas in 1 percent there is an exchange of more than 40 ml (Cohen, Zuelzer, Gustafson, & Evans, 1964). Fetal-maternal transfusions can be documented by the presence of fetal cells in maternal circulation, with the use of the Kleihauer acid elution test for the presence of fetal hemoglobin in maternal blood. Any increase in number would suggest the contamination of maternal blood by fetal blood. This test is useful in the identification of fetal red blood cells in the mother's blood, provided that no underlying condition exists that increases the amount of fetal hemoglobin in the mother's blood. A mother who receives a sudden and substantial amount of fetal blood during a transplacental hemorrhage may experience a transfusion reaction.

Twin-to-Twin Transfusion. This phenomenon, which can be both acute and chronic, occurs in 15 to 33 percent of all monochorionic (monozygotic) twins, in which the placentas tend to be fused. The anastomosis is usually between an artery of one placenta and the vein of the other (Oski & Naiman, 1982a, 1982d), although vascular connections may be artery to artery or vein to vein. In the chronic form of twin-to-twin transfusion, the size difference between twins can be helpful in determining the donor and the recipient. When the weight difference exceeds 20 percent, the smaller twin is always the donor (Tan, Tan, Tan, & Tan, 1979). When the weight difference is less than 20 percent, either twin may be the donor. In such cases, hematocrit values can help differentiate donor and recipient. The donor twin is anemic, with a blood cell count reflecting increased hematopoiesis, as evidenced by an elevated reticulocyte count and increased numbers of immature RBCs.

The recipient exhibits polycythemia but can show signs of congestive heart failure and pulmonary or systemic hypertension. On analysis of laboratory data, there is usually a 5-g/dl difference between donor and recipient hemoglobin values. Stillbirths are common in twin-to-twin transfusion, with both twins being at risk.

Obstetric Accidents. Many obstetrical problems, especially those occurring before labor and delivery, can result in chronic as well as acute blood loss. Long-standing problems, such as placenta previa or partial abruption, usually result in anemia. However, acute hemorrhage rather than anemia is the case in problems occurring at the time of delivery. A tight nuchal cord can also decrease blood volume in a newborn by approximately 20 percent (Cashore & Usher, 1973). Holding a newly delivered infant above the placenta can also result in a lower hematocrit and blood volume, owing to the gravitational drainage of blood from the newborn into the placenta.

Internal Hemorrhage. A drop in hematocrit during the first 24 to 72 hours that is not associated with hyperbilirubinemia is usually attributed to internal hemorrhage. Bleeding can occur in various parts of the body secondary to birth trauma or pre-existing anomalies. The areas of potential hemorrhage in the head include the subdural, subarachnoid, intraventricular, intracranial, and subperiosteal spaces. Infants can lose an estimated 10 to 15 percent of their blood during an intraventricular or intracranial hemorrhage. In cases of traumatic delivery or vacuum extraction, extensive scalp bleeding may occur, causing a significant blood loss that can be estimated by measuring the increase in the head circumference. Each centimeter of increase represents an estimated 38 ml of blood lost from the intravascular compartment. Hemorrhage into the liver, kidneys, spleen, or retroperitoneal space can also occur and is associated with traumatic and breech deliveries. Hepatic rupture occurs in 1.2 to 5.6 percent of stillbirths and neonatal deaths, with one half of the hemorrhages being subcapsular. The condition of these infants tends to be stable for 24 to 48 hours and then suddenly deteriorates. This deterioration seems to coincide with rupture of the capsule and hemoperitoneum. Hepatic rupture carries a very poor prognosis, but rapid surgery preceded by multiple transfusions can save the infant. Splenic rupture is associated with severe EBF and should be suspected at the time of exchange transfusion, when the central venous pressure is low rather than elevated. Signs of splenic rupture include scrotal swelling and peritoneal effusion without free air. Adrenal hemorrhage has been seen more frequently in the infant of a diabetic mother or of a prediabetic mother and is characterized by the presence of a flank mass with bluish discoloration of the overlying skin.

RBC Destruction and Hemolysis

Maternal-Fetal Blood Group Incompatibilities. Isoimmunization, as in ABO and Rh incompatibility, is responsible for the majority of cases of neonatal hemolysis. Decreased erythrocyte life span as the result of hemolysis is usually associated with a rise in bilirubin level, with 1 g of hemoglobin yielding an equivalent of 35 mg of bilirubin (Lemberge & Legge, 1949).

Acquired Defects of the RBC. This problem is seen in bacterial sepsis and viral infections, especially of the TORCH variety. Drug-induced RBC destruction, due to either maternal ingestion or direct administration to the newborn, is another common cause of hemolysis.

Congenital Defects of the RBC. Defects can involve the RBC membrane, enzymatic system, or hemoglobin component, as in such conditions as glucose-6-phosphate dehydrogenase deficiency, thalassemia, and hereditary spherocytosis. These conditions, although causes of hemolysis in the newborn period, occur infrequently in comparison with the previous two entities.

Blood Sampling

Blood loss secondary to sampling is one of the two most frequent causes of chronic anemia in infants, the other being physiologic anemia of the newborn. Among a group of preterm infants admitted to one neonatal intensive care unit, the estimated average blood loss from sampling during the first 4 to 6 weeks of life was 46 to 50 ml/kg, with severity of illness correlating with the amount of blood removed for sampling (Blanchette & Zipursky, 1984; Obladen, Sachsenweger, & Stahnke, 1988).

HISTORY

Acute and chronic anemia can often be distinguished from each other, and from other problems, by analyzing the family history for the presence of anemia or jaundice.

LABORATORY DATA

The type of anemia can often be identified on the basis of laboratory studies that evaluate RBC content and morphology:

- Hematocrit and hemoglobin levels can define the type as well as the degree of anemia.
- Elevated reticulocyte counts and increased numbers of immature RBCs reflect the degree of hematopoietic activity in response to anemia.
- Peripheral blood smears are helpful in evaluating iron content and the size and shape of the red cell, which vary in different forms of anemia.
- Blood typing, Rh determination, and Coombs testing can help identify blood group incompatibilities as causes of anemia.

TREATMENT

Management of Acute Anemia

Stabilization of an infant with acute anemia includes the following:

- Basic resuscitation of the infant experiencing precipitous blood loss often includes stabilization of the airway, requiring intubation and ventilation.
- Rapid line placement for fluid replacement, volume expansion, and blood sampling may necessitate use of the umbilical vein or artery. Central venous pressure can be helpful in assessing the degree of volume loss and the quantity of needed replacement.
- If acute volume expansion is required, low-titer type O-negative blood,

plasma, albumin, or saline can initially be used in 10- to 20-ml/kg increments until a type and crossmatch is available. If the infant does respond to bolus infusion, this usually indicates that hemorrhage was of an obstetrical nature, but failure to respond may indicate ongoing internal hemorrhage. A good response may also justify repetition of another 10- to 20-ml/kg fluid bolus. An aliquot of 3 ml/kg of RBCs raises the hemoglobin level by 1 g/dl (Oski & Naiman, 1982a).

- Laboratory tests and physical examination should be initiated after stabilization of the infant to determine the cause of the anemia and to rectify the problem.
- Examination of the placenta, and a maternal blood sample testing for the presence of fetal hemoglobin, may prove useful in determining the cause of the blood loss.

Collaborative Management
Acute Anemia

After initial stabilization, nursing care must include modifications that either eliminate recurrence of precipitous events or prevent further blood loss.

Chronic Anemia

The major focus of therapy in the infant with chronic anemia is control or elimination of its cause. Several forms of anemia in term and preterm infants are linked to dietary deficiencies that can be eradicated by replacement therapy. Chronic forms of anemia requiring symptomatic therapy can also be treated with transfusion therapy and erythropoietin.

Dietary Supplementation

Three major dietary factors affecting RBC production are iron, folic acid, and vitamin E. Because all three increase in amount with increasing gestational age, premature birth predisposes such an infant to anemia owing to insufficiency.

In the newborn without benefit of iron supplementation, the hematopoiesis necessary to maintain a normal hemoglobin depletes iron reserves by the time birth weight is doubled. Various factors can further contribute to subsequent iron deficiency anemia, such as low birth weight, low initial hemoglobin levels, and blood loss through trauma, hemorrhage, or sampling. In the term infant, exhaustion of iron reserves normally occurs by 20 to 24 weeks of postnatal age, but this happens much earlier in the preterm infant. Because iron stores needed for hemoglobin production are present in insufficient quantities at birth in the premature infant, these infants require supplementation during the first 2 to 4 months to prevent iron deficiency anemia.

Iron depletion, in any gestational age group, initially becomes evident in decreased serum ferritin levels, a measure of accumulated iron stores, and in the disappearance of stainable iron from the bone marrow. Subsequent decrease in mean corpuscular volume of the RBC (i.e., the size of the RBC) is then followed by a drop in hemoglobin level. Although prophylactic iron supplementation will not prevent the initial fall in hemoglobin, administration of 2 to 3 mg/kg/day of supplemental iron should supply term and preterm infants with adequate reserves; 4 mg/kg/day is recommended in the very low birth weight infant.

Folic acid is a component of the B-complex vitamins involved in the maturation of RBCs, particularly, the synthesis of DNA, which controls nuclear maturation and division. Because bone marrow is among the body's most rapidly growing and proliferative tissue, its ability to produce RBCs is reduced during folic acid deficiency, producing a megaloblastic anemia. Folic acid is present in high quantities at birth in both term and preterm infants, but levels drop rapidly, especially in the low birth weight infant. It is estimated that approximately 68 percent of infants less than 1700 g have subnormal levels of folic acid at 1 to 3 months of age (Oski & Naiman, 1982a). However, only a few infants actually develop anemia. Human milk and soy-based products contain an adequate amount of folic acid, but commonly used commercial products must be artificially enriched. Because folic acid is absorbed in the duodenum and jejunum, any disease condition or medication that impacts on the absorptive surface of these areas can impair folic acid absorption. A dosage of 50 mg/day of folacin is recommended to prevent folic acid deficiency (Goetzman & Wennberg, 1991).

Vitamin E, an antioxidant, is valuable in protecting the RBC membrane from destruction due to lipid peroxidation (Brown, 1988). Deficiency of this nutrient shortens the life span of the cell by exposing the unprotected, unsaturated membrane lipids to peroxidation and hemolysis. Administration of iron supplementation in the presence of this deficiency intensifies the hemolytic response. Signs and symptoms include edema of the feet, lower extremities, and scrotal area. The RBC morphology may vary, but abnormalities usually include fragmented or irregularly shaped cells, presence of spherocytes, and thrombocytopenia. Treatment consists of 25 IU of vitamin E per day for 6 to 8 weeks for preterm infants (Goetzman & Wennberg, 1991). This usually results in an increased hemoglobin level with a decrease in the reticulocyte count.

Transfusion Therapy

The benefits of transfusion therapy remain controversial. Although the critically ill infant requiring ventilator support is generally maintained with a hematocrit of greater than 40 percent (Dear, 1984), the elimination of symptoms by transfusion therapy in the convalescent infant does not seem consistent. In premature infants with a hematocrit of less than 30 percent, the presence of apnea and bradycardia, dyspnea, feeding difficulties, poor weight gain despite good caloric intake, lethargy, tachypnea, tachycardia, and increased cardiac output and oxygen consumption appears to be relieved by transfusion therapy in several studies (DeMaio, Harris, & Spitzer, 1986; Joshi et al., 1987).

Recombinant Human Erythropoietin Therapy

The principal action of human erythropoietin is on the hematopoietic stem cells housed in the bone marrow that have been designated as the colony-forming units–erythrocyte, the precursors of the RBC. Studies on preterm infants have demonstrated that human erythropoietin maintains the hematocrit level during the phase of normal anemia of the premature infant, with good proliferation of erythroid progenitor cells (Rhondeau et al., 1988; Ross et al., 1989; Shannon et al., 1987).

Preliminary data suggest that preterm infants less than 34 weeks' gestation respond to human erythropoietin with increased blood levels of erythropoietin, increased reticulocyte formation, and a slight increase in hematocrit 2 to 3 weeks after the introduction of therapy (Halperin et al., 1989). In this study, the doses to which infants best responded were 75 to 150 U/kg/wk. Because clinical trials are in progress, ideal dosages and time of initiation of therapy are not yet established.

Serum ferritin levels are noted to decrease rapidly after the initiation of therapy in infants with normal pretreatment ferritin levels, in spite of prophylactic iron supplementation of 2 mg/kg/day. This marks the potential for development of iron deficiency anemia and the need for increased iron supplementation in infants treated with human erythropoietin. Transient thrombocytosis shortly after the initiation of therapy and transient neutropenia lasting as long as 2 months after the discontinuation of therapy have also been documented. It has been postulated that this phenomenon is due to a stimulant effect of human erythropoietin on megakaryocyte progenitors and a negative effect on granulocyte-monocyte progenitor cells. If human erythropoietin proves effective in raising hematocrits without causing significant untoward effects, it is projected that it may eliminate the need for one third of all transfusions in premature infants (Brown, Berman, & Luckey, 1990).

PHYSIOLOGIC ANEMIA OF THE NEWBORN

The drop in hemoglobin, prompting the postnatal rise in erythropoietin, is directly correlated with the infant's gestational age and birth weight. The smaller and more immature infant reaches a lower nadir at an earlier postnatal age. The hemoglobin level in the term newborn reaches a nadir of 11.4 g/dl ± 0.9 in the first 2 to 3 months of life (Stockman, 1988). It remains at this level for approximately 2 more months and then gradually increases. Although there is no significant difference in cord blood hemoglobin levels between term infants and preterm infants born after 32 weeks' gestation, the drop in hemoglobin level occurs earlier in the preterm infant, is more precipitous, and reaches a lower nadir. Starting at 2 weeks of age, the preterm infant has a drop in hemoglobin level of 1 g/dl/wk for the first several weeks, with the nadir at 6 to 8 weeks of age being 2 to 3 g/dl lower than that of the term infant. An infant weighing 1000 to 1500 g at birth will have a low mean hemoglobin of 8 g/dl at 4 to 6 weeks of age.

Infants who have undergone exchange transfusion or multiple transfusions also have a greater fall in hemoglobin level in the first 3 months of life. This phenomenon may theoretically be due to improved oxygen delivery to tissue, associated with the replacement of fetal with adult hemoglobin (Stockman, 1988). Adult hemoglobin has less affinity for oxygen because of the structural difference of the globin portion of the hemoglobin molecule. This, coupled with the increased amount of 2,3-diphosphoglycerate present in the blood, allows adult hemoglobin to release oxygen to the tissue more easily. Improved tissue oxygenation effectively lowers serum erythropoietin levels, resulting in decreased RBC production. Although erythropoietin levels are decreased in the early newborn period, the erythroid progenitor cells in the bone marrow are exceedingly sensitive to erythropoietin and respond rapidly as blood levels increase. The normal erythropoietin level in infants beyond the newborn period is 21 to 23 mU/ml.

Physiologic anemia usually does not require any form of treatment. With good nutrition, the hemoglobin level in the term infant should start to rise by 3 months of age.

Polycythemia

PATHOPHYSIOLOGY

Polycythemia, defined as a peripheral venous hematocrit of more than 65 percent, occurs in 4 to 5 percent of the total population of newborns, in 2 to 4 percent of term infants who are appropriate for gestational age, and in 10 to 15 percent of infants who are small for gestational age and large for gestational age. It has not been observed, however, in infants less than 34 weeks' gestation. Although the fetus lives in a low Po_2 environment that should induce a polycythemic response, it protects itself by limiting hematocrit levels to less than 60 percent. This may be a function of slower fetal hepatic response to hypoxia, in comparison with rapid renal response after birth. The average hematocrit on the first day of life is approximately 50 percent in the term infant and the preterm infant greater than 32 weeks' gestation. During the first 4 to 12 hours of life, hemoglobin and hematocrit values tend to rise and then equilibrate, especially in infants receiving large placental transfusions.

Polycythemia impairs peripheral circulation by increasing the viscosity of blood, thereby decreasing the flow rate. As blood viscosity increases, vascular resistance increases, not only in the peripheral circulation but also in the microcirculation of the capillaries throughout the body. Decreased peripheral perfusion impairs blood flow, which can alter results of peripheral samples. In comparison with venous samples, capillary samples are 5 to 15 percent higher and umbilical vessel or arterial samples are 6 to 8 percent lower.

Three major factors determine blood viscosity: hematocrit, plasma viscosity (osmolality), and deformability of the RBC. With hematocrit levels less than 60 to 65 percent, blood viscosity increases in a linear fashion, but viscosity exponentially increases at higher hematocrit levels. Small vessels can be occluded and enhance sludging in the microcirculation, leading to thrombosis and tissue ischemia.

Active Polycythemia

Tissue hypoxia, regardless of cause, elicits an increase in erythropoietin that, in turn, stimulates RBC production. In the fetus, erythropoietin is produced initially by the liver and then by the kidney, mimicking the adult production site. The kidney's potential to release erythropoietin is effective by 34 weeks' gestation (Halvorsen & Finne, 1968). At this time, a renal erythropoietic factor reacts with a substance in the plasma to produce the RBC stimulating factor erythropoietin. Tissue hypoxia adjacent to the renal tubules, where erythropoietin is theorized to be produced, is the potent stimulator of this factor's release.

Many factors can lead to tissue hypoxia associated with the active form of polycythemia. Some of them are listed below:

- Maternal factors resulting in decreased placental blood flow:
  - Pregnancy-induced hypertension
  - Increased maternal age
  - Maternal renal or heart disease
  - Severe maternal diabetes. Hematocrit values of 64 percent or more are found in 42 percent of infants of diabetic mothers and 30 percent of infants of mothers with gestation diabetes.
  - Oligohydramnios
  - Maternal smoking. The mechanism is theorized to be production of carbon monoxide that crosses the placenta and induces a state of tissue hypoxia in the fetus.
- Placental factors
  - Placental infarction
  - Placenta previa
  - Viral infections, especially TORCH syndrome
  - Postmaturity
  - Placental dysfunction resulting in small for gestational age infant
- Fetal syndromes
  - Trisomies 13, 18, and 21
  - Beckwith-Wiedemann syndrome

Passive Polycythemia

Passive polycythemia is a result of increased fetal blood volume that occurs as a result of maternal-fetal transfusion; twin-to-twin transfusion, with one twin being polycythemic and the other anemic; or delay in cord clamping. A diagnosis of maternal-fetal transfusion can be considered when (1) the infant's blood is found to contain larger amounts than expected of adult hemoglobin, IgA, or IgM; (2) RBCs in the infant's blood have maternal blood group antigens, if maternal and infant blood groups are different; or (3) XX cells are found in an XY infant. In twin-to-twin transfusion, morbidity and mortality are comparable in both groups of affected infants, with one twin being anemic and the other polycythemic. By far, however, the most common cause of fetal transfusion is delayed cord clamping with positioning of the newborn below the level of the placenta. Delayed cord clamping can increase the circulating volume by as much as 60 percent and can raise the hematocrit value by 10 percent (Oski & Naiman, 1982d).

CLINICAL MANIFESTATIONS

The signs and symptoms of passive polycythemia include the following:

- Central nervous system
  - Lethargy
  - Hypotonia
  - Tremulousness

- Exaggerated startle
- Poor suck
- Vomiting
- Seizures
- Apnea
- Cardiovascular
  - Plethora
  - Cardiomegaly
  - Electrocardiographic changes: right and left atrial
  - Hypertrophy, right ventricular hypertrophy
- Respiratory
  - Respiratory distress
  - Central cyanosis
  - Pleural effusions
  - Pulmonary congestion and edema
- Hematologic
  - Thrombocytopenia
  - Elevated reticulocytes
  - Hepatosplenomegaly
- Metabolic
  - Hypocalcemia
  - Hyperbilirubinemia
  - Hypoglycemia

A venous hematocrit of 65 percent or more should be considered for treatment by partial exchange transfusion.

Five percent albumin or crystalloid is suggested as replacement for the removed aliquot of blood. With the advent of stricter precautions for prevention of viral transmission by blood products, use of fresh-frozen plasma would not seem advisable.

COLLABORATIVE MANAGEMENT

The care of any newborn should include a screening hematocrit before 6 hours of age. The infant should be kept adequately hydrated, with glucose and calcium levels being closely monitored. A hematocrit value of greater than 65 percent should prompt careful observation of the infant for any symptoms associated with hyperviscosity. If symptoms appear, the infant should undergo partial exchange transfusion. During the partial exchange, the same care given during a single- or double-volume exchange transfusion should be provided.

Coagulopathies in the Newborn Period

Bleeding disorders affecting the newborn can be classified as (1) intensification of existing transient deficiencies of the coagulation mechanism, (2) disturbances of coagulation associated with certain disease states, (3) inherited deficiencies, or (4) abnormalities of platelets or vascular structures.

When vascular integrity is destroyed or interrupted there are four hemostatic parts that interact:

1. *Vascular components.* The components of the vascular wall affect the structure and function of damaged blood vessels. Vascular spasm is the first mechanism by which hemostasis is achieved in a damaged vessel.
2. *Platelets and their activating substances.* Formation of a platelet plug is the second mechanism of hemostasis after vascular injury has occurred.
3. *Coagulation or plasma factors.* These factors consist of procoagulants and anticoagulants (inhibitors). Coagulation completes the hemostatic mechanism by strengthening the platelet plug.
4. *Fibrinolytic pathway.* This pathway contributes to disintegration of the clot and re-establishment of normal circulatory flow. It consists of fibrinolytics (substances that lyse a fibrin clot) and inhibitors.

COAGULATION

When bleeding cannot be controlled merely with a platelet plug, circulating plasma coagulation factors are triggered to form a network of fibrin that turns the existing plug into a hemostatic seal. In the presence of normal coagulation factors, a clot can develop in 15 to 20 seconds if vascular trauma is severe and in 1 to 2 minutes if trauma is minor. Within 3 to 6 minutes after vascular rupture, the entire opening is occluded by a clot; and within 30 to 60 minutes, the clot begins to retract, pulling the injured vascular portions together and further sealing the vascular end. This coagulation reaction involves several plasma proteins and three distinct phases. The first phase involves the formation of thromboplastin, the second involves the activation of prothrombin to thrombin, and the third involves the conversion of soluble fibrinogen to fibrin.

Phase I: Formation of Prothrombin Activator

There are two separate pathways by which prothrombin activator can be generated: the intrinsic and extrinsic pathways. The intrinsic pathway is triggered by trauma or damage occurring inside the vessel or to the blood itself, and the extrinsic pathway is triggered by the production of tissue thromboplastin that is generated by vessel wall damage. This bimodal pathway can be interrupted or negated by a deficiency in platelets or any of the plasma coagulation factors or by the presence of inhibitors (anticoagulants) in the plasma. Selective activation of one of these pathways is dependent on the site of injury and the extent of its severity.

The steps of intrinsic activation of coagulation are as follows:

1. An activator (blood trauma, injury within the vessel, or contact with collagen) activates factor XII, converting it to XIIa, while simultaneously damaging platelets, which causes a release of platelet phospholipids.
2. Factor XIIa activates factor XI, converting it to XIa.
3. Factor XIa activates factor IX, converting it to IXa.
4. Factor IXa, platelet phospholipid, and factor VIII combine to activate factor X, converting it to Xa.
5. Factor Xa combines with factor V and platelet phospholipids to form prothrombin activator (prothrombinase), which releases thrombin

from prothrombin. Calcium is required for this and the preceding two steps.

The extrinsic pathway can generate thrombin in a matter of seconds when injury occurs outside the vascular space. Tissue thromboplastin, composed of glycoproteins and phospholipids, is produced when tissue is injured. When plasma comes into contact with this substance, the initial intrinsic phases are bypassed and the following responses occur:

1. Tissue thromboplastin (factor III) activates factor VII to VIIa. These two factors then form a complex with glycoprotein that activates factor X, converting it to factor Xa.
2. Factor Xa complexes with phospholipids and factor V, in the presence of calcium, to form prothrombin activator.
3. From this point on, the intrinsic and extrinsic pathways are identical, with both proceeding to phase II.

Phase II: Formation of Thrombin

Prothrombin activator from either of the two pathways continues the clotting cascade by further influencing the breakdown of the unstable plasma protein prothrombin. Prothrombin (factor II) is synthesized by the liver, under the influence of vitamin K, along with the other factors that form the prothrombin complex (factors VII, IX, and X). When acted on by prothrombin activator, prothrombin forms the potent coagulant thrombin. The newly formed thrombin stimulates completion of the third and final phase of coagulation.

Phase III: Formation of the Fibrin Clot

Thrombin promotes the conversion of fibrinogen (factor I), a protein produced by the liver, into fibrin by splitting off two peptides from the soluble fibrinogen molecule. This exposes two sites to which other split fibrin molecules can link, forming an insoluble fibrin chain. Fibrin stabilizing factor (factor XIII) further strengthens the tight bond of this developing fibrin mesh. Fibrin stabilizing factor is naturally found in the plasma and is also secreted by entrapped platelets. The forming fibrin clot begins to contract and retract with the help of platelets that have actin–myosin action, the same action by which a muscle works. Extension of the clot into the surrounding circulating blood promotes further thrombosis. Thrombin from the clot has the ability to cleave prothrombin into more thrombin and enhances the production of prothrombin activator, thus acting as a potent biofeedback system for perpetuation of the clotting cascade.

There are three main anticoagulant actions: (1) fibrin threads that are formed during clot formation absorb thrombin, thus removing it from circulation along with its potential for further coagulation; (2) antithrombin III combines with thrombin, blocking the activation of fibrinogen into fibrin; and (3) heparin, along with antithrombin III, removes several activated procoagulants. Both antithrombin III and heparin are produced in the precapillary connective tissue of the lungs and liver.

Fibrinolysis

Once a clot has developed, either it can be invaded by fibroblasts that lay down connective tissue throughout the clot or it can be dissolved. The process of dissolution occurs via activation of naturally occurring factors that lyse the clot. This system is activated simultaneously with stimulation of the coagulation system, actually having a powerful but inactivated anticoagulant built right into the clot. This anticoagulant known as plasminogen is manufactured by the liver, kidneys, and eosinophils. Plasminogen, under the influence of thrombin, activated factor XII, and other factors, is converted into plasmin, a proteolytic enzyme that breaks down fibrin into fibrin split products. Plasmin not only digests the fibrin chains but also deactivates fibrinogen, factors V, VII, and XII, and prothrombin.

COMMON COAGULATION DISORDERS IN THE NEWBORN

Hemorrhagic Disease of the Newborn

Hemorrhage occurring during the early neonatal period that can be attributed to a deficiency of vitamin K–dependent factors is classified as hemorrhagic disease of the newborn. This disease entity usually occurs during the first 2 days of life and manifests as generalized and occasionally dramatic bleeding. The most common sites are the gastrointestinal tract, umbilicus, circumcision site, skin, and internal organs. Definitive diagnosis includes a history of lack of vitamin K prophylaxis at birth and a prolonged prothrombin time that measures the prothrombin complex clotting factors consisting of factors II, VII, IX, and X.

Because these factors are gestational age dependent, the more premature the infant, the lower the levels at birth. The exaggerated drop after birth is probably due to immature liver function and delayed synthesis by the bowel. These factors slowly rise but do not reach normal adult levels until approximately 9 months of age. Administration of approximately 25 μg (0.025 mg) of vitamin K can prevent this decline and normalize the prothrombin time (Aballi & DeLamerens, 1962).

The most obvious predisposing factor is failure of an infant to receive prophylactic vitamin K postnatally. Other risk factors include maternal ingestion of anticonvulsants and coumarin anticoagulants, which interfere with the action of the prothrombin complex factors, and breastfeeding. Human milk contains a lower vitamin K content than cow's milk. Infants receiving a commercial formula for 24 hours have similar prothrombin times in comparison with those of infants receiving vitamin K after birth (Keenan, Jewett, & Glueck, 1971). Infants having hepatic dysfunction or bowel malabsorption can develop vitamin K deficiency in spite of having received prophylaxis at birth. Such disorders as chronic diarrhea, biliary atresia, hepatitis, cystic fibrosis, and prolonged parenteral nutrition do not allow for adequate vitamin K production, resulting in low prothrombin complex factors. These infants benefit from weekly vitamin K supplementation of 1 mg intramuscularly (Goetzman & Wennberg, 1991). This dosage is also the recommended American Academy of Pediatrics dosage for postnatal newborn prophylaxis.

Active bleeding due to hemorrhagic disease of the newborn may require blood replacement or the utilization of fresh-frozen plasma for immediate clotting factor replacement.

Hemophilia

Classic hemophilia (hemophilia A) is the most commonly inherited coagulation abnormality, accounting for 90 percent of all genetically linked coagulopathies and 85 percent of all hemophilias. It is passed from mother to son as an X-linked trait and is caused by factor VIII deficiency. Factor VIII has two components: a large glycoprotein called von Willebrand factor, which is required for proper platelet adhesion, and a small procoagulant protein, the antihemophilic factor, which is defective in hemophilia A. The defect involves the production of structurally and functionally ineffective clotting factors, as opposed to a deficiency in quantity.

The concentration of circulating antihemophilic factor in the serum determines the severity of the disease. Levels of 1 to 2 percent are associated with severe disease, 2 to 5 percent with moderate disease, and more than 5 percent with mild disease, a level at which active bleeding rarely occurs.

Infants affected with hemophilia have a prolonged partial thromboplastin time but the prothrombin time, thrombin time, and platelet count are relatively normal. The major symptom is bleeding, with the most common areas being the circumcision site, scalp, umbilicus, and brain (Baehner & Strauss, 1966).

Diagnosis

Prenatal diagnosis is feasible, but results are not always accurate. Diagnosis involves the measurement of the ratio of factor antigen to coagulant antigen on blood samples of fetuses of more than 20 weeks' gestation.

Treatment

Treatment consists of raising the defective or deficient factor to a level that will prevent bleeding. The suggested mode of therapy is the use of cryoprecipitate in the dose of 10 units/kg. Each unit per kilogram raises the antihemophilic factor level by 1.5 to 2 percent with a bag of cryoprecipitate containing 80 units. Another method of treatment that raises all components of the factor VIII system twofold to threefold is the use of desmopressin. Its route of administration is intravenous or intranasal, but its effectiveness and applicability to the newborn are still unknown.

Thrombocytopenia

The normal range of platelets is 150,000 to 450,000/mm^3, with the average count in the newborn being approximately 250,000/mm^3 (Aballi, Puapondh, & Desposito, 1968). Platelet counts less than 150,000/mm^3 are considered abnormal and subject to investigation for possible pathologic processes.

Thrombocytopenia is the most common bleeding disorder in the newborn, with 20 percent of all admissions to neonatal intensive care units having platelet counts of less than 50,000/mm^3 and 80 percent of sick infants having counts of less than 100,000/mm^3. However, the pathogenesis of the thrombocytopenia can be determined in only 60 percent of these infants.

Infants with a platelet count of less than 20,000/mm^3 are at particularly high risk for bleeding.

Maternal Factors

Maternal factors associated with thrombocytopenia are as follows:

- Maternal drug ingestion such as chloramphenicol, hydralazine, tolbuta-mide, and thiazides
- Maternal eclampsia and hypertension
- Placental infarction
- Maternal platelet antibodies

In immune-mediated thrombocytopenia, in which maternal antibodies cause destruction of platelets, 80 percent of these cases are due to the immune form or maternal idiopathic thrombocytopenic purpura. Idiopathic thrombocytopenic purpura is a pre-existing condition in a pregnant woman in whom IgM or IgG is attached to the platelets. These antibodies are specifically directed at platelet antigen and cause destruction of platelets. Because IgG can cross the placenta, fetal platelets can be destroyed by the transplacental passage of platelet antibodies, resulting in thrombocytopenia in the fetus and newborn. The mortality rate is 7 to 10 percent in these affected infants, with postnatal persistence of this condition for as long as 4 months (Plunket, 1987).

Antenatal Treatment

Antenatal treatment consists of administration of corticosteroids 1 to 2 weeks before delivery by cesarean section. Postnatal treatment consists of platelet transfusion, exchange transfusion with blood less than 2 days of age, and steroid therapy (prednisone, 1 to 5 mg/kg/day) (Goetzman & Wennberg, 1991).

Other Causes of Immune-Mediated Thrombocytopenia

The remaining 20 percent of immune-mediated thrombocytopenias are caused by an isoimmune reaction in which maternal antibodies are produced against foreign fetal platelets. This occurs when fetal platelets possessing an antigen not found on maternal platelets pass into maternal circulation. The mother develops IgG antibodies that eventually cross into fetal circulation, resulting in platelet destruction. This phenomenon occurs in approximately 3 percent of all pregnancies. The mortality rate of 14 percent in isoimmune thrombocytopenia is higher than that in idiopathic thrombocytopenic purpura because bleeding tends to be more severe. The treatment consists of transfusion of maternal platelets, exchange transfusion, and the use of intravenous immune globulin in the dosage of 400 mg/kg over 5 days (Suarez & Anderson, 1986). Platelets will usually normalize in the newborn by 4 weeks of age.

Neonatal Factors

Neonatal factors associated with thrombocytopenia include the following (Mehta et al., 1980):

- Asphyxia
- Apgar scores of less than 7 in 70 percent of infants

- Dissemination intravascular coagulation—16 percent
- Exchange transfusion—12 percent
- Infection—52 to 77 percent (Mondanlou & Ortiz, 1981; Zipursky & Jaber, 1978)
- Small for gestation age
- Necrotizing enterocolitis—90 percent (Hutter, Hathaway, & Wayne, 1976)
- Hyperbilirubinemia and phototherapy
- Meconium aspiration
- Cold injury
- Polycythemia
- Pulmonary hypertension

Treatment of thrombocytopenia due to neonatal factors consists initially of amelioration of the underlying problem, followed by symptomatic treatment using platelet transfusion. Transfusion therapy should be considered if platelet counts are in the range of 40,000 to 100,000/mm³ and active bleeding is present. Platelet transfusion should be considered at levels of less than 40,000/mm³ even if active bleeding is not present. In estimating the rise in platelets after transfusion, the following formula is a helpful calculation: 1/10 of the volume (in milliliters) of a unit of platelets per kilogram of weight raises the platelet count by 50,000/mm³.

Disseminated Intravascular Coagulation

Disseminated intravascular coagulation is marked by a generalized deficiency in coagulation factors and platelets that leaves the infant predisposed to hemorrhage. Because this condition is triggered by a pre-existing illness and does not occur independently, treatment consists of identification and resolution of the underlying problem. The most common factors associated with bleeding that occurs secondary to disseminated intravascular coagulation are obstetrical complications, respiratory distress syndrome, hypoxia, hypotension, and sepsis. Occasionally, thrombosis of large vessels can trap platelets and consume an amount of clotting factors sufficient to cause this disorder. Mortality rates reach 60 to 80 percent in infants with disseminated intravascular coagulation who experience severe bleeding (Oski & Naiman, 1982a, 1982c, 1982d).

The hematologic picture reflects a depletion of platelets, prothrombin, fibrinogen, and factors V, VIII, and XIII. The prothrombin time and partial thromboplastin time are prolonged and are not corrected with the addition of fresh-frozen plasma to the blood sample. The fibrinolytic system is also stimulated and is evident by the presence of degradation products of fibrinolysis (i.e., fibrin degradation products or fibrinolytic split products).

Successful treatment of disseminated intravascular coagulation depends on alleviation of the underlying cause. Palliative treatment consists of replacement of deficient clotting factors and platelets and exchange transfusion. Heparin is infrequently used and only with the occurrence of large vessel thrombosis. It is administered as a constant infusion of 0.5 to 2 units/ml of intravenous fluid, or a bolus of 50 units/kg followed by 15 to 25 units/kg/hr (Young & Magnum, 1990).

DIFFERENTIAL DIAGNOSIS OF NEWBORN COAGULOPATHIES

Analysis of multiple factors can often help in identifying a specific coagulopathy affecting an infant. Careful evaluation of these factors can pinpoint the correct diagnosis and influence the choice of therapy or intervention to be used. Some factors that aid in the differential diagnosis are listed below:

- Familial history of a bleeding disorder such as hemophilia
- Maternal history of a bleeding disorder, as in idiopathic thrombocytopenic purpura
- Obstetrical history suggesting a possible abnormality, as in maternal isoimmunization or hypofibrinogenemia
- Adverse neonatal history, such as the presence of hypoxia or asphyxia
- Failure to administer prophylactic vitamin K at birth
- Physical manifestations of a bleeding disorder. Note obvious bleeding, sites where bleeding occurs, presence or absence of petechiae or ecchymosis, and the overall condition of the infant
- Laboratory data that identify specific abnormalities, such as specific coagulation factor deficiencies, thrombocytopenia, and prolonged prothrombin, partial thromboplastin, and clotting times.

COLLABORATIVE MANAGEMENT OF A COAGULOPATHY

Prevention of injury to fragile tissue and limitation of blood drawing from sites other than central catheters are of great importance in the infant who lacks adequate clotting factors to control bleeding. Appropriate administration of platelets, clotting factors, or blood products requires the correct equipment, the correct method of administration, and conscientious monitoring of vital signs to ensure effective therapy without causing further harm to the infant. Wise decisions regarding replacement blood products are quite important in light of the severe and potentially lethal sequelae of acquired infection. Monitoring laboratory tests to determine ongoing needs and the efficacy of therapy continues to be an important need throughout the infant's entire course of therapy.

Blood and Blood Component Therapy
Commonly Used Blood Products

Whole Blood. This product is not used for routine volume expansion because of the hematocrit dilution that occurs. It is used in surgical procedures requiring large volumes of blood for replacement, for exchange transfusions, and for priming heart–lung oxygenators for extracorporeal membrane oxygenation.

Packed Red Blood Cells (PRBCs). Blood is "hard spun" to concentrate cells and allow the supernatant to be removed. As the result of this form of preparation, less volume can be administered. PRBCs can be reconstituted with normal saline, 5 percent albumin, or fresh-frozen plasma. PRBCs can be used in exchange transfusions or in the treatment of anemia in the acutely ill or symptomatic convalescent infant.

Washed Red Blood Cells (WRBCs). For additional protection, RBCs can be washed to remove as much of the plasma, nonviable RBCs, WBCs, and metabolic wastes as possible. To further eliminate the possibility of a graft-versus-host reaction, cells can be irradiated with 5000 rad of radiation. This prevents T-lymphocyte proliferation and, when done in conjunction with washing, can remove up to 95 percent of T lymphocytes.

Frozen Deglycerolized Red Cells. Frozen storage of glycerolized RBCs allows for preservation of rare units of blood, but the cost of preparation increases considerably. In addition, this product tends to have a higher potassium content and hemoglobin concentration. Centrifuging it, removing the supernatant, and diluting it to the desired hematocrit tend to control these problems.

Fresh-Frozen Plasma. A whole unit of fresh-frozen plasma can be thawed but, once entered, is only good for 6 hours. If, however, it is packaged in aliquots such as a quad pack before freezing and then thawed, the quad pack unit is good for 24 hours once it is thawed. Fresh-frozen plasma provides a rich source of coagulation factors, containing 1 IU/ml of all clotting factors; 10 to 15 ml/kg raises the overall level of clotting factor activity by 20 to 30 percent. Fresh-frozen plasma can often normalize a prolonged prothrombin time and partial thromboplastin time in the newborn having a generalized deficiency in quantity and activity of available clotting factors.

Platelets. The number of platelets available for circulation after transfusion depends on the storage time. In transfusions using platelet bags less than 7 days of age, the rise in platelet levels is comparable with the use of fresh platelets. Use of packs older than 7 days achieves only 70 percent of the rise seen with the use of fresh platelets. Platelets can also be concentrated by centrifuge if smaller volumes are required. One caveat to remember is that platelets cannot be filtered when given.

Granulocytes. Granulocytes, used for infusion in septic infants with severe neutropenia, are prepared from fresh donor blood through the process of plasmapheresis. WBCs are removed from the unit of blood, but a large number of RBCs remain. For this reason, the donor unit needs to be typed and crossmatched to the infant for type and Rh compatibility. WBCs are usually irradiated to eliminate donor T cells to prevent graft-versus-host responses.

Cryoprecipitate. This form of plasma preparation is rich in factors VIII, XIII, and fibrinogen and is very useful in the treatment of hemophilia. Because it is a single donor collection, the risk of infection is lower than in pooled substances.

Factor Concentrates. Factor concentrates are used as specific therapy for identified factor deficiencies. They are obtained from pooled plasma and expose the recipient to multiple donors, thereby increasing the potential for infection, especially with hepatitis B, cytomegalovirus infection, and acquired immunodeficiency syndrome. Eighty percent of hepatitis B can be identified by the third-generation screening tests, and blood screening for cytomegalovirus is also available. Because the risk of transmission of human lymphotropic virus-III is increased by pooled concentrates, it is now recommended that concentrates be treated with heat, solvent, steam, detergent, or ultraviolet light to kill any potential virus. It is unclear if such treatment alters or inactivates the clotting activity of factor concentrates.

REFERENCES

Aballi, A., & DeLamerens, S. (1962). Coagulation changes in neonatal period and early infancy. *Pediatric Clinics of North America, 9,* 785–817.

Aballi, A., Puapondh, A., & Desposito, F. (1968). Platelet counts in thriving premature infants. *Pediatrics, 42,* 685–689.

Aranda, J., & Sweet, A. (1977). Alterations in blood pressure during exchange transfusion. *Archives of Disease in Childhood, 52,* 545–548.

Baehner, R., & Strauss, H. (1966). Hemophilia in the first year of life. *New England Journal of Medicine, 275,* 524–528.

Barnard, D. R., Chapman, R. G., Simmons, M. A., & Hathaway, W. E. (1980). Blood for use in exchange transfusion in the newborn. *Transfusion, 20,* 401–408.

Baumgart, S., & Kim, H. (1988). Blood component therapy in the neonate. In J. Stockman & C. Pochedly (Eds.), *Developmental and neonatal hematology* (pp. 199–222). New York: Raven Press.

Blanchette, V., & Zipursky, A. (1984). Assessment of anemia in newborn infants [Review]. *Clinics in Perinatology, 11,* 489–510.

Bowman, J. (1978). The management of Rh-isoimmunization. *Obstetrics and Gynecology, 52,* 1–16.

Bowman, J. (1988). Alloimmune hemolytic disease of the neonate. In J. Stockman & C. Pochedly (Eds.), *Developmental and neonatal hematology* (pp. 223–248). New York: Raven Press.

Bowman, J., & Pollock, J. (1965). Amniotic fluid spectrophotometry and early delivery in the management of erythroblastosis fetalis. *Pediatrics, 35,* 815–835.

Brown, M. (1988). Fetal and neonatal erythropoiesis. In J. Stockman & C. Pochedly (Eds.), *Developmental and neonatal hematology* (pp. 39–56). New York: Raven Press.

Brown, M., Berman, E., & Luckey, D. (1990). Prediction of the need for transfusion during anemia of prematurity. *Journal of Pediatrics, 116,* 773–778.

Cashore, W., & Usher, R. (1973). Hypovolemia resulting from a tight nuchal cord at birth. *Pediatric Research, 7,* 399.

Christensen, R., & Rothstein, G. (1979). Pitfalls in the interpretation of leukocyte counts of newborn infants. *American Journal of Clinical Pathology, 72,* 608–611.

Cohen, F., Zuelzer, W., Gustafson, D., & Evans, M. (1964). Mechanics of isoimmunization: I. The transplacental passage of fetal erythrocytes in homospecific pregnancies. *Blood, 23,* 621–646.

Dear, P. (1984). Blood transfusion in the preterm infant. *Archives of Disease in Childhood, 59,* 296–298.

DeMaio, J., Harris, M., & Spitzer, A. (1986). The response of apnea of prematurity to transfusion therapy. *Pediatric Research, 20,* 389A.

Edgar, W. M., & Hamblin, M. H. (1977). Rubella vaccination and anti-D immunoglobulin administration in the puerperium. *British Journal of Obstetrics and Gynaecology, 84,* 754–757.

Glader, B. E., & Naiman, J. L. (1991). Erythrocyte disorders in infancy. In H. W. Taeusch, R. A. Ballard, & M. E. Avery (Eds.), *Schaffer and Avery's diseases of the newborn* (6th ed., pp. 798–827). Philadelphia: W. B. Saunders.

Goetzman, B. W., & Wennberg, R. P. (1991). Neonatal intensive care handbook (2nd ed.). St. Louis: Mosby–Year Book.

Gold, W., Queenan, J., Woody, J., & Sacher, R. (1983). Oral desensitization in Rh disease. *American Journal of Obstetrics and Gynecology, 146,* 980–981.

Govoni, L. E., & Hayes, J. E. (1988). *Drugs and nursing implications* (5th ed.). Norwalk, CT: Appleton & Lange.

Graham-Pole, J., Barr, W., & Willoughby, M. (1977). Continuous-flow plasmapheresis in management of severe rhesus disease. *British Medical Journal, 1,* 1185–1188.

Guyton, A. (1996a). Blood groups: Transfusions, tissue and organ transplantation. In A. Guyton. *Textbook of medical physiology* (9th ed., pp. 457–462). Philadelphia: W. B. Saunders.

Guyton, A. (1996b). Hemostasis and blood coagulation. In A. Guyton. *Textbook of medical physiology* (9th ed., pp. 463–472). Philadelphia: W. B. Saunders.

Halperin, D. S., Wacher, P., Lacourt, G., et al. (1989). Response of premature anemic infants to subcutaneous recombinant erythropoietin [Abstract]. *Molecular Biotherapy, 1,* 64.

Halvorsen, S., & Finne, P. (1968). Erythropoietin production in the human fetus and newborn. *Annals of the New York Academy of Sciences, 149,* 576–577.

Hathaway, W., & Bonnar, J. (1978). Coagulation and hemostasis: General considerations. In W. Hathaway & J. Bonnar (Eds.), *Perinatal coagulation* (pp. 1–26). New York: Grune & Stratton.

Hutter, J. J. Jr., Hathaway, W. E., & Wayne, E. R. (1976). Hematologic abnormalities in severe neonatal necrotizing enterocolitis. *Journal of Pediatrics, 88,* 1026–1031.

Jones, W. R. (1969). The application of the Kleihauer technique to fetal blood. *Australia and New Zealand Journal of Obstetrics and Gynaecology, 9,* 33–36.

Joshi, A., Gerhardt, T., Shandloff, P., & Bancalari, E. (1987). Blood transfusion effects on the respiratory pattern of preterm infants. *Pediatrics, 80,* 79–84.

Keenan, W. J., Jewett, T., & Glueck, H. I. (1971). Role of feeding and vitamin K in hypoprothrombinemia of the newborn. *American Journal of Diseases of Children, 121,* 271–277.

Lackner, T. (1982). Drug replacement following exchange transfusion. *Journal of Pediatrics, 100,* 811–814.

Lemberge, R., & Legge, J. (1949). *Hematin compounds and bile pigments.* New York: Intersciences Publishers.

Maisels, M. (1990). Hyperbilirubinemia. In N. M. Nelson (Ed.), *Current therapy in neonatal-perinatal medicine, No. 2* (pp. 258–262). Philadelphia: B. C. Decker.

McEvoy, G. K. (Ed.). (1990). *American Hospital Formulary Service (AHFS) drug information.* Bethesda, MD: American Society of Hospital Pharmacists.

Mehta, P., Vasa, R., Neumann, L., & Karpatkin, M. (1980). Thrombocytopenia in the high-risk infant. *Journal of Pediatrics, 97,* 791–794.

Mollison, P. (1984). *Blood transfusion in clinical medicine* (7th ed., p. 675). Oxford: Blackwell Scientific.

Mondanlou, H. D., & Ortiz, O. B. (1981). Thrombocytopenia in neonatal infection. *Clinical Pediatrics, 20,* 402–407.

Obladen, M., Sachsenweger, M., & Stahnke, M. (1988). Blood sampling in very low birth weight infants receiving different levels of intensive care. *European Journal of Pediatrics, 147,* 399–404.

Oski, F., & Naiman, J. (1982a). Anemia in the neonatal period. In F. Oski & J. Naiman (Eds.), *Hematologic problems in the newborn. Vol IV. Major problems in clinical pediatrics* (3rd ed., pp. 56–86). Philadelphia: W. B. Saunders.

Oski, F., & Naiman J. (1982b). Erythroblastosis fetalis. In F. Oski & J. Naiman (Eds.), *Hematologic problems in the newborn. Vol IV. Major problems in clinical pediatrics* (3rd ed., pp. 283–346). Philadelphia: W. B. Saunders.

Oski, F., & Naiman, J. (1982c). Normal blood values in the newborn period. In F. Oski & J. Naiman. *Hematologic problems in the newborn. Vol IV. Major problems in clinical pediatrics* (3rd ed., pp. 1–31). Philadelphia: W. B. Saunders.

Oski, F., & Naiman., J. (1982d). Polycythemia and hyperviscosity in the neonatal period. In F. Oski & J. Naiman. *Hematologic problems in the newborn. Vol*

IV. Major problems in clinical pediatrics (3rd ed., pp. 87–96). Philadelphia: W. B. Saunders.

Phibbs, R. (1970). Response of newborn infants to leukocyte depletion during exchange transfusion. *Biology of the Neonate, 15,* 112–122.

Plunket, D. (1987). Bleeding syndromes of the newborn. In D. Kaprisin & N. Luban (Eds.), *Pediatric transfusion medicine* (Vol. I, pp. 53–68). Boca Raton, FL: CRC Press.

Rhondeau, S. M., Christensen, R. D., Ross, M. P., et al. (1988). Responsiveness to recombinant human erythropoietin of marrow erythroid progenitors from infants with the "anemia of prematurity." *Journal of Pediatrics, 112,* 935–940.

Ross, M. P., Christensen, R. D., Rothstein, G., et al. (1989). A randomized trial to develop criteria for administering erythrocyte transfusions to anemic preterm infants 1 to 3 months of age. *Journal of Perinatology, 9,* 246–253.

Sacher, R., & Queenan, J. (1987). Hemolytic disease of the newborn: Antenatal and prophylactic management. In D. Kaprisin & N. Luban (Eds). *Pediatric transfusion medicine* (Vol. 1, pp. 23–42). Boca Raton: CRC Press.

Scanlon, J. W., & Krakaur, R. (1980). Hyperkalemia following exchange transfusion. *Journal of Pediatrics, 96,* 108–110.

Sell, E. J., & Corrigan, J. J., Jr. (1973). Platelet counts, fibrinogen concentrations and factor V and factor VIII levels in healthy infants according to gestational age. *Journal of Pediatrics, 82,* 1028–1032.

Shannon, K. M., Naylor, G. S., Torkildson, J. C., et al. (1987). Circulating erythroid progenitors in the anemia of prematurity. *New England Journal of Medicine, 317,* 728–733.

Stockman, J. (1988). Physiology of the neonate as it relates to transfusion therapy. In D. Kaprisin & N. Luban (Eds.), *Pediatric transfusion medicine* (pp. 1–22). Boca Raton: CRC Press.

Suarez, C. R., & Anderson, C. (1986). High-dose intravenous gamma globulin in neonatal immune thrombocytopenia. *Pediatric Research, 20,* 393A.

Tan, K. L., Tan, R., Tan, S. H., & Tan, A. M. (1979). The twin transfusion syndrome: Clinical observations on 35 affected pairs. *Clinical Pediatrics, 18,* 111–114.

Tuchmann-Duplessis, H., David, G., & Haegel, P. (1975). Circulatory system. In H. Tuchmann, G. David, & P. Haegel (Eds.), *Illustrated human embryology: Vol 2. Organogenesis* (pp. 104–137). New York: Springer-Verlag.

Usher, R. H., Saigal, S., O'Neil, A., et al. (1975). Estimation of red blood cell volume in premature infants with and without respiratory distress syndrome. *Biology of the Neonate, 26,* 241–248.

Valaes, T. (1963). Bilirubin distribution and dynamics of bilirubin removal by exchange transfusion. *Acta Paediatrica Scandinavica, 52*(Suppl), 604–605.

Woodrow, J. (1970). Rh immunization and its prevention. In K. Jensen & S. Killman (Eds.), *Series Haemologica* (Vol. 3, pp. 29–46). Baltimore: Williams & Wilkins.

Young, T., & Magnum, B. (1995). *Neofax* (3rd ed.). Columbus: Ross Laboratories.

Zaizov, R., & Matoth, Y. (1976). Red cell values on the first postnatal day during the last 16 weeks of gestational age. *American Journal of Hematology, 1,* 276–278.

Zipursky, A., & Jaber, H. M. (1978). The haematology of bacterial infection in newborn infants. *Clinics in Haematology, 7,* 173–193.

CHAPTER 17

Assessment and Management of Neurologic Dysfunction

ANENCEPHALY

Anencephaly is caused by failure of the anterior neural tube to fuse in the cranial area.

INCIDENCE

The incidence of anencephaly has been declining with the advent of perinatal diagnosis and folic acid therapy. The overall frequency is 1 per 1000 live births (Paidas & Cohen, 1994).

PHYSIOLOGY

Genetic and environmental factors seem to be involved in the development of this defect. Many infants have other anomalies, the most consistent being adrenal hypoplasia secondary to pituitary dysfunction. Three fourths of these infants are stillborn; the remainder die during the neonatal period, with less than 20 percent still alive at 1 week (Volpe, 1995).

COLLABORATIVE MANAGEMENT

Management of infants with anencephaly is supportive, with provision of warmth and comfort until the infant dies. Families require emotional support and assistance in coping with their grief over the birth of an infant with a defect and the death of their infant. Anencephalic infants have been considered candidates for organ donation and kept alive for this purpose.

ENCEPHALOCELE

INCIDENCE

Encephalocele has an incidence of 1 in 2000 births (Bellig, 1989).

PHYSIOLOGY

Encephaloceles, including craniomeningomyelocele, encephalomyelocele, and other forms of cranium bifidum, arise from failure of closure of a portion of the neural tube in the anterior region. Although this defect can occur in any region, approximately three fourths occur in the occipital region. The sac protrudes from the back of the head or base of the neck. The next most common area is the frontal region, with involvement of the orbit, nose, and/or nasopharynx (Volpe, 1995; Volpe & Hill, 1987).

The protruding sac varies considerably in size. The size of the external sac does not correlate with the presence of neural elements. In general, prognosis for these infants is poor if the sac contains significant brain tissue. Mortality rate and later outcome are significantly better for infants with anterior rather than posterior defects (Brown & Sheridan-Pereira, 1992).

COLLABORATIVE MANAGEMENT

Collaborative management includes prevention of infection and trauma and positioning to avoid pressure on the defect. Promotion of normothermia is essential, especially in infants with cerebrospinal fluid (CSF) leakage, because these infants are at risk for thermoregulatory problems owing to evaporative losses.

Postoperative management includes the following:

- Assessment of ventilation and perfusion
- Comfort measures
- Monitoring of neurologic and motor function
- Promotion of normothermia
- Prevention of infection
- Positioning to prevent pressure on the operative site
- Monitoring of the site for CSF leakage

Families of infants with an encephalocele need initial and ongoing support and counseling. Initial parental care involves assisting parents with the shock of the defect and its appearance, their grief over having an infant with an anomaly, and dealing with the outcome implications of this defect. Nursing care also involves enhancing parent–infant interaction and involving the parents in the infant's care when they are ready. Education of the parents before discharge includes skin care, positioning, exercises, handling and feeding techniques, and provision of activities to promote growth and development.

SPINA BIFIDA

Spina bifida is a general term used to describe defects in closure of the neural tube associated with malformations of the spinal cord and vertebrae. Defects range from minor malformations with minimal clinical significance to major disorders that result in paraplegia or quadriplegia and loss of bladder and bowel control. The degree of sensory and motor neurologic deficit depends on the level and severity of the defect.

INCIDENCE

Spina bifida occulta occurs in 10 to 30 percent of the population.

PHYSIOLOGY

A vertebral defect at L5 or S1, or both, arises from failure of the vertebral arch to grow and fuse between 5 weeks of gestation and the early fetal period (Moore & Persaud, 1993). *Spina bifida occulta* is a defect in formation of the caudal portion of the spinal cord (secondary neurulation).

Spina bifida cystica is a generic term for neural tube defects characterized by a cystic sac containing meninges or spinal cord elements, or both, along with vertebral defects. The sac is covered by epithelium or a thin membrane. This defect occurs in approximately 1 in 1000 live births, with a decrease in incidence noted in recent years, similar to that for anencephaly. The three main forms of spina bifida cystica are meningocele, myelomeningocele, and myeloschisis (Fig. 17–1). Spina bifida cystica can occur anywhere along the spinal column but most often occurs in the lumbar or lumbosacral area.

A *meningocele* involves a sac that contains meninges and CSF, but the spinal cord and nerve roots are in their normal position. These infants usually have minimal residual neurologic deficit if the defect is covered with skin and if appropriate management is instituted early. A meningocele arises at 6 to 8 weeks' gestation (O'Rahilly & Muller, 1994).

Myelomeningocele is the most common form of spina bifida cystica. The sac contains spinal cord or nerve roots, or both, in addition to meninges and CSF. Infants with myelomeningocele have a neurologic deficit below the

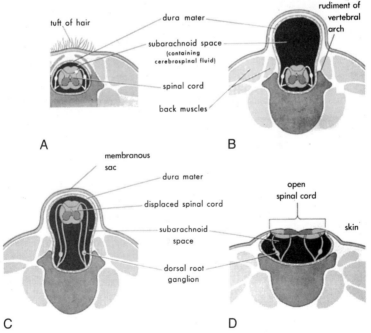

FIGURE 17–1. Different types of spina bifida. *A,* Spina bifida occulta. *B,* Spina bifida cystica: meningocele. *C,* Spina bifida cystica: myelomeningocele. *D,* Spina bifida cystica: myeloschisis. (From Moore, K. L. & Persaud, T. V. N. [1993]. *Before we are born: Essentials of embryology and birth defects* [4th ed., p. 284]. Philadelphia: W. B. Saunders. Reprinted with permission.)

level of the sac. Approximately 80 percent of these malformations occur in the lumbar area, which is the final area of neural tube fusion.

Myeloschisis is a severe defect in which there is no cystic covering, so the spinal cord is open and exposed. Myeloschisis is thought to arise from a local overgrowth of the neural plate, which prevents neural tube closure. The spinal cord in the affected infants is a flattened mass of neural tissue. These infants have significant neurologic deficits and are at great risk for infection. This defect can involve the entire length of the spinal cord and can occur in association with anencephaly (Moore & Persaud, 1993). Most infants with this defect are stillborn.

Another spinal cord defect is a *spinal dermal sinus.* A dermal sinus is a tract of squamous epithelium that connects to the dura mater. This defect is found in the midline and corresponds to the location of the caudal or rostral neuropores. The more common defect occurs in the lumbosacral area and may be associated with a sacral dimple. Dermal sinus is occasionally recognized at birth but is more often diagnosed later, following repeated episodes of meningitis (Milhorat & Miller, 1994).

CLINICAL SIGNS ASSOCIATED WITH NEUROLOGIC DYSFUNCTION

Clinical manifestations of neurologic dysfunction can be specific or nonspecific or subtle. However, five types of clinical signs are commonly seen in infants with neurologic problems:

- Central nervous system (CNS) depression
- Hyperirritability
- Increased intracranial pressure (ICP)
- Seizure activity
- Movement alterations

DIAGNOSTIC TECHNIQUES

Diagnostic techniques include neurophysiologic studies, radiographic assessment, structural brain imaging, measurement of cerebral blood flow, and measurement of ICP. Laboratory tests are performed to assist in the diagnosis of specific neurologic disorders and to identify underlying causes. CSF is examined for signs of hemorrhage (increased red blood cells, increased protein, decreased glucose, and xanthochromia) and to rule out infection (Table 17–1). Xanthochromia is often a late sign and may reflect increased protein rather than blood (Clancy, 1983). If ICP is increased, this may be reflected by the pressure of the CSF on needle insertion. Other laboratory evaluations include hematocrit; serum glucose, electrolyte, and blood gas values, and acid–base status. A sepsis work-up or screen for TORCH syndrome should be done if intrauterine infection or neonatal sepsis and meningitis is suggested. A genetic work-up and other metabolic studies should be done if there is a suggestion of inborn errors of metabolism or other inherited disorders.

Transillumination of the head has been used less frequently with the

TABLE 17–1. Evaluation of Cerebrospinal Fluid

CSF Finding	Appearance
Normal	Clear and colorless
Xanthochromia	Yellowish discoloration that may be due to ICH (discoloration by RBC pigments seen as early as 12 hr after hemorrhage), hyperbilirubinemia, with CSF protein content >150 mg/dl, or a normal variation
Turbidity or cloudiness	Presence of cell counts >400/mm³
Pink or bloody	RBC count >6000 mm³

CSF Finding	RBC Count
Normal	30 mm³ (range up to 100 mm³) with a nontraumatic tap
Abnormal	>100 mm³, associated with increased protein (protein increased 1 mg/dl per every 1000 RBC)

Normal CSF Findings in Noninfected High-Risk Infants	Term	Preterm
WBC count (cells/mm³)		
Range	0–32	0–29
Mean	8.2	9.0
Protein (mg/dl)		
Range	20–170	65–150
Mean	90	115
Glucose (mg/dl)		
Range	34–119	24–63
Mean	52	50
Ratio of CSF to blood glucose		
Range	44–248	55–105
Mean	81	74

CSF, cerebrospinal fluid; ICH, intracranial hemorrhage; RBC, red blood cell; WBC, white blood cell.
Modified from Sarff, L. D., Platt, L. H., & McCracken, G. H. (1976). Cerebrospinal fluid evaluation in neonates: Comparison of high risk infants with and without meningitis. *Journal of Pediatrics, 88,* 473. In Clancy, R. R. (1983). Neonatal seizures. In R. A. Polin & F. Berg (Eds.), *Workbook in practical neonatology* (pp. 125–152). Philadelphia: W. B. Saunders. Reprinted with permission.

advent of ultrasonography and computed tomography. Abnormal diffusion of light with a ring of illumination around the light source, translucence of the entire skull, or a ring of light around the source in a localized area occurs when there is (1) an abnormal collection of fluid in the ventricles, subdural space, or scalp (intracranial hemorrhage, hydrocephalus, cephalhematoma, scalp edema) or (2) cerebral atrophy or cysts (hydranencephaly, ventricular enlargement with cortical mantles < 1 cm thick, porencephaly). Small anomalies may result in negative findings on transillumination (Amiel-Tison & Larroche, 1988; Brann & Schwartz, 1987). If a flashlight is used, the ring of light should be less than 1 cm (< 1.5 cm in frontal area of preterm). Gestational age norms are available for use with findings from Chun-gun transillumination (Vyhmeister, Schneider, & Cha, 1977).

TYPES OF NEUROLOGIC DYSFUNCTION

Seizures

Seizures are the most frequent neurologic sign seen during the neonatal period. Seizures are not a disease but a sign of underlying disease processes that have resulted in an acute disturbance within the brain (Volpe, 1995). If left untreated, these disorders can lead to permanent damage of the CNS or other tissues. Disease processes associated with seizures in the neonate include primary CNS disorders, asphyxia, systemic diseases, and metabolic insults.

INCIDENCE

The reported incidence of neonatal seizures ranges from 0.15 percent in term infants to up to 22.7 percent in preterm infants (Bernes & Kaplan, 1994).

PHYSIOLOGY

Seizure activity may be an acute, recurrent, or chronic phenomenon. Neonatal seizures are usually acute and disappear within the first few weeks after birth. Recurrent or continuous seizures increase the risk of neurologic damage from the seizure activity itself (Bernes & Kaplan, 1994).

RISK FACTORS

Seizures are a clinical manifestation associated with a variety of underlying pathologic processes. The two events that most often place the neonate at risk for seizures are perinatal asphyxia and metabolic disturbances such as hypoglycemia and hypocalcemia. Other problems increasing the risk for seizures in the neonate include the following:

- Intracranial hemorrhage
- Infection (meningitis, congenital viral infections, viral encephalopathy)
- Congenital anomalies of the CNS
- Other metabolic disturbances (e.g., alkalosis, hypomagnesemia, hypernatremia, and hyponatremia

Less frequent causes of seizures are drug withdrawal from opiates or barbiturates, genetic disorders of amino and organic acid metabolism, kernicterus, hyperviscosity, and local anesthetic intoxication.

CLINICAL MANIFESTATIONS

Recognition of seizures in the neonatal period requires careful, ongoing assessment by the nurse of all infants at risk. Clinical manifestations of seizures in the neonate differ from those seen in older children and adults owing to immaturity of the CNS. As a result, seizure manifestations tend to be subtler. Clinical manifestations may include abnormal movements or alterations in tone of the trunk or extremities; abnormal facial, oral, tongue, or ocular movements; and respiratory problems (Clancy, 1983; Gale, 1981). Status epilepticus in the neonate is defined as seizures that recur frequently within a short time interval before the infant recovers consciousness or as a prolonged single seizure (Amiel-Tison, Korobkin, & Klaus, 1986).

TYPES OF SEIZURES

The types of seizures seen in the neonate are, in order of decreasing frequency, subtle, tonic, clonic (multifocal and focal), and myoclonic (Bernes & Kaplan, 1994; Volpe, 1995).

Subtle Seizures

Subtle seizures are the most common type of seizure seen in neonates, particularly among preterm infants. This type of seizure is often missed because the clinical manifestations are often difficult to recognize and distinguish from other events. The most common behaviors seen with subtle seizures are listed below (Bernes & Kaplan, 1994; Volpe, 1995):

- Tonic, horizontal deviations of the eyes with or without nystagmoid jerking
- Repetitive blinking or fluttering of the eyelids
- Drooling, sucking, and/or tongue thrusting
- Swimming or rowing movements of the arms with occasional bicycling movements of the legs

Apnea may occur but is usually due to the underlying cause of the seizure rather than to the seizure per se.

Tonic Seizures

The most common form of tonic seizures are generalized tonic seizures, which usually involve tonic extension of all of the extremities but are sometimes limited to one extremity or manifested by tonic flexion of all limbs. Generalized tonic seizures can be confused with decorticate or decerebrate posturing. Other signs may include eye deviations, apnea, and occasional clonic movements. This type of seizure is seen most frequently in preterm infants, especially those with intraventricular hemorrhage and hypoxic-ischemic insults. Generalized tonic seizures are often accompanied by apnea or decerebrate-type postures or both. Occasionally, focal tonic seizures may occur that are characterized by sustained asymmetrical posturing of the limbs, trunk, and/or neck. Focal tonic seizure activity may be difficult to differentiate from voluntary movement (Bernes & Kaplan, 1994; Goldbarg & Yeh, 1991).

Clonic Seizures

Clonic seizures may be multifocal or focal. Because multifocal clonic (migratory) seizures involve the cortex, they are more characteristic of term infants but may occasionally be seen in older preterm infants. This type of seizure involves rhythmic, jerky clonic movements of one or more limbs that migrate to other parts of the body in a random fashion. Multifocal clonic seizures can be confused with jitteriness. These seizures are associated with diffuse hyperexcitability of the cortex such as occurs with metabolic derangements (Bernes & Kaplan, 1994). Focal clonic seizures are also seen more frequently in term than in preterm infants. This relatively uncommon form of seizure is characterized by localized clonic jerking that is usually confined to one limb or the face. Focal clonic seizures may be associated with focal traumatic CNS injuries such as cerebral contusions and infarcts or may be a response to a severe metabolic disturbance or asphyxia. These seizures are often seen in combination with other seizure types (Bernes & Kaplan, 1994; Goldbarg & Yeh, 1991).

Myoclonic Seizures

Myoclonic seizures are uncommon in infants and rarely seen in preterm infants. These seizures are characterized by single or multiple sudden jerks with flexion of the upper (most frequent) or lower extremities and occasionally the trunk and neck. Myoclonic seizures are most often seen with inborn errors of metabolism or other metabolic problems.

COLLABORATIVE MANAGEMENT

Management of neonatal seizures has two goals: (1) to determine and treat the underlying cause of the seizures and (2) to protect the infant from injury during and after the seizure. Determining etiology involves assessment of the perinatal and neonatal history, physical examination, laboratory evaluation, and other diagnostic studies. Previous events that may indicate the underlying etiology include delivery history, bleeding, birth trauma, perinatal asphyxia, exposure to infectious agents and other teratogens, maternal substance abuse, and postbirth illnesses.

Physical examination includes evaluation of general health and neurologic status. Routine laboratory studies include electrolytes, glucose, calcium, magnesium, hematocrit, blood gases, pH, and blood urea nitrogen. A blood culture and lumbar puncture is also often done. The lumbar puncture helps to rule out both infection and CNS bleeding. Other laboratory and diagnostic studies may include computed tomography, ultrasonography, magnetic resonance imaging, skull radiography, TORCH screen, amino acid screen (for inborn errors of metabolism), or electroencephalography. An electroencephalogram (EEG) may or may not be useful in determining the cause of seizures, especially in preterm infants, but can be used to localize the origin or to validate subtle seizure manifestations (Bernes & Kaplan, 1994). The results of an interictal EEG can provide information on prognosis, more so in a term than in a preterm infant. The timing of seizure onset and type of seizure can also help in determining the etiology. An EEG for prognosis is often recommended 24 hours after seizure onset and again 5 days later (Amiel-Tison, Korobkin, & Klaus, 1986; Amiel-Tison & Larroche, 1988; Volpe, 1995).

Ongoing monitoring of blood gases, acid–base status, serum glucose level, and fluid and electrolyte status is important for any infant with seizures. Infants who are having seizures, regardless of their cause, need intravenous glucose because seizure activity depletes brain glucose and energy supplies (Wasterlain & Duffy, 1975). Alterations in oxygenation and acid–base status can occur as a complication of the apnea associated with a seizure or the physiologic consequences of seizure activity. Fluid and electrolyte management should be appropriate to the underlying cause of the seizures. For example, fluids are restricted initially in infants with cerebral edema and perinatal asphyxia.

Issues of when to treat with anticonvulsant drugs and for how long are controversial. Some clinicians favor early aggressive therapy, whereas others do not, because neonatal seizures often abate spontaneously. Recurrent or prolonged seizures require treatment with anticonvulsants to reduce the risk of brain injury. The most common anticonvulsant used in the neonate is phenobarbital. Other anticonvulsants used include phenytoin (Dilantin), diazepam, and lorazepam. Table 17–2 summarizes loading and maintenance doses for treatment of neonatal seizures. Blood levels of these drugs must be monitored carefully to ensure therapeutic levels and prevent toxicity. Cardiovascular status and respiratory function must also be monitored. Anticonvulsants may or may not be discontinued before discharge. Volpe (1995) indicates that anticonvulsants can be discontinued if the infant has a normal neurologic examination and EEG and there are no brain lesions seen on cranial imaging. If infants are discharged on anticonvulsant therapy they should be re-evaluated in about 1 month.

Nursing Management

Nursing management focuses on recognizing and documenting seizure activity and protecting and supporting the infant during and after the seizure. Observing and documenting seizure activity involves noting and recording the following: the time the seizure began and ended, body parts involved (e.g., extremities, eyes, head), description of motor movement, eye deviations, pupillary reactions, respiratory status, color, state and level of consciousness, and postictal status (Gale, 1981).

During the seizure, the nurse must ensure the following:

- Ensure maintenance of airway
- Monitor vital signs
- Assess for adequacy of respiration and heart rate to maintain ventilation and perfusion

To protect the infant from injury during the seizure, the nurse should not force anything into the infant's mouth or try to restrain the extremities and should try to turn the infant's head to the side if possible. After the seizure, the infant's condition should be monitored and supportive care should be provided to maintain ventilation, oxygenation, adequate fluids, glucose, and warmth. The infant should be assessed for signs related to the various events that can cause seizure activity to help determine the cause of the seizure and prevent further seizures.

Care also involves administering and monitoring anticonvulsants and interventions aimed at treating the underlying cause of the seizures. Because

TABLE 17–2. Treatment of Seizures with Anticonvulsant Drugs

Drug	Dose	Comments
Phenobarbital (drug of choice for neonatal seizures)	Loading: 10–20 mg/kg IV to maximum of 40 mg/kg Maintenance: 5–7 mg/kg in 2 divided doses beginning 12 hr after last loading dose	Therapeutic level: 20–25 μg/ml (obtain levels any time 1 hr after dose); respiratory depressant; incompatible with other drugs in solution
Phenytoin (added if seizures not controlled by phenobarbital alone)	Loading: 10–20 mg/kg IV (no more rapidly than 10–20 mg/min) Maintenance: 5–7 mg/kg in 1–2 doses/day beginning 12 hr after last loading dose	Therapeutic level: 15–20 μg/ml (obtain levels 1–10 hr after last loading or maintenance dose, incompatible with all other drugs, glucose, and pH <11.5; give slowly directly into vein; too-rapid administration causes dysrhythmias, bradycardia, hypotension, cardiovascular collapse, and/or respiratory distress
Diazepam	0.3 mg/kg IV (0.1–0.3 mg/kg/dose)	Sodium benzoate competes with bilirubin for albumin binding sites—potentiates jaundice, so kernicterus is possible at lower serum bilirubin levels
Pyridoxine	50–100 mg IV bolus	Pyridoxine (vitamin B_6) deficiency as etiology of neonatal seizures is rare; seizures will cease within 5 minutes after vitamin B_6 injection if deficient
Lorazepam (Ativan)	0.05 mg/kg/dose IV over 2–5 min	Use justified in severely ill newborns with seizures nonresponsive to other drugs
Primidone	Loading: 15–20 mg PO Maintenance: 12–20 mg/kg/day	Use justified for refractory seizures; close monitoring of phenobarbital levels is necessary, because levels rise after primidone loading and fall precipitously with phenobarbital discontinuance
Valproic acid	Initial dose: 15–30 mg/kg/day PO, PR Maintenance: 15–60 mg/kg/day PO q12h	Anticonvulsant for refractory neonatal seizures; complications include neutropenia, hepatic damage, and hyperammonemia

From Merenstein, G. B., & Gardner, S. L. (1993). *Handbook of neonatal intensive care* (3rd. ed.). St. Louis: C. V. Mosby. Reprinted with permission.

anticonvulsants can be respiratory or myocardial and CNS depressants or can compete with bilirubin for albumin binding, cardiorespiratory status, color, and neurologic status are monitored in addition to drug effectiveness. Parent teaching includes helping the family to understand the cause and significance of the seizure or seizures and any diagnostic tests that are planned. Discharge teaching of parents includes recognition of seizure manifestations, care of the infant during and after a seizure, and administration of anticonvulsants (dosage and side effects) if these drugs are to be continued after discharge.

Periventricular/Intraventricular Hemorrhage

Periventricular/intraventricular hemorrhage (P/IVH) is the most common type of intracranial hemorrhage seen in the neonatal period. P/IVH has been described as the most common and serious neurologic disorder of preterm infants. This type of hemorrhage occurs almost exclusively in preterm infants, particularly those born at less than 32 weeks' gestation, those weighing less than 1500 g, or both.

CLINICAL MANIFESTATIONS

More than 90 percent of infants with P/IVH bleed within the first 72 hours after birth, with 50 percent of hemorrhages occurring in the first 24 hours (Volpe, 1995). Ten to 20 percent of infants followed serially with cranial ultrasonography after a hemorrhage demonstrate progressive increases in the size of the hemorrhage over a 24- to 48-hour period (de Vries, Larroche, & Levene, 1988b). Late hemorrhages are seen after a few days or weeks in about 15 percent of infants. Late hemorrhages occur primarily in preterm infants with severe, prolonged respiratory problems. These infants may develop a new hemorrhage or extension of a previous one. Some infants may also develop a P/IVH before birth (Wigglesworth, 1989).

Signs and symptoms of P/IVH are often nonspecific and subtle. Clinical signs that correlate most closely with CT evidence of hemorrhage include the following (Volpe, 1995):

- A falling hematocrit or failure of the hematocrit to rise after a transfusion
- Full anterior fontanelle
- Changes in activity level
- Decreased tone

Other clinical signs that are associated with the presence of P/IVH include impaired visual tracking, increased tone of the lower limbs, neck flexor hypotonia, and brisk tendon reflexes (de Vries, Larroche, & Levene, 1988b).

P/IVH is classified into different types according to the location and severity of the hemorrhage.

Laboratory evidence suggestive of P/IVH, in addition to a falling hematocrit, includes CSF findings indicative of hemorrhage: increased red blood cell levels, increased protein, decreased glucose levels, and xanthochromia (often a later finding and due to increased protein). Extremely low CSF glucose levels, or hypoglycorrhachia, can be found several days to a week (usually 5 to 15 days) after the hemorrhage in some infants. The CSF glucose level remains depressed for up to 2 to 3 months. The basis for this finding is unclear, but it may be due to inhibition or alteration in glucose transport between the CNS and CSF (Volpe, 1995).

There are wide variations in the patterns of clinical manifestations seen in individual infants. Three clinical syndromes have been described: silent, catastrophic, and saltatory (Volpe, 1995). At one end of the continuum are the majority of infants. These infants have only silent, subependymal hemorrhages with no clinical signs. The hemorrhage is discovered during routine ultrasonographic screening.

Catastrophic deterioration usually involves major hemorrhages that evolve rapidly over several minutes or hours. Clinical findings include stupor progressing to coma, respiratory distress progressing to apnea, generalized tonic seizures, decerebrate posturing, fixation of pupils to light, and flaccid quadriparesis. This clinical presentation is associated with a falling hematocrit, bulging fontanelle, hypotension, bradycardia, alterations in temperature, hypoglycemia, and syndrome of inappropriate secretion of antidiuretic hormone. Infants with catastrophic hemorrhages have a high mortality and, if they survive, a poor prognosis for later development.

The saltatory pattern is associated with small hemorrhages that develop over hours to days. Signs and symptoms are usually subtle or silent and present irregularly. Clinical manifestations, if present, include alterations in level of consciousness or stupor, hypotonia, abnormal eye movements or positions, and altered mobility. An unexplained fall in hematocrit by 10 percent or more or failure of the hematocrit to rise after a transfusion, even in the absence of other symptoms, suggests the possibility of a hemorrhage. These infants generally survive. Later developmental outcome is variable, depending on the severity of the hemorrhage.

COLLABORATIVE MANAGEMENT

Screening can identify infants with silent hemorrhages or hemorrhages associated with nonspecific, subtle symptoms. By identifying these vulnerable infants, interventions can be instituted to prevent new hemorrhages or extensions of existing ones. Management of P/IVH involves prevention of hemorrhage in infants at risk, acute care of infants with current hemorrhages, pharmacologic therapies, and management of posthemorrhagic ventricular dilation (Volpe, 1995).

Prompt resuscitation at birth minimizes hypoxemia and hypercarbia, which can alter cerebral autoregulation. Hypertonic solutions and volume expanders are administered slowly, with careful monitoring of vital signs and color. This may be particularly important during delivery resuscitation and early stabilization efforts. Activities that can increase ICP or cause wide swings in arterial or venous pressure are avoided or minimized when possible, especially during the first 72 hours of life. Because seizures can alter cerebral blood flow and ICP, they must be recognized promptly and treated. Acute care of infants with hemorrhages focuses on monitoring and maintaining oxygenation and perfusion to prevent further damage or extension of the hemorrhage. Institution of guidelines to avoid factors associated with development of P/IVH were reported by Szymonowicz and colleagues (1986) to reduce the incidence of this disorder by nearly one half.

Pharmacologic therapies, including phenobarbital, indomethacin, and vitamin E, have been tried prophylactically to reduce the incidence of hemorrhage or prevent more severe hemorrhages, neurologic damage, or both (Cooke, 1989; Kaempf et al., 1990; Ment et al., 1994a, 1994b).

Management of Progressive Ventricular Dilation

Progressive posthemorrhagic ventricular dilation is a frequent complication in infants with P/IVH. Therefore, all infants with a history of P/IVH are followed with serial cranial ultrasonography. In most infants, ventricular dilation occurs slowly without increased ICP (normopressive hydrocephalus). Ventricular growth spontaneously arrests in approximately half of these infants within about 30 days. The remaining infants continue to demonstrate ventricular dilation and increased ICP (Volpe, 1995).

Initial management of infants with normopressive hydrocephalus involves observation because many will arrest spontaneously without treatment. Clinicians may use serial lumbar punctures to remove CSF and decrease ventricle size. Fifteen to 20 ml of CSF may be removed, with daily taps over a 1- to 3-week period. When the volume of CSF decreases to less than 5 ml for several days, the frequency of taps is gradually decreased and then discontinued (Amiel-Tison, Korobkin, & Klaus, 1986; Volpe, 1995). Drugs to decrease CSF production have also been used, with variable results. These agents include carbonic anhydrase inhibitors such as acetazolamide (Diamox) and furosemide or osmotic agents such as isosorbitol and glycerol. These agents require careful monitoring of serum potassium, acid–base status, renal function, and hydration (Amiel-Tison & Larroche, 1988).

Progressive ventricular dilation with increasing ICP is managed with a ventriculoperitoneal shunt or, if the infant is too ill or small for surgery, or both, with temporary ventricular drainage. Ventricular drainage can be accomplished by an external ventricular drain or a tunneled catheter attached to a subcutaneous reservoir (Volpe, 1995).

Nursing Management

Nursing management involves recognition of factors that increase the risk of P/IVH, interventions to reduce the risk of bleeding, and supportive care of infants with acute hemorrhages or posthemorrhagic ventricular dilation. Prevention and risk reduction activities include interventions to avoid or reduce hypoxic or asphyxial events, avoid rapid alterations in cerebral blood flow, prevent fluctuations in systemic blood pressure, prevent hyperosmolality, and prevent or minimize fluctuations in ICP. Specific nursing interventions to accomplish these goals are listed in Table 17–3.

These interventions are based on analysis of pathophysiologic events that are thought to be involved in the pathogenesis of P/IVH. There have been few investigations to examine the effectiveness of specific interventions. Als and associates (1994) found that infants managed with individualized developmental care had a significantly decreased incidence of P/IVH and fewer severe hemorrhages than infants managed with conventional care.

TABLE 17–3. Nursing Interventions to Reduce the Risks of Periventricular/ Intraventricular Hemorrhage*

Nursing Care	Rationale
1. Position with head in midline and head of bed slightly elevated.	ICP is lowest with head in midline and head of bed elevated 30 degrees Turning the head sharply to the side causes an obstruction of the ipsilateral jugular vein and can increase ICP.
2. Avoid tight, encircling phototherapy masks.	Pressure on the occiput can increase ICP by impeding venous drainage.
3. Avoid rapid fluid infusions for volume expansion. a. Know normal BP for infant's weight and age. b. Suggest dopamine therapy to maintain BP if infant is not hypovolemic.	Rapid increase in intravascular volume can cause rupture of capillaries in germinal matrix. Risk may be increased if a history of hypoxia and hypotension exists. Even modest, abrupt increases in BP may cause P/ IVH.
4. When NaHCO$_3$ therapy is necessary to correct a documented metabolic acidosis, slowly give dilute solution.	Role of NaHCO$_3$ unclear, but rapid infusions may cause elevations in CO$_2$, which could dilate cerebral vessels and contribute to a pressure-passive cerebral circulation.
5. Monitor BP diligently. Note fluctuating pattern in arterial pressure tracing in high-risk ventilated infants and inform physician.	Blood flow velocity in the anterior cerebral artery is reflected by the pattern of simultaneously recorded arterial BP. A fluctuating pattern is associated with the development of P/ IVH and can be stabilized by pancuronium bromide.
6. Monitor closely for signs of pneumothorax: a. Increased mean BP, especially increases in diastolic BP (early) b. Increased heart rate c. Changes in breath sounds, which may or may not be appreciated d. Decreased Pao$_2$ e. Increased Paco$_2$ f. Shift in cardiac point of maximum impulse g. Hypotension and bradycardia (late)	Pneumothorax frequently precedes P/ IVH. The sum of hemodynamic changes caused by pneumothorax is flow under increased pressure in the germinal matrix capillaries. Changes in vital signs can be early indicators of pneumothorax.
7. Maintain temperature within neutral thermal range.	Hypothermia has been associated with P/IVH.
8. Suction only as needed.	Even brief (20-sec) suctioning episodes can increase cerebral blood flow velocity, increase BP, increase ICP, and decrease oxygenation.

TABLE 17–3. Nursing Interventions to Reduce the Risks of Periventricular/ Intraventricular Hemorrhage* Continued

Nursing Care	Rationale

9. Avoid interventions that cause crying.
   a. Consider long-term methods of achieving venous access to avoid frequent venipunctures.
   b. Critically evaluate all manipulations and handling.
   c. Use analgesics for stressful procedures.
	Crying can impede venous return, increase cerebral blood volume, and compromise cerebral oxygenation in sick infants.

10. Maintain blood gas values within a normal range.
   a. Use continuous noninvasive monitoring of oxygenation.
   b. Adjust FiO_2, as needed, to maintain $TcPO_2$ or pulse oximeter values within desired range.
   c. Avoid interventions that cause hypoxia.
	Hypoxia and hypercapnia are associated with the development of P/IVH. These events increase cerebral blood flow and may impair the neonate's already limited ability to autoregulate the cerebral blood flow. Hypoxia can injure the germinal matrix capillary endothelium.

....

*Premature neonates are most vulnerable to P/IVH during the first 4 days of life, with approximately 50% of hemorrhages occurring in the first 24 hours. Attempts to minimize the risk of P/IVH should begin immediately after birth, even before the infant has reached the special care nursery.

ICP, intracranial pressure; BP, blood pressure; P/IVH, periventricular/intraventricular hemorrhage.

From Kling, P. (1989). Nursing interventions to decrease the risk of periventricular-intraventricular hemorrhage. *Journal of Obstetric, Gynecologic, and Neonatal Nursing, 18,* 457. Reprinted with permission.

Acute management of infants with P/IVH includes the following:

- Provision of physiologic support
- Maintenance of oxygenation
- Maintenance of perfusion
- Normothermia
- Normoglycemia
- Minimal physical manipulations and handling
- Reduced environmental stress
- Placement prone or side-lying
- Positioning of head in midline or to the side but without neck flexion
- Slight elevation of head of the bed
- Avoidance of Trendelenburg position
- Frequent monitoring of vital signs, blood pressure, tone, activity, and level of consciousness

Other Types of Intracranial Hemorrhage

PRIMARY SUBARACHNOID HEMORRHAGE

Primary subarachnoid hemorrhage (SAH) is the most prevalent form of intracranial hemorrhage in neonates and the least clinically significant for most infants. SAH occurs in both preterm and term infants but is more common in preterm infants. SAH may occur alone (primary SAH) or as a secondary event with other forms of intracranial hemorrhage. For example, with P/IVH, blood moves into the subarachnoid space through the fourth ventricle.

Clinical Manifestations

The clinical features of SAH are as follows:

- Preterm infants with a minor SAH are asymptomatic.
- Term or preterm infants may present at 2 to 3 days of age with isolated seizure activity or occasionally with apnea.
- Between seizures, the infant appears and acts healthy. Infants in both these groups survive and usually do well developmentally.
- Infants with a massive SAH have a rapid and fatal course. This is very rare and is often associated with both a severe asphyxial event and birth trauma.

Collaborative and Nursing Management

The management of an infant with SAH includes the following:

- Observation for seizures and other neurologic signs
- Supportive care
  - Maintenance of oxygenation and perfusion
  - Provision of warmth
  - Provision of fluids
  - Provision of nutrients

SUBDURAL HEMORRHAGE

Subdural hemorrhage (SDH) is more common in term infants than preterm infants.

Clinical Manifestations

Clinical signs relate to the site of bleeding and severity of the hemorrhage. Three patterns are seen in infants with bleeding over the cerebral hemispheres (Volpe, 1995; Volpe & Hill, 1987). The first pattern is seen in most infants with SDH; they have a minor hemorrhage and are asymptomatic or have features such as irritability and hyperalertness. The second group develops seizures during the first 2 to 3 days of life. These seizures are usually focal. Other neurologic signs may include hemiparesis, pupils that are unequal and respond sluggishly to light, a full or tense fontanelle, bradycardia, and irregular respirations. The third pattern is seen in a few infants who have no or nonspecific signs in the neonatal period but who develop them at 4 weeks to 6 months of age. These infants generally present with increasing head size owing to continued hematoma formation, poor feeding, failure to thrive, altered level of consciousness, and, occasionally, seizures from the chronic subdural effusion.

Infants with bleeding over the posterior fossa with tentorial lacerations usually present with abnormal neurologic signs from birth. Signs include the following:

- Stupor or coma
- Eye deviation
- Asymmetrical pupil size
- Altered pupillary response to light
- Tachypnea
- Bradycardia
- Opisthotonos

As the clot enlarges, these infants rapidly deteriorate, with signs of shock appearing over minutes to hours. The infant becomes comatose, with fixed, dilated pupils and altered respirations and heart rate culminating in respiratory arrest.

Infants with small tears of the posterior fossa may have no clinical manifestations for the first 3 to 4 days of life. During this time, the clot is gradually enlarging until signs of increased ICP appear. As the brain stem becomes compressed, the infant's condition deteriorates, with oculomotor abnormalities, altered respiration, bradycardia, and seizures (Volpe, 1995).

Collaborative and Nursing Management

The management of SDH is as follows:

- SDH can often be prevented or its severity reduced by reducing trauma during the perinatal period.
- Management of infants with bleeding over the cerebral hemispheres is supportive.
- If the history is suggestive, observation is done for seizures and other neurologic signs.
- Care is primarily supportive and includes the following:
  - Maintenance of oxygenation
  - Maintenance of perfusion
  - Provision of warmth
  - Provision of fluids
  - Provision of nutrients

Symptomatic infants with bleeding over the temporal convexity and increased ICP may be managed with subdural taps to relieve the pressure. SDH is first located by ultrasonography or computed tomography to determine if the hematoma is accessible. Massive posterior fossa hemorrhage requires craniotomy and surgical aspiration of the clot (Amiel-Tison, Korobkin, & Klaus, 1986; de Vries, Larroche, & Levene, 1988a). Infants at risk for SDH should be monitored carefully over the first 4 to 6 months after birth for late signs of bleeding and hematoma formation. Monitoring of these infants includes following head size, growth, feeding, activity, and level of consciousness and observing for seizures.

INTRACEREBELLAR HEMORRHAGE

Intracerebellar hemorrhage is rare and thought to be due to hypoxia. These hemorrhages occur in both term and preterm infants but are more common in preterm infants. Intracerebellar hemorrhage is seen at autopsy in infants with a history of perinatal asphyxia, severe respiratory distress syndrome, or both and P/IVH. Intracerebellar hemorrhage also occurs secondary to trauma, especially in infants with very low birth weight. Mechanical deformation of the occiput during forceps or breech delivery and compression of the compliant skull during fixation of the head for caregiving procedures or with use of constrictive head bands are thought to be predisposing factors (Pape, Armstrong, & Fitzhardinge, 1976).

Many infants are critically ill from birth, with rapidly progressive apnea, falling hematocrit, and death within 24 to 36 hours. Other infants are less ill initially and develop symptoms at 2 to 3 weeks of age.

Clinical manifestations include the following:

- Apnea
- Bradycardia
- Hoarse or high-pitched cry
- Eye deviations
- Opisthotonos
- Seizures
- Vomiting
- Hypotonia
- Decreased or absent Moro reflex

Hydrocephalus may develop as early as the end of the first week. The prognosis is poor.

HYPOXIC-ISCHEMIC ENCEPHALOPATHY

Hypoxic-ischemic encephalopathy (HIE) occurs with injury to the brain from a combination of systemic hypoxemia and decreased cerebral perfusion leading to ischemia (de Vries, Larroche, & Levene, 1988c). The hypoxemia and ischemia may occur simultaneously or sequentially. In the preterm infant of less than 32 to 34 weeks of gestational age, hypoxic–ischemic damage is usually associated with P/IVH.

Incidence

The incidence of severe forms of HIE has decreased markedly with advances in perinatal care. The incidence of perinatal asphyxia in term infants ranges from 2.9 to 9 in 1000 births, with moderate to severe postasphyxial encephalopathy seen in approximately 1 in 1000 births (Levene, 1988).

Clinical Manifestations

Most term infants with HIE demonstrate a characteristic pattern of neurologic findings over the first 72 hours of life. Neurologic findings are listed below:

- Seizures
- Altered level of consciousness
- Altered tone
- Altered activity

- Irregular respirations
- Apnea
- Poor or absent Moro reflex
- Abnormal cry and poor suck
- Altered pupillary responses and eye movements

Sarnat and Sarnat (1976) developed a clinical grading system for infants with HIE (Table 17–4) that can be useful in evaluating infants and following the progression of their symptoms. Seizures occur in 30 to 60 percent of these infants, with usual onset at 12 to 14 hours of age. The most common types of seizures are multifocal-clonic in term infants. Three clinical states (hyperalert, lethargy, and stupor or coma) have been described in these

TABLE 17–4. Clinical Grading System for Postasphyxial Encephalopathy in the Full-Term Newborn Infant

Neurologic Features	Stage 1	Stage 2	Stage 3
Level of consciousness	Hyperalert	Lethargic or obtunded	Stuporous
Neuromuscular control			
Muscle tone	Normal	Mild hypotonia	Flaccid
Posture	Mild distal flexion	Strong distal flexion	Intermittent decerebration
Stretch reflexes	Overactive	Overactive	Decreased or absent
Segmental myoclonus	Present	Present	Absent
Complex reflexes			
Suck	Weak	Weak or absent	Absent
Moro	Strong; low threshold	Weak, incomplete, high threshold	Absent
Oculovestibular	Normal	Overactive	Weak or absent
Tonic neck	Slight	Strong	Absent
Autonomic function	Generalized sympathetic	Generalized parasympathetic	Both systems depressed
Pupils	Mydriasis	Miosis	Variable, often unequal, poor light reflex
Heart rate	Tachycardia	Bradycardia	Variable
Bronchial and salivary secretions	Sparse	Profuse	Variable
Gastrointestinal motility	Normal or decreased	Increased; diarrhea	Variable
Seizures	None	Common: focal or multifocal	Uncommon (excluding decerebration)
Electroencephalographic findings	Normal (awake)	Early: low-voltage continuous delta and theta Later: periodic pattern (awake) Seizure: focal 1 to 1.5 Hz spike and wave	Early: periodic pattern with isopotential phases Later: totally isopotential
Duration	Less than 24 hr	2–14 days	Hours to weeks

From Sarnat, H. B., & Sarnat, M. S. (1976). Neonatal encephalopathy following fetal distress. *Archives of Neurology, 33,* 696. Copyright 1976, American Medical Association. Reprinted with permission.

infants and correlated to outcome (Finer et al., 1981; Sarnat & Sarnat, 1976). Development of stupor or coma at any time or lethargy for more than 7 days was associated with the poorest prognosis.

Collaborative Management

Acute management of infants with HIE focuses on delivery room resuscitation; stabilization and management of the primary problem, usually perinatal asphyxia; and related alterations in the cardiovascular, pulmonary, gastrointestinal, and renal systems. Seizures are treated promptly to prevent further alterations in ICP and cerebral blood flow.

Management focuses on the following:

- Eliminating the original hypoxia
- Alleviating tissue hypoxia
- Promoting adequate cerebral perfusion and brain oxygenation (Brann & Schwartz, 1987)
- Establishing ventilation
- Providing adequate perfusion
- Preventing or minimizing the following:
  - Hypotension
  - Hypoxia
  - Acidosis
  - Severe apneic and bradycardic episodes
- Avoiding hyperoxia. Hyperoxia can result in cerebral vasoconstriction and decreased perfusion.
- Managing fluids. This is critical not only in relation to the cerebral edema but also because of alterations in renal function and problems such as acute tubular necrosis.
- Avoiding institution of hypothermia to decrease metabolic rate, which is not recommended
- Monitoring and documenting neurologic status
- Monitoring serum and urinary electrolytes and osmolality, blood urea nitrogen, serum creatinine, glucose, and fluids and electrolytes

Blood glucose deviations should be treated promptly. Volpe and Hill (1987) recommend that blood glucose levels be maintained between 75 and 100 mg/dl.

Acute intracranial hypertension may be managed with osmotically active agents such as mannitol or furosemide, barbiturates, or corticosteroids, as well as fluid restriction. During the initial cytotoxic edema, management is directed toward decreasing localized increases in pressure with fluid restriction and decreasing energy requirements. Osmotically active agents such as mannitol (0.25 to 1.0 g/kg of a 10 to 20 percent solution intravenously every 6 hours) or furosemide (1.0 mg/kg intravenously) may be used in the first 24 hours to reduce cerebral edema. Barbiturates and corticosteroids are usually not particularly effective during this period.

During the period of vasogenic edema, management is directed toward reducing the elevated ICP by fluid restriction, osmotic and diuretic agents, and possible use of steroids and barbiturates (Brann & Schwartz, 1987). If used, dexamethasone is often started soon after birth, but it is not effective for 12 to 24 hours. This corticosteroid is given intramuscularly or intravenously, with a priming dose of 0.50 mg/kg, followed by 0.25 to 0.50 mg/kg/day for 5 to 7 days (Amiel-Tison & Larroche, 1988).

Barbiturates have also been proposed as a therapeutic measure to decrease cerebral metabolic rate, cerebral blood flow, and cerebral edema and to promote consumption of oxygen free radicals and modification of cell physiology. Barbiturates seem most effective when used before the hypoxic-ischemic event. Usefulness of these agents is debatable (Brann & Schwartz, 1987).

Nursing Management

Care activities include the following:

- Avoidance or reduction of hypoxic or asphyxial events
- Avoidance of rapid alterations in cerebral blood flow
- Prevention of fluctuations in systemic blood pressure
- Prevention of hyperosmolality or minimizing fluctuations in ICP

The interventions listed in Table 17–3 to alter ICP and promote oxygenation in infants at risk for P/IVH can also be used with infants with HIE.

Periventricular Leukomalacia

Periventricular leukomalacia (PVL) is a form of hypoxic-ischemic injury and the most common ischemic brain lesion seen in preterm infants. *Leukomalacia* means "softening of the white matter" (de Vries, Larroche, & Levene, 1988c). PVL is often associated with P/IVH but is a separate lesion that may also occur in the absence of P/IVH. PVL is a symmetrical, nonhemorrhagic lesion due to ischemia from alterations in arterial circulation. As the IVH moves from the germinal matrix area into the surrounding white matter, periventricular hemorrhagic infarction associated with intraparenchymal echodensities develops. Periventricular hemorrhagic infarction differs from PVL in that it is an asymmetrical, hemorrhagic lesion primarily arising from alterations in the venous circulation (Volpe, 1995).

COLLABORATIVE MANAGEMENT

Initial management focuses on treatment of the primary insult and its attendant complications and prevention of further hypoxic-ischemic damage. This management involves preventing or minimizing hypotension, hypoxia, acidosis, and severe apneic and bradycardic episodes. Ultrasonography or computed tomography is used serially on infants at risk to diagnose PVL and follow its progression. Specific evidence of PVL on ultrasonography or computed tomography may not be seen before cavitation, cerebral atrophy, and ventricular enlargement (Bennett, Silver, Leung, & Mack, 1990).

Early changes may be transient in some infants and resolve over a few weeks. In other infants, areas of increased density appear within 2 to 4 weeks, followed by development of cystic lesions. Magnetic resonance imaging can also be used to predict cystic changes (Bozynski et al., 1985; de Vries, Larroche, & Levene, 1988c). Later management involves care related to residual problems such as spastic diplegia and hydrocephalus.

Nursing Management

Interventions focus on acute management of the primary problem and supportive care for the infant and parents. Any signs of hypoxia and asphyxia are identified and interventions instituted to prevent further ischemic damage. Developmental and environmental interventions are an important aspect of nursing care.

Parents need initial and ongoing support in dealing with their infant's illness and risk of later neurologic problems. Parent teaching focuses on promoting an understanding of the infant's health status and care, as well as providing anticipatory guidance and follow-up care.

Birth Injuries

Traumatic injury to the central or peripheral nervous system can occur during the perinatal or postnatal periods. Most of these injuries happen during the intrapartum period and may co-occur with perinatal asphyxia.

INCIDENCE

Birth injury occurs in an incidence of 2 to 7 in 1000 live births, with the incidence of neural injury being 0.22 in 1000 live births (Tudehope & Vacca, 1988).

RISK FACTORS

Perinatal events that are most frequently associated with birth injury include midforceps delivery, shoulder dystocia, low forceps delivery, weight more than 3500 g, and second stage of labor longer than 60 minutes (Levine et al., 1984).

Injuries that arise before the intrapartum period are usually due to compression or pressure injuries from an unusual fetal position. The risk of injury to the central or peripheral nervous system is increased with malpresentation (especially breech), malposition, prolonged or precipitate labor, prematurity, multiple gestation, shoulder dystocia, macrosomia, and instrumental delivery. The most prevalent types of injury to the nervous system are extracranial hemorrhage, intracranial hemorrhage, skull fractures, spinal cord injury, and peripheral nerve injury.

EXTRACRANIAL HEMORRHAGE

Caput succedaneum and cephalhematoma are the most frequent types of birth injury, as well as the most benign. *Caput succedaneum* is characterized by soft, pitting, superficial edema that is several millimeters thick and overlies the presenting part in a vertex delivery. This edematous area lies above the periosteum and thus crosses suture lines. The edema consists of serum, blood, or both. Infants with caput succedaneum may also have ecchymosis, petechiae, or purpura over the presenting part. Caput succedaneum occurs in infants after a spontaneous vertex delivery or after use of a vacuum extractor. This type of extracranial hemorrhage requires no care other than parent teaching regarding its etiology and significance. It resolves within a few days after birth with no sequelae.

Cephalhematoma occurs in 0.2 to 2.5 percent of newborns (Andre & Vert, 1987; Brann & Schwartz, 1987). It involves subperiosteal bleeding, usually over the parietal bone, but may occur over other cranial bones. Cephalhematoma is usually unilateral but can be bilateral. This type of hemorrhage is seen most frequently in males; following the use of forceps; after a prolonged, difficult delivery; and in infants born to primiparas. The characteristic finding is a firm, fluctuant mass that does not cross the suture lines. The mass often enlarges slightly by 2 to 3 days of age. Ten to 25 percent will have a linear skull fracture underlying the mass. Rarely, an infant may have a subdural or subarachnoid hemorrhage.

A cephalhematoma can be distinguished from a caput succedaneum by the following characteristics (Brann & Schwartz, 1987):

- Limitation to the periosteal area
- Does not cross suture lines
- Absence of ecchymosis
- Increase in size over first several days
- Longer time to resolve

Infants with a cephalhematoma generally have no symptoms. Management includes parent teaching and monitoring for development of hyperbilirubinemia. Generally, cephalhematomas resolve between 2 weeks and 6 months (most by 6 weeks). Calcium deposits occasionally develop, and the swelling remains for 1 to 1½ years.

SKULL FRACTURE

Two forms of skull fractures are seen in newborns: linear and depressed.

Clinical Manifestations

Linear fractures usually occur over the frontal or parietal bones. Linear fractures are often associated with extracranial hemorrhage and underlie 10 to 25 percent of cephalhematomas (Axton, 1966). This type of fracture is usually asymptomatic. Skull radiographs are required to make the diagnosis.

Rarely, a linear fracture occurs in the occipital bone at the base of the skull. This type of fracture is seen primarily after breech deliveries with traction on a hyperextended spine (Brann & Schwartz, 1987). An occipital fracture is associated with intracranial hemorrhage and meningeal tears. Infants present with shock, neurologic abnormalities, and leakage of CSF through their nose, ears, or both.

A depressed skull fracture presents as a visible and palpable depression or "dent" in the skull, usually over the parietal area. These fractures are often described as resembling a ping-pong ball because the depression does not involve any loss of bone continuity. Unless there is underlying cerebral contusion or hemorrhage, no other signs or symptoms are seen.

Collaborative and Nursing Management

Cranial ultrasonography or computed tomography is performed to identify cerebral contusions or hemorrhage. Nursing assessment includes monitoring these infants for signs of neurologic dysfunction, intracranial hemorrhage, meningitis, and seizures. These findings are rare.

Infants with uncomplicated linear fractures require no special management. Follow-up skull radiographs are usually recommended to rule out a growing fracture and development of leptomeningeal cyst. Infants with basal fractures are managed for shock and hemorrhage. If the infant has leakage of CSF, antibiotics are usually given prophylactically to prevent meningitis.

In some infants with a depressed fracture, the fracture will elevate spontaneously within the first week. Most clinicians recommend manually elevating an uncomplicated depressed fracture that does not elevate spontaneously within a few days (Brann & Schwartz, 1987; Minarick & Beachy, 1989; Tudehope & Vacca, 1988). After this time, manual elevation is more difficult or impossible. Manual elevation can be accomplished by three methods:

- The thumbs of the clinician are placed on opposite margins of the depression, and gentle pressure is applied toward the middle.
- Elevation can also be accomplished with a breast pump or vacuum extractor. A hand breast pump, with petroleum jelly around the rim to ensure a good seal, is placed over the depression, and gentle pressure is applied. Use of a vacuum extractor involves placing it over the depression and applying pressure at a setting of 0.2 to 0.5 kg/cm^2 for about 4 minutes (Brann & Schwartz, 1987).
- Surgical interventions will be necessary if bone fragments are present or other methods failed. If surgery is done early, the procedure can be performed by passing a blunt instrument through the anterior fontanelle. The instrument is passed extradural to the site of the fracture and applied to the base of the fracture to "pop" the area back into alignment. If surgery is delayed until after 10 days, craniotomy may be needed (Tudehope & Vacca, 1988).

SPINAL CORD INJURY

Spinal cord injuries usually occur in the mid to lower cervical and upper thoracic areas. Injury can occur at any point along the cord. Lower cervical to midthoracic injuries are usually seen associated with breech deliveries; mid to high cervical injuries occur with vertex deliveries.

Clinical Manifestations

Infants with partial spinal cord injury have subtle neurologic signs and variable degrees of spasticity. Infants with high cervical or brain stem injuries are either stillborn or die shortly after birth of respiratory depression, shock, and hypothermia. Infants with mid or upper cervical injury may be stillborn, born with marked respiratory depression, or present with respiratory depression with the neurologic injury unrecognized until flaccidity, immobility of the legs, or urine retention (or all three) is noted. If born alive, these infants usually die within the first week, following development of progressive central respiratory depression often complicated by pneumonia.

Other clinical findings include the following:

- Relaxation of the abdominal wall
- Absent sensation in the lower half of the body
- Absent deep tendon and spontaneous reflexes
- Brachial plexus injury (20 percent)
- Constipation

This group also includes injuries at the C8 to T1 level. These infants usually survive. Infants with this type of injury may have a transient paraplegic paralysis at birth. Infants with mild injury may recover most or all of their function. Infants with moderate to severe damage are paraplegic or quadriplegic with permanent neurologic damage.

Initially, the clinical manifestations are those of spinal cord shock:

- Hypotonia
- Weakness
- Flaccid extremities
- Sensory deficits
- Relaxed abdominal muscles
- Diaphragmatic breathing
- Horner's syndrome (ipsilateral ptosis, anhidrosis, miosis)
- Distended bladder

Infants with low cervical lesions have shallow, paradoxical respirations and do not sweat. The skin over the affected area is dry and warm, and pinprick and deep tendon reflexes are absent.

Areflexia may be noted over the upper and lower extremities. After several weeks or months, a paraplegic autonomic hyperreflexia develops characterized by periodic mass reflex response. This results in tonic spasms of extremities, spontaneous micturition, and profuse sweating over the paralyzed area.

Collaborative Management

At birth, the infant may be in shock and require delivery room resuscitation. Initial management focuses on stabilization, treatment of associated problems such as perinatal asphyxia or hemorrhage, and management of respiratory depression. Infants with mid to upper cervical or brain stem lesions require assisted ventilation at birth or by 1 to 2 days (Tudehope & Vacca, 1988). The parents will be upset initially and need time to grieve. They will need ongoing support and teaching regarding care of the infant. Ongoing management of these infants and their families requires a multidisciplinary team that includes nursing, medicine, neurology, neurosurgery, physical therapy, orthopedics, urology, social work, and psychology. Ultrasonography, computed tomography, or magnetic resonance imaging may be done to determine the level and extent of injury. Laminectomy is rarely useful and may affect later stability of the spine (Andre & Vert, 1987).

Nursing Management

Care of the infant in the delivery room and neonatal intensive care unit involves initial stabilization, management related to accompanying perinatal asphyxia or hemorrhage, and promotion of ventilation. Ongoing management of these infants presents a major challenge to the nurse to support the infant and prevent further complications.

- Skin integrity over the paralyzed area must be maintained.
- Thermoregulation may be a problem because of evaporative loss.
- The infant should be positioned and repositioned regularly to promote normal alignment of body parts.
- A soft foam, sheepskin, lambskin, or similar material is used, or the infant is placed on a waterbed.
- The position should be changed every 2 to 3 hours.
- Affected areas should be kept clean and dry and massaged with gentle, passive range-of-motion exercises.
- Meticulous bowel and bladder care is required to prevent urinary tract infection and skin excoriation.
- Glycerin suppositories at regular intervals can help normalize bowel function.
- Monitoring is done for signs of respiratory infection and pneumonia.
- Parental teaching focuses on normal infant care issues as well as the special needs of a paralyzed infant.

FACIAL NERVE PALSY

Facial nerve palsy is one of the most common types of peripheral nerve injuries. The incidence ranges from 1.3 to 7.5 in 1000 live births (Levine et al., 1984).

Clinical Manifestations

Clinical manifestations vary, depending on whether the injury is to the central nerve, peripheral nerve, or peripheral nerve branch. The complete peripheral nerve injury results in a unilateral inability of the infant to close the eye or open the mouth. The lower lip on the affected side does not depress with crying nor does the forehead wrinkle. The affected side appears full and smooth, with obliteration of the nasolabial fold. These infants dribble milk while feeding.

Central injury usually results in a spastic paralysis of the lower portion of the face contralateral to the side of CNS injury, without involvement of the eyes or forehead. Peripheral nerve branch injury results in varying degrees of paralysis of the forehead, eye, or lower face, depending on the branch involved. The paralysis is apparent at birth or within 1 to 2 days.

Collaborative and Nursing Management

Nursing management involves parent counseling and teaching and prevention of complications. The eye on the affected side is patched, and 1 percent methylcellulose eye drops are instilled every 3 to 4 hours to prevent corneal damage. Dribbling with sucking can be a transient problem. If there is no improvement noted by 7 to 10 days or there is further loss of function, a neurosurgical consultation is usually recommended (Tudehope & Vacca, 1988). In infants with partial degeneration, physical therapy, massage, or electrical stimulation, or all three, may be used. Usefulness of these therapies is controversial and not well documented. Electromyography, nerve excitability, or nerve conduction latency examinations may be performed to evaluate the damage.

BRACHIAL PLEXUS PALSY

Clinical Manifestations

Clinical manifestations vary with the location and severity of the injury. Signs of injury are usually apparent from birth but may be delayed for several days to a few weeks in some infants. The three major types of injury and their relative frequencies are (1) Erb-Duchenne palsy (85 to 90 percent), (2) Klumpke's palsy (1 to 3 percent), and (3) Erb-Duchenne–Klumpke palsy (7 to 9 percent).

Erb-Duchenne palsy results from injury to the C5 and C6 nerve roots. The shoulder and upper arm are involved, with denervation of the deltoid, supraspinous, biceps, and brachioradial muscles. The arm lies passively at the infant's side, abducted and internally rotated, with the forearm pronated. The wrist and fingers are flexed. This posture is referred to as the "waiter's tip" position. The Moro reflex is absent, and biceps and radial reflexes are diminished or absent on the affected side; the grasp reflex is normal. Occasionally, C4 roots are also affected, with an associated phrenic nerve (diaphragmatic) paralysis.

Klumpke's palsy involves the C8 to T1 roots, affecting the lower arm and hand, with denervation of the intrinsic muscles of the hand and flexors of the wrist and fingers. Cervical sympathetic fibers may also be affected, with absence of sweating and sensation in the affected hand and arm. The infant holds the affected arm at the side of the thorax in a clawhand posture. The Moro and grasp reflexes are absent, and the triceps reflex is diminished or absent on the affected side; biceps and radial reflexes are present. If the T1 root is affected, the infant will manifest Horner's syndrome (ipsilateral ptosis, anhidrosis, and miosis).

Erb-Duchenne–Klumpke palsy involves the entire arm and hand owing to injury of the nerve roots of the brachial plexus from C5 to T1. This form of paralysis involves all the nerve fibers, with complete paralysis of the upper and lower arm and hand, flaccidity, and accompanying sensory, trophic, and circulatory changes (Tudehope & Vacca, 1988). Deep tendon and Moro's reflexes are all absent. If C4 roots are also affected, there will be an associated phrenic nerve (diaphragmatic) paralysis. Involvement of the T1 root leads to Horner's syndrome in about one third of these infants.

Collaborative Management

Initial management focuses on protection of the arm until localized edema and pain are diminished. The affected arm is immobilized with shoulder and elbow splints to prevent contractures and further stretching of the plexus. After edema subsides, at 7 to 10 days, physical therapy is gradually instituted to as much as the infant can tolerate. Initially, this may involve gentle, passive range-of-motion exercises. These infants will have continued physical therapy with massage and exercise over the first months until recovery (total or partial) occurs. Infants with brachial plexus injury should be evaluated for associated problems, including fractures and respiratory difficulty secondary to phrenic nerve paralysis.

If improvement is not noted within the first few months, electromyography and nerve conduction studies are done to determine the extent of the damage, to follow recovery, and to determine if surgical intervention is needed (Brann & Schwartz, 1987). Radicular ruptures can be repaired with microsurgical reconstruction, tendon transfers, and nerve grafts (Boome & Kaye, 1988). Surgery is considered if no improvement is seen by 3 months of age. Avulsion cannot be repaired.

Nursing Management

Infants with brachial plexus injuries often experience considerable pain with movement of the affected arm during the first few weeks. Nursing management is directed at reducing passive and active movement of the arm and at comfort measures. Splints are removed intermittently to reduce the risk of abduction contractures. The paralyzed arm is supported in a position of relaxation. Parent teaching regarding positioning, prevention of contractures, and exercise is essential.

PHRENIC NERVE PALSY

Clinical Manifestations

Infants with mild to moderate phrenic nerve injury may present with early respiratory difficulty, suggestive of hypoventilation, that stabilizes or improves. The infant may have recurrent episodes of cyanosis and dyspnea. The breathing pattern is altered. Breathing involves primarily thoracic movement with minimal or no abdominal excursions. Infants with complete avulsion or bilateral injuries will have severe respiratory distress from birth with tachypnea, apnea, and a weak cry (Brann & Schwartz, 1987).

Collaborative Management

Management focuses on promotion of ventilation and oxygenation. Infants may be placed on NPO status initially, with feeding instituted as the infant's respiratory status improves. Infants with severe distress require positive-pressure ventilation or constant positive airway pressure for support until recovery occurs. The effectiveness of electrical pacing of the diaphragm is unclear and controversial. Some infants require prolonged assisted ventilation and may develop hypostatic pneumonia. Surgical plication of the diaphragm will be done if no improvement is noted or if the infant is still ventilator dependent at 4 to 6 weeks.

Nursing Management

The infant is positioned on the affected side. If the infant cannot be fed, adequate fluid and calories must be provided. Feeding is instituted gradually. Initially, the infant may need to be gavage fed. When oral feeding is started, the infant is fed slowly, with ample opportunity for rest and monitoring of respiratory status. Because recovery will take several months, parents must be taught feeding, positioning, and comfort techniques. Nursing management of infants with respiratory problems is similar to that for any infant with respiratory distress. Developmental needs of infants requiring prolonged hospitalization must be met with provision of sensory input and play activities appropriate to their maturity and health status.

Neurologic Structural Dysfunction

NEURAL TUBE DEFECTS

Incidence

Neural tube defects (NTDs) of the CNS occur in 2 to 3 in 1000 births, with a decreasing incidence in the United States (Yen et al., 1992). Eighty percent of these defects result from failure of closure of the neural tube at either the cranial or the caudal ends (Moore & Persaud, 1993). NTDs include anencephaly, encephalocele, and spina bifida. This section focuses on assessment and management of spina bifida cystica, especially myelomeningocele.

NTDs can be diagnosed prenatally by analysis of alpha-fetoprotein (AFP) and acetylcholinesterase (AChE) levels in amniotic fluid and via fetal ultrasonography. AFP is a major fetal glycoprotein, similar to albumin, produced in the fetal liver from 6 weeks of gestation. Concentrations of AFP peak at 13 to 15 weeks. AFP is found in fetal serum, CSF, and amniotic fluid. Normally, AFP concentrations in CSF are 100 times higher than amniotic fluid concentrations, so when CSF leaks into the amniotic fluid, as occurs with an open NTD, amniotic fluid AFP levels are increased.

Most women with NTDs have AFP values greater than 3.0 MoM (Cuckle, 1994). False-positive results are generally due to blood contamination of the sample, fetal death, or severe malformation. Elevated AFP levels may also be found with open lesions (abdominal wall or skin defects), reduced amniotic fluid production (from renal agenesis or urethral obstruction), altered fetal swallowing (intestinal atresia), or altered protein breakdown (nephrosis) (Cuckle, 1994).

Amniocentesis is generally done only if there is a specific indication, such as a family history of NTDs or advanced maternal age. If the maternal serum AFP level is elevated, an amniocentesis and/or fetal ultrasonography is done to confirm the diagnosis. If the diagnosis can be confirmed by ultrasound, amniocentesis may not be done, unless chromosome analysis or other studies are also warranted.

Leakage of CSF from the defect can lead to maternal hydramnios. Overdistention of the uterus by excessive accumulation of amniotic fluid can stimulate preterm labor. Thus, infants with NTDs may be preterm.

Clinical Manifestations

The defect may vary greatly in size but is apparent on examination of the infant. The protruding sac is usually in the lumbosacral area and covered with skin or meninges. Fluid may be leaking from a partially or completely ruptured sac. Infants with this defect have altered tone and activity of the lower extremities and may assume a frog-like posture. If there is bowel and bladder involvement, dribbling of urine and feces may be noted. The neurologic deficit will vary with the level of the defect. Sensory level generally tends to approximate the motor level but may be several segments lower owing to differences in the pattern of innervation between sensory and motor fibers. Sensory level can be useful in predicting prognosis (Brann & Schwartz, 1987).

Infants with NTDs may have evidence of hydrocephalus at birth. Ultrasonography, computed tomography, or magnetic resonance imaging can be used to determine the size of the ventricular system, to rule out aqueductal stenosis and/or an Arnold-Chiari malformation, and to monitor ventricular status and the development of hydrocephalus. Renal dysfunction may develop from recurring urinary tract infections. Hydronephrosis may be present at birth. An intravenous pyelogram may be obtained to evaluate renal status and the presence of hydronephrosis (Brann & Schwartz, 1987).

Collaborative Management

Management of infants with NTDs, especially severe defects, is controversial and raises many ethical issues. Decisions must be made in the immediate neonatal period regarding whether to close the defect surgically and how aggressively the infants will be managed. If all infants with NTDs are managed aggressively at birth, a proportion of them will survive with severe neurologic, motoric, renal, bowel, and bladder problems, with significant psychological and economic stress to the family (Brann & Schwartz, 1987). Some clinicians believe that immediate surgical closure is not justified with open, draining defects, severe hydrocephalus, or multiple anomalies, and they recommend conservative, supportive care (Milhorat & Miller, 1994). Considerations in these decisions include the size and location of the defect, prognosis, presence of other anomalies, availability of facilities for long-term care, suffering of the infant, and family dynamics and wishes (Brann & Schwartz, 1987). If the decision is made not to close the defect surgically, care is supportive. Some of these infants will die in a few days to weeks, often secondary to infection, whereas others may survive for months or years, requiring long-term care.

For many infants with NTDs, immediate closure and aggressive care of the infant is the appropriate management. Unless the defect is severe or associated with multiple life-threatening anomalies, over 90 percent of infants with myelomeningocele will survive the neonatal period. If untreated, 15 to 30 percent will survive and be left with increased deficit. Thus, immediate closure is the treatment of choice for most infants.

Immediate closure reduces the risk of infection and improves the prognosis by reducing further deterioration of the spinal cord and nerve tracts. Early closure also facilitates caregiving. Surgical closure is done within the first 24 to 48 hours and often in the first few hours after birth. A large defect may require several surgical procedures to achieve complete closure. If the defect is completely covered by epithelium, surgery may be delayed for a short period to further evaluate function. All infants with NTDs are evaluated and monitored for hydrocephalus. Function of the urologic and renal systems is also assessed on an ongoing basis. All infants with involvement of the spinal cord or nerve roots, or both, will require multidisciplinary follow-up and continuing care to deal with ongoing neurologic, urologic, orthopedic, and psychological problems.

Nursing Management

Immediate nursing management includes stabilization and prevention of trauma or infection of the sac and its contents. Monitoring is done for signs of infection. This includes signs of sepsis or meningitis and localized infection with redness or discharge from the sac. These infants are at increased risk for hypothermia and dehydration from the open lesion, which lacks the normal protective skin covering.

The infant is positioned prone or on the side to reduce tension on the sac. A roll between the legs at hip level assists in maintaining abduction of the legs; a foot role is used to maintain the feet in a neutral position. Change of position from prone to side-lying or side to side, as well as range-of-motion exercises, helps to prevent skin breakdown and contractures. Low Trendelenburg position may be used to reduce CSF pressure on the sac. If the infant must be temporarily placed in a supine position for a procedure, a donut roll can be used to prevent pressure on the sac. Positioning postoperatively also involves use of the prone or side-lying position, maintenance of body alignment, prevention of hip abduction, and prevention of pressure on the operative site with holding.

The sac must be kept sterile and free of fecal or urine contamination. Warm sterile saline dressings are often used on the sac itself. An alternative approach is to cover the sac with Telfa pads or another nonadherent dressing soaked in warm saline. Telfa pads are less likely to adhere to the lesion. The Telfa pad can be covered by dry pads and a sterile plastic drape (Silver, Marzocchi, Farrell, & McLone, 1989). Meticulous skin care by keeping the skin clean and dry and removing urine and stool helps prevent skin breakdown as well as infection. The timing and characteristics of urination and stool excretion are observed to assist in determining the degree of deficit.

Tone, spontaneous movement, range of motion, and reflex activity are assessed. Head circumference is monitored serially, and signs of increasing ICP are noted. The infants have an intravenous drip and are placed on NPO status initially because surgery is usually performed within the first hours after birth. Postoperatively, the infants are also placed in a prone position initially until the surgical site heals. Skin care to prevent excoriation and contamination of the excision site continues to be critical during this period, as does prevention of contractures.

Families of infants with NTDs will need initial and ongoing support and counseling. Initial parental care involves assisting parents with the shock of the defect and its appearance and their grief over having an infant with an anomaly. Nursing care also involves enhancing parent–infant interaction and involving the parents in the infant's care when they are ready. Teaching before discharge includes skin care, positioning, exercises, handling and feeding techniques, and provision of activities to promote development. Many areas have spina bifida associations and parent-to-parent support programs to which parents can be referred for peer support.

Care of untreated infants is supportive, with provision of warmth, hydration, and comfort. Decisions not to treat these types of infants, however, are controversial. A case of an infant with NTD was the basis for the Baby Doe regulations. In any case, the birth of an infant with NTD is a difficult situation for the family as well as nurses and other staff and requires mutual understanding, support, and discussion of feelings.

HYDROCEPHALUS

Incidence

Hydrocephalus is the most common cause of head enlargement in the neonate. The incidence of this disorder is 3 to 4 in 1000 live births (Punt, 1988).

Physiology

Hydrocephalus is due to an abnormal accumulation of CSF in the ventricles and subarachnoid space. It arises from alterations in circulation or production of CSF owing to a congenital defect or after postbirth problems such as infection or hemorrhage.

Clinical Manifestations

Enlargement of the head may be noted at birth in infants with congenital hydrocephalus, or it may develop gradually. Posthemorrhagic and infection hydrocephalus develop after birth at varying times after the initial insult. Head size can increase without increases in ICP (normopressive hydrocephalus), owing to the neonate's soft, malleable skull and open sutures and fontanelles (Brann & Schwartz, 1987). A tense fontanelle may be noted when the infant is placed in an upright position. Progressive ventricular dilation may initially cause compression and damage to the cortex without any change in head size. The developing hydrocephalus may be apparent only on ultrasonographic examination. Transillumination is generally negative unless the cortical mantle is less than about 1 cm thick (Milhorat & Miller, 1994).

Head appearance may be altered, especially in congenital hydrocephalus with prominent frontal bones, a wide anterior cranium, or, in infants with Dandy-Walker syndrome, a large head with a prominent occiput (Amiel-Tison & Larroche, 1988).

With aqueductal stenosis, the cranial vault is expanded with a small posterior fossa, whereas in communicating hydrocephalus, the entire head is enlarged with separation of all the sutures (Milhorat & Miller, 1994).

Signs of increased ICP include the following:

- Bulging anterior fontanelle
- Setting-sun sign
- Dilated scalp veins
- Widely separated sutures (late sign)
- Separation of the squamosal suture above the ear between the temporal and parietal bones. This is a good indicator of markedly increased ICP.
- "Cracked pot" sound (Macewen's sign) on percussion of the head (Milhorat & Miller, 1994)

Collaborative Management

Serial head circumference measurements are plotted on all infants at risk for progressive ventricular enlargement and hydrocephalus (Fig. 17–2). The most accurate measurements are made using a metal tape marked in centimeters (rather than inches) (Amiel-Tison & Larroche, 1988). The rate of head growth is more critical than the absolute circumference.

Management can involve either surgical or medical therapy. Surgical management involves placement of a shunt to drain excess CSF. Other, less common surgical procedures include removal of arachnoidal cysts or tumors or fenestration procedures for infants with Dandy-Walker syndrome.

A ventriculoperitoneal shunt is generally the shunt of choice in infants and children because this type is easier to insert, revise, and lengthen and has a lower risk of infection than a ventriculoatrial shunt. One end of a radiopaque catheter is placed into the lateral ventricle, usually on the right side, and the other end is placed into the peritoneal cavity. The catheter contains a one-way valve palpable on the side of the head near the ear (Fig. 17-3).

In a term infant, revision of the shunt for growth can be anticipated at 3 to 4 years of age and at 10 to 13 years of age, when a permanent adult-length system is implanted. Preterm infants usually require an additional revision for growth at about 1 year of age (Milhorat & Miller, 1994). Major complications of ventriculoperitoneal shunts are infection and obstruction. Too rapid drainage of CSF immediately after shunt insertion can lead to herniation of the brain or subdural hematoma.

The role of medical management is controversial. Infants with uncomplicated hydrocephalus may not need shunting if the hydrocephalus arrests. These infants are managed by close follow-up and monitoring of ventricular size and cortical mantle thickness with serial cranial ultrasonography. Medical therapy is used primarily with posthemorrhagic hydrocephalus, which is associated with spontaneous arrest in about 50 percent of infants. Serial lumbar punctures or pharmacologic agents (see section on P/IVH) to reduce CSF may be used while monitoring these infants for cessation of progressive ventricular dilation (Volpe, 1995). These therapies may also be used in infants who are too ill to tolerate surgery and shunt placement (Milhorat & Miller, 1994; Punt, 1988).

Nursing Management

The nursing management of these infants is as follows:

- Monitor head circumference serially.
- Monitor for signs of progressive ventricular enlargement and increased ICP.
- Provide skin care.
- Use soft foam, sheepskin, lambskin, or other materials that minimize pressure and excoriation.
- Change infant's position regularly.
- Provide additional head support, with repositioning and holding
- Provide small, frequent feedings if infant feeds poorly

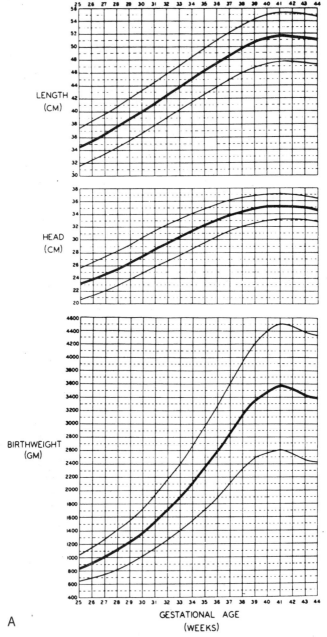

A

FIGURE 17–2 See legend on opposite page

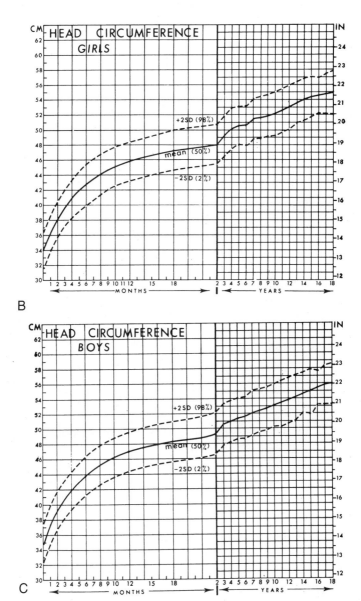

FIGURE 17–2. Charts for plotting head circumference. *A,* Intrauterine growth curves. *B* and *C,* Head circumference records for girls and boys, respectively. (*A,* from Klaus, M. H., & Fanaroff, A. A. [1986]. *Care of the high-risk neonate* [3rd ed., p. 424]. Philadelphia: W. B. Saunders; as compiled from Usher, R., & McLean, F. [1969]. Intrauterine growth of liveborn Caucasian infants at sea level: Standard obtained in 7 dimensions of infants born between 25 and 44 weeks of gestation. *Journal of Pediatrics, 74,* 901; *B* and *C,* from Nellhaus, G. [1968]. Head circumference from birth to eighteen years: Practical composite international and interracial graphs. *Pediatrics, 41,* 106. Reprinted with permission.)

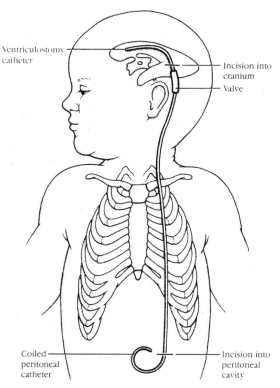

FIGURE 17–3. Ventriculoperitoneal shunt placement. (From Servonsky, J., & Opas, S. R. [1987]. *Nursing management of children* [p. 1297]. Boston: Jones & Bartlett. Reprinted with permission.)

Postoperatively, the following are recommended:

• Positioning on the side opposite the shunt
• Maintenance of head of the bed flat or slightly elevated to prevent rapid loss of CSF and decompression
• No pumping of valve unless specifically ordered
• Rotation of position to supine every few hours
• Maintenance of clean and dry skin
• Placement on sheepskin or lambskin to prevent skin breakdown

Shunted infants are observed for the following:

• Signs of localized or systemic infection
• Ileus
• Shunt obstruction
  • Enlargement of the head
  • Signs of increased ICP
  • Infection of the shunt
  • Localized redness or drainage around the incision

- Temperature instability
- Altered activity
- Poor feeding
- Monitor fluid status and intake and output.
- Monitor for signs of dehydration.
- Monitor for signs of too rapid decompression.
  - A sunken fontanelle
  - Agitation or restlessness
  - Increased urine output
  - Electrolyte abnormalities

Parent teaching before discharge is as follows:

- Care of the infant and shunt, including positioning and skin care
- Education as to signs of shunt malfunction, increased ICP, infection, and dehydration
- Referral to parent groups for peer support

Cerebral Palsy

Cerebral palsy (CP) has been described as a "non-progressive, chronic disability, characterized by aberrant control of movement and posture, and appearing in early life" (Fawer & Calame, 1988).

INCIDENCE

The incidence of CP is 5 in 1000 births, with approximately 50 percent having mild, 40 percent moderate, and 10 percent severe disability.

CLINICAL MANIFESTATIONS AND PROGNOSIS

This disorder is not diagnosed in the neonatal period. Manifestations become apparent over the first 3 to 18 months of age. Generally, the more severe the involvement, the earlier a specific diagnosis can be made. Thus, infants with quadriplegia are likely to be diagnosed within the first 3 to 6 months, whereas children with mild spastic diplegia affecting the legs may not be diagnosed until 12 to 18 months. Infants at risk or with subtle signs are treated with a high index of suspicion and observed carefully. Transient dystonia is seen in many infants with birth weights less than 1500 g during the first year. In a little over half of these infants, this resolves by about 12 months of age with no sequelae. In the remainder of infants with this problem, the dystonia either disappears but returns later or persists with later diagnosis of CP. Transient dystonia has also been associated with later learning problems and hyperactivity (Amiel-Tison, Dube, Garel, & Jequier, 1983; Taeusch & Yogman, 1987).

COLLABORATIVE AND NURSING MANAGEMENT

Early recognition through careful monitoring of infants at risk for CP is critical for prompt diagnosis as evidence of this disability presents. Physical therapy is a primary discipline in providing ongoing assessment of motor behavior, movement patterns, postures, tone, reflex patterns, and motor development appropriate to the child's age. Treatment is directed at developing alternative pathways to achieve desired motor function, preventing development of contractures and other deformities, and preventing the child from using and thus learning abnormal movement patterns.

REFERENCES

Als, H., Lawhon, G., Duffy, F. H., et al. (1994). Individualized developmental care for the very low birthweight preterm infant: Medical and neurofunctional effects. *Journal of the American Medical Association, 272,* 853.

Amiel-Tison, C., Dube, R., Garel, M., & Jequier, J. C. (1983). Late outcome after transient neuromotor abnormalities within the first year of life. In L. Stern, H. Bard, & B. Friis-Hansen (Eds.), *Intensive care IV* (pp. 247–258). New York: Masson Publishing.

Amiel-Tison, C., Korobkin, R., & Klaus, M. H. (1986). Neurologic problems. In M. H. Klaus & A. A. Fanaroff (Eds.), *Care of the high-risk neonate* (3rd ed., pp. 356–378). Philadelphia: W. B. Saunders.

Amiel-Tison, C., & Larroche, J. C. (1988). Brain development and neurological survey during the neonatal period. In L. Stern & P. Vert (Eds.), *Neonatal medicine* (pp. 245–267). New York: Masson Publishing.

Andre, M., & Vert, P. (1987). Birth injury. In L. Stern & P. Vert (Eds.), *Neonatal medicine* (pp. 176–190). New York: Masson Publishing.

Axton, J. H. (1966). Depressions of the skull in the newborn. *Nursing Mirror and Midwives Journal, 123*(5), 123–124.

Bellig, L. L. (1989). A window on the neonate's brain. *Neonatal Network, 7*(4), 13–20.

Bennett, F. C., Silver, G., Leung, E. J., & Mack, L. A. (1990). Periventricular echodensities detected by cranial ultrasonography: Usefulness in predicting neurodevelopmental outcome in low-birth-weight, preterm infants. *Pediatrics, 85*(3 pt. 2), 400–404.

Bernes, S. M., & Kaplan, A. M. (1994). Evolution of neonatal seizures. [Review]. *Pediatric Clinics of North America, 45,* 1069–1104.

Boome, R. S., & Kaye, J. C. (1988). Obstetric traction injuries of the brachial plexus: Natural history, indications for surgical repair and results. *Journal of Bone and Joint Surgery, British Volume, 70,* 571–576.

Bozynski, M. E., Nelson, M. N., Matalon, T. A., et al. (1985). Cavitary periventricular leukomalacia: Incidence and short term outcome in infants weighing ≤ 1200 grams at birth. *Developmental Medicine and Child Neurology, 27,* 572–577.

Brann, A. W., & Schwartz, J. F. (1987). Developmental anomalies and neuromuscular disorders. In A. A. Fanaroff & R. J. Martin (Eds.), *Neonatal–perinatal medicine* (5th ed., pp. 734–752). St. Louis: C. V. Mosby.

Brown, M. S., & Sheridan-Pereira, M. (1992). Outlook for a child with a cephalocele. *Pediatrics, 90,* 914–919.

Clancy, R. R. (1983). Neonatal seizures. In R. A. Polin & F. Berg (Eds.), *Workbook in practical neonatology* (pp. 125–152). Philadelphia: W. B. Saunders.

Cooke, R. (1989). The prevention and management of germinal layer hemorrhage and intraventricular hemorrhage. In J. S. Wigglesworth & K. Pape (Eds.), *Perinatal brain lesions* (pp. 191–217). Boston: Blackwell Scientific Publications.

Cuckle, H. S. (1994). Screening for neural tube defects. *CIBA Foundation Symposium, 181,* 253–269.

de Vries, L. S., Larroche, J. C., & Levene, M. I. (1988a). Intracranial haemorrhage and intraventricular haemorrhage. In M. I. Levene, M. J. Bennett, & J. Punt (Eds.), *Fetal and neonatal neurology and neurosurgery* (pp. 303–311). Edinburgh: Churchill Livingstone.

de Vries, L. S., Larroche, J. C., & Levene, M. I. (1988b). Germinal matrix haemorrhage and intraventricular haemorrhage. In M. I. Levene, M. J. Bennett, & J. Punt (Eds.), *Fetal and neonatal neurology and neurosurgery* (pp. 312–325). Edinburgh: Churchill Livingstone.

de Vries, L. S., Larroche, J. C., & Levene, M. I. (1988c). Cerebral ischemic lesions. In M. I. Levene, M. J. Bennett, & J. Punt (Eds.), *Fetal and neonatal neurology and neurosurgery* (pp. 326–338). Edinburgh: Churchill Livingstone.

Fawer, C. L., & Calame, A. (1988). Assessment of neurodevelopmental outcome. In M. I. Levene, M. J. Bennett, & J. Punt (Eds.), *Fetal and neonatal neurology and neurosurgery* (pp. 71–88). Edinburgh: Churchill Livingstone.

Finer, N. N., Robertson, C. M., Richards, R. T., et al., (1981). Hypoxic-ischemic encephalopathy in term infants: Perinatal factors and outcome. *Journal of Pediatrics, 98*, 112–117.

Gale, E. (1981). Neonatal seizures. In R. Perez (Ed.), *Protocols for perinatal nursing practice* (pp. 385–390). St. Louis: C. V. Mosby.

Goldbarg, H., & Yeh, T. F. (1991). Seizures. In T. F. Yeh (Ed.), *Neonatal therapeutics* (pp. 313–325). St. Louis: Mosby–Year Book.

Kaempf, J. W., Porreco, R., Molina, R., et al. (1990). Antenatal phenobarbital for the prevention of periventricular and intraventricular hemorrhage: A double-blind, randomized, placebo-controlled, multihospital trial. *Journal of Pediatrics, 117*, 933–938.

Levene, M.I. (1988). The asphyxiated newborn infants. In M. I. Levene, M. J. Bennett, & J. Punt (Eds.), *Fetal and neonatal neurology and neurosurgery* (pp. 371–382). Edinburgh: Churchill Livingstone.

Levine, M. G., Holroyde, J., Woods, J. R., Jr., et al. (1984). Birth trauma: Incidence and predisposing factors. *Obstetrics and Gynecology, 63*, 792–795.

Ment, L. R., Oh, W., Ehrenkranz, R. A., et al. (1994a). Low dose indomethacin and prevention of intraventricular hemorrhage: A multicenter randomized trial. *Pediatrics, 93*, 543–550.

Ment, L. R., Oh, W., Ehrenkranz, R. A., et al. (1994b). Low dose indomethacin therapy and extension of intraventricular hemorrhage: A multicenter randomized trial. *Journal of Pediatrics, 124*, 951–955.

Milhorat, T. H., & Miller, J. I. (1994). Neurosurgery. In G. B. Avery, M. A. Fletcher, & M. G. MacDonald (Eds.), *Neonatology: Pathophysiology and management of the newborn* (4th ed., pp. 1139–1163). Philadelphia: J. B. Lippincott.

Minarick, C. J., & Beachy, P. (1989). Neurologic disorders. In G. B. Merenstein & S. L. Gardner (Eds.), *Handbook of neonatal intensive care* (2nd ed., pp. 501–530). St. Louis: C. V. Mosby.

Moore, K. L., & Persaud, T. V. N. (1993). Before we are born: Essentials of embryology and birth defects (4th ed.). Philadelphia: W. B. Saunders.

O'Rahilly, R., & Muller, F. (1994). Neurulation in the normal human embryo. [Review]. *CIBA Foundation Symposium, 181*, 70–82.

Paidas, M. J., & Cohen, A. (1994). Disorders of the central nervous system. [Review]. *Seminars in Perinatology, 18*(4), 266–282.

Pape, K. E., Armstrong, D. L., & Fitzhardinge, P. M. (1976). Central nervous system pathology associated with mask ventilation in the very low birthweight infant: A new etiology for intracerebellar hemorrhage. *Pediatrics, 58*(4), 473–483.

Punt, J. (1988). Hydrocephalus. In M. I. Levene, M. J. Bennett, & J. Punt (Eds.), *Fetal and neonatal neurology and neurosurgery* (pp. 586–591). Edinburgh: Churchill Livingstone.

Sarnat, H. B., & Sarnat, M. S. (1976). Neonatal encephalopathy following fetal distress: A clinical and electroencephalographic study. *Archives of Neurology, 33*(10), 696–705.

Silver, R. K., Marzocchi, M., Farrell, E. E., & McLone, D. G. (1989). The perinatal management of central nervous system anomalies. [Review]. *Clinics in Perinatology, 16*(4), 939–953.

Szymonowicz, W., Yu, V., Walker, A., & Wilson, F. (1986). Reduction in periventricular hemorrhage in preterm infants. *Archives of Diseases in Childhood, 61,* 661–665.

Taeusch, H. W., & Yogman, M. W. (1987). *Follow-up and management of the high risk infants.* Boston: Little, Brown.

Tudehope, D. I., & Vacca, A. (1988). Traumatic injuries to the nervous system. In M. I. Levene, M. J. Bennett, & J. Punt (Eds.), *Fetal and neonatal neurology and neurosurgery* (pp. 393–404). Edinburgh: Churchill Livingstone.

Volpe, J. J. (1995). *Neurology of the newborn* (3rd ed.). Philadelphia: W. B. Saunders.

Volpe, J. J., & Hill, A. (1987). Neurologic disorders. In G. B. Avery (Ed.), *Neonatology: Pathophysiology and management of the newborn* (3rd ed., pp. 1073–1132). Philadelphia: J. B. Lippincott.

Vyhmeister, N., Schneider, S., & Cha C. (1977). Cranial transillumination norms of the premature infant. *Journal of Pediatrics, 91,* 980–982.

Wasterlain, C. G., & Duffy, T. E. (1975). Neonatal status epilepticus: Decrease in brain glucose without decrease in blood glucose. *Neurology, 25,* 365.

Wigglesworth, J. S. (1989). Current problems in brain pathology in the perinatal period. In J. S. Wigglesworth & K. Pape (Eds.), *Perinatal brain lesions* (pp. 1–23). Boston: Blackwell Scientific Publications.

Yen, I. H., Khoury, M. J., Erickson, J. D., et al. (1992). The changing epidemiology of neural tube defects. United States, 1968–1989. *American Journal of Diseases of Children,* 146, 857–861.

CHAPTER 18

Assessment and Management of Musculoskeletal Dysfunction

TYPES OF MUSCULOSKELETAL DYSFUNCTION

Osteogenesis Imperfecta

Osteogenesis imperfecta (OI) is a connective tissue disorder with genetic etiology. The primary pathophysiologic defect involves the collagen structure. Collagen (the major extracellular protein) formation fails to progress beyond the reticulin fiber stage. Further significant disruption in the collagen formation in OI includes a defect in cross-linking that results in decreased collagen stability (Francis, Smith, & Bauze, 1974). Although osteoblastic activity appears normal, there is typically no collagen production (Follis, 1952). Any tissue containing collagen, such as sclerae, bones, ligaments, and teeth, may be affected.

TYPES

Type I

Type I is an autosomal dominant disorder. Severe forms of OI present as early-onset fractures, and the frequency of fractures is increased. Another clinical feature is severe hearing impairment, which has an incidence of 40:1. A majority of the affected individuals (75:1) report a predisposition to bruising. The sclerae are often bluish as well.

Type I is subdivided into types IA and IB. Type IA occurs without dentinogenesis imperfecta, whereas patients with type IB present with dentin abnormalities.

The incidence of OI type I is 1 in 30,000 (Sillence, Rimoin, & Danks, 1979).

The disorder is evident in the neonatal period in 10 percent of affected individuals. Fractures are the primary sign in neonates. Affected neonates typically have normal height and weight for their gestational age. However, owing to the progressive nature of kyphoscoliosis, a component of OI disorders, the majority of persons are of short stature.

Type II

Type II is an autosomal recessive disorder. It is an extremely severe OI disorder and results in death in either the prenatal or neonatal period. Prenatal diagnosis is possible with this condition. Death occurs through damage to vital organs (brain, liver, and lungs) not protected by the fragile bony structures.

437

The incidence OI type II has been reported as 1 in 62,487 (Sillence, Senn, & Danks, 1979).

Neonates affected with this disorder are typically small for gestational age and present with dwarf-like appearance (Baraitser & Winter, 1996). The extremities are deformed and short as a result of multiple fractures and crumbling of the long bones. Chest radiographs exhibit beaded ribs with numerous fractures, both old and new. Blue sclerae are characteristic features in both type I and type II. However, blue sclerae can be a normal finding in neonates and cannot serve as a diagnostic criterion for this age group (Gertner & Root, 1990).

Trauma of birth exacts a further toll on the appearance of these infants, contributing to the maceration of the head and limbs. This form of OI is also referred to as the perinatal lethal form.

Type III

Type III is a rare, yet severe, disorder with autosomal recessive inheritance patterns. Fractures may be present at birth, and the clinical course may simulate OI type II. Variations between types II and III are identified on physical examination. Neonates affected with OI type III have normal height and weight for gestational age at birth. Although there may be multiple rib fractures on chest radiograph, there is an absence of the beaded rib appearance. The long bones in type II are crumbled, whereas in type III the bones have multiple fractures and calcifications. The extremities do not usually appear deformed as in type II. However, individuals affected with OI type III have the shortest stature for all OI disorders. Mortality rates for children with type III are high, owing to severe kyphoscoliosis (Sillence, 1981).

Type IV

Type IV is similar to type I in that it is an autosomal dominant disorder with variable penetrance. Type IV is subdivided into types IVA and IVB, depending on the absence or presence of dentinogenesis imperfecta. OI type IV resembles types I and III in clinical presentation and course. Incidence rates for OI types III and IV have not been established.

DIAGNOSIS

All forms of OI can be present at birth, although severity varies among the different types. In the milder cases, fractures in the neonatal period may result from birth trauma. Fractures are most abundant in the arms, legs, clavicles, and ribs. As the infant ages, the lower extremities are affected more frequently as a result of increased weight-bearing trauma.

Calcification is rapid in neonates, with callus formation usually occurring within 10 days. There does not appear to be a deficiency in callus formation in OI disorders, but the callus is weaker than in normal individuals and predisposes the bone to further fractures in that area.

Multiple rib fractures in a neonate may prompt respiratory compromise, because the pain from the fracture thwarts the infant's breathing attempts. Difficulty in weaning from ventilatory support, when other pathologic causes have been ruled out, may lead one to suspect the presence of OI. Chest radiographs should be closely inspected for rib fractures or callus formation, or both, in such cases.

Case reports in the literature have identified newborns sustaining fractures of the femurs during routine examination of the hip for dysplasia.

TREATMENT

There is no treatment for the underlying pathology of OI disorders. Therefore, management centers on support and promoting independence in terms of mobility, function, and social integration. Rehabilitation techniques include active range of motion, strengthening exercises, stretching, and coordination exercises. Water activities appear well tolerated even in severely affected patients. Outcome appears enhanced when physical and occupational therapies are instituted promptly after birth, condition allowing.

COLLABORATIVE MANAGEMENT

In the neonatal period, affected infants are managed according to clinical presentation and protocol for that particular gestational age.

- The infant must be handled carefully.
- Padded splints for the extremities may help reduce the incidence of accidental fractures.
- Signs are posted on the infant's bed to warn all individuals of the consequences of improper handling.
- As the infant grows, padded orthotic devices provide support to the trunk and extremities in an effort to reduce the incidence of skeletal deformities.
- Vascular checks of the casted or splinted extremity are required.
  - The capillary bed should be pink.
  - White (or pallor) symbolizes decreased or poor arterial flow.
  - Cyanosis of the extremity indicates venous stasis. By the time a pulse is absent, irreparable harm has probably occurred.
- Skin care in terms of positioning should be provided.
- Bedding that discourages decubitus formation should be supplied.
- Splints placed beside the chest stabilize the thoracic wall and potentiate effective ventilation. These may be in the form of rolled blankets or sandbags.
- Pain relief through medication as well as supportive measures should be considered.
  - Watch for signs of grimacing and crying when infant is moved.
  - Note any alterations in vital signs (tachycardia, tachypnea, hypertension), irritability, and restlessness.
  - Educate the family on proper handling of the infant.

Achondroplasia

Although the term was once used to describe any form of dwarfism, achondroplasia is now recognized as one distinct type of dwarfism having characteristic features. It is the most common type of dwarfism and has an autosomal dominant pattern of inheritance. The majority of cases occur by spontaneous mutation.

INCIDENCE

Achondroplasia occurs in 3 in 1 million live births (Gardner, 1977).

DIFFERENTIAL DIAGNOSIS

The differential diagnosis of an infant presenting with dwarfism includes achondroplasia, OI type II, thanatophoric dwarfism, and achondrogenesis. Although achondroplasia presents with markedly shortened limbs and often bowing of the lower limbs, radiographic studies do not show evidence of multiple fractures and long-bone crumbling as seen in OI type II. Thanatophoric dwarfism and achondrogenesis, both typically fatal in the neonatal period, are characterized by an extremely narrow chest and marked defective ossification, respectively.

CLINICAL MANIFESTATIONS

Achondroplasia is apparent at birth, unlike hypochondroplasia, which becomes clinically significant at 5 to 6 years of age. Characteristic features of achondroplasia include dwarfism, with a disproportionately large head size due to an increased anteroposterior skull diameter; flattened nasal bridge with a prominent frontal region; short, broad hands; and a flattened anterior chest wall with costal flaring. Later, an exaggerated lumbar lordosis and increased muscular development become obvious. Intelligence is usually normal; however, a positive self-esteem may be difficult to establish.

COLLABORATIVE MANAGEMENT

Respiratory or ventilatory management of the severely affected achondroplastic dwarf is the primary concern. Mildly affected infants may be able to compensate for decreased lung volume with a mild to moderate increase in the work of breathing. As the infant grows, this compensation becomes more difficult.

Compensatory mechanisms such as increased work of breathing in the mildly affected achondroplastic dwarf require that meticulous attention be paid to nutrition to support the increased energy that is being used. There is a need for increased caloric intake in an infant exhibiting tachypnea or retractions if positive growth is to occur. However, if growth is allowed to proceed too rapidly, the infant's body mass may exceed the pulmonary capacity and decompensation may occur. For this reason, nutritionists may provide additional insights in daily management concerning how to provide calories but not add to the work of the infant.

Parental and family needs may be satisfied through education and collaboration with social services. Support groups specifically for parents of dwarfed infants are found in many cities. From these groups, parents can gain a better perspective of the long-term development of their infant.

LONG-TERM CONSEQUENCES

Complications of achondroplasia are primarily of a neurologic nature involving the spinal nerves. Anatomic configuration of the intraspinal canal results in pressure on the cord and spinal nerves. This pressure produces chronic backache and, in the most severe scenario, paraplegia. Referrals to physical and occupational therapists along with long-term orthopedic follow-up can reduce some of the complications. If these changes in the spinal column do occur, the child is at greater risk for developing increased respiratory difficulties, mobility problems, self-concept and self-esteem concerns, physical pain, and central or peripheral nervous system neuropathies.

Because with this condition the child looks different from peers, any exaggeration of the condition has the potential for adding to a faulty self-concept. As the child grows, it is important for both parents and health care professionals to assess continually the personal image that is being formed in the child's mind. Positive support of parents during the neonatal period through comments about what the infant is doing and how the infant looks may provide a role model of positive behavior that the parents can emulate with the child.

Arthrogryposis

Historically, the term *arthrogryposis* (curved, hooked joint) has been used not only to provide a description of a clinical appearance but also as a diagnosis for various conditions. The one common denominator for conditions termed *arthrogryposis* is the presence of multiple congenital joint contractures. There are over 150 known conditions in which multiple congenital contractures are the dominant feature, many of which are syndromes unrelated to a chromosomal or genetic problem (Clark & Eteson, 1991; Moessinger, 1983). The most common forms are autosomal dominant distal arthrogryposis, amyoplasia, multiple pterygium syndrome, and cerebro-oculofacioskeletal syndrome (Clark & Eteson, 1991). Another, less common form that is being examined by geneticists in more detail is Pena-Shokeir syndrome. Therefore, the name arthrogryposis multiplex congenita is often used.

PHYSIOLOGY

Arthrogryposis is a condition involving congenital, nonprogressive limitation of movement in two or more joints in different body areas (Hall, 1981). The deformity is primarily a result of fibrous and fatty changes in muscles secondary to decreased fetal movement. Although muscles undergo normal embryologic development, they are replaced by fibrous and fatty tissue after a reduction of normal fetal movement. The physiologic muscle changes subsequently produce contracted joints. Ultimately, any process resulting in limited intrauterine movement by the fetus can lead to multiple congenital contractures (Hall, 1983). The severity of such contractures increases with a longer duration of limited movement. Also, the earlier in fetal development the limitation is imposed, the greater the severity of contractures.

INCIDENCE AND INHERITANCE PATTERNS

The incidence of multiple congenital contractures is 1 in 3000 live births (Hall, 1989). Hall (1981) examined 350 infants and divided them into three categories based on the body areas affected by the contractures. This classification system, still in use today, can provide a prognostic indicator for the clinician.

The first category primarily involves the limbs. The majority of infants fall into this category. These infants are otherwise normal. The second category primarily involves contractures in the limbs but also involves other organ systems, predominantly the visceral organs. The third category involves multiple congenital contractures concurrent with central nervous system (CNS) dysfunction.

Two types of arthrogryposis have an autosomal recessive inheritance pattern. The first is multiple pterygium syndrome, which consists of webbed, contracted fingers with later development of camptodactyly; micrognathia; low-set rotated ears; palpebral fissures that appear to have a downward slant; ptosis; rocker-bottom feet much like those of an infant with trisomy 13 or 18; possibly neck webbing; and possibly cleft palate (Clark & Eteson, 1991). The second type is cerebro-oculofacioskeletal syndrome. It is associated with failure to thrive postnatally, microcephaly, intracranial calcifications, shortened palpebral fissures, and congenital cataracts (Clark & Eteson, 1991). These children usually die by school age.

Another form of arthrogryposis, which is very rare, is Pena-Shokeir syndrome. The infant with this syndrome presents with a short umbilical cord, pulmonary hypoplasia, intrauterine growth retardation, ankyloses, and camptodactyly (Clark & Eteson, 1991). The maternal history includes oligohydramnios and fetal akinesia or decreased fetal movement. This condition may have an autosomal recessive inheritance pattern, but this has not been confirmed. It is the second most common condition involving multiple congenital contractures of the limbs.

CLINICAL MANIFESTATIONS

On physical examination, amyoplasia has a typical appearance with symmetrical joint involvement, usually of all four limbs. There is decreased muscle mass. Frequency of joint involvement increases from proximal to distal joints. Therefore, there is almost universal severe equinovarus deformity, and the wrists are typically flexed. The elbows and knees can be in a flexed or extended position; however, most cases present with both upper and lower extremities in extension. There may be notable dimpling at the elbows and knees. Shoulders are internally rotated. Hips are frequently dislocated. Normal skin creases overlying the joints are absent, and the skin is tense and glossy.

The facies of an infant with amyoplasia are characterized by a round face and mild micrognathia. A midline hemangioma involving the eyes, nasal bridge, and forehead may be present that usually fades with time.

Newborns affected with amyoplasia are usually active but with decreased limb movement. They feed well, although positioning of the infant during feeding and routine baby care presents a challenge. Distal arthrogryposis primarily involves the hands and feet. On physical examination, the hands of the newborn with distal arthrogryposis are typical and thus easily recognized. Hands are clenched, with the thumb flexed into the palm. Fingers cross over the thumb and palm, usually overlapping each other. This hand position resembles that of an infant diagnosed with trisomy 18.

COLLABORATIVE MANAGEMENT

Excluding those infants having concurrent CNS dysfunction, infants with multiple congenital contractures have excellent prognoses. The goal of collaborative management is to achieve and maintain an acceptable range of motion in the affected joints. Independent living is a reality for many individuals with appropriate management.

Physical therapy should be initiated early in the neonatal period. Collaboration with physical and occupational therapists should begin in the neonatal intensive care unit. In the past, infants with multiple congenital contractures were casted; however, this therapy was found to produce additional muscle atrophy secondary to the immobilization. Therefore, physical therapy is now used in conjunction with splinting when necessary.

Physical therapy is a lifelong process, and parents are taught the techniques that they must use with their child daily. Therefore, parental or family involvement is a key factor in the success of the physical therapy for these infants. Creativity on the part of the health care professional as well as the parents complements efforts to manipulate the rather rigid infant during feedings, sleeping, holding, and daily care activities. Parents may need referrals to agencies that can provide respite care or assistance from volunteers to carry out these physical therapies on a daily basis. Financial assistance for such services may fall into the realm of nursing, because the nurse can collaborate with social workers and financial counselors.

PROGNOSIS

The long-term prognosis depends on the extent of involvement. Hall (1981) reported a mortality rate of only 1 percent for those infants affected primarily with limb involvement. Those infants with limb and other organ involvement had a 7 percent mortality rate, whereas those with limb and CNS involvement experienced a 50 percent mortality rate.

Certain characteristics have placed the fetus in a high-risk category. These characteristics include decreased fetal movements, contractures, micrognathia, hydramnios, and thin ribs on radiographs (Bianchi & Van Marter, 1994).

Congenital Dislocation of the Hip

Congenital dislocation, or dysplasia, of the hip (CDH) refers to any manifestation of hip instability, ranging from subluxation to complete dislocation. CDH remains a common problem despite almost universal neonatal screening. Reports indicate success rates as high as 100 percent for the diagnosis of CDH in the neonatal period, yet these same reports also suggest that neonatal screening programs are ineffective (Robertson, 1984). Although controversy surrounds the usefulness of neonatal screening programs for the diagnosis of CDH, these programs have led to earlier diagnosis and treatment of many infants. Because some infants possess normal hip movement, findings of some examinations may initially be normal and yet later indicate abnormal hip development. Dysplastic hip screenings should be performed at routine health visits at 2 weeks and 2, 4, 6, 9, and 12 months of age.

INCIDENCE RATES AND RISK FACTORS

There is an increased incidence of CDH in first-born children (Carter & Wilkinson, 1964). This increase may be due to the unstretched uterine and abdominal muscles, oligohydramnios, and the high association of fetal breech positioning in primigravidas. There is a definite preponderance toward CDH in female children. The ratio of occurrence of CDH in girls to boys is 6:1 (Bennett & MacEwen, 1989). Females account for 80 percent of all cases of CDH. Factors that may contribute to this finding include the fact that twice as many females as males present in the breech position. Also, in females, there appears to be a heightened laxity in response to maternal relaxin hormones.

The breech position remains a major factor contributing to the development of CDH. Authors have reported that from 16 to 25 percent of affected infants are born in the breech presentation (Tachdijian, 1990a). Specific incidences of CDH in relationship to positioning are 0.7 percent for cephalic, 2 percent for footling, and 20 percent for single breech. The incidence of CDH for infants in the breech presentation is not altered by delivery methods. Breech-positioned infants delivered by cesarean section have the same predisposition to hip dislocation as those delivered vaginally (Artz et al., 1975).

The left hip is involved three times more frequently than the right hip. Approximately 60 percent of CDH is on the left side, 20 percent on the right side, and 20 percent bilateral (Tachdijian, 1990a). This finding is attributed to the tendency of the fetus to lie with its left thigh against the maternal sacrum. This position forces the left hip into a posture of flexion and adduction. Thus, the femoral head is covered more by the joint capsule than by the acetabulum.

CDH is a dynamic disorder that may improve or deteriorate with or without treatment. Thus, the joint may spontaneously dislocate and reduce (return to normal position) with normal neonatal movement. At the initial phase of the disorder seen during the neonatal period, there is no other significant pathology. With time, this simple mechanism progresses in complexity secondary to adaptive changes. CDH can eventually progress to either permanent reduction, complete dislocation, or dysplasia (abnormal development). For those infants noted to have hip instability, more than 60 percent will stabilize within the first week of life and 88 percent will stabilize within the second month postnatally. Only 12 percent of infants with initial hip instability will be considered to have congenital dysplastic hips with the potential for progressive pathology.

In those instances in which complete dislocation occurs, pathologic changes occur to the femoral head, acetabulum, and ilium. This complete dislocation is due to the adaptive changes that occur in the adjacent tissue and bone. The long-term complication of dislocation, when adequate treatment has not occurred, is degenerative change of both the femoral head and the acetabulum. Once adaptive changes occur, there is an increased risk for progressive degeneration despite treatment.

The subluxated hip, when not diagnosed in the neonatal period, is generally diagnosed at adolescence, when the strain of puberty and rapid growth spurts occur. With subluxation, the femoral head is laterally displaced and pushed upward into the joint; it is not completely out of the acetabulum. As the child grows and there is increased weight bearing, the femoral head slides around and moves to the joint's edge. Degenerative changes result from this continual sliding. Sclerosis of the underlying bone, loss of cartilage, and the formation of degenerative cysts are the most common degenerative changes.

DIAGNOSIS AND CLINICAL MANIFESTATIONS

In the neonatal period, diagnosing CDH can be facilitated through the Ortolani and Barlow maneuvers. The Ortolani test determines dislocation in the hip of a newborn, whereas the Barlow test is used to determine whether the hip is dislocatable (Barlow, 1962; Ortolani, 1976). In practice, both procedures are done in sequence. For examination, the infant is placed on a firm surface in the supine position. The infant should be relaxed and quiet. Only one hip should be examined at a time.

To perform the Ortolani test, the pelvis is stabilized with one hand and, with the other hand, the thigh is grasped on the side to be tested. The middle finger is located over the greater trochanter (lateral aspect of the upper thigh), and the thumb is across the knee. The hip is flexed to 90 degrees while bending the knee. The leg is then gently abducted with an anterior lift. A positive Ortolani test would reveal a "clunk" with abduction. This clunk occurs as the dislocated femoral head slides over the posterior rim of the acetabulum and into the hip's socket. Next, the hip is adducted, and for the infant with CDH, a second clunk can be observed as the femoral head is displaced out of the acetabulum.

False-positive diagnoses of CDH have occurred when the examiner misinterprets a normal "click" (high-pitched sound) for a "clunk." A click is not a sign of CDH. Clicks may be heard as a result of snapping of ligaments or tendons and are normal.

Barlow's test determines instability of the hip and identifies those hips that can be dislocated on manipulation. Both hips and knees are flexed, with the hip to be tested in slight adduction. The middle finger remains positioned as for the Ortolani test, over the greater trochanter. However, the thumb is now located over the medial aspect of the lower thigh. Gentle pressure is exerted by the thumb posteriorly and laterally (down and out). For the infant with CDH, the femoral head can be felt to move out of the acetabulum with the typical clunk. The hip can then be reduced by the Ortolani maneuver or simply by releasing thumb pressure and abducting and flexing the hips.

In cases in which the femoral head is subluxated, one might note a sliding motion in the hip joint on physical examination. This sliding motion can be characteristic of an unstable hip joint. The majority of these unstable hips spontaneously resolve without treatment. There is no way to determine which hips will reduce and stabilize without treatment; therefore, it is best to treat all hips that are determined to be unstable.

Ultrasonography has proved valuable for CDH detection. Radiographic examination has not been reliable, owing to the cartilaginous composition of the neonatal pelvis.

COLLABORATIVE MANAGEMENT

The goal is to achieve and maintain reduction of the unstable hip. The sooner treatment is implemented, the greater the chance for successful outcome. Various splinting devices are used to treat infants with CDH. Examples of splints include the (1) Pavlik harness, (2) von Rosen splint, (3) Denis Browne hip adduction splint, and (4) Frejka pillow splint. The most commonly used splint for neonates is the Pavlik harness.

The Pavlik harness is a device that allows for spontaneous hip and lower extremity movement while maintaining reduction of the hip joint. It can be worn comfortably during all aspects of normal newborn care, including diaper changes. This device can be adjusted for growth and is indicated for use in newborns and infants up to 6 months of age. Use of the Pavlik harness is contraindicated for infants able to stand and for those infants in whom the hip joint is not reducible by manipulation, specifically the Ortolani procedure, because the infant may actually attempt to bear weight with the harness on, potentially pushing the hip out of alignment. This movement would defeat the purpose of reduction of the hip joint. The greatest danger, however, is that the child will become entangled in the parachute-like straps as he or she attempts to push up to a standing position: there is the possibility that a child could hang himself or herself in the straps.

A major factor influencing the success of the Pavlik harness is parental compliance with the treatment.

PARENT AND FAMILY EDUCATION AND SUPPORT

In addition to providing information regarding the pathology and treatment goals of CDH, the nurse should provide the parents an opportunity to remove and reapply the harness while under supervision. Parental support groups can help parents adjust to the infant's temporary awkward condition. Parents should also be educated in the procedure used to reduce the dislocated hip, because complete reduction must be achieved before the harness is applied.

LONG-TERM CONSEQUENCES AND COMPLICATIONS

As with most therapeutic treatments, the potential for iatrogenic complications exists. Complications observed after CDH treatment include (1) avascular necrosis, (2) redislocation, and (3) acetabular dysplasia. Complications can result from either inadequate or overly aggressive treatment.

If the hip does not reduce after 2 to 3 weeks of splinting, alternative treatment modalities must be considered. Such alternatives include closed reduction with traction or open reduction with casting. A hip spica cast is most often used with these infants. Care then includes observance for poor pedal pulses, decreased peripheral circulation, pain, skin excoriation or abrasions, and possible development of respiratory infections due to decreased mobility. Parents will need to learn cast care, because the child will go home with the cast in place.

Clubfoot

The classic clubfoot, talipes equinovarus, refers to a dysmorphic-appearing foot with hindfoot equinus, forefoot adduction, and midfoot supination. The term *clubfoot* may also be used to describe milder talipes conditions, including talipes calcaneus and talipes varus.

INCIDENCE

Foot deformities are among the most commonly occurring birth defects. Clubfoot has an incidence of 1 in 1000 live births. Males are affected nearly twice as often as females; and in those with unilateral presentation, the majority appear on the right (Palmer, Conneally, & Yu, 1974; Wynne-Davies, 1964).

CLINICAL MANIFESTATIONS

Clubfoot deformities are apparent at birth. The skin overlying the lateral aspect of the foot may be taut, whereas the medial aspect may present with increased skinfolds. The affected foot may be smaller in size than a normal foot. In older children, the calf muscle may be noticeably decreased in size. Milder talipes conditions may be returned to the neutral position by manipulation.

COLLABORATIVE MANAGEMENT

Early diagnosis and treatment is essential. In the early newborn period, joints, muscles, and ligaments may be more compliant to corrective manipulation without surgical intervention. This may involve serial casting as frequently as 2- to 4-day intervals. As many as 50 percent of clubfoot deformities may require surgery. Difficulty with skin closure has been reported as a complication after correction of severe clubfoot. This is especially true if there has been prior surgery on the affected foot.

Parental education includes implementation of routine newborn care for an infant wearing either splints or bilateral casts. Problems and solutions associated with clothing, sleeping, feeding, and bathing should be addressed. Compliance by parents in using splints may vary. Because consistent treatment is necessary for a favorable outcome, health care professionals must explore parental feelings while providing anticipatory guidance.

Syndactyly

Fusion, or webbing, between two digits is referred to as syndactyly. This condition is the most common anomaly of the hand, with an incidence of 1 in 2250 live births (Tachdijian, 1990b). Males are affected slightly more than females. Half of the time, both hands are involved in a symmetric presentation. Syndactyly of the fingers may be accompanied by syndactyly of the toes.

ETIOLOGY

Although most occurrences appear to be through spontaneous mutation, there have been reports of a familial predisposition, indicating an autosomal dominant pattern (Tachdijian, 1990b). Syndactyly may also be associated with a specific syndrome such as Apert's syndrome.

There are four classifications of syndactyly. Complete syndactyly is when the fusion is from the base to the tip of the digit. Fusion not extending to the tip of the digit is considered incomplete. Simple syndactyly refers to digits connected by skin and soft tissue. Fusion of digits involving an osseous connection is considered complex. Abnormal nerve and vessel configurations may accompany complex syndactyly.

TREATMENT

The type and timing of treatment depend on the classification. Surgery is directed toward promoting normal function and appearance. Fingers of unequal length should be separated within 6 to 12 months of age to prevent curvature of the longer finger deviated toward the shorter finger. If more than two adjacent digits are involved, surgery should be performed in stages so as to prevent vascular compromise of the middle digits.

COLLABORATIVE MANAGEMENT

Parents are instructed in physical therapy, specifically in massage of the interconnecting skin. This allows the webbed area to be stretched, thus providing for easier repair.

Polydactyly

Polydactyly is any duplication of digits beyond the normal five. It is the second most common hand anomaly. Polydactyly is believed to be caused by duplication of a single embryonic bud. Blacks are affected 10 times more often than whites. Blacks more often have postaxial polydactyly (duplication of the little finger), whereas preaxial polydactyly (duplication of the thumb) occurs primarily in whites. In blacks, postaxial polydactyly is typically an isolated incidence, whereas in whites it is associated with syndromes and chromosomal anomalies. Central axial polydactyly is the duplication of the ring, long, or index finger. It is often associated with complex syndactyly.

Polydactyly may be further classified into three types. Type I is merely a rudimentary soft tissue mass connected by a pedicle. Treatment of this type involves simple excision, which is often done in the newborn nursery before discharge. Type II is a partial duplication with involvement of the phalanges. Type III, a rare occurrence, involves complete duplication of the metacarpal and phalanges.

COLLABORATIVE MANAGEMENT

Treatment of types II and III centers on functional capacity first and appearance second. The infant is observed for which duplication is the dominant and most functional, and efforts are made to remove the least functional counterpart. If both duplicated digits appear to be equally functional, surgery should then be used to promote aesthetic appearance. Reparative surgery should be completed by 3 years of age.

Amniotic Band Syndrome

INCIDENCE AND PHYSIOLOGY

Amniotic band syndrome, with an incidence ranging from 1 in 5000 to 1 in 15,000 live births, is characterized by uncommon, asymmetrical fetal deformities (Ossipoff & Hall, 1977). Deformities that have been attributed to the amniotic band syndrome include congenital limb amputation, syndactyly, constriction bands, clubfoot, craniofacial defects such as cleft lip and palate, and visceral defects such as gastroschisis and omphalocele.

DIAGNOSIS

Many clinicians believe that amniotic bands must be present for the diagnosis of amniotic band syndrome to be made. However, others believe that the presence of fetal deformities in a nonanatomic pattern, without obvious bands, is sufficient to establish the diagnosis of the syndrome. Congenital deformations, such as the visceral and craniofacial types, in the absence of amniotic bands may go undiagnosed as amniotic band syndrome because they could represent a faulty midline developmental pattern during the first trimester of pregnancy instead of the production of amniotic bands that constricted or restricted growth. Therefore, the true incidence of this syndrome may be much higher than it generally appears, not only because of the difficulty establishing a diagnosis but also owing to the high mortality rate during gestation. Amniotic band syndrome has been implicated in fetal deaths secondary to cord compression by the constricting bands (Kalousek & Bamfort, 1988).

COLLABORATIVE MANAGEMENT

Constricting bands are usually associated with edema distal to the band. The resulting edema and vascular compromise contribute to complications such as skin breakdown, necrosis, thromboemboli formation due to venostasis, and infection. Care should include frequent vascular checks to assess perfusion. Trauma and tissue breakdown are discouraged through positioning and skin care. Observation for localized areas of necrosis is stressed.

As with other aesthetically disappointing musculoskeletal disorders, the family requires emotional and psychological support as adjustment to and acceptance of the infant are allowed to occur. They may be fearful that an extremity is going to be lost from necrotic tissue formation or infection. These fears may be justified, and the parents need to be prepared for such a possibility. Complete surgical repair may not be possible during the infant's initial hospitalization, necessitating frequent hospitalizations during the early developing years. The delay in repair may necessitate teaching parents how to observe the vascular perfusion of an extremity, signs of infection, and even dressing changes over open or healing areas. Preparation for discharge requires a multidisciplinary approach. The family may need surgical supplies, follow-ups by a home-visiting nurse, orthopedic or surgical consultations, pediatrician visits for general well-child care, and support of social or financial services to meet the long-term responsibilities of caring for their infant.

In addition, the nurse, working with the perinatal social worker, must attempt to provide opportunities for parent–infant bonding if the parents are to feel somewhat prepared for discharge. While the infant is still in the hospital, the parents must be encouraged to touch and talk to the infant and to participate in the infant's care. They must also be encouraged to verbalize their own feelings about their infant's condition. Every attempt should be made to attend to their fears, concerns, or misconceptions about the cause of their infant's problem. Only then will positive transition to home be possible.

Congenital Muscular Torticollis

INCIDENCE AND PHYSIOLOGY

Congenital muscular torticollis, with an incidence of 0.4 percent of all live births, is another musculoskeletal deformity with unknown pathogenesis (Coventry & Harris, 1959). It is known to be primarily a disorder of the sternocleidomastoid muscle.

DIAGNOSIS

Congenital torticollis can present within the neonatal period. Presentation may include a 1- to 3-cm, hard, palpable mass in the neck on the affected side accompanied by abnormal positioning of the head. Infants with congenital torticollis tilt the head to the affected side, and the chin is pointed upward in the opposite direction. Facial asymmetry may be a later-appearing sign. The face and skull on the affected side appear smaller.

In children with untreated congenital torticollis, or in cases with torticollis unresponsive to therapy, the shoulder on the affected side is raised in an effort to compensate for the abnormal head positioning. This form of compensation may lead to cervical and lumbar scoliosis as well as chronic back pain.

COLLABORATIVE MANAGEMENT

Traditionally, physical therapy is instituted immediately. Because congenital torticollis may resolve naturally within the first year of life, surgery is typically delayed until after 1 year of age. Persistent congenital torticollis past 1 year of age should be surgically treated to prevent the compensatory complications described.

Physical therapists and orthopedic surgeons should be consulted to assist in the management and subsequent follow-up of these infants. Family members should be taught home physical therapy, which should be performed at least twice daily. Parents should be counseled regarding the possibility of a neck brace to be worn by the infant postoperatively. It will most likely be the nurse's responsibility to coordinate consultations and to prepare the family with discharge instructions. In addition, the nurse must determine if the family lives in an area accessible to follow-up care. If not, a referral to social services or financial counseling may be needed for the family to be able to participate in follow-up physically and financially.

REFERENCES

Artz, T. D., Lim, W. N., Wilson, P. D., et al. (1975). Neonatal diagnosis, treatment, and related factors of congenital dislocation of the hip. *Clinical Orthopedics and Related Research, 110,* 112–136.

Baraitser, M., & Winter, R. M. (1996). *Color atlas of congenital malformation syndromes.* St. Louis: Mosby-Wolfe.

Barlow, T. G. (1962). Early diagnosis and treatment of congenital dislocation of the hip. *Journal of Bone and Joint Surgery, British Volume, 44,* 292–301.

Bennett, J. T., & MacEwen, G. D. (1989). Congenital dislocation of the hip: Recent advances and current problems. [Review.] *Clinical Orthopedics and Related Research, 247,* 15–21.

Bianchi, D. W., & Van Marter, L. J. (1994). An approach to ventilator-dependent neonates with arthrogryposis. *Pediatrics, 94,* 682–686.

Carter, C. O., & Wilkinson, J. A. (1964). Genetic and environmental factors in the etiology of congenital dislocation of the hip. *Clinical Orthopedics and Related Research, 33,* 119–128.

Clark, D. R., & Eteson, D. J. (1991). Congenital anomalies. In H. W. Taeusch, R. A. Ballard, & M. E. Avery (Eds.), *Schaffer and Avery's diseases of the newborn* (6th ed., pp. 159–191). Philadelphia: W. B. Saunders.

Coventry, M. B., & Harris, I. E. (1959). Congenital muscular torticollis in infancy. *Journal of Bone and Joint Surgery, 41,* 815.

Follis, R. H. (1952). Osteogenesis imperfecta congenita: A connective tissue diathesis. *Journal of Pediatrics, 41,* 713–721.

Francis, M. J., Smith, R., & Bauze, R. J. (1974). Instability of polymeric skin collagen in osteogenesis imperfecta. *British Medical Journal, 1,* 421–424.

Gardner, R. J. M. (1977). A new estimate of the achondroplasia mutation rate. *Clinical Genetics, 11,* 31–38.

Gertner, J. M., & Root, L. (1990). Osteogenesis imperfecta. *Orthopedic Clinics of North America, 21,* 151–162.

Hall, J. G. (1981). An approach to congenital contractures (arthrogryposis). [Review.] *Pediatric Annals, 10,* 15–26.

Hall, J. G. (1983). Arthrogryposes (congenital contractures). In A. E. Emery & D. L. Rimoin (Eds.), *Principles and practice of medical genetics* (pp. 58–69). New York: Churchill Livingstone.

Hall, J. G. (1989). Arthrogryposis. [Review.] *American Family Physician, 39,* 113–119.

Kalousek, D. K., & Bamfort, H. S. (1988). Amnion rupture sequence in previable fetuses. *American Journal of Medical Genetics, 31,* 63–73.

Moessinger, A. C. (1983). Fetal akinesia deformation sequence: An animal model. *Pediatrics, 72,* 857–863.

Ortolani, M. (1976). Congenital hip dysplasia in the light of early and very early diagnosis. *Clinical Orthopedics and Related Research, 119,* 6–10.

Ossipoff, V., & Hall, B. D. (1977). Etiologic factors in the amniotic band syndrome: A study of 24 patients. *Birth Defects, 13,* 117–132.

Palmer, R. M., Conneally, P. M., & Yu, P. L. (1974). Studies of the inheritance of idiopathic talipes equinovarus. *Orthopedic Clinics of North America, 5,* 99–108.

Robertson, N. R. C. (1984). Screening for congenital hip dislocation. *Lancet, 1,* 909–910.

Sillence, D. (1981). Osteogenesis imperfecta: An expanding panorama of variants. *Clinical Orthopedics and Related Research, 159,* 11–25.

Sillence, D. O., Rimoin, D. L., & Danks, D. M. (1979). Clinical variability in osteogenesis imperfecta: Variable expressivity or genetic heterogeneity. *Birth Defects, 15,* 113–129.

Sillence, D. O., Senn, A., & Danks, D. M. (1979). Genetic heterogeneity in osteogenesis imperfecta. *Journal of Medical Genetics, 16,* 101–116.

Tachdjian, M. (1990a). Congenital dysplasia of the hip: Embryology. In M. Tachdjian (Ed.), *Pediatric orthopedics* (Vol. 1, 2nd ed., pp. 297–312). Philadelphia: W. B. Saunders.

Tachdjian, M. (1990b). Syndactyly. In M. Tachdjian (Ed.), *Pediatric orthopedics* (Vol. 1, 2nd ed., pp. 222–236). Philadelphia: W. B. Saunders.

Wynne-Davies, R. (1964). Family studies and cause of congenital clubfoot. *Journal of Bone and Joint Surgery, 46B,* 445–465.

CHAPTER 19

Assessment and Management of Genitourinary Dysfunction

ASSESSMENT OF THE UROGENITAL SYSTEM

History

The history should focus on any family members with anomalies of the genitourinary system, cystic kidney disease, renal failure, or renal transplants or who have undergone dialysis. Do any family members have the fragile X syndrome or Turner's syndrome? Are there any abnormalities of the external genitalia, such as hypospadias, ambiguous genitalia, or undescended testes? Do any members have low-set ears or were they born with a single umbilical artery, both of which may indicate renal disorders?

The prenatal history should include whether there was polyhydramnios or oligohydramnios or an increased fetal abdominal area on an ultrasonogram, which may indicate renal impairment or anomalies.

The neonatal history should include the following questions:

- Has the infant undergone any hypoxic episodes that may result in delayed voiding? (The first voiding may occur in the delivery room or by 24 hours of life.)
- Is the infant feeding? If so, is the fluid intake sufficient (120 to 160 ml/kg/day in the term infant)? (Requirements for the premature infant may be greater, but this amount may not be achieved during the first 48 hours of life.)
- Is the infant under treatment for jaundice? (Phototherapy increases fluid losses.)
- Is the infant under a radiant warmer that increases insensible water loss?
- Is the infant experiencing any frank hemorrhaging or increased gastrointestinal losses such as are caused by nasogastric suctioning, vomiting, or diarrhea?
- What is the specific gravity of urine? (Normal range is 1.003 to 1.015.)
- How old is the infant?
- What is the gestational age?
- Has micturition taken place? If so, at what age?

Physical Assessment

INSPECTION

Observation of the abdominal region is an important place to start. Is there distention? If so, is it unilateral or generalized? Is there urine from the

453

umbilicus? Does the bladder appear distended? Abdominal asymmetry is an abnormal finding.

Next the genital area is inspected. Peritoneal tissue leading to the anal opening should be intact and smooth. Any abnormal openings, depressions, or swellings should be noted. The anus is normally located midline and should be tested for patency by gently inserting a gloved, well-lubricated small finger. The anal wink, which indicates muscle tone, may be tested by gently stroking the anal tissue and observing for anal sphincter constriction. Inspection is also made for meconium or stool.

Male

If this is a full-term male infant, is the scrotal sac full, with rugae present? The premature male exhibits a generally flaccid, smooth scrotal sac. The coloration of the scrotal sac is important. It is generally darkly pigmented without any bluish discoloration. A blue color may denote disruption of circulation to the area, and when coupled with dimpling, torsion of the testes must be suspected. The scrotum that is enlarged or very edematous may accompany a hydrocele (a trapping of fluid in the tunica vaginalis), or it may result from pressure on this tissue during the birth process, which is especially true in a breech birth. If a hydrocele is suspected, transillumination of the scrotum with a good light source such as a transilluminator or flashlight helps determine the presence of fluid. On transillumination, fluid allows light to pass through it, showing as a highly lightened area.

The penis should be observed for length. Is it abnormally large or small in proportion to the gestational age and the rest of the body parts? If the penile structure is enlarged, a renal problem may be present. The penis generally is straight. Any downward incurvation, bowing, or chordee most often is associated with hypospadias. Priapism, a constantly erect penis, is also an abnormal finding. The position of the urinary meatus is usually on the ventral portion, midline, of the glans penis. Alterations of this position result in dorsal or ventral placement anywhere along the shaft of the penis. With epispadias, the urinary meatus is on the dorsum of the penis, and with hypospadias the opening is displaced along the ventral penile surface. If the male is uncircumcised, the foreskin is gently retracted for accurate observation. This foreskin must be returned to its unretracted state after inspection; otherwise, swelling with associated decreased circulation to the glans penis will occur. The urinary stream should be straight.

Female

In the full-term female, are the labia majora present and extending beyond the labia minora? Are the labia minora well formed? Is the clitoris present? (The clitoral tissue may be enlarged in both the full-term and premature neonate.) If this is a premature female, the labia majora may well be smaller than the minora. The urinary meatus should be patent and anterior to the vaginal orifice. The vagina should be inspected for patency and any vaginal secretions noted. A white milky vaginal secretion in the first few days of life followed by pseudomenses or slight vaginal bleeding is a normal finding.

Both Sexes

The urine is most often straw colored. Hematuria is a significant finding in either sex, which may denote infection, urinary obstruction, renal necrosis, renal thrombosis, trauma, traumatic suprapubic tap, or administration of hyperosmotic or nephrotoxic drugs. A urine dipstick test may be performed to determine the presence of blood in the urine as well. This test also indicates the presence of urinary protein. Blood is a protein, so if blood is present, a positive protein test should also be expected. This test requires only one to two drops of urine be placed on the dipstick by a dropper, or the stick may be dipped into a specimen of urine. The results are obtained within 30 seconds to 1 minute after the stick is wet with urine. The exact timing for the most accurate reading is found on the bottles of dipstick materials, based on the manufacturer's suggested clinical timing cycle.

It is important to observe the genital and peritoneal regions to make certain that a clear differentiation of the sexes is possible. If it is not, a genetics consultation should be made.

PALPATION

This portion of the physical examination is upsetting to the newborn, so it is best left until last. On palpation, the infant is best placed in a supine position. Drawing the legs up with knees bent in the fetal position usually puts the infant at ease. In this position, gentle palpation of the abdomen is done gradually, moving downward, anteriorly to posteriorly. Kidneys may be felt on deep palpation. If palpation is not possible in this position, or if the infant starts crying, thus tensing the abdominal musculature, the palpation should be stopped and the infant repositioned.

Another technique that is sometimes successful is placing the infant again in the supine position, with one hand placed along the flank area posteriorly while the other hand is poised anteriorly to gently begin palpation. This technique allows the examiner a chance to trap the kidney's pole between the two hands (ballottement).

The kidneys, located in the flank area, are bilaterally equal in size. The right kidney may be slightly lower than the left kidney, owing to the position of other abdominal organs. Ureters are not palpable unless they are grossly enlarged (Scanlon, Nelson, Grylack, & Smith, 1979). No masses should be felt; however, if one is encountered, its position, mobility on palpation, and contour (either flat, lumpy, or depressed) must be accurately described. If Wilms' tumor is suspected, palpation should *not* be performed, because this may break the tumor into small fragments, leading to tumor seeding. Inguinal hernias may be found in either sex, although they are less frequent in females. Bladder distention or ureterocele sometimes exhibits a mobile mass.

Male

The scrotal sac may be palpated by gently pressing the tissue between two fingers, one located on the anterior surface and the other on the posterior surface. Gentle movement of the fingers upward over the scrotum until the testes are detected bilaterally will indicate if one or both testes are descended and where they are in relationship to the internal ring in the inguinal canal. The cremasteric reflex may be elicited at the same time by gently stroking the upper thigh or scrotal sac. A positive reflex is elicited when the testes recoil toward the inguinal canal (Scanlon, Nelson, Grylack, & Smith, 1979).

PERCUSSION

If bladder distention is palpated or observed, percussion should be done. This technique is useful in determining whether fluid is filling the bladder, denoted by a somewhat tympanic sound; if a solid mass is present, dullness is noted. Percussion may also be used over the entire abdominal region. Dullness is a normal finding at the right costal margin, indicating the liver. Tympany is the high-pitched sound noted over the gastric bubble just at the left costal margin. Over the intestines a semitympanic or more resonating sound is produced, depending on whether the neonate has been fed yet. If feeding has taken place, some intestinal gas may cause a tympanic sound; otherwise, if the infant is several days old and the gastrointestinal tract has begun to colonize with bacteria, feces may be present, causing a duller sound on percussion. Even with the newly born neonate, meconium may be present in the intestines in sufficient quantities to produce a duller sound. This finding alone does not necessarily indicate a problem. The intestines should be palpated and the abdomen inspected as well.

RELATED FINDINGS

Low-set ears and abnormal facies often accompany syndromes that have renal disorders as a component (Smith, 1988). A minor anomaly such as a single umbilical artery is a common finding when renal problems are present (Smith, 1988).

Meningomyelocele and other neural tube defects may result in decreased or absent innervation to the bladder. The result may be a neurogenic bladder characterized by bladder distention.

DIAGNOSTIC WORK-UP

Urinalysis

Although leukocytes may be present from vaginal drainage, infection should not be assumed unless bacteria are also present. Laundau, Turner, Brennan, and Majd (1994) found that a urinalysis is an effective method for initial screening for a differential diagnosis between acute pyelonephritis and lower urinary tract infection in neonates displaying a fever. Variables normally assessed in urinalysis include the following:

- pH
- Color
- Specific gravity
- Cells
- Odor
- Blood
- Protein

URINE COLLECTION

Urine collection is a relatively simple procedure in the neonate. Care is taken not to include the rectum or scrotum within the opening of the bag. Alternative collection systems can be used if sterile specimens are not required and accurate measurement of output is not needed. Cotton balls can be placed inside diapers to catch a small specimen for dipstick analysis or for measurement of specific gravity. In the male, test tubes or syringe barrels may be secured to the penis to collect small specimens. In the female, a disposable diaper can be placed plastic side toward the infant to obtain a small pool of urine. For long-term collections, the use of a collection bag with connecting tubing can be used to drain into a collection bottle.

Blood Urea Nitrogen and Creatinine

During the first few days of life, blood urea nitrogen levels may not reach beyond 20 mg/dl. Placental function has maintained normal serum fetal levels, which remain stable in the early newborn period. In many cases, dehydration can cause dramatic rises in serum levels in comparison with adult norms. Ingestion of high protein loads may affect levels in infants with normal renal function. Creatinine levels in the newborn are near adult levels at birth, then decline by 1 month of age. These levels, unless significantly elevated, may not be a clear indicator of renal disease.

Renal Clearance Tests

Renal clearance tests are of little value in the newborn. Although inulin clearance tests may be performed, other measurements may be more diagnostic in the newborn period.

Serum Chemistries

Dehydration, fluid overload, metabolic disorders, fluid and electrolyte losing disorders, and respiratory compromise all lead to alterations in serum electrolyte levels. High serum sodium levels may reflect severe dehydration, excessive fluid loss, or administration of high solute loads. Low sodium levels can occur with overhydration, the use of large amounts of free water, or inappropriate antidiuretic hormone secretion (Schreiner & Bradburn, 1988). Potassium losses are apparent in diuretic use and with episodes of diarrhea.

Urine Chemistries

In looking at serum electrolytes, urine chemistries are helpful in determining fluid and electrolyte balance. If urine sodium levels are outside normal values, serum levels may still be normal. In this instance, the infant may be struggling to retain or secrete sodium to maintain homeostatic balance.

Adrenocorticosteroid Levels

In the infant with adrenogenital syndrome, adrenocorticosteroid levels can be helpful in determining the specific disorder and treatment. The most common form is deficiency of 21-hydroxylase. In addition to physical evidence of deficiency on external genitalia examination, urine or plasma levels of 17-ketosteroids, pregnanediol, and 17α-hydroxyprogesterone are deficient (Goodman & Gorlin, 1983).

Urine Culture

In many cases, clean-catch specimens are obtained using either sterile or clean infant specimen collectors. When organisms appear on a culture report, a repeat culture is usually performed. The presence of leukocytes may not be an indication of infection, especially in the female, owing to vaginal secretions.

Latex Agglutination Test

The latex agglutination test is used to detect antigens produced by bacteria such as group B streptococci (Goetzman & Wennberg, 1991). It should be used in conjunction with other tests such as urine cultures to aid in accurate identification of a specific organism.

Suprapubic Tap

The performance of the suprapubic tap involves minimal equipment and time. The lower abdomen is prepped with an antimicrobial solution and allowed to dry. Palpation of the bladder is attempted, although it may not be felt in the neonate. If the infant has voided within the last hour, the attempt should be delayed until the infant has a full bladder. If severe dehydration, distention, or abdominal congenital anomalies are present, a suprapubic tap may not be warranted. A 3-ml syringe with an 18-gauge straight needle may be used. The needle is placed midline 1 to 1.5 cm above the symphysis pubis and inserted perpendicularly or at a slight angle pointing toward the head (Bradburn & Schreiner, 1988). Entry into the bladder is determined when resistance decreases as the needle is inserted. A slight traction on the plunger may be all that is necessary to aspirate urine into the syringe. If no urine is obtained on the first attempt, a second attempt should be delayed until sufficient urine build-up has occurred. Pressure should be applied over the puncture site until all evidence of bleeding has ceased.

Uterine and bowel perforations, trauma to other portions of the renal system, and infection are known complications. Suprapubic tap is not recommended for any neonate with clotting disorders or known disseminated intravascular coagulation.

Specific Gravity

Normal levels often fall in the range of 1.003 to 1.015. A low specific gravity may appear normal yet not be an accurate reflection of renal functioning, because the infant has a decreased ability to concentrate urine. High specific gravities often reflect dehydration versus high solute excretion. Excretion of glucose and protein in the urine may artificially increase the specific gravity in the newborn.

Radiologic Examination

The injection of contrast medium can be used to visualize kidney mass and ureter and bladder outline and to help in determining the amount of functioning kidney. In the premature infant, contrast medium should be used selectively, because the solution is hyperosmolar and may lead to further renal compromise. In instances when an intravenous pyelogram is ineffective in determining structure outlines, retrograde instillation of dye may be used.

Radionuclide Evaluation

Radionuclide evaluation may be necessary if pyelographic studies do not indicate accurate renal mass. The amount of uptake and timing of excretion both may indicate renal deficiencies.

Another radionuclide test is diuretic renography, which is used most often if hydronephrosis is suspected. A radioisotope injection is given, followed 15 minutes later by a diuretic injection. The diuretic facilitates the movement of the radioisotope through the renal system. The isotope's movement is tracked by a gamma computer. If there is a urinary obstruction, the isotope's progress is slowed or impeded, showing retention of the radioactive substance. If a dilation exists along the renal system, urine is retained at the uteropelvic junction, until overflow occurs with diuretic action. The stretching of the muscle fibers at this point causes strong contractions to begin. Soon the urine is released, thus rapidly moving the isotope along (about 20 minutes) and showing a sharp, immediate decline in isotope concentration. In a normal kidney, about 25 minutes is required to clear the system, showing a gradual decline in the isotope concentration. Institutional variations in selection of the diuretic and isotope are possible.

Renal Ultrasonography

Analysis can often determine differences in normal versus cystic tissue. Solid tumors and masses may be readily apparent. In most institutions, ultrasound examinations are performed before invasive studies are performed. In many cases, accurate and specific diagnosis may be determined from ultrasonography alone. Ultrasound evaluation also has been found useful in cases of scrotal swelling that were assumed to be torsion of the testes but were really due to an adrenal hemorrhage (Liu, Ku, Cheug, & Chan, 1994).

Another instance in which renal ultrasonography should be used as a screening tool is in the case of a single umbilical artery (Bourke et al., 1993). Some affected infants (with about a five times increase in renal anomalies over the general population) have renal anomalies that often result in vesicoureteric reflux. These anomalies are megaureter and abnormal positioning of one or both kidneys, dilation of ureters, and other morphologic abnormalities (Bourke et al., 1993). Renal ultrasonography is also helpful in determining ureteric reflux because this dysfunction will show as a ballooning of the renal pelvis (Hiraoka, Kasuga, Hori, & Sudo, 1994).

Computed Tomography

Computed tomography can be helpful in locating major structures. Its use is limited in providing specific diagnoses, and the cost may be prohibitive in relation to other available testing methods.

Genetic Consultation

Genetic consultation is an important part of the care for the infant with genital abnormalities. Chromosome banding and karyotyping should be performed if there is a positive family history of genitourinary anomalies or if a visible neonatal genitourinary malformation is present.

COLLABORATIVE AND NURSING MANAGEMENT

General Principles

ELECTROLYTE BALANCE

Prevention of hyperkalemia is most important in the management of renal failure. Potassium should never be added to an intravenous solution until an appropriate urine output has been established. When urine output declines, serum electrolytes should be frequently monitored to prevent the overload of fluids and potassium. Excess potassium, whether through excess administration or extracellular shift, can often be controlled through the use of an exchange resin (Kayexalate). Urine and serum chemistries should be monitored at least twice daily. Special attention should be paid to the serum potassium levels, because hyperkalemia is a consequence of renal failure. If sodium polystyrene sulfonate or Kayexalate is given by rectal suppository to reduce the potassium level, the nurse should observe for cardiac arrhythmias. One milliequivalent of potassium is exchanged for each 2 to 3 mEq of sodium. The usual dosage is 1 g/kg repeated every 4 to 6 hours (Kim & Mandell, 1988). If the serum potassium level is 7 mEq/L or more, Kim and Mandell (1988) suggest that 10 percent calcium gluconate, 0.5 to 1.0 ml/kg, be given intravenously slowly over 1 to 3 minutes. Continuous electrocardiographic monitoring is required. This should be followed by 2 to 3 mEq/kg of sodium bicarbonate intravenously, then 2 g/kg of 25 percent dextrose, and, finally, 0.5 to 1.0 unit/kg of insulin intravenously (Kim & Mandell, 1988, p. 73). Placement of the infant on a cardiorespiratory monitor is essential. Electrocardiograms are necessary to detect any abnormal rhythms or patterns that result from alterations in potassium levels. Dialysis can be used to return the body to normal potassium levels, but the use of long-term dialysis in the neonate is limited. Hypokalemia may result if diuretics such as furosemide (Lasix) are used. Again, close observation is critical.

Furosemide is used to treat congestive heart failure as well as fluid balance problems due to genitourinary problems. One experimental therapy aimed at decreasing the incidence of electrolyte imbalance is the use of nebulized furosemide. A single dose of 1 mg/kg of inhaled furosemide appears to be more effective than the intravenous route, with fewer side effects (Keszler, 1995). Whereas this therapy is experimental, if side effects such as hypokalemia can be diminished it certainly merits further investigation.

FLUID VOLUME AND NUTRITIONAL MANAGEMENT

Aggressive fluid management may lead to fluid overload and hypertension, which are often problems because of attempts to maintain adequate blood pressure levels, since sepsis and shock may precipitate oliguria. The use of antihypertensive agents and diuretics may be necessary to control blood pressure. Hydralazine, 0.2 to 0.5 mg/kg, intravenously or intramuscularly every 4 to 8 hours, or nitroprusside, 0.5 µg/kg/minute, or diazoxide, 1 to 3 mg/kg/dose, may be given (Kim & Mandell, 1988). The latter two drugs should be used with extreme caution in the neonate because they are very potent medications. Sodium levels should be checked because excess fluid dilutes the extracellular sodium. No treatment is needed if the neonate is showing no signs of hyponatremia. Hypertonic saline solution should be used with caution because it can raise the intracranial pressure. The sodium is increased by using the following formula (Kim & Mandell, 1988, p. 73):

$$\text{Dose of sodium (mEq)} = \text{weight (kg)} \times 5 \times 0.65$$

Nursing management involves the assessment and reporting of signs and symptoms. Fluid volume excess can be a problem. Daily or twice-daily weights should be obtained and recorded for baseline determination of any excessive fluid retention or loss. Accurate intake and output must be measured. This output may include the weighing of diapers. Urine specific gravity is checked every 4 hours. Fluid restriction may be important if hypovolemia is not a causative factor. This fluid restriction is based on insensible water loss in addition to the urinary output of the previous 24 hours (Ingelfinger, 1985). Alterations in fluids and electrolytes are another neonatal problem. Sodium, protein, and phosphorus restrictions may also be imposed, although if the infant is asymptomatic such electrolyte restrictions are not necessary. A formula low in phosphorus may be given in the form of Similac PM 60/40 or SMA. However, the formula should be checked for the amount of potassium present, because additional potassium may not be tolerated by the neonate who is already hyperkalemic (Ingelfinger, 1985). Aluminum hydroxide, 60 mg/kg, can be used to bind phosphate in the intestines and lower the phosphorus levels to the normal range of 5 to 6 mg/dl (Kim & Mandell, 1988). Use of aluminum hydroxide to bind phosphorus in the intestines may be helpful. Calcium supplements can be used after phosphorus level is lowered. The calcium often stabilizes on its own. However, calcium supplementation may also be needed because the calcium level is affected by the phosphorus level. These levels are inversely proportional—as one goes up, the other drops. Calcium gluconate (10 percent) or carbonate intravenously or orally may be given at a dose of 50 to 100 g/kg/day (Kim & Mandell, 1988). Such supplementation should be instituted when the calcium level drops below 6 mg/dl (Kim & Mandell, 1988). Calcium carbonate may help correct acidosis. One caveat, however, is that rapid administration of calcium can precipitate a cardiac arrest, thus requiring close observation by the nurse.

Dihydrotachysterol or vitamin D supplementation is also a useful adjunct to correct calcium levels, because under its influence, calcium is shifted from the bones, freed, and absorbed by the body.

In addition to these concerns, there is the problem of positive growth and nutrition. If a fluid restriction has been imposed, it is necessary to increase the caloric consumption without increasing fluid volume. MCT oil can be used to increase the fat content, or Polycose or Controlyte can be added to increase the carbohydrates. Hyperalimentation is a mode of nutrition needed by those infants no longer capable of enteral feedings. The overall goal of nutritional therapy is to preserve a positive nitrogen balance and to avoid increases in nitrogenous waste products that can lead to further increases in urea nitrogen levels and uremia (Kim & Mandell, 1988).

Close monitoring of serum electrolyte and phosphorus and calcium levels is necessary whether or not oral or intravenous electrolyte supplementation is being used. In addition, fluid shifts may occur secondary to fluid overload or a change in electrolyte balance, resulting in edema. Assessment for the presence of edema includes observation for periorbital edema, observation of dependent surfaces, and examination of the hands, feet, and scrotum. Pitting should be determined by gently depressing a fingertip into the suspected edematous site. Caution should be taken around the ocular area, since direct pressure on the eyeball may precipitate bradycardia. If ascites is present, the infant is gravely ill, because this is a late sign of renal failure.

SKIN MANAGEMENT

The infant's position should be changed every 2 hours, because swelling may accumulate in the dependent regions. Skin around any operative site should be inspected with every dressing change for any signs of irritation or infection. The skin must be kept dry and clean to prevent skin breakdown and infection.

RESPIRATORY MANAGEMENT

During fetal life, insufficient amniotic fluid is linked to a decreased development of the respiratory tree. The chest may be small in comparison with the distended abdomen.

The ability to use accessory muscles that help achieve effective respiration is lacking. This can lead to a decrease in ventilatory effort. In some cases, lung hypoplasia may result. Before extensive therapy is initiated to treat renal anomalies, careful evaluation of respiratory status should be performed. Measures to improve renal function should not be undertaken if there is insufficient respiratory capacity to support life.

General Preoperative Management

Preoperatively, the goal is to maintain the stability of the fluid and electrolyte balance and the hemodynamic status of the infant. Assessment for any signs of urinary tract infection such as poor feeding, temperature instability, cyanosis, or any other detectable subtle change from the infant's baseline norm should be done, because it is imperative to have the infant infection free, if possible, before surgery.

General Postoperative Management

Postoperatively, the nursing management is again focused on careful assessment and monitoring of the fluid and electrolyte status as well as the hemodynamic system, including blood pressure, pulse, and respiration of the infant. Accurate measurement of fluid intake and output is again critical. If an infant develops poor renal function in one kidney, surgical placement of a nephrostomy tube is needed (Sugar & Firlit, 1988). This tube's insertion site is covered with a sterile dressing.

The renal system is a highly vascular system, so the chance for bleeding or infection is great. After the insertion of a nephrostomy tube or tubes, it is not uncommon to have pink-tinged urine or even urine with visible bloody streaks. These tubes should *not* be irrigated because they are located within the renal pelvis. The tubes should be connected to a closed drainage system to maintain sterility. A clean dressing surrounding the tube to maintain the position and protect the underlying skin is important. On removal of such tubes, urine leakage for as long as 48 hours is not unusual.

Maintenance of an aseptic suture line is important. Any dressings, especially over a nephrostomy site, should be closely observed for bleeding or drainage. An infant with a nephrostomy tube or who has undergone other renal surgery is at risk for infection. Although broad-spectrum antibiotics such as ampicillin and gentamicin are useful, use of trimethoprim-sulfamethoxazole (Bactrim) is appropriate in the infant older than 2 months of age and without severe renal impairment. This drug is specific to the bacteria that most often cause urinary tract infections.

A urinary stent may also be placed in the ureter to splint the site of the anastomosis that has been performed. Although no drainage is expected through this stent, a closed drainage system is necessary to protect the neonate from infection. The infant may have a Foley catheter as well. Eventually the neonate may require a ureterostomy, followed by a nephrectomy if kidney function cannot be restored.

When urinary stents or suprapubic or nephrostomy tubes are used, it may be necessary to maintain the infant's position by placement in traction. Bryant's traction, a type of skin traction, may be used (Spindel, Winslow, & Jordan 1988).

Support to Parents

Collaboration among the neonatologist, pediatric urologist, nurse, clergy, social worker, and financial counselor helps the parents adjust to this frightening neonatal problem. If the infant is dying, early involvement by the clergy or other social support network—other parents, family or friends—can ease the pain of realizing that their child will not go home.

GENITOURINARY DISORDERS
Urinary Tract Infection
PATHOPHYSIOLOGY

Urinary tract infections in neonates are not common and are usually due to iatrogenic factors or urinary malformations/obstructions. Bacteria may be introduced during procedures such as suprapubic bladder taps.

Common infectious agents are gram-negative bacteria. These are most often introduced during urinary catheterization procedures. *Escherichia coli* and group B *Streptococcus* also may cause urinary tract infections. Seventy percent of all urinary tract infections are attributable to *E. coli*. This pathogen along with group B *Streptococcus* is normally found in the female genital tract, especially in the vagina. Thus, infants are exposed to these agents during the birth process. These organisms may be found on the neonatal skin surface; thus, if a good cleansing prep of the pubic area is done before a suprapubic tap, for instance, the pathogens may be removed. *Klebsiella, Pseudomonas,* and *Proteus* have also been implicated in urinary tract infections (Ingelfinger, 1985).

Fungal infections are becoming more common in those neonates with long-term health problems who have required invasive procedures, and they may cause pyonephrosis.

CLINICAL MANIFESTATIONS

Characteristics of urinary tract infections, if demonstrated, include the following (McCracken & Freij, 1987):

- Temperature instability
- Poor feeding
- Cyanosis
- Abdominal distention
- Poor weight gain
- Hepatomegaly
- Jaundice
- Thrombocytopenia purpura
- Fever
- Proteinuria

DIFFERENTIAL DIAGNOSIS

In any neonate suspected of having a urinary tract infection, a blood culture should be obtained, because overwhelming septicemia may be present (Ingelfinger, 1985). Positive diagnosis of a urinary tract infection is made when a urine culture grows the causative agent.

PROGNOSIS

The prognosis is directly dependent on the cause of such an infection.

COLLABORATIVE MANAGEMENT

Intravenous antibiotics are the drugs of choice. Because they are broad-spectrum antibiotics, ampicillin and gentamicin are preferred, unless the causative organism is not sensitive to these medications. The dosage of ampicillin is 100 mg/kg/day, and that of gentamicin is 3.5 to 7.5 mg/kg/day. These standardized neonatal dosages are dependent on functional kidneys and adequate urine output (1 ml/kg/hr). The physician should be notified immediately if urinary output is diminished. Another drug that is particularly useful for urinary tract infections is trimethoprim-sulfamethoxazole (Bactrim). It is especially effective in infections stemming from group A beta-hemolytic streptococci and *Staphylococcus, E. coli, Proteus mirabilis, Klebsiella,* and *Enterobacter.* This sulfonamide is not recommended in infants younger than 2 months of age or in those with severe renal dysfunction (Deglin & Vallerand, 1988).

An intravenous pyelogram and a voiding cystourethrogram should be done to ensure that no damage to the urinary tract exists. After the infection is cleared, radiologic tests and a renal ultrasonogram should be performed to determine if there is an obstruction or deformity (Ingelfinger, 1985). Otherwise, the infant will experience recurrent urinary tract infections.

Nursing Management

A review of the maternal and newborn history is essential. Maternal infections, especially of the genital tract, should be noted. Neonatal procedures such as suprapubic bladder taps should be noted along with the dates such procedures were performed. These dates give an estimation of the incubation time for possible pathogens.

A neonate with hepatomegaly, jaundice, or thrombocytopenic purpura may actually be exhibiting associated symptoms of urinary tract infections. This infant should be monitored closely for any baseline deviations and considered as potentially having a urinary tract infection.

Familial pyelonephritis is a risk factor for the development of neonatal renal dysfunction. Yet, pyelonephritis is not a common finding in the newborn period.

Careful assessment of the infant must include observation of fluctuations in temperature or the presence of fever. Temperature should be checked at least every 4 hours. If wide fluctuations are present or if there is a persistent temperature higher than 37.5°C measured rectally, temperature checks should be made every 1 to 2 hours. If fever is present, tachycardia greater than 160 beats per minute or tachypnea greater than 60 breaths per minute may also occur. For the premature infant whose temperature is consistently lower than the 36.5°C to 37°C range, the baseline norm should be used for each individual infant. If the temperature is consistently higher than previous temperatures, a fever should be suspected.

If the infant has an indwelling urinary catheter, observation of the urine for cloudiness or hematuria should be noted. A urine specimen should be sent for culture any time a urinary tract infection is suspected. Hematuria alone is not a good indicator of a urinary tract infection. A urine dipstick test may or may not be helpful, because proteinuria can indicate the presence of urinary bacteria. However, if hematuria is present, this finding is essentially useless because blood is a protein.

Especially worrisome is a neonate who begins to progressively lose weight or does not feed as well as in the past. Gastrointestinal disturbances such as vomiting and diarrhea may also suggest a urinary tract infection (Ingel-finger, 1985).

Circumcision

The removal of the prepuce, or foreskin, covering the glans penis may be done in the delivery room or in the newborn nursery. The actual decision to circumcise is usually based on parental cultural values and beliefs.

Circumcision does make the cleansing of the penis and removal of smegma (the whitish secretions generally found lying underneath the fore-skin) easier.

Neonatal local anesthesia should be used to reduce the discomfort (Stang et al., 1988). Parents should be taught to observe the penis for any drainage or bleeding. They should have an explanation about the Plastibell if it is left in place, including how long it will be on the penis and the fact that it will fall off. They need to be shown how to cleanse the penis without introducing bacteria.

Acute Renal Failure

PATHOPHYSIOLOGY

Acute renal failure is a diminished or complete stoppage of kidney function. Any condition that potentially interferes with kidney function can lead to acute renal failure. It is most often associated with an accelerated production of vasoconstrictor prostaglandins, which result in vasoconstriction of the renal vessels. Thus, the blood flow through the kidneys is diminished, as is the glomerular filtration rate (Sadler, 1995). Acute renal failure has been estimated to affect as many as 25 percent of all neonates admitted to an intensive care unit (Brion, Satlin, & Edelmann, 1994).

Acute renal failure occurs in three forms: prerenal, intrarenal, and postrenal. Prerenal failure results from congenital conditions such as cystic disease, aplasia, or nephrosis; acquired conditions such as clotting or necrosis; ischemia due to hypotension or hypoxia; nephrotoxic exposure due to drug therapy (e.g., aminoglycosides, methicillin, or indomethacin); high technology therapies such as extracorporeal membrane oxygenation or use of contrast dye in radiologic testing; and miscellaneous conditions such as acidosis, polycythemia, or urinary tract infections (John & Yeh, 1985; White, Richardson, & Raibstein, 1990).

In the prerenal type of renal failure, urine output in the neonate is directly influenced by the perfusion of the kidneys. Prerenal failure causes hypovolemia and hypoperfusion. Reversing the effects of hypovolemia and hypotension may prevent the occurrence of renal damage.

Intrarenal causes such as acute tubular necrosis, use of maternal or neonatal nephrotoxic drugs, renal agenesis, pyelonephritis, nephritis, hypoplasia or dysplasia, or birth trauma may result in renal failure (Fanaroff & Martin, 1992).

Postrenal failure is usually caused by congenital anomalies that obstruct flow of urine. A back-up of urine into the kidney pelvis inhibits the ability of the kidneys to function. If this condition persists, fluid permanently fills the tissue spaces. Damage can occur as early as the 16th to 18th weeks of gestation (Inturrisi, Perry, & May, 1985). Hydronephrosis may be nonreversible, leading to renal failure in one or both kidneys. Oliguria of the fetus leads to oligohydramnios, which may be detected on maternal physical examination. Familial tendency for some renal disorders may suggest antenatal testing for fetal renal disease in identified groups.

Persistent acute renal failure after the initial insult is related to tubular obstruction from cell debris. This decrease in blood flow leads to tubular damage and loss of sodium, resulting in release of renin, thereby decreasing the glomerular filtration rate. The lack of renin release leads to a loss of sodium and water, which accounts for high output failure (John & Yeh, 1985).

Acidosis may readily follow acute renal failure.

RISK FACTORS

Risk factors for acute renal failure are listed below:

- Treatments such as mechanical ventilation and umbilical and femoral vessel catheterization
- Birth injury
- Hypovolemia
- Hypoxemia
- Aplastic kidney
- Polycystic renal disease
- Necrosis
- Maternal ingestion of nephrotoxic agents
- Prematurity
- Respiratory distress syndrome
- Prenatal exposure to indomethacin
- Maternal use of acetaminophen in excess (potentially nephrotoxic)
- Lithium use (potentially nephrotoxic)

DIFFERENTIAL DIAGNOSIS

The specific diagnostic tests are determined by what the practitioner suspects is the contributing process.

CLINICAL MANIFESTATIONS

Clinical features of acute renal failure may include the following:

- Decreased urine output—oliguria
- Edema
- Lethargy
- Hematuria
- Proteinuria
- Abdominal distention
- A flank mass

LABORATORY/ASSESSMENT CONSIDERATIONS

The maximum fetal urine electrolytes considered within normal limits are sodium, 100 mEq/L; chloride, 90 mEq/L; and osmolality, 210 mOsm/kg

(Grupe, 1987). Levels higher than these values indicate renal failure and a poor prognosis.

- Blood urea nitrogen and serum creatinine levels are elevated.
- Urine output should be at least 1 ml/kg/hr.
- Shock and volume depletion should always be evaluated when oliguria results.
- In the presence of open or draining congenital anomalies, hidden fluid losses may occur.
- Surgery to repair defects can lead to "third spacing" of fluids.

COMPLICATIONS

Complications of acute renal failure are as follows:

- Hyperkalemia
- Volume overload
- Hyponatremia
- Hypertension
- Acidosis
- Hypocalcemia
- Hyperphosphatemia
- Nutritional problems
- Sepsis
- Anemia
- Azotemia

The blood pressure may at first be hypotensive, then rebound to an above-normal level. Hypertension, greater than 90/65 mm Hg in term infants, is often due to fluid overload or increased secretion of renin and aldosterone.

PROGNOSIS

The prognosis of acute renal failure is solely dependent on the ability to treat the underlying problem.

COLLABORATIVE MANAGEMENT

Symptomatic treatment is carried out until a definitive cause is determined and treated.

- Intravenous isotonic solution, 10 to 20 ml/kg given over 1 hour, is administered if there are no signs of heart failure.
- Mannitol and furosemide are given to prevent acute renal failure.
- Dopamine may also be tried in low doses (John & Yeh, 1985).
- Fluid replacement is limited to insensible loss and replacement of renal output.
- If acidosis is present, sodium bicarbonate is used instead of sodium chloride in the solution but with caution (hypertonic).
- For hyponatremic acute renal failure, fluids are restricted.
- Peritoneal dialysis or hemodialysis should be used only in infants with

severe congestive heart failure, fluid overload, or uremia. Peritoneal dialysis seems to be the method of choice.

- Drugs with high sodium levels, such as carbenicillin, penicillin G, ampicillin, and cephalothin, or drugs diluted in sodium chloride should be used with caution.

Nursing Management

Nursing care is aimed at maintaining fluid and electrolyte balance. It is also necessary to accurately calculate fluid intake and output to guard against fluid overload and resultant hypertension and edema. Nurses must remember, too, that potassium affects cardiac conduction. Therefore, because these neonates may experience hyperkalemia, all intake of potassium must be eliminated. This includes use of only fresh blood for transfusions, because the older the blood, the more likely the cells are to have broken down, releasing potassium. Calcium gluconate (10 percent) or calcium carbonate helps decrease the effect of potassium on the heart.

Increased phosphorus and decreased calcium levels are treated by restricting protein. Calcium supplementation and phosphorus-binding substances may be needed. The infant's hematocrit and hemogloblin level must be measured at least daily.

Hypertension, secondary to fluid overload, may be treated by sodium and fluid restriction. Antihypertensive agents may also be tried. Dialysis may be indicated if the condition is severe.

Signs of infection should be watched for and reported to the physician or neonatal practitioner so that treatment is begun immediately.

Metabolism of drugs is altered when renal failure occurs. Aminoglycosides, penicillins, cephalosporins, theophylline, indomethacin, tolazoline, and magnesium should all be used with caution.

Nutritional needs for the infant are 1 to 1.5 g/kg/day of protein with 30 to 50 cal/kg/day. Vitamin D, vitamin B complex, and folic acid supplements may be needed. Vitamin A should be avoided. Breast milk, Similac PM 60/40, and SMA are recommended by some institutions because of their decreased sodium, potassium, and phosphorus loads.

If the infant's condition continues to deteriorate and high blood urea nitrogen levels coupled with increasing ammonia levels are present, dialysis may be necessary. This procedure may be performed in the neonatal intensive care unit and requires one-on-one nursing care. The dialyzing cycle is dependent on medical treatment and the severity of the condition. Nursing responsibility includes monitoring the equipment, monitoring the cycles if done manually, doing clotting studies, and administering heparin and other drugs via the dialysis setup. Either hemodialysis or peritoneal dialysis may be performed.

Catheter care includes maintenance of aseptic technique, prevention of hemorrhage and clotting, and observation of the insertion site for signs of infection or dislodgment. Signs and symptoms of chemical imbalances should be observed for during the entire dialysis procedure. Fluid shifts affecting blood pressure and electrolyte balance can occur rapidly, causing cardiac arrhythmias, muscle spasms, seizures, and shock.

Potter's Association (Syndrome)

PATHOPHYSIOLOGY

Potter's association is an association of defects that begins with bilateral renal agenesis. For this reason, the term *syndrome* is generally being replaced by the word *association*. It occurs when the uretic bud fails to divide and develop, culminating in bilateral renal agenesis. Renal agenesis is the complete absence of the kidney. Because fetal urine is a major component of amniotic fluid, oligohydramnios is present. In the severest form, no amniotic fluid may be present. The developing fetal structures are compressed because of this lack of fluid, leading to the characteristic Potter facies.

CLINICAL MANIFESTATIONS

The signs and symptoms of Potter's association are listed below:

- Ears—low set and malformed
- Micrognathia
- "Senile" appearance
- Wrinkled skin
- Parrot-beak nose
- Wide-set eyes with obvious epicanthal folds
- Abnormal genital development
- Leg deformities
- Gastrointestinal defects
- Arthrogryposis, a condition associated with contractures of the extremities
- Breech delivery
- Small for gestational age

RISK FACTORS

The incidence is 1 in 10,000 births, with the condition being found predominantly in males (Goodman & Gorlin, 1983). Although no strong genetic predisposition exists, siblings of infants with Potter's association have a higher than average incidence of neural tube defects.

DIFFERENTIAL DIAGNOSIS

Potter's association is usually readily identifiable on direct observation because of its characteristic facies. Most often no other diagnosis is even questioned. Potter's association is also a part of the XYY syndrome.

PROGNOSIS

The infant may die within the first several days of life because of lack of kidney tissue to support life. Because of the association of renal agenesis with lung hypoplasia, death often occurs as the result of respiratory insufficiency.

COLLABORATIVE AND NURSING MANAGEMENT

Focus is placed on the parents. The nurse must offer the parents the chance to see and hold their child, but some parents may fear attachment. It is often helpful even after the infant's death to allow siblings to see and touch the infant for incorporation of the infant into a small child's reality.

Aplastic Kidney

PATHOPHYSIOLOGY

When the uretic bud fails to form in utero, aplasia or absence of the kidney occurs. One kidney develops while the other kidney does not. This is also called unilateral renal agenesis.

RISK FACTORS

The rate of occurrence may be as high as 1 in 500 births (Kaplan, 1994). It is most often associated with other structural defects.

CLINICAL MANIFESTATIONS

The infant may be asymptomatic. The exact symptoms exhibited are directly associated with the type of renal problem the infant is experiencing.

DIFFERENTIAL DIAGNOSIS

The differential diagnosis centers on the confirmation of the presence of a single kidney by renal ultrasonography.

PROGNOSIS

The prognosis for survival with a single kidney is excellent if the remaining kidney is disease free.

COLLABORATIVE AND NURSING MANAGEMENT

If kidney function is not compromised, no nursing care beyond normal newborn care may be necessary. If kidney disease is found, management is specific to the cause.

Cystic Kidney Disease

PATHOPHYSIOLOGY

Cystic disease of the kidney involves the replacement of normal kidney mass with cysts. Cystic disease includes a variety of disorders such as polycystic disease and multicystic disease.

Infantile polycystic disease is a genetic autosomal recessive disease. The cystic lesions occur in the collecting tubules. Cystic lesions may also occur in the liver, bile duct, and pancreas. The disease generally involves both kidneys and has a poor prognosis. Adult-type polycystic disease is an autosomal dominant disease that is rarely seen in infants. When it occurs, it leads to serious renal compromise and death.

Multicystic kidney disease is a noninherited disorder. It usually follows an obstructive uropathy in utero and is most often unilateral. Back-up of urine causes the fluid-filled kidney mass to develop into cystic lesions.

RISK FACTORS

There are no specific risk factors.

CLINICAL MANIFESTATIONS

The abdomen may be enlarged with an apparent palpable mass. The mass may not be perceived as a kidney, because the cystic lesions distort its normal shape. In single-kidney cystic disease, normal urine output is maintained. The affected kidney has a high potential for infection owing to urinary stasis. Albuminuria occurs in polycystic kidney disease.

DIFFERENTIAL DIAGNOSIS

Ultrasonography and pyelograms are necessary to differentiate between normal renal mass and cystic lesions. These tests should be delayed until age 48 hours to allow the neonate to become hydrated and restore fluid balance after birth. A voiding cystogram should be done with those infants who are highly suspect for having cystic disease. With cystic kidney disease, if one kidney is functional, the serum and urine chemistries may be normal. A renal scan helps differentiate between ureteropelvic junction obstruction and multicystic kidney disease. The radioactive isotope will be concentrated in a mass, whereas in ureteropelvic junction obstruction, the isotope will continue on into the renal pelvis (King, 1988; Radhakrishnan, 1990).

PROGNOSIS

The prognosis is poor for infantile polycystic disease. The prognosis for multicystic disease is directly dependent on the severity of kidney damage. It also has been noted that infants with multicystic disease are at greater risk for later development of Wilms' tumor, a malignancy with a relatively poor prognosis. More research is needed in tracking this possible relationship.

Tissue hypertrophy in the contralateral, normal kidney begins at birth. Thus, the body compensates for the loss of one kidney.

COLLABORATIVE MANAGEMENT

Treatment for single-kidney cystic disease is complete nephrectomy, because the diseased kidney may continue to harbor infection. This infection may spread to the unaffected kidney. A partial nephrectomy may be performed if sufficient unaffected renal mass is found. If the cystic disease is the result of a ureteropelvic junction obstruction, pyeloplasty has been successful.

Nursing Management

If Wilms' tumor is suspected, no palpation should be done, because the tumor can break up and may be spread in this fashion. If urine output is normal, careful consideration of the fluid intake and output may not be necessary; but for the infant with compromised renal function, strict attention must be paid to fluid balance. Electrolyte status must be checked at least daily. Urine should be checked for the presence of albumin. Because hydronephrosis may be present, hematuria is also a consideration.

Before surgery a complete blood cell count with differential and a urine culture should be obtained, because the infant is at risk for a urinary tract infection.

Hypertension is related to decreased arterial renal perfusion with concomitant elevations in renin levels (King, 1988). A nephrectomy reverses this trend.

If the infant undergoes a complete nephrectomy, strict adherence to aseptic technique must be followed. The infant is prone to infection, so vital signs should be monitored at least every 2 to 4 hours after the immediate postoperative period. Any dressings should be inspected for the presence of bloody drainage or secretions. Initially, a small amount of bleeding at the site is common, but it should be short-lived. No urine drainage should be noted on the dressing, because the entire kidney has been removed. Abdominal decompression is often necessary to prevent distention that could cause pressure and pull the suture line apart. If a nasogastric tube is in place, it should be irrigated with 2 ml of saline or air every 2 to 4 hours to maintain patency.

Feedings may be resumed once bowel sounds can be auscultated and the nasogastric tube has been removed. Feedings are usually tolerated 2 to 3 days after surgery.

Prune-Belly Syndrome (Eagle-Barrett Syndrome)

PATHOPHYSIOLOGY

A congenital lack of appropriate abdominal musculature, undescended testes, and urinary tract malformations are the classic characteristics. The abdominal muscles may be so weakened that the abdominal region actually appears wrinkled, much like a prune's surface. It typically affects males; in the female, the true syndrome does not exist (Short, Groff, & Cook, 1985). Pseudohermaphroditism may be associated.

The incidence rate is approximately 1 in every 50,000 births (Goodman & Gorlin, 1983).

The associated urinary problems include an enlarged bladder and dilated, curved ureters (megaureter). A patent urachus may also be associated. Other associated problems include hip and feet deformities, respiratory insufficiency, imperforate anus, and cardiac anomalies. Owing to an imbalance of muscle pull, spinal deformities may occur.

No clear etiology is known for prune-belly syndrome, but the defect may occur between the 23rd day and the 10th week of fetal development.

RISK FACTORS

No clear risk factors are known to precipitate this syndrome. Maternal use of cocaine, however, has been documented as a known teratogen resulting in prune-belly syndrome, among other genitourinary anomalies (Chasnoff, Chisum, & Kaplan, 1988; Rosenstein, Wheeler, & Heid, 1990).

CLINICAL MANIFESTATIONS

The musculature defect may be small or may cover the entire surface of the abdomen. Although all layers of musculature are present, the degree of development of these muscle layers varies. A thin layer of subcutaneous tissue coupled with distention gives the abdomen a wrinkled appearance. Cryptorchidism (undescended testes), prostatic urethral dilatation, bladder distention, patent urachus, abdominal distention or protuberance, malrotation of the intestines, varying cardiac defects, congenital hip dysplasia and associated "click," and clubfoot (talipes equinovarus) are some of the other associated clinical findings.

DIFFERENTIAL DIAGNOSIS

Underlying renal disease must be distinguished from abdominal muscle defects with accompanying renal dysfunction. What must be determined is the exact nature of the renal problem, the degree to which renal function is compromised, and what other deformities might also be present. The exact diagnosis can be made only when a demonstrable lack of abdominal musculature is present.

Appropriate diagnostic tests for determination of definitive renal disease would include abdominal radiographs and renal ultrasonography, intravenous pyelography, voiding cystography, and blood urea nitrogen and creatinine analysis (Brueggemeyer, 1988).

PROGNOSIS

The prognosis is directly related to the degree of severity of the underlying renal dysfunction. As many as 50 percent of infants afflicted with prune-belly syndrome may die within the first 2 years of life if severe renal dysfunction or chronic renal failure is present (Goodman & Gorlin, 1983).

COLLABORATIVE MANAGEMENT

This triadic anomaly leads to severe urinary tract complications. The condition of the kidney can range from normal kidney mass to complete atresia. In many cases, dilatation of the ureter, bladder, and urethra occurs, which may be caused by a lack of muscle fiber in the lining of the structures. The lack of muscle in the ureters leads to their elongation and distention. If obstruction occurs as a result of the tortuous nature of the ureters, surgical intervention may be necessary. Reimplantation or diversion may be necessary to prevent urine stasis and renal failure.

Obstruction of the urethra may be caused by angulation, owing to a lack of musculature in the urethra or by an obstructive action due to distention of the enlarged prostatic urethra (Tank & McCoy, 1983). Surgical correction may not achieve bladder functioning, because bladder atonia persists.

This syndrome is accompanied by undescended testes. Orchiopexy may be performed.

Bladder decompression is necessary to prevent stasis. Any severe abdominal distention and insufficient urinary output in the first day of life observed by the nurse should be evaluated by other members of the health care team to rule out the possibility of this syndrome. Renal dysplasia is an abnormal development of the kidney or its associated structures. It is most commonly seen as aplastic kidneys and multicystic disease (Fanaroff & Martin, 1992).

If urine drainage is compromised, nephrostomy or ureterostomy diversion should be undertaken. Peristalsis may be absent or deficient. A vesicostomy may allow temporary drainage until extensive surgical intervention is tolerated by the infant. Long-term use of antimicrobial therapy may be necessary to prevent sepsis. In the presence of a patent urachus (fetal communication between the bladder and umbilicus), closure may not be necessary in the neonatal period if adequate drainage and prevention of infection can be maintained. If the bladder is distended, reduction cystoplasty is done to relieve the tension on the bladder and promote emptying (Hanna, 1989).

Long-term therapy includes exercise, the use of abdominal binders, and reconstructive surgery. Although not curative, these methods provide some palliative benefit to the appearance and function of the distended and sagging abdomen.

The effects of renal damage that occur in the early stages of life require careful attention to fluid and electrolyte balance, removal of wastes, and adequate nutrition for growth and development.

Nursing Management

Fluid intake and output should be strictly measured and recorded. If an appliance is used, skin surfaces must be kept clean and dry. The use of adhesives may be necessary to prevent leakage around the stoma, owing to skin folds and wrinkling. Turning and repositioning every 2 hours also helps decrease skin breakdown. Bladder decompression may be accomplished by intermittent catheterization or the Credé method. The use of the Credé method may be sufficient to empty the bladder. This method involves placing both hands under the infant's flank area and bringing the practitioner's thumbs together at the umbilicus. Pressure is gently applied and the thumbs are rolled downward from the umbilicus to the symphysis pubis.

Parents must be taught the signs and symptoms of a urinary tract infection. If a vesicostomy or other urinary diversion has been performed, specific instructions are necessary to prevent bladder contamination. Stoma care is another aspect of parent education and discharge planning.

Lack of abdominal musculature also can lead to constipation. Suppository use and bowel training may be necessary. Feedings should not promote distention and respiratory compromise. Parents should be well informed of dietary approaches to aid in management of this disorder.

Exstrophy of the Bladder

PATHOPHYSIOLOGY

In exstrophy of the bladder, the anterior abdominal wall fails to close at the point of the bladder. During the first 4 weeks of gestation, the abdominal wall begins to fuse. When the mesenchymal cells fail to migrate over the abdomen, exstrophy results. A thin membrane forms over the abdominal contents, which may later rupture, leaving the bladder exposed.

RISK FACTORS

The incidence of this defect is 1 in 24,000 to 40,000 live births, with males being affected more than females (King, 1980; O'Donnell, 1984). Exact risk factors are not known.

CLINICAL MANIFESTATIONS

This condition is obvious on visual inspection. The bladder region appears open or uncovered. Because of the failure of the abdominal and anterior bladder wall to close, the posterior wall of the bladder is then exposed. The implantation of the ureters may be visible as urine continues to pass from the orifices. This defect occurs most frequently in the male, with a concomitant defect in the genitalia. In the male, the penis may be short, flat, and angulated. Epispadias may occur to the extent that proper sex identification may be difficult. In the female, the labia do not meet in the midline, and there is a divided clitoris. The defect may also include a prolapse of the rectum. This prolapse may occur through the abdominal wall defect, requiring an intestinal diversion. The failure of the pubic bones to meet anteriorly may lead to hip and leg deformities. Neurospinal defects, omphalocele, and other chromosomal abnormalities may occur with this defect.

DIFFERENTIAL DIAGNOSIS

The diagnosis of exstrophy of the bladder may be done on visual inspection.

PROGNOSIS

The exact prognosis is directly related to the presence of other deformities.

COLLABORATIVE MANAGEMENT

Before surgical correction, the defect is covered with a petrolatum dressing and sufficient gauze to absorb urine flow. This dressing should be changed when it becomes saturated. The skin should be observed for extreme dryness. Addition of humidification in the incubator helps prevent the drying. Diapers should be kept folded well below the defect.

Urinary tract infection is not common if abdominal dressings are changed regularly.

Primary closure of the defect is usually performed in the neonatal period.

Some institutions perform a staged approach to closure and correction of genital defects. Closure in some cases may be delayed for a year or longer without serious complications. Before surgery is performed, broad-spectrum antibiotics (ampicillin and gentamicin) are started to add protection against infections. These are continued for at least 7 days postoperatively, because 42 percent of wound dehiscence is due to infections (Mesrobian, 1988). Strict observation of aseptic technique when working with these infants is essential. If infection is suspected, aggressive treatment should be started.

Surgical correction of the defect does not guarantee continence. In some cases, urinary diversion or the use of ileal conduits may be necessary. In the infant with concomitant neurospinal defects, continence might never be achieved (O'Donnell, 1984). The nurse may need to coordinate follow-up by surgical, medical, and neurosurgical teams. Long-term follow-up may include the use of social services and financial counseling.

Nursing Management

Petrolatum-impregnated gauze should be used to protect the moist surface from trauma or drying. Preweighed gauze dressings can be used to collect and measure urine output. If accurate output measurement is not necessary, diapers may be used to collect urine drainage. If rectal prolapse has occurred through the abdominal defect, separate dressings should be maintained if possible.

Hydronephrosis

PATHOPHYSIOLOGY

Hydronephrosis is the accumulation of urine within the renal pelvis and calices to the point of overdistention. Hydronephrosis often follows obstruction of urine flow at the junction of the ureteropelvis, ureterovesical valve, or urethrovesical valve. The build-up of fluid that then accumulates in the kidney leads to distention of the renal pelvis and damage of the kidney mass. If only one ureter is affected, then damage occurs to that kidney only, leaving the other capable of supporting life. In some cases, hydronephrosis can be treated by removing the obstruction before permanent damage has occurred.

Prevention of hydronephrosis is possible in some circumstances. Fetal surgery may be done, which can relieve the obstruction in utero by placing a catheter into the bladder to drain the urine, thus preventing the infant from being born with permanently damaged kidneys. After birth, definitive surgery is performed to correct the obstructive defect or provide diversion of urine flow.

RISK FACTORS

Any factor or condition that potentially obstructs renal or urinary flow may contribute to the development of hydronephrosis.

CLINICAL MANIFESTATIONS

In the newborn, hydronephrosis may be detected as a large, solid palpable smooth mass at the region of the kidney. Urine output may be decreased or normal. Urinary tract infection often accompanies hydronephrosis, making fever and discomfort observable signs. Gross hematuria may be present and must be differentiated from hematuria associated with Wilms' tumor and renal vein thrombosis.

DIFFERENTIAL DIAGNOSIS

Clinical diagnostic studies include pyelograms, ultrasonograms, and computed tomograms. Intravenous pyelograms may not be definitive in that interpretation of the results could indicate nonexistence of the kidney because the fluid-filled mass does not readily pick up the dye. Kidney outline can be determined with a retrograde pyelogram. Before attempting drastic reparative procedures, respiratory status must be assessed.

PROGNOSIS

The prognosis for this condition depends on the underlying causative factor and the degree of severity of the permanent renal damage.

COLLABORATIVE MANAGEMENT

Hydronephrosis is managed according to its cause.

Nursing Management

Presence of cyanosis, grunting, nasal flaring, and retractions is important, because the lungs may not have fully developed. The chest should be observed for any alterations in the anteroposterior diameter or asymmetry. Vital signs, including blood pressure, must be monitored at least every 4 hours and more frequently if the infant's condition is unstable. The blood pressure is especially important, because hypertension is not uncommon in the hydronephrotic infant. If hypertension is severe, antihypertensive agents may be given. Some institutions use intravenous hydralazine, intravenous diazoxide, or methyldopa. Use of any of these drugs requires extremely close monitoring of the cardiorespiratory system. Fluid and electrolyte status also must be carefully watched. Fluid intake and output should be recorded at least every 2 to 4 hours. Specific gravity may be checked every 4 to 8 hours. A urine dipstick may be useful to determine the presence of protein or hematuria. Assessment of the hydration status is important. The fontanelles should be observed to determine if they are sunken, dehydrated, or bulging. Skin turgor should demonstrate instant recoil.

The presence of any dependent or pitting edema should be checked for and recorded. Palpation of the abdomen is also helpful to determine if a mass is present.

Postoperatively, a nephrostomy or urinary stent may be placed. These are connected to a closed drainage system.

Ureteral Obstruction

PATHOPHYSIOLOGY

Ureteral obstruction occurs when the developing ureter fails to form a tube or the junction of the kidney pelvis or bladder is constricted. Most commonly, the obstruction occurs at the ureteral junction of the kidney pelvis; the second most common site is the junction of the bladder. Unilateral or bilateral obstructions may occur. The result is a back-up of urine into the affected kidney, resulting in a fluid-filled kidney. In some instances, complete obstruction does not occur, and minimal functioning persists until the child is older and symptomatology increases. Recurrent infection of the urinary tract should be investigated in the young child. The presence of static fluid in the kidney leads to permanent damage of renal tissue. The fluid may be contained in a sac or cyst-like lesion on the ureter.

RISK FACTORS

Cystic kidney disease, polycystic kidney disease, ureteropelvic junction obstruction, and urethral atresia are among the most common causes of this entity.

CLINICAL MANIFESTATIONS

An infant may be asymptomatic unless complete obstruction is present. Delayed voiding or failure to void may be a sign. Hematuria may or may not be present. Because the presence of a blocked ureter may lead to hydronephrosis, an enlarged, palpable kidney may be the first indication of a problem.

DIFFERENTIAL DIAGNOSIS

A radiologic examination after a renal scan or ultrasonogram will help to determine the cause.

PROGNOSIS

The prognosis is directly dependent on the severity of kidney damage. The lesser the damage, the greater the chances for survival if no other lethal conditions are present.

COLLABORATIVE MANAGEMENT

Correction or repair of the blocked ureter may lead to reversal of hydronephrosis. If permanent damage has occurred, nephrectomy may be performed. Once surgical correction is completed, long-term medical care is essential for early detection of chronic renal problems.

Nursing Management

The nurse must observe for signs of decreasing urine output. The infant may be edematous, making good skin care a high priority. Infection may be present and should be treated before surgical intervention.

Hydrocele

PATHOPHYSIOLOGY

Hydrocele is the collection of fluid in the scrotal sac.

RISK FACTORS

The premature infant and the infant who experiences increased abdominal pressure secondary to manual resuscitation and high ventilatory pressures are at risk for hydrocele.

CLINICAL MANIFESTATIONS

Fluid accumulation in the scrotum readily transilluminates with the use of a good light source. Palpation reveals no masses. Some infants may have a mass in the groin that fades when abdominal pressure is decreased, such as after an infant stops crying. This mass is most often associated with a hernia, but a hydrocele may also exist. If the defect is large enough, fluid may continue to shift from the abdomen into the scrotal sac and back into the abdomen. As abdominal pressure rises, the shift of fluid becomes unidirectional into the scrotal sac. When the defect is large, abdominal contents may also pass into the scrotal sac. This condition would be called a congenital herniation or inguinal hernia.

In rare instances, female infants may have fluid accumulation in the labia, causing edema. They may also experience herniation into the patent passageway, the processus vaginalis.

DIFFERENTIAL DIAGNOSIS

Because the hydrocele may be asymptomatic, if it does not occur in conjunction with an inguinal hernia and is not large enough to create observable scrotal swelling, it may be difficult to detect. The "silk glove" test is useful in an older infant but generally is not useful in the neonatal period. In this test, the examiner places pressure on the peritoneal surfaces by rubbing gently on the scrotal tissue following the inguinal canal. If a hydrocele is present, the two distinct open layers of tissue should be felt sliding over each other. If the hydrocele is palpable, it will feel smooth and be painless. In the neonate, direct observation and transillumination with a strong light source should reveal a lightened area of scrotum where the fluid has accumulated. Observation of the infant during a crying episode, in which the intra-abdominal pressure is the greatest, may also demonstrate a hydrocele or scrotal swelling. If scrotal swelling is detected, the nurse should report this finding immediately to the medical team.

The most important differential diagnosis is distinguishing a hydrocele from an incarcerated inguinal hernia. This distinction can best be made by rectal examination and simultaneous palpation of the inguinal canal. If the examiner encounters loops of intestine near the vas deferens or ductus deferens within the scrotal sac, an inguinal hernia is present.

PROGNOSIS

The prognosis is excellent.

COLLABORATIVE MANAGEMENT

The treatment involves removal of the fluid. The fluid may be aspirated, or actual tissue removal may be necessary to close the freely communicating space. It is often not attempted until the infant reaches 1 year of age. Until the hydrocele is corrected, the nurse must observe closely for signs of herniation. If any herniation is suspected or the bowel is believed to be incarcerated, surgical intervention is needed immediately.

Nursing Management

Hydrocele repair is usually not performed in the newborn stage, because resolution often occurs spontaneously. Parents must be taught the signs of herniation and incarceration before discharge. These signs are the presence of a lump found in the groin, which is especially noticeable when the infant is crying, and increased irritability on the part of the infant. They must understand the need to seek immediate medical attention if either of these symptoms appears. Careful attention must be paid to skin care of the edematous scrotum.

Postoperatively, the infant may experience abdominal distention that could place pressure on the suture line, pulling it apart. Therefore, the use of a nasogastric tube attached to low intermittent suction may be necessary. If a nasogastric tube is used, patency must be maintained by irrigation with 2 ml of air or saline every 2 to 4 hours. The infant should be placed in the side-lying or supine position with the head turned to the side to prevent rubbing or pressure on the suture line. The bed should be flat. Maintenance of a dry sterile or waterproof occlusive dressing over the operative site is essential to prevent infection and skin breakdown. The perineum should be carefully cleaned after every void and stool.

Torsion of the Testis

PATHOPHYSIOLOGY

Torsion of the testis occurs when the testes or spermatic cord twists, restricting circulation to the testis. If circulation is allowed to remain compromised, permanent damage to the testis results. In the newborn, permanent damage may have resulted in utero, with consequent necrosis of the testis. In the female, torsion of the fallopian tube may result in compromised circulation to the ovary.

Torsion in the neonate results when the descent of the testis into the scrotal sac is complicated by the twisting of the tunica vaginalis. This can be unilateral or bilateral.

RISK FACTORS

No specific risk factors are known. Torsion of the testis is a common finding in the newborn period.

CLINICAL MANIFESTATIONS

Common to many scrotal problems are enlargement and edema. In torsion, the scrotum is firm to the touch and is very tender. The mass itself does not transilluminate. The scrotum and surrounding abdomen may show significant discoloration, being either plethoric or cyanotic.

DIFFERENTIAL DIAGNOSIS

The diagnosis is usually made on the basis of the presence of the discoloration of the scrotum and the nontransilluminating consistency of the scrotal sac.

PROGNOSIS

The prognosis for survival is very good; however, maintenance of testicular function to the affected testis may not be possible.

COLLABORATIVE MANAGEMENT

The treatment is aimed at surgical relief of the twisting of the testis. Correction can be performed either transscrotally or inguinally. Usually if the torsion is severe a simple orchidopexy may be performed (Kaplan, 1994). In certain instances, the twisted testis has been left in place to atrophy and necrose, in an attempt to preserve the function of Leydig cells to avoid testosterone therapy. This method of treatment is done only sporadically in the neonate (Kaplan & Silber, 1988).

Nursing Management

The focus of nursing care is on keeping the infant comfortable and as quiet as possible. The abdominal girth should be measured every 4 hours for any signs of distention. The scrotum must be inspected for the presence of edema, any discoloration, and the skin temperature. If the infant is experiencing vomiting owing to abdominal distention, the use of a nasogastric tube attached to intermittent low suction may be necessary. The tube should be irrigated every 2 to 4 hours with 2 ml of saline or air to maintain patency. Positioning of the infant should be only on the back with the head turned to the side or in a side-lying position, because otherwise too much pressure may be placed on the abdominal and scrotal areas.

Postoperatively, the nursing care is centered on stability of the vital signs and prevention of infection. The respiratory status must be carefully assessed, because abdominal distention may compromise the respiratory function. Nasopharyngeal suctioning may be necessary. The suture line is generally small but still requires aseptic technique. The site should be assessed for the presence of edema, drainage, or discoloration. A urinary drainage bag may be necessary to protect the skin and to prevent infection if excessive drainage is present.

Inguinal Hernia

PATHOPHYSIOLOGY

Inguinal hernia occurs when the small intestine and gonads pass through the open processus vaginalis. In the female, the herniation may occur into soft tissue of the labia. Small hernias without complications may be allowed to close on their own. Often, hernia repair is deferred until the infant is older and can tolerate anesthesia. The matured premature infant must be closely observed for respiratory and cardiac compromise in the postoperative period, because he or she is prone to apnea and bradycardia. When the intestines are caught within the processus, incarceration can occur. Vomiting and abdominal distention may indicate obstruction of the herniated intestine. Strangulation of the bowel and gonads occurs when the circulation becomes compromised. Necrosis may follow in a few hours.

RISK FACTORS

Right-sided hernias occur more often than those on the left, with bilateral hernias making up only a small percentage of the occurrences. Males are commonly affected more than females, with a high incidence in the premature population. There is a rare genetic syndrome called deficiency of mullerian inhibition substance that results in a phenotypic male; however, a uterus and fallopian tube can be found in the scrotal sac (Snyder, 1988).

CLINICAL MANIFESTATIONS

The inguinal hernia can be felt as a mass in the groin. In many cases, crying or increased abdominal pressure can exaggerate the hernia. In reducible hernias, the intestine can be gently manipulated back into the abdomen. Transillumination may not be helpful in diagnosis, because bowel air may be difficult to differentiate from a hydrocele.

DIFFERENTIAL DIAGNOSIS

The differential diagnosis is concerned with distinguishing an inguinal hernia in isolation or one accompanying a hydrocele. Some experts do not believe such a distinction is possible (Filston & Izant, 1985). A distinction should be made between undescended testes by scrotal examination for the presence of testes. A hydrocele may or may not be palpated, but a hernia will appear as a lump or swelling within the groin. Another concern is whether the hernia is incarcerated. It is then necessary to perform a rectal examination and palpate the scrotum simultaneously. This examination will reveal if an intestinal loop is present in the scrotal sac versus a fluid-filled hydrocele.

A reducible hernia may be easily "popped" back into place, whereas an incarcerated hernia is thick and nonreducible. Radiologic studies may demonstrate the presence of intestinal gas within the scrotal sac (Filston & Izant, 1985).

PROGNOSIS

The prognosis for survival is excellent.

COLLABORATIVE MANAGEMENT

Surgery is indicated in all inguinal hernias that do not resolve spontaneously. Surgical intervention is also required if strangulation or incarceration occurs. It involves repair of the hernia and separation of the hernia from the inguinal canal.

Nursing Management

The nurse must instruct the parents in recognizing symptoms of intestinal obstruction or protrusion of bowel loops through the hernia that will not reduce easily or become discolored. These symptoms would indicate need for immediate surgery.

The focus of nursing care preoperatively is on keeping the infant quiet and comfortable. If vomiting has occurred, the infant should be assessed for dehydration and the fluid and electrolyte status monitored closely. Postoperatively, the aim is adherence to aseptic technique with regard to suture line maintenance. The infant should be placed in a side-lying or supine position with the head turned to the side to prevent disruption of the suture line. If abdominal distention is present, a nasogastric tube for decompression may be necessary. Operative dressings should be observed for any drainage and bleeding. They should be kept dry and the underlying skin should be inspected for irritation or breakdown.

Nephroblastoma

PATHOPHYSIOLOGY

The occurrence of malignant tumor in the neonate is rare. Wilms' tumor does occur in the young infant. Associated with Wilms' tumor are aniridia, genitourinary tract defects, and hemihypertrophy. The presence of these signs in the neonate should alert the health care professional to the potential development of Wilms' tumor beyond the neonatal period.

RISK FACTORS

When hemihypertrophy is present, the infant may be at risk for nephroblastoma (Brion, Satlin, & Edelmann, 1994).

CLINICAL MANIFESTATIONS

The usual finding is a smooth, solid abdominal or flank mass that is actually a renal mass. It is accompanied by hypertension, owing to the possibility of renal artery stenosis. Fever is another common symptom with Wilms' tumor.

DIFFERENTIAL DIAGNOSIS

The diagnosis may be made on the basis of an intravenous pyelogram showing distorted renal calices; and on abdominal radiograph, the mass will appear coarse (Filston & Izant, 1985). A chest radiograph should be taken to determine the presence of any lung metastatic lesions.

PROGNOSIS

Although the prognosis is generally considered good, this may be due to the mislabeling of mesoblastic nephroma, a benign tumor, as Wilms' tumor. Metastasis may occur in the newborn period, making treatment difficult.

NURSING MANAGEMENT

One very important consideration is that there should be no palpation of the mass because of the danger of seeding the tumor to other areas of the body. The major focus of nursing management, at least initially, is support of the parents. They may fear attachment to the infant. Otherwise the neonatal nurse may not see an infant with Wilms' tumor, because this is often not diagnosed in the newborn period.

REFERENCES

Bourke, W. G., Clarke, T. A., Mathews, T. G., et al. (1994). Isolated single umbilical artery—the case for routine screening. *Archives of Disease in Childhood, 68,* 600–601.

Bradburn, N. C., & Schreiner, R. L. (1988). Infectious diseases. In R. L. Schreiner & N. C. Bradburn (Eds.), *Care of the newborn* (2nd ed., pp. 119–131). New York: Raven Press.

Brion, L. P., Satlin, L. M., & Edelmann, C. M., Jr. (1994). Renal diseases. In G. B. Avery (Ed.), *Neonatology: Pathophysiology and management of the newborn* (4th ed., pp. 792–886). Philadelphia: W. B. Saunders.

Brueggemeyer, A. (1988). Alterations in genitourinary system. In C. Kenner, J. Harjo, & A. Brueggemeyer (Eds.), *Neonatal surgery: A nursing perspective* (pp. 191–217). Orlando, FL: Grune & Stratton.

Chasnoff, I. J., Chisum, G. M., & Kaplan, W. E. (1988). Maternal cocaine use and genitourinary tract malformations. *Teratology, 37,* 201–204.

Deglin, J. H., & Vallerand, A. H. (1988). *Davis's drug guide for nurses.* Philadelphia: F. A. Davis.

Fanaroff, A. A., & Martin, R. J. (1992). *Neonatal-perinatal medicine: Diseases of the fetus and infant.* 5th ed. St. Louis: C. V. Mosby.

Filston, H. C., & Izant, R. (1985). *The surgical neonate: Evaluation and care* (2nd ed.). New York: Appleton-Century-Crofts.

Goetzman, B. W., & Wennberg, R. P. (1991). *Neonatal intensive care handbook.* St. Louis: C. V. Mosby.

Goodman, R., & Gorlin, R. (1983). *The malformed infant and child* (p. 154). New York: Oxford University Press.

Grupe, W. E. (1988). The dilemma of intrauterine diagnosis of congenital renal disease. *Pediatric Clinics of North America, 34*, 629–638.

Hanna, M. K. (1989). Megaureter. In L. R. King (Ed.), *Urologic surgery in neonates and young infants* (pp. 160–203). Philadelphia: W. B. Saunders.

Hiraoka, M., Kasuga, K., Hori, C., & Sudo, M. (1994). Ultrasonic indicators of ureteric reflux in the newborn. *The Lancet, 343*, 519–520.

Ingelfinger, J. R. (1985). Renal conditions in the newborn period. In J. P. Cloherty & A. R. Stark (Eds.), *Manual of neonatal care* (2nd ed., pp. 377–394). Boston: Little, Brown.

Inturrisi, M., Perry, S. E., & May, K. A. (1985). Fetal surgery for congenital hydronephrosis. *Journal of Obstetric, Gynecologic, and Neonatal Nursing, 14*, 271–276.

John, G., & Yeh, T. F. (1985). Renal failure. In T. F. Yeh (Ed.), *Drug therapy in the neonate and small infant* (pp. 277–298). Chicago: Year Book Medical Publishers.

Kaplan, G. W. (1994). Structural abnormalities of the genitourinary system. In G. B. Avery, M. A. Fletcher, & M. G. MacDonald. (Eds.), *Neonatology: Pathophysiology and management of the newborn* (4th. ed., pp. 887–913). Philadelphia: J. B. Lippincott.

Kaplan, G. W., & Silber, I. (1988). Neonatal torsion—To pex or not? In L. R. King (Ed.), *Urologic surgery in neonates and young infants* (pp. 386–395). Philadelphia: W. B. Saunders.

Keszler, M. (1995). Nebulized Furosemide. Personal Communication via NICU-Net. Washington, DC: Georgetown University.

Kim, M. S., & Mandell, J. (1988). Renal function in the fetus and neonate. In L. R. King (Ed.), *Urologic surgery in neonates and young infants* (pp. 59–76). Philadelphia: W. B. Saunders.

King, L. (1980). Exstrophy of the bladder and epispadias. In J. Raffensperger (Ed.), *Pediatric surgery* (pp. 753–768). New York: Appleton-Century-Crofts.

King, L. R. (1988). The management of multicystic kidney and ureteropelvic junction obstruction. In L. R. King (Ed.), *Urologic surgery in neonates and young infants* (pp. 140–154). Philadelphia: W. B. Saunders.

Laundau, D., Turner, M. E., Brennan, J., & Majd, M. (1994). The value of urinalysis in differentiating acute pyelonephritis from lower urinary tract infection in febrile infants. *Pediatric Infectious Disease Journal, 13*, 777–781.

Liu, K. W., Ku, K. W., Cheung, K. L, & Chan, Y. L. (1994). Acute scrotal swelling: A sign of neonatal adrenal haemorrhage. *Journal of Paediatric Child Health, 30*, 368–369.

McCracken, G., & Freij, B. T. (1987). Bacterial and viral infections of the newborn. In G. B. Avery (Ed.), *Neonatology: Pathophysiology and management of the newborn* (3rd. ed., pp. 917–943). Philadelphia: J. B. Lippincott.

Mesrobian, J. G. J. (1988). Exstrophy of the bladder. In L. R. King (Ed.), *Urologic surgery in neonates and young infants* (pp. 265–290). Philadelphia: W. B. Saunders.

O'Donnell, B. (1984). The lessons of 40 bladder exstrophies in 20 years. *Journal of Pediatric Surgery, 19*, 547–549.

Radhakrishnan, J. R. (1990). Obstructive uropathy in the newborn. *Clinics in Perinatology, 17*, 215–239.

Rosenstein, B. J., Wheeler, J. S., & Heid, P. L. (1990). Congenital renal abnormalities in infants with in utero cocaine exposure. *Journal of Urology, 144*, 110–112.

Sadler, T. W. (1995). *Langman's medical embryology* (7th ed.). Baltimore: Williams & Wilkins.

Scanlon, J. W., Nelson, T., Grylack, L. J., & Smith, Y. F. (1979). *A system of newborn physical examination.* Baltimore: University Park Press.

Schreiner, R. L., & Bradburn, N. C. (Eds.). (1988). *Care of the newborn* (2nd ed.). New York: Raven Press.

Short, K. L., Groff, D. B., & Cook, L. (1985). The concomitant presence of gastroschisis and prune belly syndrome in a twin. *Journal of Pediatric Surgery, 20,* 186–187.

Smith, D. L. (1988). *Recognizable patterns of malformations in development.* Philadelphia: W. B. Saunders.

Snyder, H. M. (1988). Management of ambiguous genitalia in the neonate. In L. R. King (Ed.), *Urologic surgery in neonates and young infants* (pp. 346–385). Philadelphia: W. B. Saunders.

Spindel, M. R., Winslow, B. H., & Jordan, G. H. (1988). The use of paraexstrophy flaps for urethral construction in neonatal girls with classical exstrophy. *Journal of Urology, 140,* 574–576.

Stang, H., Gunnar, M. R., Snellman, L., et al. (1988). Local anesthesia for neonatal circumcision. *Journal of the American Medical Association, 259,* 1507–1511.

Sugar, E. C., & Firlit, C. F. (1988). Management of cloacal exstrophy. *Urology, 32,* 320–322.

Tank, E., & McCoy, G. (1983). Limited surgical intervention in the prune belly syndrome. *Journal of Pediatric Surgery, 18,* 688–691.

White, C., Richardson, C., & Raibstein, L. (1990). High-frequency ventilation and extracorporeal membrane oxygenation. *AACN Clinical Issues in Critical Care, 1,* 427–444.

CHAPTER 20

Assessment and Management of Integumentary Dysfunction

ASSESSMENT AND PHYSIOLOGIC VARIATIONS

Much can be learned about an infant's physiological state by systematically assessing the skin, including color, turgor, and quality. Important variations are described here.

Acrocyanosis, or peripheral cyanosis involving the hands, feet, and the circumoral area, occurs from sluggish blood flow that results from an immature peripheral capillary system. Acrocyanosis usually resolves within the first few days of life but may reappear with cold stress.

Pallor is most commonly a sign of anemia, hypoxia, or poor peripheral perfusion due to hypotension or infection.

Meconium staining is caused by the passage of meconium in utero and usually requires at least 6 hours of meconium contact to stain the skin.

Jaundice, which occurs in 50 to 70 percent of newborns (Ziai, Clark, & Merritt, 1984), is a yellowing of the skin that develops because of the presence of indirect bilirubin in the blood. For visible staining of the skin and sclera, a level of at least 5 mg/dl is required. The head-to-toe progression of jaundice over the body gives a crude estimate of the level of bilirubin.

Linea nigra is a line of increased pigmentation from the umbilicus to the genitalia. This benign pigmentation may become less noticeable as skin darkens.

Mongolian spots are the pigmented lesions of the skin most frequently seen at birth. They are blue-gray, irregular, bruise-like spots seen primarily over the sacrum and buttocks but may extend over the back and shoulders. They are caused by the presence of pigmented cells deep in the dermis. Most commonly seen in newborns with darkly pigmented skin, they are found in 90 percent of black, Asian, and Native American infants. They occur in 1 to 5 percent of white infants (Margileth, 1994). Although they look like bruises, they are harmless.

Lanugo is the fine, downy hair most common over the back, shoulders, and facial areas of a premature newborn. It is shed at the seventh to eighth month of gestation and is one criterion used to estimate gestational age.

Milia are tiny epidermal cysts that develop in connection with the follicle and sebaceous gland. They are small, white pinhead-sized bumps scattered over the chin, cheeks, nose, and forehead of 25 to 40 percent of full-term infants (Avery, Fletcher, & MacDonald, 1994). They spontaneously resolve within the first month of life. Mothers should be instructed not to squeeze or prick this pimple-like spot. Milia can develop on the foreskin of infant boys, called *epidermal inclusion cysts,* or on the palate, called *Epstein's pearls.*

Miliaria are caused by the retention of sweat as a result of edema of the stratum corneum blocking eccrine pores. This results in four types of miliaria: rubra (prickly heat), crystallina, pustulosa, and profunda (Arndt, 1978). Miliaria pustulosa and miliaria profunda are rarely seen in temperate climates. Miliaria rubra is commonly observed in infants exposed to excessive environmental temperatures with humidity. It appears as pink or white pimples with a little redness around them. They resolve when the infant is moved to cooler temperatures. Miliaria crystallina presents as clear, 1- to 2-mm superficial water blisters without inflammation (Margileth, 1994). The distribution and grouping of vesicles that contain no eosinophils help to differentiate them from erythema toxicum.

Harlequin color change is a dramatic but benign phenomenon in which the color on the dependent half of an infant in a side-lying position turns deep red while the upper half is pale. The color reverses when the infant is turned. Attributed to a temporary imbalance in the autonomic regulatory mechanism of the cutaneous vessels, this phenomenon is more common in the low birth weight infant whether well or sick (Solomon & Esterly, 1973).

Vernix caseosa is a gray-white, cheesy substance that is protective to the fetal skin while in utero and helps the infant slide through the birth canal. The vernix covering diminishes as the fetus reaches term and is one determinant of gestational age dating.

Cutis marmorata, or mottling, is a normal physiologic vascular response to cool air. This generalized mottling reflects the infant's vasomotor instability (Esterly & Spraker, 1985). The marbling disappears with rewarming and is uncommon after several months of age. Mottling is often very prominent in infants with Cornelia de Lange's syndrome and Down syndrome (Jones, 1988).

Erythema toxicum, the most common rash of newborns, usually occurs within 5 days of birth and affects 30 to 70 percent of term infants. It appears as small, firm, white or pale yellow pustules with an erythematous margin. It is most commonly found on the trunk, arms, and diaper area. It is less likely to occur on the face and is never found on the palms of the hands or soles of the feet (Moschella & Hurley, 1985).

A smear and Wright's stain of the pustules reveal numerous infiltrates of eosinophils devoid of bacteria. The differential diagnosis includes transient neonatal pustular melanosis, candidiasis, staphylococcal pyoderma, and miliaria.

The cause of erythema toxicum is unknown, although a sensitivity to the environment is suspected. No treatment is necessary.

Acne neonatorum, or infantile acne, is caused by the stimulation and dysfunction of the immature oil-producing (sebaceous) glands of the infant's face. The glands are stimulated by maternal hormones. Acne develops during the first or second postnatal month and is seen more frequently in boys.

Most infants require no treatment for the acne; daily cleansing with a mild soap and water is sufficient. Petrolatum, baby oils, and lotions should be avoided because the underlying problem centers in the production of oily skin (Margileth, 1994).

Transient neonatal pustular melanosis is a lesion similar to miliaria but present at birth, usually causing the infant to be unnecessarily isolated. It occurs most frequently on the face, palms of the hands, and soles of the feet. It is most commonly seen in black infants. If the lesions are ruptured, smeared on a slide, and stained, the contents will be found to be amorphous debris. It is neither infectious nor contagious and is self-limiting and requires no treatment.

Sucking blisters containing sterile, serous fluid may be seen on the thumb, index finger, or lip. Presumably, they are the result of vigorous sucking in utero and resolve without treatment.

Pigmentary Lesions

The causes of skin coloration are listed in Table 20–1 (Nasemann, Sauerbrey, & Burgdorf, 1983).

Café au lait spots are irregularly shaped, oval lesions. Their color resembles coffee to which milk has been added. They should be noted on the newborn's initial physical examination; and if they are larger than 4 to 6 cm or if there are more than six, neurofibromatosis should be considered (Korones, 1986).

Hyperpigmentation that presents in a diffuse pattern is unusual in the newborn. It may be caused by congenital Addison's disease, hepatic or biliary atresia, metabolic disease (Hartnup's disease, porphyria), nutritional disorders (pellagra, sprue), hereditary disorders (lentiginosis, melanism), or unknown causes, such as the bronze discoloration seen in Niemann-Pick disease. Hyperpigmentation of the labial folds with clitoral hypertrophy may result from the transplacental passage of androgens (Margileth, 1994).

Hypopigmentation presenting as a diffuse or localized loss of pigment in the neonate may be the result of metabolic (phenylketonuria), endocrine (Addison's), genetic (vitiligo, piebaldism, tuberous sclerosis, albinism), traumatic, or postinflammatory causes (Avery, Fletcher, & MacDonald, 1994).

Piebaldism, or partial albinism, an autosomal dominant disorder present at birth, is easily detected in the dark-skinned infant. Off-white macules are seen on the scalp, widow's peak, and forehead, with extension to the base of the nose, trunk, and extremities. Differential diagnoses are Klein-Waardenburg syndrome, vitiligo, nevus anemicus, Addison's disease, and white mac-

TABLE 20–1. Materials That Contribute to Skin Color

	Exogenous	
Endogenous	*External*	*Internal*
Melanin	Tattoos	Carotene—yellow
Blood	Other foreign objects (e.g.,	Atabrine—yellow
Bile products	dirt from accidents)	Clofazimine—reddish
	Silver nitrate, gentian violet	Silver, other metals—gray
	(dermatologists and	Phenothiazines—gray
	patients)	

From Nasemann, T., Sauerbrey, W., & Burgdorf, W. (1983). *Fundamentals of dermatology* (p. 19). New York: Springer-Verlag. Reprinted with permission.

ules of tuberous sclerosis. When illuminated with a Wood's light, the amelanotic areas of piebaldism exhibit a brilliant whiteness (Margileth, 1994).

Albinism is a lack of pigmentation and may occur in any race. The incidence is approximately 1 in 5,000 to 1 in 15,000, and it is caused by an autosomal recessive gene (Margileth, 1994).

White leaf macules are the earliest cutaneous manifestations of tuberous sclerosis, an autosomal dominant neurocutaneous syndrome. They vary in size and shape but most often resemble a mountain ash leaflet. They may be difficult to see and may be more readily observed by examination with a Wood's lamp, which heightens the contrast between the macule and the normal skin. Normal infants occasionally have a single lesion, but the presence of one or more of these macules in an infant with neurologic problems strongly suggests the diagnosis of tuberous sclerosis. Skin biopsy is nondiagnostic. A careful family history, physical examination, and, when appropriate, additional diagnostic studies are indicated in infants with these lesions (Ziai, Clark, & Merritt, 1984).

DERMATOLOGIC DISEASES

Diseases of the skin in newborns often present patterns that are very different from the presentation of the same disease in adults. All lesions should be described and their location and pattern noted.

Lesions can be classified as either primary or secondary. A *primary lesion* is the initial or principal lesion that is identified when the disease begins. A *secondary lesion* is one that ordinarily develops from a primary lesion.

A reduction in the newborn's cellular and humoral immune response easily explains their increased susceptibility to infectious diseases.

Terminology

Ecchymoses appear as black and blue bruises of varying sizes anywhere over the body. They are caused by hemorrhage into the superficial skin layers. They do not disappear with blanching because the blood is contained in the tissues. Primarily seen over the presenting part in a difficult vertex delivery or a vaginal breech delivery, ecchymosis is most frequently due to trauma associated with labor and delivery. It occurs more commonly in the fragile premature infant. This bruising, however, can be indicative of serious infection or bleeding disorders.

Petechiae are pinpoint hemorrhagic areas, less than 1 mm in size, scattered over the upper trunk and face as a result of pressure during the descent and rotation of birth. Their incidence is increased when the umbilical cord has been around the neck or when the cervix clamps down after the delivery of the head. Like ecchymoses, there are purple discolorations caused by hemorrhage into the superficial skin layers. They do not disappear with blanching because the blood is trapped in the tissues. They usually fade within 24 to 48 hours. If they continue to develop or are unusually numerous, a complete work-up for infection or bleeding disorders should be done (Ziai, Clark, & Merritt, 1984).

Intracutaneous hemorrhage may be caused by thrombocytopenia, inherited disorders of coagulation, transient deficiency of vitamin K, disseminated intravascular coagulation, and trauma. Disseminated intravascular coagulation should be suspected in an acutely ill infant who develops intracutaneous hemorrhage. Both thrombocytopenia and disorders of coagulation generally occur in infants who seem well otherwise. Thrombocytopenia should be suspected when the infant presents with general cutaneous petechiae. It frequently accompanies neonatal infections and is most commonly associated with the TORCH diseases (toxoplasmosis, rubella, cytomegalovirus, and herpes simplex) (Moschella & Hurley, 1985).

Ecchymoses and petechiae are both purple discolorations caused by hemorrhage into the superficial skin layers. They do not disappear with blanching because the blood is contained in the tissues.

Macules are nonpalpable, nonraised lesions less than 1 cm in diameter that are identified only by color change (Nasemann, Sauerbrey, & Burgdorf, 1983). They are seen in measles, rubella, scarlet fever, roseola, typhoid fever, and drug reactions.

Papules are superficial elevated solid lesions less than 1 cm in diameter. They are firm and not fluid filled (Nasemann, Sauerbrey, & Burgdorf, 1983). They may follow the macular stage in many eruptive diseases.

Vesicles are skin elevations containing serous fluid (blisters). They are common with herpes simplex, insect bites, and poison ivy.

Pustules are localized accumulations of pus in or just beneath the epidermis. They are often centered around appendageal structures (e.g., hair follicles) and are usually caused by bacterial infections or skin abscesses. When a pustule breaks, the degree of crusting is more marked than with the rupture of a vesicle (Nasemann, Sauerbrey, & Burgdorf, 1983).

Nodules are deep solid lesions larger than 1 cm in diameter. They are similar to papules but larger. Because of their size, they are more likely to have a dermal component.

Developmental Vascular Abnormalities

Angiomas or vascular nevi are very common cutaneous congenital malformations seen during early infancy. Two major groups seen in children are the involuting and the noninvoluting vascular lesions, which may be flat (telangiectatic) or raised (hemangiomatous). The common involuting types include salmon patch, spider nevi (telangiectases), and strawberry and cavernous hemangiomas. Noninvoluting lesions, rare in newborns, are the portwine stain and the pyogenic granuloma (Margileth, 1994).

Pigmented Nevi

Pigmented nevi are benign tumors of the skin containing nevus cells. Nevus cells can produce melanin and are closely related to melanocytes. In contrast to melanocytes, they tend to lie in groups or nests. Congenital pigmented nevi are different from pigmented nevi arising later in that they are usually larger and more extensive. As the infant grows, the area becomes thicker and darker (Margileth, 1994).

Flat, junctional nevi are seen in about 1 percent of newborns. They are brown or black, and their size varies from 1 to several centimeters. When present at birth, they may be associated with neurofibromatosis, tuberous sclerosis, or bathing trunk nevi. Therapy is rarely needed, but lesions larger than 3 cm should be removed.

Giant Hairy Nevus

A *giant hairy nevus* is characterized by a pigmented, hairy, and softly infiltrated area. Their color varies from pale brown to black. When they are large they tend to have a dermatome distribution, and their location and size give them their name (e.g., bathing trunk nevus, vest nevus, shoulder stole nevus). On histologic examination of a biopsy specimen, the nevus cells are seen penetrating deeply into the dermis and subcutaneous tissue (Ziai, Clark, & Merritt, 1984).

When a giant nevus is situated on the head or neck, it may be associated with mental retardation, epilepsy, or hydrocephalus. Spina bifida or meningocele may occur when this nevus is present over the spine (Margileth, 1994). Other abnormalities sometimes associated with a giant pigmented nevus are clubfoot, hypertrophy or hypotrophy of the affected limb, and von Recklinghausen's disease (neurofibromatosis).

Besides being a cosmetic problem, there is also a higher incidence of malignancy associated with the giant nevus. As many as 15 percent of these patients develop malignant melanomas.

COLLABORATIVE MANAGEMENT

Management involves surgical excision of the entire giant hairy nevus at or near puberty to prevent the development of skin cancer in the lesion (Rosen, Lanning, & Hill, 1983; Walton, 1971). Plastic surgical reconstruction may be needed if the excision was extensive.

Hemangiomas

Hemangioma of infancy is an angiomatous disorder characterized by the proliferation of capillary endothelium, with multilamination of the basement membrane and the accumulation of mast cells, fibroblasts, and macrophages (Ezekowitz, Mulliken, & Folkman, 1992). Hemangioma is the most common tumor of infancy, occurring in up to 22 percent of preterm infants weighing less than 1000 g and in 10 to 12 percent of whites. Hemangiomas appear on 1 to 3 percent of infants at birth and develop on another 10 percent, usually within the first 3 to 4 weeks of life. When examined microscopically, hemangiomas are one of two kinds, either capillary or cavernous (Korones, 1986). They most often appear in the skin as a single tumor, but multiple cutaneous lesions also occur, often with involvement of other organ systems.

The natural history of the hemangioma is characterized by the appearance during the first few weeks of life, rapid postnatal growth for 8 to 18 months (proliferative phase), followed by very slow but inevitable regression for the next 5 to 8 years (involutive phase). There is complete resolution of hemangiomas in over 50 percent of children by the age of 5 years and in over 70 percent by 7 years of age, with continued improvement in the remaining children until the age of 10 to 12 years. The rate of regression does not seem related to sex or age of the infant, the site, size, or appearance of the hemangioma, or the duration of the proliferative phase (Ezekowitz, Mulliken, & Folkman, 1992).

Strawberry hemangiomas consist of a dilated mass of capillaries in the dermal and subdermal layers that protrude above the skin surface. They are bright red, soft, compressible tumors that can appear anywhere on the body. These marks require no treatment, and no permanent scars will occur if they are left alone. However, when these lesions interfere with vital functions, such as vision, feeding, or respiration, intervention is required (Ziai, Clark, & Merritt, 1984).

Cavernous hemangiomas are more deeply situated in the skin than strawberry hemangiomas. They appear bluish red and feel spongy when touched.

Most hemangiomas are small, harmless birthmarks that involute to leave either normal or slightly blemished skin. Even a small hemangioma can obstruct the airway or impair vision. A large hemangioma in the liver or an extensive cutaneous hemangioma can divert a considerable volume of blood through the extensive labyrinth of capillaries and produce high-output heart failure. The increased capillary endothelial surface that characterizes a giant hemangioma can also trap platelets and may cause thrombocytopenic coagulopathy (Kasabach-Merritt syndrome) (Ezekowitz, Mulliken, & Folkman, 1992).

A few hemangiomas grow to an alarming size or proliferate simultaneously in several organs, causing life-endangering conditions, such as soft tissue destruction, deformation or obstruction of vital structures, serious bleeding, congestive heart failure, and sepsis (Morad, McClain, & Ogden, 1993; Rosen, Lanning & Hill, 1983). Large lesions can expand the skin, and even after regression they can result in excess slack skin, pigment changes, and a fibrofatty residuum (Enjolras, Riche, Merland, & Escade, 1990).

In general, visceral hemangiomas denote a poor prognosis (Enjolras, Riche, Merland, & Escade, 1990). Death is usually caused by heart failure. Laryngeal hemangiomas are the most frequent visceral vascular manifestation. Liver and gastrointestinal hemangiomas are extremely rare. Flow through extensive hemangiomas increases the total blood volume, causes hemodeviation, and disturbs the hemodynamic equilibrium. The hyperdynamic cardiovascular state, with hypoperfusion of other tissues, may cause brain hypoxia and acidosis, predisposing to seizures seen in some cases. Close surveillance of the cardiovascular system is necessary to determine the proper time to begin digitalization (Enjolras, Rich, Merland, & Escade, 1990).

COLLABORATIVE MANAGEMENT

Management of both strawberry and cavernous hemangiomas consists of a detailed history; close scrutiny of the lesion or lesions, including three-dimensional measurements; and evaluation of the growth pattern of the hemangioma. As involution progresses, the color gradually changes from a grayish pink to a white or pink color, and the lesion has a decrease in tension. Ulcerated hemangiomas should be treated with topical antibiotics to prevent infection (Rosen, Lanning, & Hill, 1983).

While monitoring the cutaneous lesions, it is essential to closely follow the infant's clinical course and physical development for poor growth, altered cry, stridor, dyspnea, cyanosis, feeding difficulties, or swallowing impairment. If any abnormal sign or symptoms such as tachycardia, heart murmur, hepatomegaly, or bruit heard over the liver appear, the infant should be examined for evidence of heart failure. Ultrasound, echocardiography, and computed tomographic scans may be needed (Enjolras, Riche, Merland, & Escade, 1990).

In general, management consists of planned neglect, which is essential in avoiding disfiguring scars. Complications after therapy may be significant, but residual scarring after complete involution is uncommon. Hemangiomas located in exposed areas often cause great parental anxiety, which increases as the hemangioma grows. This anxiety often puts pressure on the physician to do something. However, the hemangioma should be left to regress spontaneously, and preconceived notions about birthmarks should be discussed with the family.

Visceral hemangiomas are associated with cervicocephalic hemangiomas or with small hemangiomas scattered over the body. About a third of these life-threatening hemangiomas respond to treatment with corticosteroids, but for the others there is no safe and effective treatment. The mortality rate can be as high as 54 percent for life-threatening visceral or hepatic hemangiomas and may be up to 30 to 40 percent with platelet-consumptive coagulopathy despite the administration of steroids (Ezekowitz, Mulliken, & Folkman, 1992).

High-dose corticosteroids are the primary means of controlling hemangiomas pharmacologically. They inhibit the activators of fibrinolysis in vessel walls, decrease plasminogen activator content of endothelium, and increase sensitivity to vasoactive amines, causing constriction of arterioles (Morad, McClain, & Orden, 1993). When steroids fail, less conventional modalities such as embolization, operative excision, and radiation therapy are used.

Port-Wine Stain

Port-wine stain is a capillary angioma consisting of dilated and congested capillaries lying directly beneath the epidermis. It appears in approximately 3 in 1000 newborns. This birthmark appears pink at birth but gradually darkens to a purple color. Most commonly found on the face and neck, it is a permanent developmental defect. Although a port-wine stain is primarily a cosmetic problem, occasionally it is an indicator of a multisystemic disorder such as Sturge-Weber syndrome or Klippel-Trenaunay-Weber syndrome. The presence of convulsions, mental retardation, hemiplegia, or intracortical calcification suggests the Sturge-Weber syndrome (Solomon & Esterly, 1973). An ophthalmologic examination is extremely important in these infants. A water-repellent cosmetic cream (e.g., Covermark, Retouch) will effectively cover the mark. Because of the inability to properly match the skin color of the normal skin and the possibility of scar formation, tattooing cannot be recommended. Plastic surgical repair may be necessary in the older child because of the development of a thickened nodular surface. Laser beam therapy appears to be effective, with the best results being achieved when the child is near puberty (Apfelberg, Maser, & Lash, 1978; Cosman, 1980).

Blistering Diseases

EPIDERMOLYSIS BULLOSA

Epidermolysis bullosa (EB) is a group of rare congenital blistering disorders, all of which are inherited (Ziai, Clark, & Merritt, 1984). They are considered mechanobullous diseases, meaning that trauma to or friction on the skin induces blister formation. The different varieties of EB are distinguished by the level of the skin at which the blister forms (Rosen, Lanning, & Hill, 1983). Pathologically, the disease is characterized by blister formation resembling that of second-degree burns after slight or innocuous trauma (Artnak, Moore, & Clements, 1981). The underlying defect appears to be a lack of cellular glue in squamous epithelium, which is responsible for maintenance of cellular integrity. Diagnostic studies should include a skin biopsy for light and electron microscopy.

This disease has been classified into two major subgroups: nonscarring and scarring EB (Watson, 1978). Four of the subtypes may occur at birth or in early infancy (Margileth, 1994). Nonscarring EB presents in two forms: epidermolysis bullosa letalis (Herlitz's disease), which is extremely rare, and epidermolysis bullosa simplex (EBS), which is common by comparison.

Epidermolysis bullosa simplex is the mildest form of EB. The lesions occur at the basal layer of epidermis and do not lead to scarring and hyperkeratosis. Usually present at birth, the vesicles and bullae appear over the joints and the bony protuberances and at sites subject to repeated trauma (Hymes, 1983). Differential diagnosis may be aided by the absence of milia, which are common in the dystrophic types of EB.

In *epidermolysis bullosa letalis,* a rare autosomal recessive type of EB, severe generalized blistering is present at birth. Subsequent extensive denudation may prove fatal in a few days to a few months owing to fluid loss or sepsis. Histopathologically, a separation occurs between the plasma membrane of the basal cells and basal lamina (Hymes, 1983).

Mild symptoms of dominant epidermolysis bullosa dystrophica may appear in early infancy but are not as severe as in the recessive forms, owing to the presence of a normal gene, which seems to reduce the severity of its manifestation. Moderately severe blisters are seen on the distal extremities and bony protuberances. Some scar formation occurs, and the nails may be mildly dystrophic. Atrophy may occur with healing. Nikolsky's sign (the external skin layer is easily rubbed off by slight friction or injury) is present. Milia, due to a functional disorder of the sweat glands, are found on the rims of the ears, the dorsal hands, and the extensor surfaces of the arms and legs. The oral, anal, and esophageal mucosae are frequently involved. Some of the associated complications are dwarfism, pseudosyndactylism, contractures, claw-like hands, partial scalp alopecia, and absence of body hair (Hymes, 1983).

Recessive epidermolysis bullosa dystrophica is the most severe form of the disease. Generalized cutaneous and mucosal blistering begin at birth. Subsequent esophageal strictures result in anemia and growth retardation. Digits of the hands and feet become fused from scarring and develop claw-like deformities. The skin is atrophic and easily blistered, with frequent flexion contractures from scarring. The lesions appear to lie at the level of the basement membrane, and the epidermis is thickened and flat with hyperkeratosis (Artnak, Moore, & Clements, 1981).

Complications include infections and hemolytic, nutritional, orthopedic, gastrointestinal, and psychiatric sequelae (Artnak, Moore, & Clements, 1981). These vary depending on the severity of the disease. However, the nursing care centers around three main issues: skin breakdown, contractures, and dysphagia.

Skin breakdown occurs after the rupture of bullae, reflecting the decrease in skin collagen. Preventive measures include the following:

- Alleviating skin excoriation
- Placing clean, soft dressings over bony pressure points
- Using bacitracin ointment after surgical soap cleansing two or three times daily for prevention of secondary infection
- Using emollients to avoid dry skin (Avery, Fletcher, & MacDonald, 1994)
- Using sterile gloves
- Diminishing insensible water loss by using cool, humidified air and maintaining accurate records of intake and output

From birth to 6 months of age, the environment is easy to control:

- Use sheepskins, loose-fitting clothes, and mittens for hands and feet.
- Use cloth diapers softened with fabric softener.
- Do not let caregivers wear jewelry.
- Always have infant wear long pants once mobile.
- Use foam rubber pads sewn in the knees to help avoid trauma during crawling.

Contractures may form quickly as scarring begins to occur. The pathologic increase in elastic skin fiber adds to this process (Hymes, 1983). Gentle range-of-motion exercises lessen the contracture formation.

Dysphagia can occur from facial and pharyngeal scarring, which is secondary to erosions on the buccal mucosa, tongue, palate, esophagus, and pharynx (Hymes, 1983).

- Feedings should be done slowly and carefully to avoid aspiration and maintain adequate nutrition.
- Metabolic needs are high, owing to the continuous sloughing of epithelium resulting in large protein, fluid, and electrolyte losses (Artnak, Moore, & Clements, 1981).
- Adding additional puncture holes to a nipple may help prevent oral mucosal trauma.
- If oral ulcerations do occur, several weeks of hyperalimentation and high-dose steroid therapy are instituted.
- Gavage feedings are discouraged owing to the possibility of trauma.

It is essential that the family receive genetic counseling regarding the inheritance pattern associated with epidermolysis bullosa; a negative family history does not exclude its occurrence.

Bacterial Infections

STAPHYLOCOCCUS AUREUS INFECTION

Infections resulting from *Staphylococcus aureus* are seen in newborns and can result in two specific types of skin lesions. *Bullous impetigo* of the newborn involves blisters that originate in the stratum corneum and are filled with clear or straw-colored fluid, which appear after the first few days after delivery. There may be few or many blisters, dispersed body wide, that rupture easily, leaving denuded areas of skin. *S. aureus* is most commonly cultured, but other bacteria such as group A *Streptococcus* or beta-hemolytic *Streptococcus* are sometimes found.

Collaborative Management

Treatment consists of either cleansing the lesions with antimicrobial solutions three or four times a day (Margileth, 1994) or using saline or sterile water compresses, followed by antimicrobial ointment (Esterly & Solomon, 1995). Antibiotics should be given if systemic infection is suggested. Fluid and electrolyte monitoring is necessary if the denuded areas cover a large surface or if the infant is of low birth weight. Isolation is necessary to prevent the spread of the infection throughout the nursery.

SCALDED SKIN SYNDROME

S. aureus can also result in a severe bullous eruption called scalded skin syndrome. Initially, the skin is bright red, resembling a scald, followed by large flaccid blisters that quickly progress to large sheets of skin being shed. The entire epidermis is frequently shed during the course of this disease. The mechanism for this involves the production of an endotoxin, called exfoliatin, that causes the skin manifestations. Usually the skin lesions do not culture positive for the responsible organism, so culturing the nasopharynx, blood, conjunctiva, and normal skin is recommended to recover the organism for appropriate sensitivity testing (Esterly & Solomon, 1995).

Collaborative Management

Management involves administration of the appropriate antibiotics and supportive measures such as fluid and electrolytic replacement, prevention of secondary infection, and comfort. Application of local antibiotic solutions or ointments is generally not necessary; keeping open areas clean and dry promotes healing and prevents secondary infection. The infant may be more comfortable in an incubator rather than in a radiant warmer; this is because the incubator is a convective heat source that does not have a direct cutaneous effect, whereas the radiant heat source heats directly through the skin. In addition, the radiant heat source may further increase the degree of insensible water loss through the damaged epidermis. Usually a flaking process is observed on the skin during the healing process.

Viral Infections

HERPES SIMPLEX INFECTION

Herpes simplex infection is one of the most serious neonatal viral infections. Vesicles with this disease may vary; there may be a few faint scars or actual vesicle formations with either one large swelling or discrete groups of vesicles. Vesicles may recede, then recur over months.

Collaborative Management

Collaborative management is centered primarily on early recognition and treatment with antiviral medication. Prognosis with systemic disease is extremely poor if encephalitis develops, with either death or severe mental retardation the sequela. An important consideration is isolation from other patients to prevent transmission.

VARICELLA-ZOSTER

This viral condition is rare, but varicella-zoster infection occurring in the first 10 days of life is generally thought to have been acquired in utero. Vesicular eruptions are the same as those in chickenpox acquired at any age. A 20 percent mortality is reported. This infection poses a significant risk for the immunocompromised infant. No systemic or topical treatment is required for these lesions. Occasionally, scarring can occur. Strict isolation is absolutely necessary to protect other infants from exposure, because this virus is airborne. Passive immunization of infants exposed to the affected infant may also be necessary.

TOXOPLASMOSIS

Toxoplasmosis, caused by an intracellular parasite, can be transmitted transplacentally and result in systemic infection. Some infants affected may have a generalized maculopapular rash as well as hepatosplenomegaly, jaundice, fever, and anemia. The rash may progress to desquamation and hypopigmentation in very severe cases. Direct topical therapy is not reported as necessary or efficacious; systemic therapy may be considered.

CYTOMEGALOVIRUS AND RUBELLA

Both *cytomegalovirus (CMV)* and *rubella* have symptoms that are manifested in the skin. Petechial lesions can occur with both. These are the result of thrombocytopenia and usually disappear in 2 to 6 weeks. In severe rubella infection, and very rarely in CMV, bluish red papules that are 2 to 8 mm in diameter can occur over the head, trunk, and extremities. This so-called blueberry muffin syndrome is the result of erythropoiesis in the dermis and usually subsides in 2 to 3 weeks. Neither of these lesions requires topical therapy.

Fungal Infections

Candida albicans is the primary fungal infection with cutaneous manifestation, although other strains such as *Malassezia furfur* can also potentially colonize the skin of the term and preterm newborn, particularly those who are hospitalized in an intensive care nursery. Infection with *Candida* can range from diaper dermatitis or other localized skin or mucous membrane eruptions to systemic candidemia resulting in significant morbidity and mortality. Candidal organisms are not normally found in the skin flora of the newborn. The gastrointestinal system is the primary reservoir, but the skin may be colonized during passage through a colonized vaginal canal. The incidence of candidal colonization is also increased with the frequent use of broad-spectrum antibiotics that alter normal skin flora in infants after delivery.

Collaborative Management

Management of infants with systemic or local *Candida* infection involves topical therapy with antifungal creams and systemic antifungal medications if evidence exists of systemic infection. There is sometimes difficulty in culturing yeast; techniques include obtaining urine to look for hyphae or budding yeast, blood cultures, and skin scrapings prepared with potassium hydroxide and examined for pseudohyphae. Observation in infants of low birth weight for evidence of the diffuse burn-like dermatitis or a spreading candidal diaper rash is essential and may expedite initiating therapy for systemic candidiasis.

Scaling Disorders

POSTMATURITY

Many term infants born between 40 and 42 weeks' gestation experience a period of shedding or desquamation that is considered a normal physiologic process. Postmature infants born after 42 weeks may also have this appearance, but there are other characteristics that are different. The postmature infant may have a lean appearance, with little subcutaneous fat; the infant's weight is low in relationship to length. The skin resembles parchment paper and may literally peel off in sheets. There may be staining of the fingernails with meconium, long fingernails, and long hair.

Skin care is not the major problem. Eventually the skin underneath the peeling layers will predominate; even during the period of desquamation, the skin functions well as a barrier, because these infants have all the layers of stratum corneum of a term infant or adult. Aside from bathing with a mild soap initially, no lubrication is necessary during the period of desquamation.

ICHTHYOSIS

The most serious cause of scaly skin in the newborn is *ichthyosis dermatosis.* There are four major types of ichthyosis: sex-linked ichthyosis, nonbullous congenital ichthyosiform erythroderma, and bullous congenital ichthyosiform erythroderma, all of which are present at birth, and ichthyosis vulgaris, which usually appears after the third month of life. Terms commonly used to describe infants with ichthyosis may include the *harlequin fetus* and *collodion baby,* but these terms do not define which form of ichthyosis is present.

In the *sex-linked type of ichthyosis,* males are affected because the disease is X linked. Some female heterozygotes may exhibit mild scaling of the arms and lower extremities. Affected male newborns have large yellow or brown plaques covering the whole body except palms, soles, midface, and over joints. At birth, some affected males may appear scaly, others are often called collodion babies.

Nonbullous congenital ichthyosiform erythroderma, also called lamellar ichthyosis, is an autosomal recessive disorder. Initially, affected newborns may have a bright red appearance, which rapidly progresses to desquamation; rarely is a collodion baby appearance present at birth. Later, scales develop that are yellow to brown and that may eventually become thick, horny plates. Although the prognosis is usually good, infants severely affected, the so-called harlequin fetus, may succumb to sepsis or require extensive plastic surgery.

In *bullous congenital ichthyosiform erythroderma,* autosomal dominance is the mode of heredity, so several family members may be affected. Large bullae are initially seen, as well as erythema and dry scaly skin; the blistering that recurs throughout childhood differentiates this form from the nonbullous type. Extensive denuded areas can present a problem as the blisters burst, because secondary infections with *Streptococcus* or *Staphylococcus* can occur and are life threatening.

Collaborative Management

Management of all forms of ichthyosis involves the continual use of topical therapies and prescription bathing techniques and prevention of infection. Bathing may be necessary as often as twice daily with a water-dispersible bath oil, avoiding soaps that are excessively drying or irritating. In the bullous form, judicious use of antimicrobial bathing may be prescribed to reduce colonization but should be carefully used to avoid toxicity from absorption of these substances through the skin. Ointments or creams that preserve moisturization, such as Aquaphor, are applied several times daily. At times, steroid ointments are used on a short-term basis, but only to treat irritant dermatitis should it occur. In cases of bullous ichthyosis, systemic oral steroids are sometimes necessary to reduce the inflammatory process.

Infants with severe skin involvement may require protective isolation, owing to the higher risk of contact with nosocomial infections. Use of an incubator may be useful for thermoregulation as well as provide a barrier to infection. Sterile linen, sterile gloves, and other measures are needed if larger areas of denuded skin are present.

Comfort is another key concern. Fussy, irritable agitation may be seen, related to pruritus or inflammation. Some form of analgesia may help, although the topical therapies prescribed have the most direct effect. A trial of diphenhydramine (Benadryl) with careful observation might be helpful in the case of a very irritable infant when other measures (e.g., topical treatment, pacifiers, feeding) are unsuccessful.

Working with the parents has many facets. The appearance of the infant, especially if severely affected, could be a shock and require careful interventions. As in parents of infants with other congenital abnormalities, there is a period of shock, denial, and grief over the loss of a perfect baby. Parents of these infants need genetic counseling as well as support and education as they come to terms with this disease.

ECZEMA

Eczema, a skin disorder that causes several degrees of skin irritation and has multiple causes, is more common after 2 months of age. It involves an eruption that proceeds to the development of microvesicles and oozing, which later turns into scaling of the epidermis as this layer tries to regenerate rapidly. Lichenification or thickening of the skin, which occurs in adult skin with eczema, is not seen in infants.

Primary irritants, such as saliva, feces, and some soaps or skin preparations, are the usual causes of eczema in the infant, rather than allergy. It is important to have a good history of all products that have been applied to the skin to sort out the causes. If external agents have been ruled out, other diagnoses are considered, such as seborrheic dermatitis or Leiner's disease, which involves a total exfoliation of the entire body.

Collaborative Management

Treatment of eczema involves prevention by avoiding the primary irritant source if identified, or protection, as in use of zinc oxide paste to the perianal area to prevent contact with feces. For more generalized eruptions, short-term therapy with topical 1 percent hydrocortisone cream may be used. Bathing should be carried out in tepid water with water-dispersible oil; irritating or drying soaps should be avoided. If large areas of skin are involved, thermoregulation may be a concern, especially in dry climates. Humidification may be desirable in some climates, especially during the summer months. Air conditioning may also be necessary.

Discomfort is also a significant concern, because these infants may experience considerable pruritus. Topical therapy is generally the first consideration, followed by the judicious use of diphenhydramine (Benadryl) in very severe cases.

SKIN CARE PRACTICES

The most basic aspects of skin care for newborns include the daily bath, lubrication with emollients, skin preparation with antimicrobial solutions, and affixing adhesives for life support devices, monitoring of vital signs, and oxygenation, if they are hospitalized. During all these practices, the skin has the potential for trauma or alterations in normal barrier function and pH (Gordon & Montgomery, 1996).

Bathing

The purpose of bathing has primarily been focused on reducing antimicrobial colonization and removing waste materials, as well as for general aesthetic reasons. Antimicrobial bathing has been the most extensively studied. Although quite effective in reducing colonization with *S. aureus* strains (Sarkany & Arnold, 1970), bathing with hexachlorophene has been abandoned or curtailed by most nurseries because of the toxicity associated with absorption (American Academy of Pediatrics, 1977). Many neonatal intensive care units (NICUs) are reluctant to risk even potential toxicity from antimicrobial bathing in very small premature infants, so bathing only once or not at all with an antimicrobial soap is common.

Other soaps commonly used in routine bathing practices for premature infants are the same as soaps used for term infants and include so-called "baby soaps," regular soaps (e.g., Ivory), neutral pH soaps (e.g., Neutrogena or Dove), and superfatted soaps (e.g., Basis or Oilatum); occasionally deodorant soaps (e.g., Dial) are recommended for their antimicrobial properties (Morelli & Weston, 1987). The degree of irritancy as well as the drying effects on the stratum corneum and alterations in skin pH are not known but may have consequences for the ability of the premature infant's skin to function as a barrier and maintain a normal acid surface. Therefore, both the type of soap and the frequency of bathing are considerations. Infrequent bathing with mild, neutral pH soaps may be beneficial.

Lubrication

Lubricants are commonly applied to the skin of premature infants in an effort to prevent or treat a dry or chapped appearance. The level of hydration in the stratum corneum is related to the ability of this layer to take up water and the capacity to retain water (Thune et al., 1988). It has been shown that the water content of the stratum corneum is low in conditions such as psoriasis or eczema and also in aged skin (Potts, Buras, & Chrisman, 1984; Tagami & Yoshikuni, 1985; Tagami et al., 1982). The water content of the stratum corneum of the premature infant is not known, nor is the effect of various lubrication methods on skin hydration.

Antimicrobial Skin Solutions

Use of solutions to decontaminate skin before invasive procedures such as venipuncture, heelstick blood sampling, and umbilical catheter insertion is considered necessary in premature and term infants in the NICU. Yet the literature contains anecdotal reports documenting negative effects from these practices. Despite these reports, alcohol pledgets are still found in any NICU and are used on premature infants.

Another common antimicrobial skin preparation used before invasive procedures is povidone-iodine solution. Instances of high iodine levels, iodine goiter, and hypothyroidism have been associated with liberal use of povidone-iodine as a prepping agent before invasive procedures (Chabrolle & Rossier, 1978; Jackson & Sutherland, 1981; Pyati, Ramamurthy, Krauss, & Pildes, 1977). However, the risk of introducing microorganisms through the skin during such procedures exists in these immunocompromised patients, and many continue to use povidone-iodine solution, advocating that it be removed completely with water as soon as possible after the procedure is completed.

Adhesive Application and Removal

Many different adhesives and products used to enhance adhesion are in use where life support and monitoring devices must be securely attached to premature infants. Solvents such as Wisk, Dermasol, and others have been used in many pediatric settings to prevent discomfort from adhesive removal but should not be used in premature infants because of the dangers of toxicity from absorption.

Use of skin barriers, products that are placed between the skin and adhesive to either promote adhesion or protect skin, has also been examined. A plastic polymer, spray-on dressing was examined by Evans and Rutter (1986) and found to reduce trauma, as measured by a lower transepidermal water loss, when used under the adhesive rings for transcutaneous oxygen monitors. Higher rates of water loss persisted for 12 to 16 hours after the standard adhesive rings were removed, and the authors noted no alterations in oxygen readings from the devices affixed in this manner. However, they did note a residue that built up over time and that was difficult to remove, and the potential absorption of this substance was not examined. Tincture of benzoin is also frequently used in adults, primarily to increase adherence of adhesives and strengthen the epidermis. However, the bond between tape and epidermis created by benzoin may, in fact, be stronger than the bond between epidermis and dermis, especially on premature infants, and result in increased epidermal stripping. Therefore, this barrier should be used judiciously, if at all, and probably not on premature infants during the early rapid phase of skin development that occurs postnatally.

Other adhesives that may have promise for reducing skin trauma on removal from premature infants include pectin-based barriers, such as those used for stoma appliances that have replaced similar karaya products, and hydrophilic gelled adhesives. The newer gelled adhesive products used in electrocardiographic leads, over temperature skin probes, and to secure phototherapy masks have seemed less traumatic with visual inspection but have not yet been studied using instrumentation to detect other important changes in skin function.

MANAGEMENT OF SKIN CARE PROBLEMS

The stratum corneum can be traumatized from a variety of insults, including epidermal stripping from removal of adhesives, burns from transcutaneous oxygen electrodes, pressure sores, infection, nutritional inadequacies such as zinc and essential fatty acid deficiency, extravasation of intravenous fluids, and diaper dermatitis. The goal should be to maintain skin integrity; however, even with meticulous care, skin breakdown can occur.

Skin Excoriations

When a skin excoriation is noted, the first step is to identify the cause before determining a treatment strategy. Infectious causes such as staphylococcal scalded skin syndrome or cutaneous candidiasis should be ruled out because these conditions may require culturing and either systemic or topical treatment.

If the skin excoriation is due to a known cause, such as adhesive removal, the care should include cleansing with sterile water and possibly some type of antimicrobial ointment or dressing. If an ointment is prescribed, Polysporin or bacitracin ointment is used sparingly over the excoriation and reapplied every 8 to 12 hours. Neosporin is another common topical ointment, but some dermatologists have noted increased sensitization from early uses of this ointment and potential allergy later in life.

Transparent adhesive dressings, such as Op-Site, Tegaderm, and Bioclusive, are made from a polyurethane film backed with adhesive impermeable to water and bacteria but allows air flow so that the skin can "breathe." They adhere well but require a rim of intact skin for attachment. Other uses for transparent adhesive dressings include securing intravenous catheters and percutaneous Silastic catheters and as a dressing for central venous lines. Another use is to prevent skin breakdown, and these dressings can be applied to bony prominences such as the knees or sacrum when there is the potential for friction burns or pressure sores.

Transparent adhesive dressings can also be applied over superficial or deep wounds; they have been shown in adult literature to promote faster, "moist" healing. The one caution is that the wound be uninfected or "clean," because bacteria and fungus will proliferate under the dressing. When these dressings are used for wound care, a milky white or yellow exudate will form under the dressing; this is often mistaken for pus, but it is actually composed of leukocytes that prevent infection during the process of healing. The dressing should remain until healing has occurred, or until it falls off, because removal may result in further skin excoriation because of the tenacious nature of the adhesive backing.

Large wounds, such as those that occur after surgery, can result in skin disruption when healing fails to progress in the normal fashion. Dehiscence of wounds is occasionally encountered in the neonate, although wound healing is generally less complicated in the NICU if the infant's nutritional status is appropriate and basic precautions against infection are taken.

Diaper Dermatitis

A common skin disruption that occurs in neonates and infants is diaper dermatitis. This term encompasses a range of processes that affect the perineum, groin, thighs, buttocks, and anal area of infants who are incontinent and wear some covering to collect urine and feces.

The pathogenesis of diaper dermatitis is, in part, related to the degree of wetness of the skin. Skin that is very moist and macerated becomes more permeable (Berg, 1987) and susceptible to injury because wetness acts to increase friction. In addition, moisture-laden skin is more likely to contain microorganisms.

Another component in the process of skin injury from diaper dermatitis is the effect of an alkaline pH. The normal skin pH is acidic, ranging between 4.0 and 5.5, but can become alkaline when exposed to urine, which generally has a higher pH. It is the resulting elevated pH of the skin that increases its vulnerability to injury and penetration by microorganisms and not the effect of ammonia in urine as previously thought (Berg, Buckingham, & Stewart, 1986; Leydon, Katz, Stewart, & Lkigman, 1977). Another aspect of the problems of increased pH of the skin is that it stimulates fecal enzyme activity (Buckingham & Berg, 1986). Specifically, both protease and lipase, which are found in stool, can injure skin, which is made up of protein and fat components. These enzymes can cause significant injury to the epidermis in a fairly brief period of contact and are responsible for the contact irritant diaper dermatitis.

Once the epidermis has been impaired or becomes a less efficient barrier, it can turn into a staphylococcal or fungal rash if this progression occurs. *S. aureus* can be found in large numbers on the skin surface, especially if it is inflamed or impaired, and can result in secondary infection. The classic presentation for *S. aureus* is pustule formation at the site of hair follicles.

Fungal rashes, primarily those caused by *Candida albicans,* may have different mechanisms of invasion. Many researchers have identified *C. albicans* as a secondary invader of skin that has been injured by other mechanisms, whereas others suggest that it is a primary causative factor in diaper dermatitis (Rasmussen, 1987). This is based on the ability of *C. albicans* to penetrate the stratum corneum, especially in a warm and moist environment such as that found under an occlusive diaper. The resulting intense inflammation is quite significant and appears as brightly erythematous, sharply marginated dermatitis, involving the inguinal folds as well as the buttocks, thighs, abdomen, and genitalia, characteristically with satellite lesions that may extend the rash over the trunk. The gastrointestinal tract is often the reservoir for *C. albicans,* and it can frequently be recovered in stool. Thus, oral therapy may be indicated, especially if evidence of oral infection, such as thrush, is apparent.

Some diaper dermatitis can be the result of a primary dermatologic condition such as psoriasis, eczema, or seborrheic dermatitis. Significant family history of these skin conditions may identify infants who are especially vulnerable to developing severe reactions to inflammations in the diaper area.

COLLABORATIVE MANAGEMENT

Prevention is the first goal and is paramount in breaking the cycle of diaper dermatitis. Frequent diaper changes result in skin that is drier with a more normal pH and thus maintain the functional barrier of the skin. Strategies to keep the skin dry also include the use of highly absorbent gelled diapers that act to "wick" moisture away from the skin (Campbell, Seymour, Stone, & Milligan, 1987; Davis, Leyden, Grove, & Raynor, 1989). Use of talcum powders has been discouraged, owing to the risk of inhalation of silicone particles into the respiratory tract. Cornstarch has been substituted for talc and has recently been shown not to promote yeast growth (Leydon, 1984); however, efficacy of this approach has not been researched.

Once diaper dermatitis occurs—and it is not completely avoidable in most infants—protection of injured skin during healing is the primary goal. Use of a generous layer of protective skin barriers containing zinc oxide prevents further trauma and allows impaired skin to heal. Opening the skin to light and air is not effective if the fecal contents are allowed to have direct contact with already injured areas. Because protective skin barriers tend to adhere very well to the skin, it is neither necessary nor desirable to completely remove them during diaper changes before application of more cream. It is best to generously apply more to the site to protect the area from further injury.

Treatment of diaper dermatitis that is solely due to invasion with *C. albicans* requires the use of antifungal creams or ointments; sometimes the addition of a steroid cream reduces inflammation and promotes healing faster. Some of the antifungal preparations include nystatin, miconazole, and clotrimazole. If the diaper dermatitis involves both fungus and a contact irritant component, alternating applications of the topical creams or ointments are effective.

Very serious diaper dermatitis is observed in infants suffering from severe malabsorption syndrome secondary to intestinal resection or mucosal injury. In this case, the stool is extremely caustic, containing a higher level of enzyme activity, lower pH as the result of rapid transit through the intestine, and significant amounts of undigested carbohydrates. In addition, stool frequency is often greatly increased. Although skin disruption frequently becomes the focus of nursing interventions, this symptom may be a significant indication of more serious physiologic concerns. These infants' stools should be carefully monitored by documentation of number, volume, pH, and carbohydrate testing. The infants must be observed for dehydration caused by extensive water losses in diarrhea. Once dietary manipulations and hydration have stabilized the general physiologic status, a program of skin protection is imperative, because some level of chronic diarrhea may be ongoing for many weeks or months. Products such as pectin-based powders or pectin-containing pastes without alcohol may prove better barriers to the caustic, constant fecal irritation if traditional zinc oxide creams do not work adequately. If yeast is present, antifungal creams may be applied in conjunction with protective barriers.

REFERENCES

American Academy of Pediatrics. (1977). *Standards and recommendations for hospital care of newborn infants* (pp. 109–129). Evanston, IL: American Academy of Pediatrics.

Apfelberg, D., Maser, M., & Lash, H. (1978). Argon laser treatment of cutaneous vascular abnormalities. *American Plastic Surgery, 1,* 14.

Arndt, K. (1978). *Manual of dermatologic therapeutics* (2nd ed.). Boston: Little, Brown.

Artnak, K., Moore, L., & Clements, C. (1981). Epidermolysis bullosa: An inherited skin disorder. *American Journal of Nursing, 81,* 1837–1840.

Avery, G. B., Fletcher, M. A., & MacDonald, M. G. (Eds.) (1994). *Neonatology: Pathophysiology and management of the newborn* (4th ed.). Philadelphia: J. B. Lippincott.

Berg, R. (1987). Etiologic factors in diaper dermatitis: A model for development of improved diapers. *Pediatrician, 14,* 27–33.

Berg, R. W., Buckingham, K. W., & Stewart, R. L. (1986). Etiologic factors in diaper dermatitis: The role of urine. *Pediatric Dermatology, 3,* 102–106.

Buckingham, K. W., & Berg, R. W. (1986). Etiologic factors in diaper dermatitis: The role of feces. *Pediatric Dermatology, 3,* 107–112.

Campbell, R. L., Seymour, J. L., Stone, L. C., & Milligan, M. C. (1987). Clinical studies with disposable diapers containing absorbent gelling materials: Evaluation on infant skin condition. *Journal of the American Academy of Dermatology, 17,* 978–987.

Chabrolle, J., & Rossier, A. (1978). Goiter and hypothyroidism in the newborn after cutaneous absorption of iodine. *Archives of Disease in Childhood, 53,* 495–498.

Cosman, B. (1980). Experience in the argon laser therapy of port wine stains. *Plastic & Reconstruction Surgery, 65,* 119–129.

Davis, J. A., Leyden, J. J., Grove, G. L., & Raynor, W. J. (1989). Comparison of disposable diapers with fluff absorbent and fluff plus absorbent polymers: Effects on skin hydration, skin pH, and diaper dermatitis. *Pediatric Dermatology, 6,* 102–108.

Enjolras, O., Riche, M., Merland, J., & Escade, J. (1990). Management of alarming hemangiomas in infancy: A review of 25 cases. *Pediatrics, 85,* 491–498.

Esterly, N. B., & Solomon, L. M. (1995). The skin. In A. A. Fanaroff & R. J. Martin (Eds.), *Neonatal-perinatal medicine: Diseases of the fetus and infant* (5th ed., pp. 1328–1358). St. Louis: C. V. Mosby.

Esterly, N., & Spraker, M. (1985). Neonatal skin problems. In S. Moschella & H. Hurley (Eds.), *Dermatology* (2nd ed., Vol. 2, pp. 1882–1903). Philadelphia: W. B. Saunders.

Evans, N. J., & Rutter, N. (1986). Reduction of skin damage from transcutaneous oxygen electrodes using a spray on dressing. *Archives of Disease in Childhood, 61,* 881–884.

Ezekowitz, R., Mulliken, J., & Folkman, J. (1992). Interferon alfa-2a therapy for life-threatening hemangiomas of infancy. *New England Journal of Medicine, 326,* 1456–1463.

Gordon, M., & Montgomery, L. A. (1996). Minimizing epidermal stripping in the very low birth weight infant: Integrating research and practice to affect infant outcome. *Neonatal Network, 15,* 37–44.

Hymes, D. (1983). Epidermolysis bullosa in the neonate. *Neonatal Network, 1,* 36–39.

Jackson, H. J., & Sutherland, R. H. (1981). Effect of povidine-iodine on neonatal thyroid function. *Lancet, 2,* 992.

Jones, K. L. (1988). *Smith's recognizable patterns of human malformations* (4th ed., pp. 10, 80). Philadelphia: W. B. Saunders.

Korones, S. (1986). *High-risk newborn infants* (4th ed., pp. 138–166). St. Louis: C. V. Mosby.

Leyden, J. J., Katz, S., Stewart, R., & Kligman, A. M. (1977). Urinary ammonia and ammonia-producing micro-organisms in infants with and without diaper dermatitis. *Archives of Dermatology, 113,* 1678–1680.

Leyden, J. J. (1984). Cornstarch, *Candida albicans* and diaper rash. *Pediatric Dermatology, 1,* 322–325.

Margileth, A. M. (1994). Dermatologic conditions. In G. Avery, M. A. Fletcher, & M. G. MacDonald (Eds.), *Neonatology: Pathophysiology and management of the newborn* (4th ed, pp. 1229–1268). Philadelphia: J. B. Lippincott.

Morad, A. B., McClain, K. L., & Ogden, A. K. (1993). The role of tranexamic acid in the treatment of giant hemangiomas in newborns. [Review]. *American Journal of Pediatrics Hematotogy-Oncology, 15,* 383–385.

Morelli, J. G., & Weston, W. L. (1987). Soaps and shampoos in pediatric practice. [Review]. *Pediatrics, 80,* 634–637.

Moschella, S., & Hurley, H. (1985). *Dermatology* (2nd ed., Vol. 2, pp. 1893–1894). Philadelphia: W. B. Saunders.

Nasemann, T., Sauerbrey, W., & Burgdorf, W. (1983). *Fundamentals of dermatology* (p. 11). New York: Springer-Verlag.

Potts, R. O., Buras, E. M. Jr., & Chrisman, D. A., Jr. (1984). Changes with age in the moisture content of human skin. *Journal of Investigational Dermatology, 82,* 97–100.

Pyati, S., Ramamurthy, R., Krauss, M. T., & Pildes, R. (1977). Absorption of iodine in the neonate following topical use of povidone-iodine. *Journal of Pediatrics, 91,* 825–828.

Rasmussen, J. (1987). Classification of diaper dermatitis: An overview. *Pediatrician, 14,* 6–10.

Rosen, T., Lanning M., & Hill, M. (1983). *The nurses' atlas to dermatology* (pp. 97–129). Boston: Little, Brown.

Sarkany, I., & Arnold, L. (1970). The effect of single and repeated applications of hexachlorophene on the bacterial flora of the skin of the newborn. *British Journal of Dermatology, 82*, 261–267.

Solomon, L., & Esterly, N. (1973). Neonatal dermatology. In A. Schaffer (Ed.), *Major problems in clinical pediatrics* (Vol. IX in series), Philadelphia: W. B. Saunders.

Tagami, H., Kanamaru, Y., Inoue, K., et al. (1982). Water sorption-desorption test of the skin in vivo for functional assessment of the stratum corneum. *Journal of Investigative Dermatology, 78*, 425–428.

Tagami, H., & Yoshikuni, K. (1985). Interrelationship between water-barrier and reservoir functions of pathologic stratum corneum. *Archives of Dermatology, 121*, 642–645.

Thune P., Nilsen, T., Hanstad, K., et al. (1988). The water barrier function of the skin in relation to the water content of stratum corneum, pH and skin lipids: The effect of alkaline soap and syndet on dry skin in elderly, non-atopic patients. *Acta Dermato-Venereologica, 68*, 277–283.

Walton, R. (1971). Pigmented nevi. *Pediatric Clinics of North America, 18*, 897–922.

Watson, W. (1978). Selected genodermatoses. [Review]. *Pediatric Clinics of North America, 25*, 263–284.

Ziai, M., Clark, T., & Merritt, T. (1984). *Assessment of the newborn* (pp. 86–111). Boston: Little, Brown.

RESOLIRCES
RESOURCES
•••••••••

ALOPECIA AREATA

National Alopecia Areata Foundation (NAAF)
714 C Street
Suite 216
San Rafael, CA 94901
(415) 456-4644
Vicki Kalabokes, Executive Director

CONGENITAL PORT-WINE STAIN

National Congenital Port-Wine Stain Foundation
125 East 63rd Street
New York, NY 10021
(212) 755-3820
Martha Woodhouse, Executive Director

ECTODERMAL DYSPLASIAS

National Foundation for Ectodermal Dysplasias (NFED)
108 North First Street
Suite 311
Mascoutah, IL 62558
(618) 566-2020
Mary Kaye Richter, Executive Director
Contact: Beverly Meier

EPIDERMOLYSIS BULLOSA

Dystrophic Epidermolysis Bullosa Research Association of America, Inc. (D.E.B.R.A.)
c/o Kings County Medical Center
451 Clarkson Avenue
Building E-6-101

Sixth Floor
Brooklyn, NY 11203
(718) 774-8700
Arlene Pessar, R.N., Executive Director

ICHTHYOSIS

Foundation for Ichthyosis and Related Skin Types, Inc. (F.I.R.S.T.)
3640 Grand Avenue
Suite Two
Oakland, CA 94610
(415) 763-9839
Charles Elchhorn, Executive Director

SCLERODERMA

United Scleroderma Foundation, Inc. (USF)
P.O. Box 350
Watsonville, CA 95077–0350
(800) 722-HOPE
(408) 728-2202
Diana Williams, Executive Director

XERODERMA PIGMENTOSUM

Xeroderma Pigmentosum Registry
UMDNJ–NJ Medical School
Department of Pathology
Medical Science Building
Room C-520
100 Bergen Street
Newark, NJ 07103
(201) 456-6255
W. Clark Lambert, M.D., Executive Director

CHAPTER 21

Assessment and Management of Auditory Dysfunction

Hearing is a prerequisite to cognitive and social/emotional development. Any impairment of hearing from birth to 18 months can have a profound effect on the auditory stimulation necessary for language development. Sensory deprivation affects the acquisition of communication skills even though correction of the hearing loss may be accomplished. To prevent or minimize the detrimental effects of hearing impairment on social, cognitive, and educational development, identification of hearing impairment at the earliest possible time is imperative.

National statistics indicate that of the approximately 3.76 million children born each year, 7 to 12 percent are at risk for hearing impairment (Mahoney & Eichwald, 1987). Moderate to profound hearing impairment is reported to be present in less than 2 percent of infants at risk (Mahoney & Eichwald, 1987). Approximately 1 in every 100 infants has been reported to be deaf at birth (Early Identification of Hearing Impairment in Infants and Young Children, National Institutes of Health Consensus Development Conference, 1994).

AUDITORY DEVELOPMENT AND MECHANISM OF FUNCTION

The ear is a singular organ that functions in both hearing and equilibrium. In the embryo, the ear develops from three different parts: internal, middle, and external ears. This development begins during the fourth week of gestation and continues throughout the pregnancy.

PHYSIOLOGY OF AUDIOLOGIC FUNCTION

External Ear

The external ear consists of the auricle (pinna) and the external auditory meatus (external canal). The primary function of the external ear is to funnel sound to the tympanic membrane.

Middle Ear

Advancing sound entering the auditory canal directly strikes the tympanic membrane. The tympanic membrane and the ossicles serve as transmitters from the outer ear to the inner ear.

The middle ear is lined by respiratory mucosa composed of ciliated

511

columnar epithelial cells, supporting cells, and secretory cells. Secretory cells secrete mucus that forms a complex mucous layer. Cilia of the middle ear interact with the mucus by transporting mastoid and middle ear secretions through the eustachian tube to the nasopharynx, where they are swallowed. This transport has a protective effect against ear infections. In addition to being an exit for secretion into the nasopharynx, the eustachian tube equalizes the pressure between the middle ear and the ambient atmosphere.

Inner Ear

When sound is transferred from the tympanic membrane to the inner ear, the stapes creates a fluid wave that is transmitted to the round window. This creates fluid waves that travel from the basal aspect of the cochlea to the apex. As the fluid wave moves, it displaces the basilar membrane. There is a maximum movement of the basilar membrane at the point that is specific to the frequency of sound entering the ear. High-frequency sounds cause minimal disturbance at the basal end of the cochlea and low frequencies at the apex.

Vibrations within the basilar membrane cause movement of the organ of Corti. This organ contains receptor hair cells that are on the basilar membrane. Vibrations of the hair on the hair cells cause either polarization or depolarization, depending on the direction of the bend. Hair cells act as transducers, converting mechanical energy into electrical impulses in the fibers of the spiral ganglion. Axons of these cells become the auditory nerve (vestibulocochlear nerve). Nerve fibers pass to medulla, pons, and midbrain and finally to the temporal lobes of the cortex, where the impulses are interpreted as sound.

Fluid moves within the vestibular labyrinth when the head moves. The semicircular canals respond to angular acceleration (rotation), and the utricle and saccule respond to linear acceleration (position). The vestibular apparatus functions in conjunction with proprioception and visual orientation to maintain balance.

PERINATAL AUDITORY DEVELOPMENT

Evidence is increasing that the fetus can perceive auditory stimulation and act on it at an early age. This evidence comes from investigation of fetal heart rate responses to sounds and from studies of audition in preterm infants. The newborn has been hearing sounds within the fluid-filled environment for a number of months before birth. Recognition of the mother's voice shortly after birth has been reported by health care professionals and parents just by observing the body movements of the newborn in response to the voice. Further maturation of the nerve fibers responsible for conduction and processing of auditory stimuli continues well into the first year of life.

HEARING IMPAIRMENT

Hearing impairment is defined by the American Speech-Language Hearing Association as "a loss of auditory sensitivity that can be measured at birth and for which intervention strategies are known and available." Hearing impairment represents a spectrum of hearing loss classified as mild, moderate, severe, or prolonged (Northern & Downs, 1984). The criterion for measuring bilateral conductive and sensorineural hearing deficit in children is the frequency range important for speech recognition, namely 1000 to 4000 Hz (Fig. 21–1).

Types of Hearing Impairment

The types of hearing impairment have been classified according to the location of the problem. Impairments may be one of three types: conductive, sensorineural, or combination.

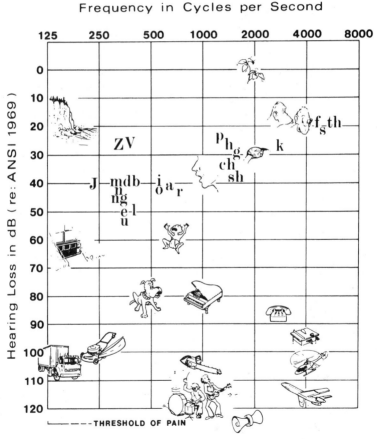

FIGURE 21–1. Frequency spectrum of familiar sounds. (From Northern, J., & Downs, M. [1984]. *Hearing in children* [p. 35]. Baltimore: Williams & Wilkins. Reprinted with permission.)

A *conductive hearing loss* exists when there is dysfunction in the outer or middle ear disrupting the normal sequence of sound localization and vibration. Common causes of this type of hearing impairment are listed below:

- Occlusion of the external auditory meatus occurring as a result of cerumen (wax)
- Otitis media, an infection of the middle ear
- Congenital deformities of the outer ear: missing pinna or atresia of the auditory canal

Disorders of conduction can be revealed by auditory pure-tone testing. Individuals with conductive hearing loss have difficulty with low-frequency sounds, that is, in the 125- to 500-Hz range.

Collaborative management includes the following:

- Early observation/detection
- Elimination of the source of infection or removal of the blockage

Sensorineural hearing impairment results from damage to the sensory nerve endings of the cochlea or dysfunction of the auditory nerve (eighth cranial nerve). A typical characteristic of inner ear dysfunction is the inability of the inner ear to interpret fluid changes in the cochlea. With sensorineural loss, hearing is normal at low frequencies. Deficits with sound are evident above 1000 Hz. Sensorineural hearing loss is caused by the following:

- Congenital inner ear abnormality, resulting in congenital deafness
- Trauma to the inner ear from injury
- Effects of certain drugs
- Prolonged exposure to loud noise
- Infections: measles
- Effects of aging

Collaborative management includes the following:

- Early identification/detection
- Restoration with amplification of sound if indicated

IDENTIFICATION OF THE HEARING-IMPAIRED INFANT

Physical Examination

Physical examinations of the infant should be performed in a quiet, warm, draft-free area to afford adequate surroundings for observation and inspection of the auditory function. Observing the infant's behavior before the actual examination of the ear will yield some valuable baseline assessments. The alert, normal newborn reacts by turning toward the sound of human speech or toward a ringing bell and is startled by the stimulus of a loud noise.

Inspection of the ear begins with the medial and lateral surface of the pinna and the surface of the scalp, face, and neck. Development of the pinna correlates with the gestational age. At term, the pinna of the newborn is well shaped and contains sufficient cartilage to maintain a normal shape and resistance. Before 34 weeks' gestation, the pinna is a slightly formed double thickness of skin.

When folded, the pinna in the term infant demonstrates instant recoil and remains erect from the head. In contrast, the premature infant will exhibit a flat, shapeless pinna that remains folded on inspection. As gestation continues, the pinna develops more cartilage, resulting in better form.

The pinna or auricle should be inspected for location as well as its relationship to other facial structures:

- Normal attachment is to the side.
- It should be level with the middle third of the face.
- It should be fixed in position to the lateral aspect of the external auditory canal.

Major convolutions of the pinna are termed the *helix, anthelix, tragus, antitragus,* and *lobule.* The lobule of the external ear contains no cartilage. The angle of the placement is almost vertical. *If the angle is more than 10 degrees from normal, this is considered abnormal.* The superior helix is located at the outer canthus of the eye, and the tragus is roughly level with the infraorbital rim.

Abnormal findings include the following:

- Low-set auricles, which are frequently associated with other abnormalities of the first and second branchial cleft and with abnormalities of the urinary system (Jones, 1988)
- Skin tags
- Sinuses or pits, which are often associated with other auditory or renal malformations
- Bruised pinna from a forceps delivery

The external auditory meatus should next be observed for patency. Atresia or stenosis of the external meatus may be observed. This abnormality results in a conductive hearing loss by blocking sound transmission and should be noted as part of the physical findings.

The next phase of the examination is directed toward inspection of the middle ear and tympanic membrane. The depths of the external meatus can be examined with a brightly illuminated pneumatic otoscope. Vernix caseosa is frequently encountered. Introduction of the otoscope into the ear canal is accomplished by gentle traction posterosuperiorly on the auricle. In the neonate, the tympanic membrane lies in a nearly horizontal plane. Visualization of the tympanic membrane through the collapsed neonatal ear is accomplished by gentle dilation of the ear canal with the speculum as the cartilaginous canal is traversed. The tympanic membrane should be examined for thickness, vascularity, and contour. All areas, including the area above the short process of the malleus (pars flaccida), should be visualized for completeness. *Normally, the tympanic membrane appears translucent.* White shadows of the ossicles can usually be seen through the membrane.

Mobility of the tympanic membrane can be assessed by applying intermittent pressure through a bulb or by blowing through a polyethylene tube connected to the otoscope.

History

Currently, the only infants screened are those identified with one or more high-risk factors associated with hearing impairment. It is of paramount importance that nurses in labor and delivery and the newborn nursery use the high-risk register as an essential part of early screening for all neonates (Table 21–1).

ASPHYXIA

Asphyxia, or anoxia, a condition in which there is a lack of oxygen with an increase in the carbon dioxide level in the tissue, is particularly damaging to the central nervous system (CNS). It is essential that an adequate supply of oxygen be available for adequate functioning of the organ of Corti. The incidence of sensorineural hearing loss in children with severe perinatal asphyxia has been reported to be approximately 4 percent (Stein, Ozdamar, Kruas, & Paton, 1983). The hearing loss is especially in the high-frequency range (Simmons, 1980).

BACTERIAL MENINGITIS

Bacterial meningitis is a common infection and sequela of bacteria in the neonate. Meningitis, a disease of the CNS, presents as an inflammation of the meninges of the brain and the cerebrospinal fluid that may extend to adjacent organs such as the brain or ear. Meningitis presents in approximately

---

TABLE 21–1. Risk Identification Criteria: Neonates (Birth–28 Days)

The risk factors that identify those neonates who are at risk for sensorineural hearing impairment include the following:
1. Family history of congenital or delayed onset childhood sensorineural impairment.
2. Congenital infection known or suspected to be associated with sensorineural hearing impairment, such as toxoplasmosis, syphilis, rubella, cytomegalovirus, and herpes.
3. Craniofacial anomalies, including morphologic abnormalities of the pinna and ear canal, absent philtrum, low hairline, etc.
4. Birth weight less than 1500 g (3.3 lb.).
5. Hyperbilirubinemia at a level exceeding indication for exchange transfusion.
6. Ototoxic medications, including but not limited to, the aminoglycosides used for more than 5 days (e.g., gentamicin, tobramycin, kanamycin, streptomycin) and loop diuretics used in combination with aminoglycosides.
7. Bacterial meningitis.
8. Severe depression at birth, which may include infants with Apgar scores of 0–3 at 5 minutes or those who fail to initiate spontaneous respiration by 10 minutes or those with hypotonia persisting to 2 hours of age.
9. Prolonged mechanical ventilation for a duration equal to or greater than 10 days (e.g., persistent pulmonary hypertension).
10. Stigmata or other findings associated with a syndrome known to include sensorineural hearing loss (e.g., Waardenburg's or Usher's syndrome).

....

From Joint Committee on Infant Hearing. (1991, March). Position statement. ASHA, pp 15–17. Reprinted with permission.

1 in 2500 live births (Feigin, Adcock, & Miller, 1992). It is acquired in most cases postnatally and is the most common cause of hearing loss in infants (Pappas, 1985).

Treatment modalities for infants with meningitis are supportive, with antibiotic therapy being an important aspect of the regimen. Antibiotic drugs such as gentamicin and kanamycin, which are widely used in treatment, are often potential ototoxic agents. Careful monitoring of drug levels is imperative to decrease the risk of hearing loss.

Sensorineural hearing loss has been reported in 7 to 35 percent of patients with bacterial meningitis (Finitzo-Hieber et al., 1981). The hearing loss is generally bilateral and ranges from mild to profound. The report that 50 percent of postmeningitic infants are subject to unstable hearing loss is significant and calls for close monitoring to ensure proper identification of at-risk patients (Pappas, 1985). Audiometry immediately after the meningitis and every 3 months until the age of 3 years is recommended (Pappas, 1985).

CONGENITAL PERINATAL INFECTION

The most common and best referenced infections are represented by the acronym TORCH, for *t*oxoplasmosis, *o*ther infections, *r*ubella, *c*ytomegalovirus, and *h*erpes. Although "other infections" does not include syphilis, this infection is discussed here in relation to its potential impact on hearing impairment. One to 5 percent of all deliveries are infected by the TORCH agents (Nahmias, 1974).

Toxoplasmosis

Toxoplasmosis is caused by the parasite *Toxoplasma gondii*. It is acquired as an active disease in 2 to 7 per 1000 pregnant women. Of these women, 30 to 40 percent will transfer the organism transplacentally to the fetus (Babson, 1980). Pathologic studies (Keleman, 1958) have demonstrated changes in the soft tissue mesenchyma and mucoperiosteum and calcium deposits in the spiral ligament of the inner ear.

Syphilis

Syphilis is caused by the *Treponema pallidum* spirochetal organism, which is transmitted in utero to the fetus from an infected mother (Feigin, Adcock, & Edwards, 1992).

Transmission of the spirochete to the fetus occurs in 70 to 100 percent of the pregnancies with untreated primary syphilis and approximately 30 percent of pregnancies with latent syphilis (Krugman & Katz, 1981). Congenital syphilis affects hearing in approximately 35 percent of children (Sando & Wood, 1971).

Early symptoms of congenital syphilis in the neonate include nasal discharge (snuffles), rash, anemia, jaundice, and osteochondritis. Late symptoms include saddle nose, saber shin, and dental abnormalities (Northern & Downs, 1984). Congenital syphilis has a profound effect on the inner ear. Pathologic changes include osteitis of all three layers of the otic capsule, with inflammatory infiltration of the membranes of the cochlea and vestibular labyrinth. Hearing impairment may be profound as a result of severe degeneration of the organ of Corti, spiral ganglion, and nerve cells along with destruction of the membranous labyrinth (Karmody & Schuknecht, 1966; Schuknecht, 1974).

Spirochetes remain visible in the perilymph of the ear despite massive therapy because penicillin does not readily cross the barrier to enter the endolymphatic fluid of the inner ear (Wiet & Milko, 1975).

Some of the complex issues surrounding hearing impairment related to congenital syphilis include the following:

- Congenital syphilis may be asymptomatic in up to 50 percent of neonatal cases (Stagno, Pass, & Alford, 1981).
- Routine hospital screenings for syphilis through the VDRL test have high false-positive and false-negative rates and may show a positive reaction in other diseases such as malaria, infectious hepatitis, infectious mononucleosis, and disseminated lupus erythematosus. In comparison, the fluorescent treponemal antibody absorption test is more sensitive but more expensive (Harner, Smith, & Israel, 1968).
- The progressive pattern of hearing impairment demonstrates variations as to the time of onset and rapidity of progression (Patterson, 1968).
- In early childhood, the onset of infantile congenital syphilis is usually between 8 and 20 years of age. Hearing loss is sudden, bilateral, symmetrical, and profound, with no accompanying symptoms (Schuknecht, 1974).
- Hearing loss as a result of congenital syphilis presents as poor function and limited use of hearing aid devices owing to neural atrophy with poor discrimination (Wilson, Byl, & Laird, 1980).
- Penicillin therapy does not prevent or retard the progressive hearing loss (Patterson, 1968).

Because syphilitic hearing impairments pose a grave threat to the future developmental milestones of the infant, early identification, testing, and lengthy follow-up are imperative.

Rubella

Congenital rubella infection is a major threat to the fetus and newborn. In the prevaccine period, before 1969, congenital rubella was the leading cause of deafness in children attending schools for the hearing impaired in the United States (Cooper et al., 1969).

Acquired rubella is a mild disease of children and adults that is transmitted by droplet contact with the virus. The virus is congenitally acquired by the fetus through placental transfer (McCracken, 1963). Clinically, the infant with congenital rubella may present with a wide range of features. Many present as normal newborns, whereas others display cardiac lesions, low birth weight, eye defects, growth retardation, thrombocytopenic purpura, hepatosplenomegaly, hepatitis, and CNS defects such as psychomotor retardation (Baley & Goldfarb, 1992). Hearing defects are the most common result of the viral insult. Congenital rubella is manifested as chronic infection in fetal tissues, causing an inhibition of fetal cell multiplication; therefore, it is not a static disease (Baley & Goldfarb, 1992). Histopathologic studies subsequent to rubella infection have revealed a degeneration of the organ of

Corti as well as anomalies of the middle ear such as fixed stapedial footplate (Sando & Wood, 1971; Scholl, Lurie, & Keleman, 1951).

Hearing deficit associated with congenital rubella syndrome is severe to profound bilateral sensorineural, with an audiometric configuration that depicts the greatest degree of loss in the midrange, from 500 to 2000 Hz (Konigsmark & Gorlin, 1976). Infants with a history of rubella or rubella exposure should be followed with serial audiograms until 18 to 24 months of age because of the potential late onset and the progressive nature of congenital rubella syndrome.

Cytomegalovirus

Cytomegalovirus (CMV), a virus of the herpes family, is the most common cause of congenital viral infection in humans. Twenty percent of pregnant women carry CMV; 2.5 percent of the infants are infected at birth, and 10 to 20 percent are at risk for latter sequelae (Baley & Goldfarb, 1992).

The virus can be transmitted to the fetus transplacentally or at the time of delivery via the cervix. CMV can also be transmitted postnatally through infected urine, saliva, breast milk, tears, feces, and blood transfusions (Weller, 1971).

The effects of CMV range from severe CNS involvement to asymptomatic carrying of the virus. Asymptomatic infants are at risk for late sequelae manifested as bilateral sensorineural hearing loss that may be mild to profound. Manifestations of CMV infection are as follows (Baley & Goldfarb, 1992):

- Hepatosplenomegaly
- Jaundice
- Petechial rash
- Chorioretinitis
- Cerebral calcifications
- Microcephaly

CMV infections of the inner ear cause either partial or total cochlear and labyrinthine end-organ destruction. The damaged cell reaction is clearly manifested among the cells of the organ of Corti and the neurons of the spiral ganglion (Stagno et al., 1977). In a follow-up study of symptomatic infants with cytomegalic inclusion disease, 30 percent were found to develop severe to profound bilateral sensorineural hearing loss (Pass, Stagno, Meyers, & Alford, 1980). The following are the basic tenets of care (Northern & Downs, 1984):

- Excretion of the CMV virus may remain active for several years after birth, contributing to degenerative hearing loss. Therefore, follow-up testing should take place at shorter time periods than for nonprogressive disease processes. Audiologic evaluation at 3-month intervals is recommended.
- In the case of cytomegalic inclusion disease, any pattern and degree of hearing loss can occur. Screening of these infants should be done with electrophysiologic testing, because the opportunity to detect a mild to moderate loss is greater with this technique.
- In the case of asymptomatic viral infection, hearing loss may manifest at a later date. This knowledge may aid in the possible cause of childhood onset of hearing loss.

Herpes Simplex Virus

Herpes simplex virus (HSV), a member of a group of DNA viruses that cause latent infection characterized by periodic recurrences, poses a threat to the health of both mother and neonate. HSV-1 infections generally occur in the oral cavity or above the waist and are most prevalent among children and young adults. Transmission is usually spread through the respiratory route from contact with family members who are asymptomatic. Recurrence of the oral lesions takes place in 20 to 45 percent of individuals with the disease (Baley & Goldfarb, 1992).

HSV-2 infections generally occur in the genital region and are transmitted by sexual contact. Isolation of the virus can be found in sexually active individuals. The majority of genital infections are asymptomatic. Patients that are symptomatic report local tenderness and burning involving the labia and vaginal mucosa. Both symptomatic and asymptomatic individuals may transmit the infection.

Although HSV infections are often asymptomatic in the adult, they are rarely so in the neonate. Vaginally contracted HSV in the neonate does not manifest initially; there is an incubation period of 6 to 12 days before clinical symptoms appear (Whitley et al., 1980). Neonatal infections are classified as disseminated with or without CNS involvement or localized. Disseminated infections may involve virtually every organ system. With CNS involvement, the majority of cases result in death; of the survivors, only 4 percent lack sequelae. Without CNS involvement, 12 percent survive free of sequelae. Of infants with localized infections, 41 percent suffer from progressive neurologic damage resulting in death; 42 percent of those who survive suffer from severe neurologic sequelae (Whitley et al., 1980).

Ventry and associates (1981), through histopathologic studies, demonstrated that herpes infects the sensory cells of the labyrinth.

DEFECTS OF THE HEAD AND NECK

Ear anomalies associated with head and neck anomalies may occur as a result of a primary regional defect, secondary to a primary defect in an area contiguous to the temporal bone, as part of an inherited defect involving the skeletal system, or as part of a chromosomal disorder.

Ear

In normal placement, the helix is located at the level of the outer canthus of the eye and the tragus is roughly level with the intraorbital rim. Low-set auricles are frequently associated with abnormalities of the urinary system (Eavey, 1989). Jaffe (1977) reported unilateral conductive hearing losses in children with normal-sized pinnas and unilateral absence of the superior crus. He also reported hearing losses in patients with fused anthelix-helix; thickened, hypertrophied earlobes; a "cup" ear; as well as a protruding pinna. The pinna may be noted to be abnormally small (microtia) or totally absent (anotia). Atresia (closure of the external auditory canal) may be observed. Atresia is classified as mild, indicating a small ear canal; medium, indicating a bony atresia plate replacing the canal with ossicular malformation; or severe, indicating a small or absent ear canal and middle ear space (Naunton & Valvassori, 1968). Multiple combinations of atresia and microtia may coexist; therefore, all children with these abnormalities should be suspect for middle ear abnormalities. Atresia is often observed with cranial, facial, mandibular, or acrofacial dysostoses. Abnormalities of the skeletal system or chromosomal aberration may also present as atresia. Aural atresia may also be associated with facial, labial, or palatal clefts. Infants with atresia often suffer conductive hearing loss related to the inability of the ear canal to transmit sound.

Preauricular abnormalities, including pits or tags and branchial fistulas, are often accompanied by external or middle ear malformations. Preauricular tags or pits usually require only cosmetic surgery or excision if draining. ·

Nose

Examination of the nose should be directed toward identification of suspicious defects such as unusual broadness with flat base and short length (saddle nose), small nostrils, and notched alae. Deformities of the nose often present as other craniofacial abnormalities.

Mouth

Defects in the oral cavity are the most common defects associated with hearing impairment. The child with cleft lip or palate displays a deficiency in palate musculature that is primarily related to the inability of the tensor veli palatini muscle to dilate the eustachian tube actively during swallowing (Doyle, Cantekin, & Bluestone, 1980).

The child is vulnerable to the effusion of fluid and, as a result, to varying degrees of hearing loss. The rate of otitis media is increased, and rates of 50 to 90 percent have been reported (Bluestone & Shurin, 1974; Doyle, Cantekin, & Bluestone, 1980). The hearing loss is generally conductive; however, there have been reports of sensorineural or combination losses (Bergstrom & Hemenway, 1971).

Eyes

A variation in eyelid configuration has been noted in which the upper lid forms an almost vertical curve at the level of the medial limit of the cornea and fuses with the lower lid. The distance of the two medial angles is increased. These findings are typically noted in Waardenburg's syndrome, an autosomal dominant disorder resulting in mild to severe sensorineural hearing loss in 50 percent of patients, which may be unilateral or bilateral and progressive (Marcus & Valvassori, 1970; Pantke & Cohen, 1971).

Epicanthal folds, true vertical folds extending from the nasal fold into the upper eyelid, are commonly noted in infants with Down syndrome. Other physical features presenting in Down syndrome, or trisomy 21, include low-set ears, small pinna, and narrow external ear canal. These infants display a strong tendency for recurrent otitis media and anomalies of the middle ear ossicles. Incidence of hearing loss is high, displaying sensorineural, conductive, or combination types (Balkany, Downs, Jafek, & Krajicek, 1979).

Hair

Observation of unusual hair texture or hairline should be regarded with suspicion when assessing for abnormalities associated with hearing loss. Twisted hair (pili torti) has been associated with sensorineural hearing loss. The hair may be twisted, dry, brittle, or easily broken. Other observations that may be significant are aberrant scalp-hair patterning.

Neck

Defects of the neck that may be associated with hearing defects are branchial cleft fistulas and mildly webbed or shortened neck (Feingold, 1982). The presence of such defects does increase the risk, however, and should be followed up in the long-term interest of the child.

INCREASED BILIRUBIN LEVEL

Hyperbilirubinemia, also referred to as neonatal jaundice, occurs when there is an excess amount of bilirubin in the blood. The condition can be neurotoxic to the infant at high concentrations. Jaundice is observed in approximately 60 percent of term infants and 80 percent of preterm infants (Behrman & Kliegman, 1992). Kernicterus, a neurologic syndrome, results from the deposit of unconjugated bilirubin in the basal ganglia of the brain, causing motor and sensory deficits, mental deficits, or death (Behrman & Kliegman, 1992).

The Joint Committee on Infant Hearing suggests that those infants with a bilirubin level that exceeds indications requiring an exchange transfusion are at risk for demonstrating hearing impairments. The Committee of the Fetus and the Newborn of the American Academy of Pediatrics (1982) suggested that the following birth weights and bilirubin levels be used as guidelines for deciding whether to place an infant on the high-risk register:

Birth Weight (g)	Bilirubin Level (mg)
>1000	10
1001–1250	10
1251–1500	13
1501–2000	15
2001–2500	17
<2500	18

FAMILY HISTORY

More than 50 types of hereditary hearing loss have been described. A significant number of hearing impairments may be classified as genetically based. The family history should include the following:

1. Determination of the cause and circumstances under which the hearing impairment was first noticed. A number of different circumstances surrounding the onset of the hearing loss may label it as congenital or hereditary or both. An example of hearing loss that is hereditary and

not congenital occurs in Alport's syndrome, an autosomal dominant inheritance resulting in deafness that appears at 8 years of age.

2. A complete family history, including a history of all previous as well as current pregnancies
3. An extended family history of data relating to hearing impairments of immediate as well as extended family members
4. A thorough physical examination, with particular inspection of the head and neck region to detect abnormalities
5. Selective testing procedures for assessing possible causes of sensorineural hearing loss

A form for identification through query of the mother is shown in Figure 21–2. This tool provides an excellent opportunity for educating the mother on normal speech and language development.

HEREDITARY HEARING LOSS

Autosomal Dominant

Autosomal dominant inheritance accounts for 10 to 25 percent of the cases of hereditary hearing impairment (Fraser, 1976; Nance & Sweeney, 1975). The hearing loss may be unilateral or bilateral, and both sexes are

---

MOTHER'S NAME:_____

ROOM NO.:_____

1. Do you know any of the baby's relatives who now have a hearing loss which started before the age of five? Think hard about all of your family and the baby's father's family . . . .
Yes _____ No _____
A. If no, proceed to question No. 2.
B. If yes, ask the following:
   (1) Who were they? (relationship to baby)
       (A)_____ (B)_____ (C)_____
   (2) Do you know what caused the loss? . . . .
       Yes _____ No _____
       (A)_____ (B)_____ (C)_____
   (3) What makes you think the onset of the hearing loss was before age five?
       (A)_____ (B)_____ (C)_____
   (4) Did he/she wear a hearing aid before age five? . . (A) _____ (B) _____ (C) _____
       Does he/she still wear an aid? . . . . (A) _____ (B) _____ (C) _____
   (5) Did he/she attend a special school for the deaf? . (A) _____ (B) _____ (C) _____
       Did the person attend public school? . . . . (A) _____ (B) _____ (C) _____
   (6) Did he/she have a speech problem? . . . . (A) _____ (B) _____ (C) _____
2. During your pregnancy, did you have 3-day measles, German measles, rubella, or a rash with a fever? . . . . Yes_____ No_____
   WHEN: 1st 3 mo._____ Middle 3 mo._____ Last 3 mo._____
3. During your pregnancy, were you around anyone who had 3-day measles, German measles, rubella, or a rash with fever? . . . . Yes_____ No_____
   WHEN: 1st 3 mo._____ Middle 3 mo._____ Last 3 mo._____
4. Do you have any reason to be concerned about your baby's hearing? . . . .
   Yes_____ No_____
   If yes, why?_____
5. What pediatrician or clinic will be caring for your baby when he/she leaves the hospital? _____

   Approximate location_____
6. Nearest relative or friend: Name:_____
                              Address:_____
                              Phone:_____

FIGURE 21–2. Mother's interview. (From Northern, J., & Downs, M. [1984]. *Hearing in children* [p. 237]. Baltimore: Williams & Wilkins. Reprinted with permission.)

affected equally. Autosomal dominant hearing disorders vary in severity ("variable expressivity") as well as in progression of hearing loss. A typical example of autosomal dominant hearing disorder is *Waardenburg's syndrome.* In this syndrome, severe profound bilateral sensorineural hearing loss presents with integumentary system involvement. Histopathologic studies indicate the absence of the organ of Corti and atrophy of the spiral ganglion (Marcus & Valvassori, 1970; Pantke & Cohen, 1971).

Treacher Collins syndrome is another example of autosomal dominant hearing loss with incomplete penetrance and variable expression. Major features include facial anomalies, small displaced or absent external ears, external auditory canal atresia, and poorly developed or malformed tympanic ossicles. Deafness is generally complete and conductive (Linsey, 1971).

Klippel-Feil syndrome, if familial, is another example of autosomal dominance with variable expression. Characteristics of this syndrome include craniofacial disorders, fusion of some or all of the cervical vertebrae, occasionally cleft palate, and severe sensorineural hearing loss (Windle-Taylor, Emery, & Phelps, 1981).

Crouzon's disease is another example of hearing loss attributed to autosomal dominance with variable expression. It is characterized by an abnormally shaped head, beaked nose, and marked bilateral exophthalmos caused by premature closure of the cranial sutures. Hearing loss may be conductive or sensorineural, owing to middle ear deformities (Baldwin, 1968).

Autosomal Recessive

Autosomal recessive inheritance accounts for about 40 percent of childhood deafness (Proctor & Proctor, 1967). It is estimated that one in eight individuals is a carrier for a recessive form of hearing impairment. Hearing loss with an autosomal recessive gene tends to be more severe than with autosomal dominant inheritance. In *Scheibe dysplasia,* the entire organ of Corti is rudimentary, with hair cells missing and the supporting cells distorted or collapsed. The vestibular membrane is usually collapsed (Konigsmark & Gorlin, 1976). *Pendred's syndrome,* a condition marked by hearing loss and goiter, is detected in the first 2 years of life (Illum, Kiaer, Hvidberg-Hansen, & Sondergaard, 1972).

X-Linked

Approximately 3 percent of hereditary deafness is due to the *X-linked mode of transmission* (Northern & Downs, 1984). The female is the carrier and has the chance to transmit the gene to 50 percent of her sons, who will manifest the disease, and 50 percent of her daughters, who will carry the abnormality. The hearing loss is characteristically *not present at birth* but develops in infancy to varying degrees.

X-linked hearing losses, with exceptions, are sensorineural, and there is often some retention of hearing in all frequencies. Recessive or *X-linked Duchenne's muscular dystrophy* is an example. Characterized by muscle wasting, the severe infantile form of muscular dystrophy is also associated with mild to moderate sensorineural hearing loss (Black, Bergstrom, & Downs, 1971).

Cytogenetic Disorders

Cytogenetic disorders are caused by structural changes in one or more of the chromosomes or by errors in the distribution of the chromosomes. *Down syndrome,* or *trisomy 21,* the most common chromosomal aberration syndrome, presenting in 1 in 600 to 800 births, is usually due to an extra chromosome 21 (Nyhan, 1983).

Balkany and associates (1979) reported on the relatively high incidence of hearing loss among children with trisomy 21. Characteristic otologic findings that have an impact on the hearing performance of these children during the early years are (1) a high incidence of stenosis of the external auditory canal, (2) a high incidence of serous otitis media, and (3) a high incidence of cholesteatoma (i.e., persistent growth of squamous epithelium from the ear canal into the middle ear or mastoid through a tear in the tympanic membrane) (Pappas, 1985).

The ear canal of infants with trisomy 21 tends to be stenotic, with an hourglass appearance. The narrowed segment is located at the junction of the cartilaginous and bony portions of the canal. With increasing age, the canal has been noted to assume a more typical appearance as the thickened tissue recedes.

The degree of hearing loss in these infants varies, but it is rarely ever profound.

Mental retardation is a clinical condition frequently observed with trisomy 21. Because of the high incidence of hearing loss in this group, it becomes imperative that early and frequent monitoring be instituted.

LOW BIRTH WEIGHT

Low birth weight (<1500 g), especially when associated with complications such as hyperbilirubinemia or perinatal asphyxia, is widely accepted as a risk factor for congenitally acquired hearing impairment.

Between 4 and 16 percent of infants with low birth weight have been reported with hearing loss (Abramovich, Gregory, Slemink, & Stewart, 1979; Anagnostakes et al., 1982). Other conditions that have been reported to enhance the risk of neurologic sequelae, including hearing impairment, are acidosis, sepsis, ototoxic drug therapy, sound trauma, and hypoglycemia (Bess, Peek, & Chapman, 1979; Perlman et al., 1980).

The hearing loss is usually sensorineural, particularly in the high-frequency range (Clark, 1978).

The higher incidence of hearing loss in low birth weight infants has been attributed to several factors (Minoli & Moro, 1985):

- Premature physiologic status
- Perinatal complications such as hyperbilirubinemia, hypoxia, acidosis, and apneic spells, which are likely to produce brain damage in low birth weight infants
- Constraints of intensive care
- Combined effects of the preceding factors

"Constraints of intensive care" refers to the iatrogenic factors common in the care of newborns admitted to the neonatal intensive care unit (NICU) that have an impact on the incidence of hearing impairment. These factors include ambient noise and exposure to ototoxic drugs (Minoli & Moro, 1985).

Ototoxic Drugs

Drugs that have been reported to be potentially ototoxic include antibiotics, diuretics, and antimalarial pharmaceutical agents (Northern & Downs, 1984). Usually they cause bilateral symmetrical hearing loss of varying degrees. A number of factors may potentially enhance the risk of ototoxicity:

- Increased drug serum levels
- Decreased renal function
- Use of more than one ototoxic drug simultaneously or in increased dose or for an extended period of time
- Age
- Health
- Heredity
- Concurrent noise

Specific aminoglycosides reported to have ototoxic potential include amikacin, clindamycin, gentamicin, kanamycin, tobramycin, and vancomycin (Pettigrew, Edwards, & Henderson-Smart, 1988). Most recent guidelines (American Speech-Language Hearing Association, 1990) suggest that aminoglycoside therapy administered for more than 5 days in combination with loop diuretics be added to the risk criteria for potential sensorineural hearing loss.

At present, neonatal nurses are urged to monitor peak and trough serum concentration of antibiotics and creatinine clearance to avoid high systemic levels in cases of impaired renal function.

Sound Trauma

Within the NICU, there is a magnitude of sound sources that constantly generate background and alarm sounds. Noise levels within the NICU have been reported to be 20 dB higher than in the well-baby nursery.

NICU sudden noises have been reported to produce hypoxemia in preterm infants, which leads to decreases in transcutaneous oxygen tension and an increase in intracranial pressure, heart rate, and respiratory rate (Long, Lucey, & Philip, 1980).

Nearly all the reported sound pressure levels of incubators are consistently below the risk levels for adults, being between 60 and 80 dB (Douek et al., 1976; Falk & Farmer, 1973; Thomas, 1989). The damage risk level of 90 dB for adults is based on intermittent exposure to noise, whereas with the neonate, exposure is continuous for weeks and months at a time (Brown & Glass, 1979). Safe noise standards have not been established for NICUs. The NICU Design Standards Task Force has made recommendations about background noise being no greater than 90 dB (White, 1996). However, when background noise is greater than 50 dB, sleep is disturbed (Robertson & Philbin, 1996). The possible potentiating effects of constant noise with other risk factors on the neonate are also not known.

Newborns at risk may be exposed to hazardous sound levels during transport procedures. In these conditions, noise levels between 90 and 110 dB can be reached in a helicopter (Despland & Galambos, 1982). Use of ear protectors during air transport has been suggested (Minoli & Moro, 1985).

SCREENING METHODS FOR IDENTIFICATION OF HEARING LOSS

Hearing screening is a method of detecting hearing impairment before the time that the deficit becomes obvious in the infant. The goal of any screening program is to accomplish the task rapidly, accurately, and economically.

Screening criteria such as the high-risk register should be the basis for any infant screening program. Infants who demonstrate no risk factors receive no audiologic follow-up unless there is some factor in the history indicating that delayed onset, degenerative disease, or intrauterine infection may present as progressive or fluctuating hearing loss.

Behavioral Measurements of Hearing Function

Early attempts at infant behavioral screening focused on observational assessments of the neonatal behavioral response to sound, using noisemakers to obtain orienting responses. A squeeze toy, bell, or rattle was employed to test for a behavioral response based on the maturational level of the subject.

Automated Screening Devices

Disappointing results from observational screening methods prompted the development of automated instrumentation methods of detecting hearing loss.

CRIB-O-GRAM

The Crib-O-Gram (Simmons & Russ, 1974) is an ingenious automated system aimed at monitoring behavioral and physiologic responses to auditory stimuli. This test is accomplished by placement of a motion-sensitive transducer under the crib mattress. The infant's state is monitored automatically by measuring crib movements before and after each sound presentation. The test sound, 92 dB, is presented by an earphone placed in the bassinet. Responses are recorded from 10 seconds before until 3.5 seconds after the stimuli onset until a statistically valid decision is made by a microprocessing unit (Marcellino, 1986).

AUDITORY RESPONSE CRADLE

The Auditory Response Cradle (ARC), designed by Bennett and Lawrence (1980), like the Crib-O-Gram, monitors behavioral and physiologic responses to auditory stimuli by an automatic, microprocessor-controlled device. The system is composed of a cradle that houses the electronic components of the device, including the microprocessor.

Four response types are monitored during the test:

1. Head and trunk movements, monitored by a pressure-sensitive mattress
2. Startle responses
3. Body movements, detected by pressure transducers beneath the mattress
4. Respiratory movements of the chest, monitored by a transducer within a band fixed around the infant's chest or abdomen

Noise stimulus is presented at 85 dB through earphones, and the analysis procedure takes into account the number of responses that occur with sound and control trials. The device assesses infant activity in the prestimulus period and defers testing if the subject is restless.

Peripheral Measurements of Hearing Function

In assessing the hearing activity of the neonate, recent focus has been directed toward a two-tiered approach, initially using a test that measures otoacoustic emissions (OAEs) with auditory brain stem response (ABR) follow-up for infants who fail the initial screening. OAEs are low-intensity sounds that can be measured by use of a sensitive microphone placed in the ear canal. Hearing screening using OAEs is quick, inexpensive, and relatively accurate. If an infant fails the OAE testing, additional testing by the ABR will confirm the validity of the OAE. The ABR test records the electrical potentials that arise from the auditory nerve system. During this measurement, disk electrodes are attached to the vertex and the mastoid areas and repetitive sounds are then presented to the ear in the form of clicks caused by a direct current pulse. The response recorded is a sequence of waves that represents the action potential of the auditory nerve. The wave latencies in infants at risk tend to show smaller and more prolonged responses. The absolute latency of the ABR waves depends on the intensity of the click stimulus. Thresholds of hearing are identified by decreasing the click stimuli from intensities of 60 dB to clicks of 30 to 40 dB. Absence of all waves indicates a peripheral lesion. An abnormal ABR may be defined as one in which there is an absence of response at 40-dB intensity or a wave V latency that exceeds the norm by two standard deviations (Cox, Hack, & Metz, 1984). Wave V responses in infants are highly repeatable and reveal little variability among normal hearing subjects; thus, they are used to determine response abnormality. The ABR appears to be a very sensitive method in that no false-negative results have been reported. Considering that any screening method should be quick, inexpensive, and easily administered and allow easy interpretation of a large number of infants, ABRs are at a disadvantage. Specialized personnel are needed to administer this test, which in the majority of cases takes from 60 minutes to 2 hours to perform. Nevertheless, the ABR can be justified as a neonatal hearing test, especially in preterm or high-risk infants. In some infants whose initial ABR testing meets risk criteria, ongoing audiologic follow-up and management may be appropriate. Infants can be fitted with hearing aids before 3 months of age.

MANAGEMENT OF THE HEARING-IMPAIRED NEONATE

For the infant with a confirmed hearing loss, efforts are directed at treatment. In accordance with Public Law 99–457, early intervention services are (1) evaluation and assessment and (2) development of an individualized family service plan. The full evaluation plan is to be completed within 45 days of referral. This plan may include various treatment modalities directed at the treatment of serous otitis media, a major cause of temporary conductive hearing loss.

For the infant with a permanent conductive hearing loss, amplification with a hearing aid may facilitate stimulation in the early critical period. Infants can be fitted with a hearing aid device as soon as the impairment is diagnosed. In addition to amplification, the family should be taught total communication skills that will enhance the interactional process between the sender and the receiver. The basic premise is to use every and all means to communicate, such as gesturing, touching, and attending to stimuli (Brewster, 1985).

Hearing screening is a task for a team of professionals—pediatricians, otolaryngologists, audiologists, and nurses. Local public health agencies may provide services such as data collection and referral. Many large metropolitan medical centers have speech and hearing centers as part of a broad base of services ranging from diagnosis to rehabilitation.

Parental Support

The mother–infant relationship is potentially damaged when the infant is hearing impaired. Reciprocal communication interaction that normally occurs between the mother and infant on both an affective and verbal level has been reported to be diminished in light of the handicap (Greenstein, Greenstein, McConnville, & Stelline, 1976). The handicapped infant may miss intended signals from its parents and may emit signals that are not understood. The parents need to capture their infant's visual attention so that their efforts will be effectively stimulating. A potential asynchrony may develop, which can retard the ability to acquire language even beyond the limits of the hearing loss itself (Luterman, 1985). The family can be taught total communication skills (gesturing, touching, and attending) to support interaction with the infant.

REFERENCES

Abramovich, S. J., Gregory, S., Slemink, M., & Stewart, A. (1979). Hearing loss in very low birth weight infants treated with neonatal intensive care. *Archives of Disease in Childhood, 54,* 421–426.

American Academy of Pediatrics (AAP). (1982). Joint Committee on Infant Hearing. Position Statement. *Pediatrics, 70,* 496–497.

American Speech-Language Hearing Association Joint Committee on Hearing. (1990). Position statement. *ASHA, 32*(3), 15–17.

Anagnostakes, D., Petmezakis, J., Papzissis, G., et al. (1982). Hearing loss in low birth weight infants. *American Journal of Diseases in Children, 136,* 602.

Babson, S. G. (1980). *Diagnosis and management of the fetus and neonate at risk.* St. Louis: C. V. Mosby.

Baldwin, J. L. (1968). Dysostosis craniofacialis of Crouzon. *Laryngoscope, 78,* 1660–1675.

Baley, J., & Goldfarb. J. (1992). Viral infections. In A. Fanaroff & R.J. Martin (Eds.), *Neonatal perinatal medicine: Diseases of the fetus and infant* (5th ed., pp. 662–682). St. Louis: C. V. Mosby.

Balkany, T. J., Downs, M. P., Jafek, B. W., & Krajicek, M. J. (1979). Hearing loss in Down's syndrome: A treatable handicap more common than generally recognized. *Clinical Pediatrics, 18,* 116–118.

Behrman, R. E., & Kliegman, R. M. (1992). Disturbances of organ systems. In R. E. Behrman (Ed.), *Nelson textbook of pediatrics* (14th ed., pp. 460–493). Philadelphia: W. B. Saunders.

Bennett, M. J., & Lawrence, R. J. (1980). Trials with the Auditory Response Cradle: II. The neonatal respiratory response to an auditory stimulus. *British Journal of Audiology, 14,* 1–6.

Bergstrom, L., & Hemenway, W. G. (1971). Otologic problems in submucous cleft palate. *Southern Medical Journal, 64,* 1172–1177.

Bess, F. H., Peek, B. F., & Chapman, J. J. (1979). Further observations on noise levels in infant incubation. *Pediatrics, 63,* 100–106.

Black, F. O., Bergstrom, L., & Downs, M. P. (1971). *Congenital deafness: A new approach to early detection through a high risk register.* Boulder, CO: Associated University Press.

Bluestone, C. D., & Shurin, P. A. (1974). Middle ear disease in children: Pathogenesis, diagnosis and management. *Pediatric Clinics of North America, 21,* 379–399.

Brewster, L. C. (1985). Interaction analysis of mother and hearing impaired child. *Ear and Hearing, 6*(1), 54–56.

Brown, A. K., & Glass, L. (1979). Environmental hazards in the newborn nursery. *Pediatric Annals, 8,* 698–705.

Clark, G. M. (1978). Cochlear implant surgery for profound or total hearing loss [Editorial]. *Medical Journal of Australia, 2,* 587–588.

Cooper, L. Z., Ziring, P. R., Ockerse, A. B., et al. (1969). Rubella: Clinical manifestations and management. *American Journal of Diseases of Children, 118,* 18–29.

Cox, L. C., Hack, M., & Metz, D. A. (1984). Auditory brainstem response abnormalities in the very low birth weight infant: Incidence and risk factors. *Ear and Hearing, 5*(4), 47–51.

Despland, P.A., & Galambos, R. (1982). The brainstem auditory evoked potential is a useful diagnostic tool in evaluating risk factors for hearing loss in neonatology. *Advances in Neurology, 32,* 241–247.

Douek, E., Bannister, L. H., Dodson, H. C., et al. (1976). Effects of incubator noise on the cochlea of the newborn. *Lancet, 2,* 1110–1113.

Doyle, W. J., Cantekin, E. I., & Bluestone, C. D. (1980). Eustachian tube function in cleft palate children. In Recent advances in otitis media with effusion. *Annals of Otology, Rhinology, and Laryngology, 89*(Suppl. 68), 34–40.

Early Identification of Hearing Impairment in Infants & Young Children, National Institutes of Health & Consensus Development Conference. (1993). *American Journal of Otology, 15*(2), 130–131.

Eavey, R. D. (1989). Management strategies for congenital ear malformations. *Recent Advances in Pediatric Otology, 36,* 1521–1540.

Falk, S. A., & Farmer, J. C. (1973). Incubator noise and possible deafness. *Archives of Otolaryngology, 97,* 385–387.

Feigin, R. D., Adcock, L., & Edwards, M. S. (1992). Fungal and protozoal infections. In A. Fanaroff & R. J. Martin (Eds.), *Neonatal-perinatal medicine: Diseases of the fetus and infant* (5th ed., pp. 683–690). St. Louis: C. V. Mosby.

Feigin, R. D., Adcock, L., & Miller, D. (1992). Postnatal bacterial infections. In A.

Fanaroff & R. J. Martin (Eds.), *Neonatal perinatal medicine: Diseases of the fetus and infant* (5th ed., pp. 619–661) St. Louis: C. V. Mosby.

Feingold, M. (1982). Clinical evaluation of a patient with a genetic birth defect syndrome. *Alabama Journal of Medical Science, 19*(2), 151–156.

Finitzo-Hieber, T., Freedman, F. J., Gerling, I. J., et al. (1981). Auditory brainstem response abnormalities in post-meningitic infants and children. *International Journal of Pediatric Otorhinolaryngology, 3,* 275–286.

Fraser, G. R. (1976). *The causes of profound deafness in childhood.* Baltimore: Johns Hopkins University Press.

Greenstein, J. M., Greenstein, B. B., McConnville, K., & Stelline, L. (1976). *Mother-infant communication and language acquisition in deaf infants.* New York: Lexington School for the Deaf.

Harner, R. E., Smith, J. L., & Israel, C. W. (1968). The FTA-ABS test in late syphilis: A serological study in 1,985 cases. *Journal of the American Medical Association, 203,* 103–106.

Illum, P., Kiaer, H. W., Hvidberg-Hansen, J., & Sondergaard, G. (1972). Fifteen cases of Pendred's syndrome: Congenital deafness and sporadic goiter. *Archives of Otolaryngology, 96,* 297–304.

Jaffe, B. F. (1977). Middle ear and pinna abnormalities. In B. J. Jaffe (Ed.), *Hearing loss in children* (pp. 294–309). Baltimore: University Park Press.

Jones, K. L. (Ed.). (1988). Smith's recognizable patterns of human malformation (4th ed.). Philadelphia: W. B. Saunders.

Karmody, C. S., & Schuknecht, H. F. (1966). Deafness in congenital syphilis. *Archives of Otolaryngology, 83,* 18–27.

Keleman, G. (1958). Toxoplasmosis and congenital deafness. *Archives of Otolaryngology, 68,* 547–561.

Konigsmark, B. W., & Gorlin, R. J. (1976). *Genetic and metabolic deafness.* Philadelphia: W. B. Saunders.

Krugman, S., & Katz, S. (1981). *Infectious diseases of children.* St. Louis: C. V. Mosby.

Linsey, J. R. (1971). Inner ear pathology in congenital deafness. *Otolaryngologic Clinics of North America, 4,* 249–290.

Long, J. G., Lucey, J., & Philip, A. (1980). Noise and hypoxemia in the intensive care nursery. *Pediatrics, 65,* 143–145.

Luterman, D. M. (1985). The denial mechanism. *Ear and Hearing, 6*(1), 57–58.

Mahoney, T., & Eichwald, J. (1987). The ups and "Downs" of high risk hearing screening: The Utah statewide program. In K. Gerkin & A. Amochaev (Eds.), *Seminars in Hearing, 8*(2), 155–163.

Marcellino, G. R. (1986). "The Crib-O-Gram" in neonatal hearing screening. In E. T. Swigart (Ed.), *Neonatal hearing screening.* Basel, Switzerland: Karger.

Marcus, R. E., & Valvassori, G. (1970). Cochleo-vestibular apparatus, radiologic studies in hereditary and familial hearing loss. *International Audiology, 9,* 95–102.

McCracken, J. S. (1963). Rubella in the newborn. *British Medical Journal, 2,* 420–422.

Minoli, I., & Moro, G. (1985). Constraints of intensive care units and follow-up studies in prematures. *Acta Otolaryngologica Supplement, 421,* 62–67.

Nahmias, A. J. (1974). The TORCH complex. *Hospital Practice, 9*(5), 65–72.

Nance, W. E., & Sweeney, A. (1975). Genetic factors in deafness of early life. *Otolaryngologic Clinics of North America, 8,* 19–48.

Naunton, R. J., & Valvassori, G. E. (1968). Inner ear abnormalities: Their associations with atresia. *Laryngoscope, 64,* 1041–1049.

Northern, J. L., & Downs, M. P. (1984). *Hearing in children.* Baltimore: Williams & Wilkins.

Nyhan, W. L. (1983). Cytogenetic diseases. *Clinical Symposia, 35*(1), 1–32.

Pantke, O. A., & Cohen, M. M. (1971). The Waardenburg syndrome. *Birth Defects, 7*(7), 147–152.

Pappas, D. G. (1985). *Diagnosis and treatment of hearing impairment in children.* San Diego: College-Hill Press.

Pass, R. F., Stagno, S., Meyers, F. J., & Alford, C. (1980). Outcome of symptomatic congenital cytomegalovirus infection: Results of long-term longitudinal follow-up. *Pediatrics, 66,* 758–762.

Patterson, M. E. (1968). Congenital luetic hearing impairment. *Archives of Otolaryngology, 87,* 378–382.

Perlman, M. A., Gartner, L. M., Lee, K., et al. (1980). The association of kernicterus with bacterial infection in the newborn. *Pediatrics, 65*(1), 26–29.

Pettigrew, A. G., Edwards, D. A., & Henderson-Smart, D.J. (1988). Perinatal risk factors in preterm infants. *Medical Journal of Australia, 148,* 174–177.

Proctor, C. A., & Proctor, B. (1967). Understanding hereditary nerve deafness. *Archives of Otolaryngology, 85,* 23–40.

Robertson, A., & Philbin, M. K. (1996). Studies of sound and auditory development. Paper presented at the Physical and Developmental Environment of the High Risk Neonate. Clearwater Beach, FL: University of South Florida College of Medicine.

Sando, I., & Wood, R. P. (1971). Congenital middle ear anomalies. *Otolaryngologic Clinics of North America, 4,* 291–318.

Scholl, L. A., Lurie, M. H., & Keleman, G. (1951). Embryonic hearing organs after maternal rubella. *Laryngoscope, 61*(2), 99–112.

Schuknecht, H. J. (1974). *Pathology of the ear.* Cambridge, MA: Harvard University Press.

Simmons, F. B. (1980). Patterns of deafness in newborns. *Laryngoscope, 90,* 448–453.

Simmons, F. B., & Russ, F. N. (1974). Automated newborn hearing screening "The Crib-O-Gram." *Archives of Otolaryngology, 100,* 1–7:

Stagno, S., Pass, K., & Alford, C. (1981). Perinatal infections and maldevelopment. *Birth Defects, 17,* 31–50.

Stagno, S., Reynolds, D. W., Amos, C. S., et al. (1977). Auditory and visual effects resulting from symptomatic and subclinical congenital cytomegalovirus and *Toxoplasma* infection. *Pediatrics, 59,* 669–678.

Stein, L., Ozdamar, O., Kraus, N., & Paton, J. (1983). Follow-up of infants screened by auditory brainstem response in the neonatal intensive care unit. *Journal of Pediatrics, 103,* 447–453.

Thomas, K. (1989). How the NICU environment sounds to a preterm infant. *MCN, American Journal of Maternal Child Nursing, 14*(4), 249–251.

Ventry, R. W., Wilson, W. R., Sprinkle, P. M., et al. (1981). Implications of virus in idiopathic sudden hearing loss: Primary infection of reactivation of latent viruses. *Archives of Otolaryngology—Head and Neck Surgery, 89,* 137–141.

Weller, T. H. (1971). The cytomegalovirus ubiquitous agents with protein clinical manifestations. *New England Journal of Medicine, 285,* 203–214.

White, R. (1996). Neonatal intensive care unit structure and design: Recommended standards. Paper presented at the Physical and Developmental Environment of the High Risk Neonate. Clearwater Beach, FL: University of South Florida College of Medicine.

Whitley, R. J., Nahmias, A. J., Bisintine, A. M., et al. (1980). The natural history of H.S.V. infection of mother and newborn. *Pediatrics, 66,* 489–494.

Wiet, R. J., & Milko, D. A. (1975). Isolation of the spirochetes in the perilymph despite prior antisyphilitic therapy. *Archives of Otolaryngology, 101,* 104–106.

Wilson, W. R., Byl, F. M., & Laird, N. (1980). The efficacy of steroids in the treatment of idiopathic sudden hearing loss: A double-blind clinical study. *Archives of Otolaryngology, 106,* 772–776.

Windle-Taylor, P., Emery, P. J., & Phelps, P. D. (1981). Ear deformities associated with Klippel-Feil syndrome. *Annals of Otology, Rhinology and Laryngology, 90,* 210–216.

CHAPTER 22

Assessment and Management of Ophthalmic Dysfunction

ASSESSMENT OF THE EYES

History

A thorough history is imperative. The interviewer should ask about the following:

- Family history of vision problems: strabismus, glaucoma, retinoblastoma, and refractive errors such as myopia
- Maternal history: exposure to infectious diseases, such as gonorrhea, chlamydia, rubella, and cytomegalovirus
- Perinatal history: difficulties resulting in hypoxia or anoxia
- Previous preterm pregnancies and prior experience with retinopathy of prematurity (ROP)

Examination

Newborns in the quiet alert state are more responsive to visual stimuli. Most important information about the eye can be obtained from inspection and observation. An examination with an ophthalmoscope is usually not indicated unless there are findings suggestive of serious problems, such as cataracts or glaucoma. The lights in the environment should be dimmed. It is important to talk to the infant and to hold the infant upright, which may facilitate natural opening of the eyes. Then assessment can be done for the following:

- Shape
- Symmetry
- Size
- Presence of eyebrows and lashes
- Clarity
- Swelling
- Discharge
- Irritation: may result from the prophylactic drops or ointment
- Lids: redness or swelling
- Colobomas
- Abnormal tumor masses
- Inability to elevate the lids or ptosis (drooping), which may lead to amblyopia or poor visual development
- Unusual folds
- Slant of the eye

- Pupils:
  - Size
  - Equality
  - Reaction to light
  - Accommodation
- Color and clarity of the red reflex (in black infants, this may be pale orange rather than red) (Johnson, 1993)
- Cornea: clarity and size. A cloudy cornea may be due to congenital glaucoma, an inborn error in metabolism, or a congenital corneal dystrophy
  - Birth trauma can give the cornea a hazy appearance
- Lens: cloudiness or opacity indicating cataract
- Leukokoria: a whitish appearing pupil almost always indicative of a serious eye problem

Examination of the posterior pole of the eye (optic nerve, macula, and blood vessels) is performed with a direct ophthalmoscope with the pupil dilated. An assistant should stabilize the head and body. The infant is given a bottle or pacifier as a calming measure. A topical anesthetic such as 0.5 percent proparacaine may be instilled to dull the corneal and conjunctival sensitivity. The assistant may separate the lids, or a small pediatric lid speculum can be employed. Care should be taken while inserting the speculum to avoid causing a corneal abrasion. Normal saline should be used to avoid corneal drying (especially under the heat of a radiant warmer).

The ability to see can be assessed by getting the newborn to fix and follow on brightly colored objects. The examiner should hold the object steady 7 to 9 inches from the eye until the newborn fixes on it (the examiner will note the reflection of the object in the middle of the newborn's pupil). Newborns should be able to follow an object about 90 degrees in either direction from a midline or central position (Algranati, 1992). Care should be taken to avoid talking or other distractions while doing this test because infants respond best to the presentation of one stimuli at a time.

Several important measurements should be obtained:

- Interpupillary distance (distance from mid pupil to mid pupil when the eyes are looking forward)
- Palpebral fissure width (distance from the medial canthus to the lateral canthus of each eye). This measure determines the appropriateness of the opening for the eye.

Determining visual acuity in a newborn is difficult. There are several methods available, including visual preference charts and visual evoked potentials. At term, newborn visual acuity ranges from 20/100 to 20/400 depending on which testing method is used. This visual acuity improves to 20/80 to 20/200 by 4 months of age, 20/40 to 20/80 by 12 months of age, and 20/20 by 2 years of age (Green, 1992).

Most infants display intermittent outward deviation (exotropia). This deviation usually disappears within the first few months of life. Any constant inward (esotropia) or outward deviation should be evaluated for a possible nerve or muscle palsy. Intermittent nystagmus (rapid movements of the eye) is a common finding in the newborn. Persistent nystagmus is abnormal and should be referred for further evaluation (Carey, 1993).

Eye Drops

Systemic absorption of eye drops, although unavoidable to some extent, can cause severe reactions, including death. Cardiovascular consequences including arterial hypertension, a predisposing factor for intracranial hemorrhage, have been reported in premature infants (Rosales, Isenberg, Leake, & Everett, 1993). Excess medications that flow out of the eyelids are easily absorbed through the porous skin of the newborn and should be wiped off to prevent systemic absorption. Absorption of the medication from the nasolacrimal system can also occur. This absorption can be minimized by applying pressure with a fingertip over the nasolacrimal duct for approximately 1 minute after instillation of the drops.

The most commonly used mydriatrics are cyclopentolate, phenylephrine, and tropicamide. To achieve maximum dilation and minimize the risk of side effects, a combination of drugs is routinely used in most clinical settings. According to Bolt and colleagues (1992), the combination of phenylephrine 2.5 percent and tropicamide 0.5 percent (one drop of each followed by a second drop of tropicamide 20 minutes later) produced a better mydriasis with no systemic side effects than the combination of cyclopentolate and tropicamide. A complete listing of ophthalmic medications commonly used in newborns can be found in Table 22–1.

After the examination, the eyes should be shielded from light until the pupils have returned to their normal size. This shielding can be achieved by covering the eyes with an occlusive eye shield such as phototherapy shields or by placing an isolette cover over the infant's incubator. Unshielded, dilated eyes are very sensitive to light. Excessive light entering a dilated pupil can result in intense pain. Systemic responses include apnea, bradycardia, cyanosis, or agitation.

NEONATAL CONJUNCTIVITIS

According to the World Health Organization (WHO), any conjunctivitis occurring in the neonatal period is classified as neonatal conjunctivitis. It may develop within the first 24 to 48 hours of life. Laboratory investigations are important to determine the exact cause. Rapid treatment in some cases of conjunctivitis is important to prevent vision loss.

Silver Nitrate Conjunctivitis

Most facilities in the United States require prophylaxis against neonatal conjunctivitis with the instillation of a 1 percent solution of silver nitrate. These drops typically cause an irritative reaction that leads to conjunctival edema, redness, and a watery discharge. The reaction starts within a few hours of the instillation of the drops and usually resolves within 48 hours.

Silver nitrate conjunctivitis is self-limiting. Laboratory cultures and smears should be obtained to rule out an infectious cause for the conjunctivitis. Parents should be informed of the benign nature of the inflammation once the proper diagnosis has been made. Any secretions from the eyes should be cleansed frequently to avoid skin irritation.

TABLE 22–1. Commonly Used Eye Medications

Generic Name	Brand Name
Topical Anesthetics	
Proparacaine hydrochloride	Alcaine, Ophthaine, Ophthetic
Tetracaine hydrochloride	Anacel, Pontocaine
Mydriatics (Dilating Drops)	
Atropine sulfate	Atropisol, BufOpto Atropine, Isopto Atropine
Cyclopentolate hydrochloride	Cyclogyl
Homatropine hydrobromide	Homatrocel Ophthalmic, Isopto Homatropine
Scopolamine hydrobromide	Isopto Hyoscine
Tropicamide	Mydriacyl
Phenylephrine hydrochloride	Mydfrin, Neo-Synephrine
Anti-inflammatory Agents	
Dexamethasone	Maxidex Ophthalmic Suspension
Dexamethasone sodium phosphate	Decadron Phosphate
Fluorometholone	FML Liquifilm Ophthalmic
Prednisolone acetate	Econopred, Pred Forte, Pred Mild
Prednisolone sodium phosphate	AK-Pred, Inflamase Forte, Inflamase, Metreton
Anti-Infectives	
Antibacterials	
Bacitracin	
Chloramphenicol	Chloromycetin, Chloroptic, Econochlor
Erythromycin	Ilotycin
Gentamicin sulfate	Garamycin
Polymyxin B sulfate	
Silver nitrate 1%	
Sulfacetamide sodium	Bleph-10, Cetamide, Sodium Sulamyd
Tetracycline hydrochloride	Achromycin
Tobramycin	Tobrex
Antivirals	
Idoxuridine	IDU
Trifluridine	Viroptic
Vidarabine	Vira-A
Miscellaneous	
Timolol maleate	Timoptic (antiglaucoma medication)
Fluorescein sodium	Diagnostic drop for corneal abnormalities

Silver nitrate is effective against *Neisseria gonorrhoeae* and most bacteria; however, it is not effective against chlamydia. Some states substitute tetracycline ointment or erythromycin ointment for routine prophylaxis. These antibiotics usually do not cause eye irritation.

Chlamydial Conjunctivitis (Inclusion Conjunctivitis)

In recent years, *Chlamydia trachomatis* has been recognized as the most common cause of conjunctivitis in the newborn. The conjunctivitis usually arises 4 to 14 days after birth. It may be mild or moderate in degree and resolves within 6 weeks with proper treatment. Clinical symptoms include swollen eyelid(s) and a mucopurulent discharge. Chronic infection can lead to more serious consequences, such as conjunctival scarring, adhesions of the eyelid, and deposits of connective tissue under the cornea (Weiss, 1993).

Diagnosis is made with laboratory studies. The conjunctiva is scraped with a spatula, and a smear is made for Giemsa staining. This classically reveals a dark-staining cytoplasmic inclusion body. Direct immunofluorescent antibody staining or enzyme immunoassay should be obtained to confirm the diagnosis.

Topical treatment to the eye should consist of sulfacetamide or tetracycline drops or ointment for 3 weeks. Although the eye infection is generally not serious, 11 to 20 percent of infected neonates develop a chlamydial pneumonitis. Systemic therapy with oral erythromycin estolate or erythromycin ethylsuccinate for 3 weeks is often necessary to eradicate the organism from the respiratory tract (Weiss, 1993).

Gonorrheal Conjunctivitis

Routine prophylaxis of neonates with silver nitrate has greatly reduced the incidence of gonorrheal conjunctivitis. Gonorrheal conjunctivitis typically presents as an acute, purulent, bilateral conjunctivitis with lid edema. If not treated appropriately, the infection may progress rapidly to corneal ulceration and endophthalmitis. Gram stains and cultures should be done routinely in all cases of neonatal conjunctivitis. The presence of *N. gonorrhoeae* confirms the diagnosis. Treatment consists of intravenous or intramuscular antibiotics and topical ointment to the eye. Irrigation of the eye with sterile saline may be necessary to cleanse the eye of drainage.

Staphylococcal Conjunctivitis

The symptoms of this bacterial infection usually appear 2 to 4 weeks after birth. The conjunctivitis is usually mild with a purulent discharge. It may progress to a corneal ulcer, endophthalmitis, or generalized skin infection. Diagnosis is made with cultures and Gram stain. Treatment involves topical bacitracin or erythromycin ointment and cleansing exudate from the lids.

Herpes Simplex Conjunctivitis

Herpes simplex infections at birth may be part of a localized or systemic disease. The conjunctivitis presents as lid swelling, conjunctival injection, corneal opacity, and epithelial dendrites. These dendrites can best be seen by staining the cornea with a fluorescein dye and then examining the cornea under the blue light of a portable slit lamp. Onset of the conjunctivitis is usually 2 to 14 days after birth. The disseminated form of the disease may also lead to cataracts and optic neuritis.

Laboratory diagnosis is based on conjunctival epithelial scrapings for Giemsa staining and tissue cultures. The Giemsa stain should reveal multinucleated giant cells and intranuclear inclusion bodies. Fluorescent antibody techniques are also helpful in the diagnosis. This disease should always be kept in mind when there is a history of maternal or paternal genital herpes.

Treatment should be instituted with the topical antiviral agent trifluridine. Systemic treatment may be helpful in disseminated cases.

LACRIMAL DYSFUNCTION

Obstructed Nasolacrimal Duct

Blockage of the nasolacrimal duct occurs in 2 percent of all newborns and is the most common cause of chronic conjunctivitis in infants. The infant will present after 1 month of age with excessive tearing and pooling in the medial canthal region and signs of infection. Pressure on the lacrimal sac area usually causes pus or mucus to exude from the puncta. Because the problem resolves spontaneously in 50 percent of affected neonates by 6 months of age, conservative treatment of lacrimal massage and topical antibiotics is recommended. Obstruction lasting beyond this point may necessitate lacrimal probing (Weiss, 1993). It is important to differentiate this problem from congenital glaucoma, a foreign body on the eye, or corneal injury/inflammation.

Mucocele

Mucoceles occur because of the one-way valve effect at the end of the nasolacrimal duct. There is an accumulation of mucus or amniotic fluid trapped in the nasolacrimal sac. The infant presents with a bluish mass in the inferior medial region of the eyelid. This swelling is most frequently confused with a hemangioma. If simple massage does not decompress the mucocele, probing of the nasolacrimal duct may be necessary.

RETINOPATHY OF PREMATURITY

Retinopathy of prematurity, a disease resulting from proliferation of abnormal blood vessels in the newborn retina, was first described by Terry in 1942. His description of a fibrous growth behind the lens and retinal detachment in premature infants gave birth to the name retrolental fibroplasia (RLF) (Weakley & Spencer, 1992). This name was changed to ROP in 1984 by an international committee to provide a uniform classification system for the disease. The classification system uses a standard description of location of retinopathy (zone, clock hours), the severity of the disease (stage), the presence of special risk factors (plus disease), and the features of regression (ICROP, 1984).

RLF was responsible for an epidemic of blindness in young children in the 1940s and early 1950s until the link to supplemental oxygen therapy was made in 1952. Subsequently, the practice of limiting oxygen administration in the care of premature infants led to the near disappearance of RLF (Phelps, 1992). Improvements in neonatal health care in the past 30 years have increased the survival of preterm infants, yet ROP remains the leading cause of blindness in premature infants (Javitt, Cas, & Chiang, 1993).

INCIDENCE

According to data from the multicenter cryotherapy trial of over 4000 infants, the greatest risk occurs in premature infants weighing less than 750 g at birth (90 percent) and in those with birth weights of 751 to 1000 g (78 percent) (Phelps, 1992). The overall incidence of ROP is increasing, with current estimates at 25 percent annually (Hunter & Mukai, 1994). Although the majority of these cases will regress, the incidence of severe disease has reached a plateau of 5 to 10 percent, with over 500 new cases of blind infants annually in the United States (Hunter & Mukai, 1994; Vander, 1994).

RISK FACTORS

Retinopathy of prematurity is a multi-factorial disease related to conceptual age that occurs primarily in premature infants. Although many risk factors have been identified, prematurity is the single most important factor leading to the development of ROP (Fielder & Levene, 1992; Hunter & Mukai, 1994; Phelps, 1992). Other risk factors include supplemental oxygen, low birth weight, intraventricular hemorrhage, sepsis, multiple births, acidosis, and blood transfusions (Todd et al., 1994; Weakley & Spencer, 1992).

Some variables linked to ROP include those for which the evidence is less conclusive or common to management of medically unstable premature infants. Often these factors are interlinked and include antioxidant deficiencies, administration of beta-adrenergic blockers late in pregnancy for preterm labor, maternal bleeding, apnea of prematurity, use of xanthines such as caffeine and theophylline, abnormal blood gases, days on mechanical ventilation, early intubation, ambient lighting, hypotension, necrotizing enterocolitis (NEC), and a patent ductus arteriosus (PDA) treated with indomethacin (Arroe & Peitersen, 1994). The impact of surfactant therapy on ROP is a major concern. Preliminary reports suggest that the incidence and severity of ROP are not altered by surfactant therapy (Holmes, Cronin, Squires, & Myers, 1994; Rankin, Tubman, Halliday, & Johnston, 1992; Repka, Hardy, Phelps, & Summers, 1993; Tubman, Rankin, Halliday, & Johnson, 1992).

Although the vast majority of ROP occurs in premature infants, there have been rare case reports of the disease in full-term infants, stillborn infants, infants with hypoxia, and infants who were not exposed to supplemental oxygen (Kushner & Gloeckner, 1984; Naiman, Green, & Patz, 1979; Stefani & Ehalt, 1974). These reports, along with the striking similarity of disease presentation from infant to infant, have led some to conclude there may be a genetic component to ROP (Flynn, 1992).

TREATMENT

Treatment of ROP can be divided into three categories: preventive, interdictive, and corrective (Weakley, 1992). Screening protocols vary from institution to institution. Several widely used, published guidelines are summarized in Table 22–2.

Preventive Treatment

Preventive strategies that have been or are under consideration are antioxidant therapy, oxygen monitoring, and modifications of environmental

TABLE 22–2. Guidelines for Screening Examinations for Retinopathy of Prematurity

Recommending Group	Infant Criteria	Exam Protocol
Cryotherapy for Retinopathy of Prematurity Cooperative Group (1988)	Birth weight <1251 g	First exam 4–6 wk after birth; continue every 2 weeks Increase to weekly exams if prethreshold disease develops
American Academy of Pediatrics (Guidelines for Perinatal Care, 1988)	Birth weight <1800 g *or* gestational age <35 wk who require oxygen All infants with birth weight <1300 g *or* gestational age <30 wk	Examine 5–7 weeks after birth or before discharge home (whichever comes first)
British College of Ophthalmologists & British Association of Perinatal Medicine (Fielder & Levene, 1992)	Infants <1500 g *or* gestational age ≤31 wk	Infants ≤25 weeks' gestation: first exam 6–7 wk after birth; continue every 2 weeks Infants 26–31 weeks' gestation: first exam 6–7 wk after birth; continue every 2 weeks

light. High doses of vitamin E, an antioxidant, gained popularity in the 1980s as a prophylactic therapy for ROP (Hittner, 1981); however, most clinical studies failed to document a protective effect (Muller, 1992). Preliminary evidence suggests penicillamine, an antioxidant used in the treatment of hyperbilirubinemia in Hungary, may lower the incidence of ROP; however, the substance has not been tested outside Hungary (Phelps, 1992). Inositol, an antioxidant found in breast milk and other dietary sources, is being investigated for a possible role in decreasing the incidence of chronic lung disease (Hallman et al., 1992).

Oxygen monitoring has been the major thrust for prevention of ROP. There are little solid data to answer the question of what is a safe level of oxygenation in infants at risk for ROP. Current practice aims at minimizing oxygen exposure while preserving optimal functioning of vital organs.

Environmental lighting in nurseries has been implicated as a contributing factor in the development of ROP (Ackerman, Sherwonit, & Williams, 1989; Robinson & Fielder, 1992). Some authorities believe there are sufficient data to warrant concern (Phelps, 1992).

Interdictive Treatment

The second strategy for treating ROP focuses on therapies aimed at minimizing or preventing blindness once the disease has developed. Interdictive therapies include cryotherapy and laser photocoagulation.

Cryotherapy is a surgical procedure involving the insertion of a probe cooled with liquid nitrogen on the medial aspect of the eye. Confluent spots on the avascular retina are ablated (destroyed by freezing), reducing the release of an angiogenic factor that appears to induce retinal vasoproliferation. Although the exact mechanism about how cryotherapy works remains unknown, there is substantial evidence that the therapy improves the outcome of ROP (CRPCG, 1988; Göbel & Richard, 1993; Javitt, Cas, & Chiang, 1993; Schulenburg & Acheson, 1992; Trese 1994).

Ocular complications include edema of the eyelid(s), laceration of the conjunctiva, intraocular hemorrhage, and late retinal detachment (Vander, 1994). Other complications reported include apnea, bradycardia, arrhythmias, increased oxygen requirement, seizures, and, in very rare cases, cardiorespiratory arrest (Batton, Ivery, & Trese, 1992; Brown et al., 1990).

Although the procedure is usually performed under local or general anesthesia, it can severely stress the infant. The oculocardiac reflex, a vagal nerve mediated reflex, may be triggered during the procedure causing bradycardia (Clarke et al., 1985). This reflex can be prevented by the preoperative administration of atropine (Phelps, 1992). It is imperative that cardiorespiratory status be closely monitored throughout the procedure and the immediate postoperative period. Analgesia during and after the procedure is also recommended. Premature infants especially those with bronchopulmonary dysplasia often experience increased oxygen requirements and apnea episodes after cryotherapy (Brown et al., 1990). Nasal stuffiness, another common side effect of cryotherapy, may be partially responsible for the increase in apnea and/or oxygen requirements postoperatively (Phelps, 1992).

Laser photocoagulation, a recent technique used in the treatment of ROP, is showing promise and may eventually replace cryotherapy (Goggin & O'Keefe, 1993; Hunter & Repka, 1993). Argon and infrared diode lasers have successfully been used to ablate the avascular retina in a similar manner to that used in cryotherapy. Advantages over cryotherapy have included technical ease to perform; usefulness in posterior ROP, which is difficult to treat with cryotherapy; less stress to the infant receiving the therapy; fewer side effects; and fewer delayed consequences of myopia and retinal detachment (Hunter & Repka, 1993; Preslan, 1993). There is some evidence that laser therapy may increase the risk of cataracts in treated infants (Christiansen & Bradford, 1995).

Corrective Treatment

The focus of corrective treatment is surgery to repair detached retinas. Scleral buckling and/or vitrectomy with or without a lensectomy are the techniques available (Trese, 1994). Scleral buckling involves the placement of a silicone or plastic band around the globe of the eye. After constricting the band, the sclera is brought into closer proximity to the retina and retinal reattachment is facilitated. This procedure is often done in conjunction with cryotherapy or laser therapy to salvage any remaining vision for the infant (Phelps, 1992).

When retinal detachment progresses beyond the point of considering a scleral buckle procedure, the ophthalmologist must consider anatomical reattachment of the retina. Vitrectomy involves surgically opening the eye, removing the lens, and gently excising the proliferative scar tissue. This process allows the retina to lie against the pigmented epithelium and reattach (Hunter & Repka, 1993; Trese, 1994). Despite the skill involved in these procedures, the functional success rate ranges from 3 to 43 percent (Hunter & Repka, 1993).

COLLABORATIVE MANAGEMENT

Parents often express concern about the development of ROP in their premature infant. General information about the relationship of ROP and prematurity can be shared at first. Once the first eye examination is performed, the information can be specific to their infant (Phelps, 1992). It is important the neonatal health care team work closely with the ophthalmologist in providing a consistent message to the family. Information shared should take into account known cultural differences such as the occurrence of severe ROP is approximately 50 percent less in black infants (Palmer et al., 1991). Parent teaching should focus on the basics of ROP, the purpose of the screening examinations, and the importance of regular vision testing in the infant after discharge.

Once ROP is diagnosed in an infant, parents may need more support than usual. Families of infants who need surgical intervention may experience increased stress from their concern for the infant's vision and the added communication with an ophthalmologist or retinal surgeon.

Information about the prognosis of ROP in the infant must be included in any discharge planning for the family. Myopia (near sightedness), strabismus (crossed eye), astigmatism, and amblyopia (lazy eye) are common sequelae. Glaucoma and late retinal detachment are common sequelae in infants with severe ROP (Hartnett et al., 1993; Quinn et al., 1992).

Many families may benefit from referral to community resources, support groups, and special programs for children with visual problems.

CONGENITAL DEFECTS

Aniridia

Aniridia is a severe ocular abnormality that presents as bilateral absence of the iris. The defect is usually accompanied by cataracts, corneal pannus, macular dysfunction, and glaucoma. Most of the infants have a significant reduction in their visual acuity to a level of 20/200 or worse. About 20 to 30 percent of children with the noninherited form of aniridia will develop Wilms' tumor of the kidney.

Persistent Hyperplastic Primary Vitreous

This condition is a unilateral disorder that affects both sexes equally. It results from persistence of the hyoid vessels connecting the optic nerve and the posterior surface of the lens. It should be considered in the differential diagnosis of leukokoria. The involved eye is invariably small, and a mature cataract is often present. Surgery may improve the integrity of the eye; however, useful vision is usually not restored.

Rubella

Congenital rubella is responsible for a wide variety of ocular complications, including pigmentary retinopathy, glaucoma, cataract, and microphthalmos. Newborns classically present with hearing, eye, and cardiac defects, although there may be a wide spectrum of clinical presentations.

Today, the incidence of congenital rubella syndrome is low; however, new information from long-term follow-up studies suggest the prevalence of ocular problems is nearly twice the previously thought rate (78 percent instead of 43 percent). Several trends have also been noted, including an increase in delayed disease and new associations of combination problems. Microphthalmia, cataracts, and glaucoma are more likely to occur in combination than as an independent problem. Pigmentary retinopathy produces a characteristic salt and pepper appearance and can result in sudden vision loss during adulthood. Poor visual acuity and diabetic retinopathy are also of concern in individuals with congenital rubella syndrome (Givens, Lee, Jones, & Listrup, 1994). Parents of infants with congenital rubella need to have their affected children screened on a regular basis.

Capillary Hemangiomas of the Lid

Capillary hemangioma of the lid, a blood vessel tumor, usually appears before the age of 6 months. It tends to enlarge, stabilize, and then regress by 5 years of age. The tumor is usually elevated and reddish purple. Capillary hemangiomas are often referred to as strawberry nevi because of their appearance.

Superficial tumors of the eyelid cause cosmetic and visual problems. Pressure on the globe from the tumor may result in significant astigmatism and subsequently amblyopia. If the tumor is large, it may cover the pupil and prevent normal visual development. Deep tumors in the orbit may present as proptosis. These tumors may be treated with surgical removal, radiation, or steroid injection. Tumors that are exclusively cosmetic should be allowed to regress on their own.

Ptosis

Ptosis refers to a drooping of one or both eyelids due to neurologic, muscular, or mechanical factors. If the ptosis is significant enough to cover the pupil, a dense amblyopia may result. If bilateral ptosis is present, the infant may have slowed motor development and delayed ambulation later in life. These problems are caused by the awkward chin-up position the child must maintain to see. Mild ptosis causing a problem with appearance is not generally repaired until the child is 4 or 5 years old because the results are usually better.

There are several familial syndromes associated with ptosis, including blepharophimosis syndrome and double elevator palsy. Significant birth trauma may result in damage to the cervical ganglion and in infantile Horner's syndrome. The infant will present with different-colored pupils, miosis, anhydrosis (lack of sweating), and a mild ptosis. Direct trauma to the lid or a tumor in the lid may also cause ptosis. Surgical repair corrects this defect easily.

Congenital Glaucoma

Congenital glaucoma occurs in approximately 1 in 25,000 births. Glaucoma is a disease in which the intraocular pressure is elevated to a sufficient level to damage the optic nerve. Because of the potential for blindness from this disease, it is important that it be detected early in the infant's life and treated properly. The neonate will present with tearing, light sensitivity, lid spasm, and a large cloudy cornea. The disease is slightly more common in males.

It is critical that congenital glaucoma be differentiated from other diseases that present with similar symptoms. Nasolacrimal duct obstruction will present with tearing but will not cause light sensitivity or a cloudy cornea. Difficult labor or a forceps injury may damage the cornea and cause temporary clouding, but the intraocular pressure will not be elevated, which is the hallmark of glaucoma. The large eyes of the infant with congenital glaucoma may appear beautiful to the parents, but health care professionals should be alert to the possibility of this disease.

The abnormality in congenital glaucoma is a maldevelopment of the filtering system within the eye that controls the level of intraocular pressure. Treatment of congenital glaucoma is surgical. The surgical results are usually good, but the parents must be educated regarding the need for continued monitoring of this condition throughout the child's life.

Congenital Cataracts

Cataracts are an important cause of blindness because they may interfere with the process of visual development early in the infant's life. For this reason, it is important that visually significant cataracts be detected and treated before they cause amblyopia, which may be unresponsive to the most persistent treatment.

Heredity is an important cause of congenital cataracts. The inheritance pattern may be autosomal dominant, autosomal recessive, or sex linked. A maternal history of diabetes, x-ray exposure, or malnutrition may be an important factor in cataract formation. In premature infants, it is common to see transient cataracts or insignificant opacities due to remnants of developmental tissues. ROP can also lead to cataracts in premature infants.

Several inborn errors of metabolism including galactosemia, Alport's syndrome, Fabry's disease, and Lowe syndrome cause cataracts. Intrauterine rubella infection is also associated with cataracts in the neonate.

Cataract surgery very early in life is critical to the infant's visual rehabilitation. Useful vision in eyes with monocular cataracts is especially difficult to achieve. It is important for nurses to work closely with the infant's parents. The parent's persistence in handling contact lenses and in amblyopia therapy often determines the outcome for their child's vision.

REFERENCES

Ackerman, B., Sherwonit, E., & Williams, J. M. (1989). Reduced incidental light exposure: Effect on the development of retinopathy of prematurity in low birth weight infants. *Pediatrics 83*, 958–962.

Algranati, P. S. (1992). *The pediatric patient: An approach to history and physical examination* (pp. 22–85). Baltimore: Williams & Wilkins.

American Academy of Pediatrics, American College of Obstetricians and Gynecologists. (1988). *Guidelines for perinatal care* (2nd ed.). Washington, DC: AAP & ACOG.

Arroe, M., & Peitersen, B. (1994). Retinopathy of prematurity: Review of a seven-year period in a Danish neonatal intensive care unit. *Acta Paediatrica 83,* 501–505.

Batton, D. G., Ivery, P., & Trese, M. (1992). Respiratory complications associated with cryotherapy in premature infants. *American Journal of Perinatology, 9,* 296–298.

Bolt, B., Benz, B., Koerner, F., & Bossi, E. (1992). A mydriatic eye-drop combination without systemic effects for premature infants: A prospective double-blind study. *Journal of Pediatric Ophthalmology & Strabismus, 29,* 157–162.

Brown, G. C., Tasman, W. S., Naidoff, M., et al. (1990). Systemic complications associated with retinal cryoablation for retinopathy of prematurity. *Ophthalmology, 97,* 855–858.

Carey, B. (1993). Neurologic assessment. In E. P. Tappero & M. E. Honeyfield (Eds.), *Physical assessment of the newborn* (pp. 121–138). Petaluma, CA: NICU Ink.

Christiansen, S. P., & Bradford, J. D. (1995). Cataract in infants treated with argon laser photocoagulation for threshold retinopathy of prematurity. *American Journal of Opthalmology, 119,* 175–180.

Clarke, W. N., Hodges, E., Noel, L. P., et al. (1985). The oculocardiac reflex during ophthalmoscopy in premature infants. *American Journal of Ophthalmology, 99,* 649–651.

Cryotherapy for Retinopathy of Prematurity Cooperative Group (CRPCG) (1988). Multicenter trial of cryotherapy for retinopathy of prematurity: Preliminary results. *Archives of Ophthalmology 106,* 339–344.

Fielder, A. R., & Levene, M. I. (1992). Screening for retinopathy of prematurity. [Review]. *Archives of Diseases in Childhood, 67*(7 Spec. No.), 860–867.

Flynn, J. T. (1992). The premature retina: A model for the in vivo study of molecular genetics? *Eye, 6*(pt. 2), 161–165.

Givens, K. T., Lee, D. A., Jones. T., & Ilstrup, D. M. (1993). Congenital rubella syndrome: Ophthalmic manifestations and associated systemic disorders. *British Journal of Ophthalmology, 77,* 358–363.

Göbel, W., & Richard, G. (1993). Retinopathy of prematurity: Current diagnosis and management. [Review]. *European Journal of Pediatrics, 152,* 286–290.

Goggin, M., & O'Keefe, M. (1993). Diode laser for retinopathy of prematurity: Early outcome. *British Journal of Ophthalmology, 77,* 559–562.

Green, M. (1992). *Pediatric diagnosis* (pp. 16–36). Philadelphia: W. B. Saunders.

Hallman, M., Bry, K., Hoppu, K., et al. (1992). Inositol supplementation in premature infants with respiratory distress syndrome. *New England Journal of Medicine, 326,* 1233–1239.

Hartnett, M. E., Gilbert, M. M., Hirose, T., et al. (1993). Glaucoma as a cause of poor vision in severe retinopathy of prematurity. *Grafes Archive for Clinical and Experimental Ophthalmology, 231,* 433–438.

Hittner, H. (1981). Retrolental fibroplasia: Efficacy of vitamin E in a double-blind clinical study of preterm infants. *New England Journal of Medicine, 305,* 1365–1371.

Holmes, J. M., Cronin, C. M., Squires, P., & Myers, T. M. (1994). Randomized clinical trial of surfactant prophylaxis in retinopathy of prematurity. *Journal of Pediatric Ophthalmology & Strabismus, 31,* 189–191.

Hunter, D. G., & Mukai, S. (1994). Retinopathy of prematurity: Pathogenesis, diagnosis, and treatment. *International Ophthalmology Clinics, 34,* 163–184.

Hunter, D. G., & Repka, M. X. (1993). Diode laser photocoagulation for threshold retinopathy or prematurity. *Ophthalmology, 100,* 238–244.

International Committee on Retinopathy of Prematurity (ICROP). (1984). An international classification of retinopathy of prematurity. *Pediatrics, 74,* 127–133.

Javitt, J., Cas, R. D., & Chiang, Y. (1993). Cost-effectiveness of screening and cryotherapy for threshold retinopathy of prematurity. *Pediatrics, 91,* 859–866.

Johnson, C. B. (1993). Head, eyes, ears, nose, throat (HEENT) assessment. In E. P. Tappero, & M. E. Honeyfield (Eds.), *Physical assessment of the newborn* (pp. 41–54). Petaluma, CA: NICU Ink.

Kushner, B. J., & Gloeckner, E. (1984). Retrolental fibroplasia in full-term infants without exposure to supplemental oxygen. *American Journal of Ophthalmology, 97,* 148–153.

Muller, D. P. (1992). Vitamin & therapy in retinopathy of prematurity [Review]. *Eye, 6*(Part 2), 221–225.

Naiman, J., Green W. R., & Patz, A. (1979). Retrolental fibroplasia in hypoxic newborn. *American Journal of Ophthalmology, 88,* 55–58.

Palmer, E. A, Flynn, J. T., Hardy, R. J., et al. (1991). Incidence and early course of retinopathy of prematurity. *Ophthalmology, 98,* 1628–1640.

Phelps, D. L. (1992). Retinopathy of prematurity. *Current Problems in Pediatrics 22,* 349–371.

Preslan, M. W. (1993). Laser therapy for retinopathy of prematurity. *Journal of Pediatric Ophthalmology & Strabismus, 30,* 80–83.

Quinn, G. E., Dobson, V, Repka, M. X., et al. (1992). Development of myopia in infants with birth weights less than 1251 grams. *Ophthalmology, 99,* 329–340.

Rankin, S. J., Tubman, T. R., Jalliday, H. L., & Johnston, S. S. (1992). Retinopathy of prematurity in surfactant treated infants. *British Journal of Ophthalmology, 76,* 202–204.

Repka, M. X., Hardy, R. J., Phelps, D. L., & Summers, C. G. (1993). Surfactant prophylaxis and retinopathy of prematurity. *Archives of Ophthalmology, 111,* 618–620.

Robinson, J., & Fielder, A. R. (1992). Light and the immature visual system. *Eye, 6*(5), 166–172.

Rosales, T., Isenberg, S., Leake, R, & Everett, S. (1981). Systemic effects of mydriatrics in low weight infants. *Journal of Pediatric Ophthalmology & Strabismus, 18*(6), 42–44.

Schulenburg, W. E., & Acheson, J. F. (1992). Cryosurgery for acute retinopathy of prematurity: Factors associated with treatment success and failure. *Eye, 6*(pt. 2), 215–220.

Stefani, F. H., & Ehalt, H. (1974). Non–oxygen-induced retinitis proliferans and retinal detachment in full-term infants. *British Journal of Ophthalmology, 58,* 490–513.

Todd, D. A., Kennedy, J., Roberts, S., et al. (1994). Retinopathy of prematurity in infants less than 29 weeks' gestation at birth. *Australian and New Zealand Journal of Ophthalmology, 22,* 19–23.

Trese, M. T. (1994). Surgery for retinopathy of prematurity. *International Ophthalmology Clinics, 34,* 105–111.

Tubman, T. R., Rankin, S. J., Halliday, H. L., & Johnston, S. S. (1992). Surfactant replacement therapy and the prevalence of acute retinopathy of prematurity. *Biology of Neonate, 61*(Suppl. 1), 54–58.

Vander, J. F. (1994). Retinopathy of prematurity: Diagnosis and management. *Journal of Ophthalmic Nursing and Technology, 13,* 207–212.

Weakley, D. R., Jr., & Spencer, R. (1992). Current concepts in retinopathy of prematurity. [Review]. *Early Human Development, 30,* 121–138.

Weiss, A. H. (1993). Chronic conjunctivitis in infants and children. *Pediatric Annals, 22,* 366–374.

Neonatal Monitoring and Evaluation

. . . .

CHAPTER 23

Monitoring Neonatal Biophysical Parameters

BIOPHYSICAL MONITORING SYSTEMS

Temperature Measurement

Neonatal body temperature is assessed by either rectal or skin surface temperature measurement. Rectal temperature is an indicator of core or "deep body" temperature. Skin temperature is widely used because unlike rectal temperature it is easily transduced to provide continuous temperature information to the caregiver. Skin temperature when coupled with core and ambient air or environment temperature can be an effective indicator of the infant's thermal balance.

Temperature is one of the most important indicators of the health status of newborns. Rectal temperature measurement using mercury-in-glass thermometers is gradually being replaced by electronic thermometers. The electronic thermometers offer a distinct advantage in that inexpensive techniques can be used to ensure sterility and prevent cross-contamination.

A common problem with all types of contact thermometry is that the indicated temperature reflects the entire contact surface the sensing element touches. Another problem is time necessary to equilibrate with its environment before a reliable temperature can be measured.

Rectal thermometers, traditionally of the mercury-in-glass type, like skin thermometers, are now also electronic. The thermistor, the platinum resistance temperature device (RTD), and the thermocouple are the most common temperature-sensing elements used in electronic thermometers.

An inherent problem in any electronic thermometer is the deterioration with age. Calibration of equipment using thermistors should be closely monitored if the thermistors are not routinely replaced.

The most common failure mode for thermistors, RTDs, and thermocouples is an open circuit or short circuit. For a thermistor, a short circuit will look like a very high temperature reading (zero resistance). Most clinical thermometers provide some type of alarm indication when catastrophic failures like this occur.

The most common problem with temperature measurement is ensuring that the sensor has good contact with the surface being measured. Otherwise, the temperature measured is greatly influenced by the environmental temperature. The sensor should be shielded from the direct radiation of the radiant warmer heating system by a reflective pad. The reflective pad is designed to reflect the incident radiation and prevent the absorption of energy, which would heat the sensor and elevate the sensed temperature.

Noncontact infrared thermometers and infrared thermographic cameras can be used to measure temperatures without contact with the surface to be measured. They offer the greatest level of sterility and protection because no physical contact is required. These noncontact thermometers work on the principle that all materials emit radiation. The intensity and the wavelength of the emitted radiation from an object are a function of the temperature of the object. As the temperature increases, so does the intensity or power at a given wavelength. For temperatures in the physiologic range, the energy is emitted in the infrared region. The infrared detectors for human body temperature measurement are designed for the 5- to 25-μm wavelengths.

When using infrared thermometers, it is important to ensure that there are no other sources of heat that can interfere with the surface being sensed. Infrared thermometers are now available for the measurement of tympanic membrane temperature. The tympanic membrane has been documented to be a good indicator of core temperature. However, the physical size of the optic head on these temperature monitors makes it difficult to position the thermometer in the ear canal to ensure good alignment with the tympanic membrane, particularly in infants. When not aligned properly, the thermometer could be reading the temperature of the ear canal and not the tympanic membrane. This type of temperature measuring device can be affected by other factors, such as the depth of the probe into the ear canal, and potentially by the presence of vernix or other debris in the ear. Some neonatal intensive care units are using tympanic temperature measurements with reportedly good results, but clinical trials need to be conducted on premature and term infants under various conditions and of different gestational ages.

Electrodes for Bioelectrical Potentials

Bioelectrical potentials are transduced from the skin surface for the electrocardiogram (ECG), electroencephalogram, and evoked potentials. The potentials on the body range from 1 μV to 1 mV. Body surface electrodes attached to the skin are used to convert the ionic potentials produced by the ionic current flow in tissue to electronic potentials.

Two electrodes are required to measure bioelectrical potentials, and the voltage measured is actually the instantaneous potentials of the two electrodes. If the two electrodes are exactly the same, then the voltage difference is dependent on the biologic ionic difference between the two electrodes. The premature infant has a poorly developed stratum corneum. This immature skin has a low resistance to current flow, and therefore it is easy to get a good electrical signal during the early postnatal period. However, as the stratum corneum develops and the skin becomes less moist, it is important to check and replace the electrodes to ensure that there is sufficient electrolyte for good electrical conduction. Difficulties with the ECG baseline can usually be attributed to drying of the electrolyte. Also, during the first week of life, the electrodes are very sensitive to motion artifact and baseline drift.

Impedance Electrodes for Respiration Rate

Impedance electrodes are used to generate an electrical field around tissue. The electrodes are the same type as those used for biopotential transduction such as with the ECG. Measured distortions or changes in the electric field can then be attributed to specific tissue effects.

Impedance is the transduction principle used to measure respiration rate and cardiac output. Two electrodes placed at the extremes of the thoracic cavity can be used to detect volume changes due to respiration. The expansion and contraction of the intervening tissue mass during each respiratory cycle cause detectable changes in the electrical conducting path. This change in the conducting path is referred to as impedance and is transducible if the changes are large enough. In the three-lead ECG configuration, impedance transduction is usually applied to two of the electrodes to determine respiration rate. Because it is the resistance to current flow that is being detected, it is extremely important to have intimate contact with the skin surface. Here also, drying of the electrolyte gel generates impedance changes that can cause baseline drift.

Pulse Oximetry (Transcutaneous Oxygen Saturation)

Measurement of transcutaneous oxygen saturation ($TcSaO_2$), referred to as pulse oximetry, is based on the principle of oximetry. Oximetry uses spectrophotometric analysis of light transmitted through or reflected back from light-absorbing substances. Light-absorbing substances will have an absorption coefficient for each wavelength. Therefore, the amount of light absorbed at any wavelength is a function of the concentration of the substances that have high absorption coefficients at that wavelength. When the distance that the light travels is kept constant, then it is only the concentration of light-absorbing substances that affects levels of transmitted or reflected light.

By irradiating a blood sample with light at a wavelength that has different absorption characteristics for oxyhemoglobin and deoxyhemoglobin (approximately 650 nm) and at a wavelength for which the absorption characteristics are the same for oxyhemoglobin and deoxyhemoglobin (805 nm), it is possible to determine the concentrations of each in blood. The percentage of hemoglobin saturated with oxygen can then be calculated from these intensities.

This same principle is used to determine the percent saturation of arterial blood in vivo, using pulse oximetry. The assumption made is that changes in the intensity of light transmitted through or reflected from tissue during the inflow phase of the cardiac cycle (systole) are due to arterial blood alone. If light intensity is measured during systole and also during the period between heart beats (diastole), then the difference between the light intensities can be attributed to arterial blood alone. Measurements of light intensities at 650 and 805 nm are taken for systole and diastole. The light intensities are corrected for tissue variations, and the pulsatile variation can then be attributed to arterial flow only. Consequently, there is no calibration required for the sensor. The ratio of the corrected light intensities gives the beat-to-beat percent saturation.

Ambient lights that have high intensities in the levels used for saturation could obviously be detected by the saturation detector if they are not adequately shielded. Also, because the absorption characteristics of fetal hemoglobin are slightly different from those of adult hemoglobin, it is important that saturation monitors used in the early postnatal period be suitably corrected to compensate for these differences. Timing for the activation of the light pulses is critical to the accuracy of the derived percent saturation. The addition of an independent source for timing the pulse wave, like an ECG, can improve the accuracy if triggering of light pulses is linked to this independent source. To compensate for poor or variable arterial perfusion, the light intensities on the transmitters of most oximeters can be adjusted so that the level of light received at the detector provides an acceptable pulse wave.

Partial Pressure of Oxygen

The partial pressure of oxygen in arterial blood ($TcPO_2$) can be measured using oxygen polarographic techniques. The polarographic cell has a cathode (usually platinum) and an anode (usually silver—silver chloride [Ag-AgCl]) whose surfaces are in contact with an electrolyte.

Transcutaneous PO_2 is based on the concept that it is possible to alter the rate of diffusion of oxygen through the skin by elevating its temperature to more than 40°C. Normally there is very low or no transport of oxygen through the skin. The skin is usually heated to 43°C to 44°C, at which point there is increased diffusion even through the outer barrier of the skin, the stratum corneum. Because heating also causes vasodilation, there is an increase in blood flow to the dermal capillaries, which makes the oxygen tension in these vessels close to the levels of the deeper arterial vessels. To protect the sensor from the effects of oxygen in the air, the probe assembly is attached to the skin with an adhesive that provides a good mechanical airtight seal. Extreme care must be taken because of the high temperatures used at the surface of the sensor, which is in contact with the very immature skin of the small premature infant. Transcutaneous PO_2 is still not an absolute measurement system. It is used primarily for trending in conjunction with absolute gas tensions measured in arterial blood with a laboratory analyzer.

Partial Pressure of Carbon Dioxide

The partial pressure of carbon dioxide in arterial blood ($TcPCO_2$) can be measured using transduction techniques based on the Severinghaus principle. This principle is based on measurement of CO_2 using an indirect transduction scheme in which the effect of CO_2 on the pH of a solution is transduced. The resultant pH is measured using standard glass pH electrodes.

CO_2 molecules are absorbed in an electrolyte (HCO_3), forming hydrogen and bicarbonate ions. A potential is generated between the pH electrode and the reference electrode. The potential is proportional to the concentration of CO_2. The CO_2 sensor must be calibrated at two points using reference gases (usually 5 percent and 10 percent CO_2). Heat is also used in the Po_2 sensor to increase the diffusion of CO_2 across the stratum corneum. Because the transduction mechanism is based on the pH glass electrode, the sensor is extremely sensitive to temperature. Both $TcPo_2$ and $TcPco_2$ are highly influenced by skin perfusion. Also, because the response time of the sensors is slow, it is difficult to use data for anything other than gross trending of gas tensions. This slow response is in contrast to the rapid response of transcutaneous oxygen saturation measurement systems.

Another type of CO_2 monitoring, a portable infrared end-tidal CO_2 monitor has been used during pediatric anesthesia and the transport of critically ill adults up to this point. The problem has been a 38-mL dead space that would potentially lead to very small infants rebreathing this air. Biochem International, in Waukesha, Wisconsin, has devised a Biochem 520 CO_2 breath indicator that is a side-stream infrared capnometer with only a 2-mL dead space. To use this form of monitoring during transport one must determine if an endotracheal tube is in proper position for ventilation.

Serum Bilirubin

Total bilirubin can be measured using a simple optical system designed to quantify the degree of yellowing of the tissue underlying the skin. Because bilirubin has unique absorption spectra, it is possible to determine the concentration of bilirubin in vivo by analyzing the reflected light from a source directed at the skin. Reflected light is split into two beams using a dichroic mirror. The light is then passed through 460-mm and 550-mm filters and is converted to electrical energy by photodetectors. The relative energies of the reflected light can be correlated to the concentration of total bilirubin at the measurement site. Measurement accuracy is ultimately dependent on the optical properties of the skin and location of sensor on body.

Pressure Monitoring

Measurement of pressure is mostly based on strain gauge transduction principles. Strain is the change in length of an object per unit length. The strain gauges are usually constructed of materials that have the ability to detect changes in electrical resistance for small changes in length. The sensitivity of the strain gauge is a function of the force necessary to cause a detectable deflection in the gauge membrane. Attaching an object to the gauge can facilitate the transduction of force. If a fluid is allowed to exert force on the active surface of the gauge, then movement of the gauge can be expressed as a pressure. Blood pressure measurement with a catheter is based on this principle. The location of the transducer at the same level as the heart helps to avoid pressure offsets.

In all direct pressure measurement systems in which a fluid-filled catheter is used to transmit the pressure wave to the strain gauge, it is important to ensure that the catheter is free of all air bubbles. If there is a significant amount of air in the system, the pressure waveform will be distorted because air, unlike saline, can be compressed. Loss of energy because of compression in the catheter can dampen the actual pressure wave. Bubbles can usually be dislodged by gently tapping the pressure transducer manifold.

Semiconductor-based strain gauges are used in catheters that have the pressure transducer at their tip. In these catheter-tipped pressure transducers, the pressure variations are transduced at the measurement site itself and not through a fluid column.

Indirect blood pressure measurement can be accomplished with an inflatable cuff placed around a major artery. These systems have automated inflation and deflation mechanisms and are designed to measure cuff pressures at the systolic and diastolic endpoints of the cardiac cycle. With the availability of small, sensitive pressure transducers and suitable plastics for the cuff, this technique has gained acceptance as a screening tool for infants. When a timer is incorporated to activate the inflation and deflation pumps at discrete intervals (e.g., every 30 minutes), this technique can be used in a semicontinuous noninvasive way to track pressure. The widespread availability of low-cost sophisticated electronics allows for the incorporation of fail-safe alarm systems to prevent overinflation or continuous inflation of the cuffs. All types of pressure monitoring, direct and indirect, are extremely sensitive to motion artifact and positioning of the pressure transducer. Pressure transducers are usually extremely temperature sensitive because they rely on the detection of small mechanical changes in metals as the transduction mechanism.

New Techniques of Monitoring the Neonate

Cerebral blood flow velocity is an area that up until recently was followed by researchers rather than clinicians. Yet cerebral blood flow velocity changes especially in the very immature neonate with routine tasks of suctioning, blood drawing from arterial lines, flushing of arterial lines, and repositioning of the infant in bed.

Cerebral blood flow can be noninvasively monitored by Doppler flow velocity monitors (e.g., Hewlett Packard Sonos 1000, Waltham, MA). Measurements are usually taken with the neonate in a supine position. A pulsed Doppler with a 7.5-mHz and continuous multifrequency scanner with a 7.5-mHz shore focus probe is used. Noise from the blood's movement in the vessel is filtered with a high pass filter of 100 Hz. The probe is positioned transcranially over the temporal bone to "catch" the vessel as it leaves the circle of Willis. Sagittal and coronal measurements are taken "through" the open fontanelle. Audio and visual signals are detectable and projected. Direct measurement can be taken with an analog output system. These measurements include the systolic velocity, diastolic velocity, and integration of the area under the curve, which is considered to be a close approximation of the blood flow volume (Aziz et al., 1995).

REFERENCE

Aziz, K., Vickar, D. B., Sauve, R. S., et al. (1995). Province-based study of neurologic disability of children weighing 500 through 1249 grams at birth in relation to neonatal cerebral ultrasound findings. *Pediatrics, 95,* 837–844.

CHAPTER 24

Diagnostic Imaging

ANATOMIC PROPORTIONS OF INFANTS

The anatomic proportions of infants are very different from those of the adult, and the younger the infant, the more marked are these differences. A thorough knowledge of these proportions is essential for accurate patient positioning for field exposure limitation and interpretation of diagnostic imaging (Gyll & Blake, 1986; Hilton & Edwards, 1994). It is important that only the area in question and the whole of it appear in the imaging field.

The neonate's head is large in proportion to the body; the cranial vault is large in proportion to the area of the face (Fig. 24–1). The neck is short; the diaphragm is high. The kidneys are low, about midway between the diaphragm and symphysis pubis. The abdomen is large due to the relative size of the liver and stomach. The pelvic cavity is very small; the bladder extends above the symphysis pubis. The chest, pelvis, and limbs are small in proportion to the abdomen (Gyll, 1985; Hilton & Edwards, 1994; Poznanski, 1976; Swischuk, 1989, 1995; Vogler, Helms, & Collen, 1986).

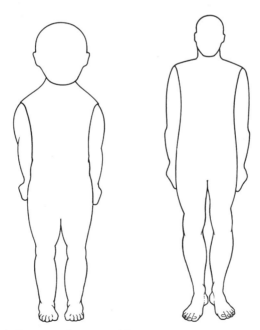

FIGURE 24–1. Proportional anatomic differences between a neonate and an adult.

In an anteroposterior (AP) projection, the neonatal anatomy causes the lungs to appear wider than they are long and much higher up in the thoracic cavity than one would normally expect (Hilton & Edwards, 1994; Swischuk, 1989, 1995; Vogler, Helms, & Collen, 1986; Wesenberg, 1973). The diaphragm is located just below the level of the nipples. On a lateral projection, the posterior aspect of the lungs may extend to twice the depth of the anterior part (Gyll & Blake, 1986; Swischuk, 1989, 1995).

The neonate's abdomen bulges laterally wider than the pelvis, and the bulge contains abdominal organs displaced by the large liver and stomach. Care must be taken so as not to eliminate this area of the abdomen from the imaging field (Gyll, 1985; Poznanski, 1976; Swischuk, 1989, 1995; Hilton & Edwards, 1994) (Fig. 24–2). The smallest possible body area should be irradiated, consistent with producing the necessary information (Fig. 24–3).

TYPES OF DIAGNOSTIC IMAGING

Diagnostic imaging methods are limited to the demonstration of pathologic features no smaller than a few millimeters in diameter, whereas biochemical and histologic methods document disease at a molecular or cellular level. It

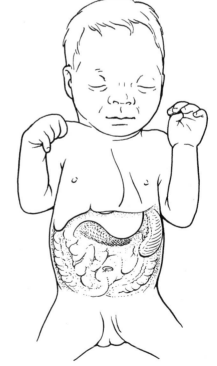

FIGURE 24–2. The organ contents of the neonatal abdomen cause it to bulge laterally. Care should be taken so as not to exclude this area from abdominal radiographs.

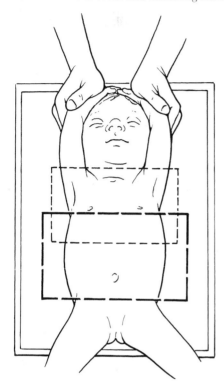

FIGURE 24–3. Neonatal radiographs should be limited to only the area of interest. Total body radiographs should be avoided. The top box *(dashed lines)* defines the area of interest for an anteroposterior chest radiograph. The bottom box *(heavy dashed lines)* defines the area of interest for an anteroposterior abdominal film. Gonad shield has been omitted for illustrative purposes.

is commonly thought that diagnostic imaging is able to provide only anatomic information; however, a significant amount of physiologic data may be derived from studies such as barium examinations or urography, as well as from dynamic radionuclide and ultrasonographic imaging. There are four major types of diagnostic imaging modalities, including x-ray (roentgenologic) imaging, radionuclide imaging, ultrasonographic imaging, and magnetic resonance imaging (Bushong, 1992; Juhl & Crummy, 1993; Horowitz, 1995; Treves, 1995).

X-ray Imaging

X-rays are one form of electromagnetic energy that travels at the speed of light (3×10^8 m/sec, or 6.7×10^8 mph). When an x-ray beam is directed toward a part of the body, there is differential absorption of the x-ray photons by different types of body tissue. A beam of x-ray photons is variously attenuated as it passes through the body tissues to produce a shadow image that is recorded on photographic film, while the absorbed x-ray photons interact with the tissue causing ionization within the body (Alpen, 1990; Bushong, 1992; Gofman, 1983; Juhl & Crummy, 1993). Bone and metal fragments absorb x-ray photons and therefore appear white, whereas air-containing structures such as lung and bowel gas absorb few x-ray photons and appear black; soft tissues and blood vessels appear as intermediate shades of gray.

A radiograph gives a two-dimensional projection of three-dimensional structures. An x-ray tube is positioned to direct the x-ray beam through the part of the neonate to be examined, so as to record different views or projections on the film. Although this type of imaging modality can distinguish between only air, fat, and tissues having densities approximately equal to those of water or metals, this simple technique continues to prove enormously valuable and is still the most commonly employed diagnostic imaging method in neonatal care.

OTHER RADIOGRAPHIC IMAGING TECHNIQUES

Xeroradiography

Xeroradiography is a radiographic imaging technique used to evaluate soft tissue. In this technique, the electrical charge of a photoconductive plate is altered in proportion to the intensity of the transmitted radiation image (Alpen, 1990; Bushong, 1992; Juhl & Crummy, 1993; Kelsey, 1985). The image is recorded on this plate rather than on x-ray film. This modality provides much better contrast than conventional radiography for soft tissue structures that differ only slightly in density. It also provides an "edge effect" at the margins of discontinuous structures and therefore is indicated for detection of nonmetallic foreign bodies and in the evaluation of complex upper airway abnormalities in the neonate (Juhl & Crummy, 1993; Kelsey, 1985; Swischuk, 1995). Despite these benefits, the risks must be considered. Radiation exposure is 6 to 12 times greater than that of conventional radiographs (Alpen, 1990).

Fluoroscopic Imaging

Fluoroscopic imaging evaluates the motion of an organ system. Fluoroscopic images can be recorded either on film or on videotape. Videotape recording of fluoroscopy has become essential. It is easier and safer to rerun a videotape several times to evaluate dysfunction rather than to prolong the radiation exposure from fluoroscopy.

During a fluoroscopic examination, the anatomic structure may also be evaluated by obtaining a spot film. This type of spot-film camera decreases the radiation dose to the infant by at least 75 percent when compared with a conventional spot-film device (Juhl & Crummy, 1993; Kelsey, 1985; Noz & Maguire, 1985). Videotapes are used to record motions, and spot films are used to document anatomy. The radiation dose of 1 minute of fluoroscopy is equivalent to more than thirty 105-mm spot films or more than eight conventional radiographs (Aplen, 1990).

Fluoroscopically guided cytologic biopsy of the lung, bone, pancreas, and lymph nodes has become possible with percutaneous needle insertion. Embolization of arteriovenous malformations may be performed, arterial stenoses may be dilated with balloon catheters, and plastic stents can be inserted to provide drainage through biliary strictures under fluoroscopy (Hilton & Edwards, 1994; Moss, Ring, & Higgins, 1984). Although at present these surgical-radiologic procedures apply to a relatively small proportion of neonates, all procedures require the cooperation between the neonatal, surgical, and radiologic teams to achieve the best results and depend on high-quality image intensification.

Conventional X-ray Tomography

Tomography is a radiologic method of imaging a slice of tissue at a specific level. A coordinated movement of the x-ray tube and film cassette gives a defined image in the two-dimensional plane of interest, whereas the structures in front or behind this plane are blurred out (Alpen, 1990; Juhl & Crummy, 1993; Kelsey, 1985; Kirks, 1984). Tomography is useful in many circumstances, but its usefulness has been overshadowed by the development of computed tomography.

Computed Tomography

Computed tomographic (CT) scanning obtains cross-sectional images rather than the shadow images of conventional radiography. In CT scanning, a fan x-ray beam from a source rotating about the infant passes through the body and the exit transmission of x-ray beam intensity is monitored by a series of detectors (Alpen, 1990; Bushong, 1992; Kelsey, 1985; Kirks, 1984). Bone is the most dense, absorbs the largest amount of x-rays, and appears white; air is the least dense and appears black; soft tissues are displayed as intermediate shades of gray. CT can detect changes in density in very small areas of tissue and permits identification of various components of soft tissue, such as subarachnoid space, white matter, gray matter, and ventricles (Alpen, 1990; Bushong, 1992; Juhl & Crummy, 1993; Kelsey, 1985; Moss, Ring, & Higgins, 1984; Squire & Novelline, 1988). Computed tomography of the body is technically more difficult than cranial examination because of cardiac and respiratory motion; however, a modern body scanner can complete a scan in 2 to 4 seconds, which decreases movement artifact. In the neonate, the rapid heart rate and respiratory rate has limited the usefulness of this technique for thoracic examination.

Computed tomography permits two-dimensional visualization of entire anatomic sections of tissue to help determine the extent of the disease or malformation. Anatomic and physiologic information can be visualized despite overlying gas and bone. Contrast enhancement can measure blood flow and help define pathologic abnormalities (Moss, Ring, & Higgins, 1984; Squire & Novelline, 1988; Swischuk, 1989, 1995). Bolus injection of contrast material permits excellent visualization of vascular structures.

As good as computed tomography is as an imaging modality, it is still not a radiologic microscope. Computed tomography does have its drawbacks. It also uses ionizing radiation, and because the computers require a cool room for proper equipment performance, there is a significant alteration in the neonate's environment, which must be considered.

Digital Radiography and Digital Vascular Imaging

Digital radiography uses techniques that use computers to produce projectional images similar to those of conventional radiography (Kelsey,

1985; Kirks, 1984). Although standard computed tomographic instruments have been designed to produce two-dimensional images of two-dimensional body slices, they can also be used to project three-dimensional structures into two-dimensional images that are similar to conventional radiographs. These projections do not have the fine detail of conventional radiographs, but because the pictorial data are stored in the computer, it is possible to manipulate the image and enhance subtle features (Bushong, 1992; Kelsey, 1985; Squire & Novelline, 1988).

Another method of digital radiography converts the image intensifier picture to digital signals that can be stored and manipulated. The most important use of this method is to obtain digital subtraction images of the heart and major arteries from data recorded before and after the injection of angiographic contrast (Bushong, 1992; Kelsey, 1985; Squire & Novelline, 1988). This method is much less invasive than catheterization, although the technique is new and the equipment is expensive.

RADIOGRAPHIC CONTRAST AGENTS

Plain radiography can differentiate only four kinds of body tissue: those containing gas (lung and bowel), fatty tissue, tissues containing calcium (bone or pathologic calcifications), and tissues of water density (solid organs, muscle, and blood). To demonstrate blood vessels within solid organs or surrounded by muscle, or to demonstrate other hollow structures, it is necessary to introduce artificial radiographic contrast agents. The contrast medium may be negative or positive and may be injected, swallowed, or administered as enemas (Gyll & Blake, 1986; Haller & Slovis, 1984; Hilton & Edwards, 1994; Squire & Novelline, 1988; Swischuk, 1989).

Negative contrast media absorb less radiation than adjacent soft tissues and so cast a darker radiographic image. Gases such as air, oxygen, or carbon dioxide can be used as negative contrast media. The amount of contrast provided by negative media for conventional radiography is limited and not readily used in medicine today (Fanaroff & Martin, 1992; Kirks, 1984; Swischuk, 1989).

Positive contrast media use elements with a high atomic number, which absorb much more radiation than surrounding soft tissues and therefore cast a lighter image. Barium and iodine are the two elements that are currently used. Barium sulfate is a relatively stable, nontoxic compound that is the major contrast agent used for outlining the walls of the gastrointestinal tract. Iodine-containing salts that are excreted by the kidneys are used for a wide variety of urographic and angiographic studies. Newer nonionic iodine-containing media, which are also excreted by the kidneys, have also been developed. These newer agents are made less painful than iodine-containing salts when injected into arteries because of their lower osmolality and are rapidly replacing the older contrast agents (Fanaroff & Martin, 1992; Hilton & Edwards, 1994).

FACTORS AFFECTING RADIOGRAPH QUALITY

There are several factors that determine technical quality of a radiograph, including film exposure, phase of respiration, motion, tube angulation, and infant positioning. If one of these factors goes awry it may lead to misinterpretation of the film. Understanding of these factors by the nurse will result in improved technical quality of radiographs.

A reasonable criterion to judge film exposure is satisfactory visualization of the dorsal intervertebral disk spaces through the entire cardiothymic silhouette (Fanaroff & Martin, 1992; Gyll, 1985; Hilton & Edwards, 1994; Kirks, 1984; Poznanski, 1976; Wesenberg, 1973). An underexposed film results in a loss of the dorsal disk spaces, and the lungs and other structures have a homogeneous "whitewashed" appearance. An overexposed film results in a progressive loss of pulmonary vascular markings, until the lungs have a black, "burned out" appearance (Hilton & Edwards, 1994; Swischuk, 1985; Wesenberg, 1973).

The phase of respiration at the time that the film was taken has considerable influence on the appearance of the radiograph. (Fig. 24–4). An expiratory film may show that the heart appears grossly enlarged and the lung fields appear opaque, which may simulate diffuse atelectasis, and the diaphragm will be located above the seventh rib (Gyll, 1985; Hilton & Edwards, 1994; Swischuk, 1989).

Inspiratory films show the diaphragm at the eighth rib, normal cardiothymic diameter, and prominent pulmonary vascularity. The right hemidiaphragm is slightly higher than the left. If the right hemidiaphragm is at or above the level of the seventh rib, the film is in an expiratory phase or the infant has hypoaeration (Gyll, 1985; Hilton & Edwards, 1994; Swischuk, 1989; Wesenberg, 1973).

Motion causes blurring of the hemidiaphragms, the cardiovascular silhouette, and all fine pulmonary detail (Hilton & Edwards, 1994; Swischuk, 1989; Wesenberg, 1973). The avoidance of movement blur on diagnostic images is achieved in one of two ways: speed and adequate immobilization.

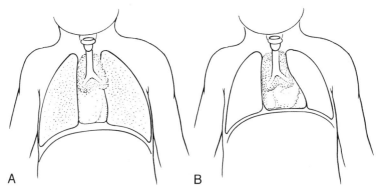

A   **B**

FIGURE 24–4. Differences in appearance between inspiration *(A)* and expiration *(B)* in a neonatal chest radiograph. On full inspiration, the diaphragm is located at the eighth rib and the lungs appear larger and darker. During expiration, the diaphragm is above the seventh rib and the lung fields appear smaller and lighter. The heart size may also appear larger on expiratory films.

IMMOBILIZATION

Proper immobilization may be less traumatic than manual restraint alone. An immobilization board may be required or may require the use of tape, foam rubber blocks and wedges, towels, diapers, or clear plastic acetate sheets (Gyll & Blake, 1986).

There are physical risks to neonates associated with immobilization. Trauma may occur as a result of restraint or use of an ill-designed immobilization device. Tape or plastic sheets may cause skin and soft tissue damage if not carefully applied and removed. In addition, there may be thermal stress encountered when placing a neonate on a noninsulated board or film cassette. The aim is to position the infant so that the technician can center the tube, position the beam, and make the exposure.

There are a number of immobilization devices on the market; however, the best method of immobilization is a pair of adequately protected adult hands.

Another factor that affects radiographic quality is x-ray tube angulation and improper field limitation. Often neonatal chest films appear mildly lordotic, with the medial clavicular ends projected on or above the dorsal vertebrae. This results in a rather peculiar chest configuration. The preossified anterior arcs of the upper ribs have a position that is superior to the posterior arcs. The lordotic projection tends to increase the apparent transverse cardiac diameter, making it difficult to determine heart size. Lordotic projections result from the x-ray tube angled cephalad, centering the x-ray beam over the abdomen, or from an irritable infant arching the back at the time of the film exposure (Gyll & Blake, 1986; Hilton & Edwards, 1994; Kirks, 1984; Swischuk, 1989; Wesenberg, 1973). Caudad angulation or centering the x-ray beam over the head results in the anterior rib arcs' being angulated sharply downward in relation to the posterior arcs (Fig. 24–5) (Hilton & Edwards, 1994; Swischuk, 1989; Wesenberg, 1973).

If the infant is rotated, there may be a false impression of a mediastinal shift. The direction and degree of rotation can be estimated by comparing the lengths of the posterior arcs of the ribs from the costovertebral junction to the lateral pleural line at a given level. The infant is rotated toward the side with the greatest posterior arc length (Kirks, 1984; Swischuk, 1989; Hilton & Edwards, 1994; Wesenberg, 1973). Another measurement to determine the degree of rotation is the distance from the medial aspect of the clavicles to the center of the vertebral body at the same level (Fig. 24–6). If the infant were properly positioned, the medial aspects of the clavicles should be equidistant from the center of the vertebral body (Poznanski, 1976; Hilton & Edwards, 1994). The measurement will be increased on the side toward which the infant is rotated. On a lateral view, rotation can be readily determined by noting the amount of offset between the anterior tips of the right and left sets of ribs.

RADIOLOGIC PROJECTIONS

Radiologic projections are the geometric views of the radiograph and vary among institutions and radiologists. They can be customized to the specific infant or clinical condition. For example, the skull may require a simple AP

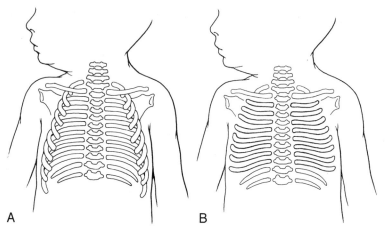

FIGURE 24–5. Skeletal position in a normally positioned radiograph *(A)* and a film taken with cephalad positioning of the x-ray tube *(B)*.

film to diagnose a fracture or a complete skull series may be necessary in the evaluation of congenital malformations. For the neck and upper airway, a lateral film in inspiration with the infant's head extended may be sufficient in the evaluation of stridor, or a xeroradiograph of the soft tissue structures of the neck may be required. Because the radiation dose of a xeroradiograph is much greater than a plain lateral neck film, the indications for this

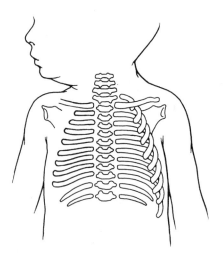

FIGURE 24–6. Skeletal configuration in a film taken with the infant rotated to the right.

examination should be clearly present (Gyll, 1985; Poznanski, 1976; Swischuk, 1995).

In the evaluation of the spine, the AP projection is most commonly used. Oblique views of the spine in the infant are usually difficult to obtain because it is difficult to position and immobilize the infant. In the evaluation of congenital hip dysplasia, an AP view of the entire pelvis and both hips is required. One should be careful to minimize gonadal exposure with proper shielding. Assessment of skeletal maturation in the infant requires an AP film of the left hemiskeleton, whereas a long bone series requires a film of the upper and lower extremities (Gyll & Blake, 1986; Hilton & Edwards, 1994; Kirks, 1984; Poznanski, 1976; Swischuk, 1989, 1995).

Chest radiographs are the most frequently performed diagnostic imaging procedure in the neonatal intensive care unit. In the vast majority of cases, an AP projection from a supine position is satisfactory to evaluate the infant's chest, heart, and lung fields. Lateral projections of the chest are often poorly positioned, have reduced technical quality, and require greater radiation exposure of the infant. For the experienced radiographer, an AP film in the supine position is sufficient in most cases. Rarely, a lateral chest film with esophageal barium contrast may be desired to evaluate the left atrium of the heart (Hilton & Edwards, 1994; Swischuk, 1989, 1995; Wesenberg, 1973).

Abdominal x-ray films are AP and cross-table lateral views (Hilton & Edwards, 1994; Poznanski, 1976; Swischuk, 1995; Wesenberg, 1973). Because the infant's abdomen is relatively cylindrical, a lateral view provides more information than in an older child or adult (Gyll, 1985). AP views define the gas pattern, intestinal displacement, some masses, and ascites, whereas the cross-table lateral view is recommended in the diagnosis of intestinal perforation, pneumoperitoneum, and portal venous air (Hilton & Edwards, 1994; Swischuk, 1995).

COLLABORATIVE CARE

Radiation Protection

Reduction of radiation exposure should be the goal for sites that are sensitive genetically (gonads) and somatically (eye, bone marrow). Although there is no evidence that somatic damage (e.g., carcinogenesis or cataract production) occurs as a result of low-dose diagnostic radiologic procedures, dose reduction should be accomplished for the site examined as well as the rest of the body (Noz & Maguire, 1985; Shapiro, 1990; Whaler & Balter, 1984). To reduce radiation exposure the following should be done:

- Perform examinations only when they are clinically indicated
- Select the appropriate imaging modality, using the lowest radiation dose that achieves an image of diagnostic quality
- Avoid repeat examinations
- Reduce the number of films obtained
- Use appropriate projections with tight field limitation
- Ensure proper positioning and immobilization
- Shield the gonads (Hilton & Edwards, 1994)

The gonads should be shielded whenever they are within 5 cm of the primary x-ray beam. Contact gonadal shields are easy to make from 0.5-mm thick lead rubber sheets and should be sized for sex and age (Fig. 24–7) (Gyll & Blake, 1986; Kirks, 1984; Shapiro, 1990; Swischuk, 1989). In males, proper positioning of the shield avoids obscuring any bony detail of the pelvis if the upper edge of the shield is placed just below the pubis and the testes have descended into the scrotum. In a female, the position of the ovaries varies with bladder distention. Because of their anatomic location, the ovaries cannot be shielded without obscuring lower abdominal and pelvic structures. The lower margin of the gonad shield should be placed at the level of the pubis, and the upper margin should cover at least the lower margin of the sacroiliac joints (Gyll & Blake, 1986; Kirks, 1984; Hilton & Edwards, 1994; Swischuk, 1989; Whaler & Balter, 1984).

Radiation Safety

There are three ways to reduce radiation exposure of personnel: (1) reduce the time of radiation exposure; (2) increase the distance from the radiation source; and (3) provide radiation shielding between the nurse and the radiation source (Alpen, 1990; Poznanski, Kanellitsas, Roloff, & Borer, 1974; Shapiro, 1990; Whaler & Balter, 1984). If certain basic radiation protection precautions are observed, it is unnecessary for nurses and other personnel in a neonatal intensive care unit to leave the room during x-ray exposures. As a precaution, staff should stay 1 foot or more away from the infant who is being radiographed. Care must be taken to be certain that if a horizontal beam film is obtained, as in a cross-table lateral projection, that no one is in the direct x-ray beam, because the radiation dose in the primary beam would be considerably higher than the scattered dose. When a horizontal beam is used, it should be directed so as not to aim it at any other patient or personnel. If an employee is within 1 foot of the incubator or is holding the infant for the exposure, lead gloves and aprons should be worn (Shapiro, 1990).

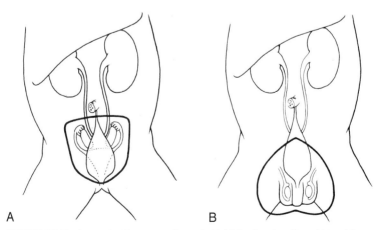

A   B

FIGURE 24–7. Anatomic placement of gonad shield for female infants *(A)* and for male infants *(B).*

The x-ray beam must be confined to within the cassette edges. There is not much scatter from an infant, but an adult's hands can easily come within the field of primary radiation and cause scatter (Gyll, 1985; Kirks, 1984; Shapiro, 1990). It is important to properly position and secure the infant as well as keep the hands out of the x-ray beam at the same time. If correct radiographic technique is employed, the dose to the nurse's lead-protected hands is about 0.01 mSv. The annual dose limit to the hands of nondesignated personnel is 500 mSv (Gyll, 1985; Shapiro, 1990).

Radionuclide Imaging

Use of radioisotopes has brought a new dimension to diagnostic imaging, because they have the advantage of yielding physiologic information as well as anatomic representations of the distribution of radioactivity, depending on the selective uptake of radionuclide by different organs of the body (Siddiqui, 1985; Treves, 1995; Walker & Margouleff, 1984). The primary disadvantage is the limited anatomic resolution to diameters greater than 2 cm.

COLLABORATIVE CARE

The care of a neonate undergoing a radionuclide scan requires knowledge about the patient's history and clinical manifestations, the type of nuclear scan requested, and the radiopharmaceutical utilized. In general, the doses of radiopharmaceuticals are based on the infant's body weight, and the total whole-body radiation dose received is considerably below that of a conventional radiograph. The infant poses no radioactivity hazard for the nursing staff or other neonates. Linen, diapers, and body excreta can be disposed of in the usual manner. The nurse should be aware of the ability of the radionuclide to concentrate in areas other than the organ of interest so that proper thyroid iodine-uptake blocking agents can be administered or diuresis can be promoted.

Ultrasonographic Imaging

Ultrasonography, unlike conventional radiography, emits no ionizing radiation. Instead, sound waves are used to evaluate tissue densities, movement of tissues, and flow of blood (Bushong, 1992; Fanaroff & Martin, 1992; Kirks, 1984; Martin, 1985; Swischuk, 1989). The images can be recorded on videotape, photographic film, or light-sensitive paper.

COLLABORATIVE CARE

The care is to ensure that any disruption of the infant's microenvironment is minimal. The infant's temperature can be maintained more easily if the ultrasound examination is performed by placing the transducer in the incubator. Although this method is technically more cumbersome for the ultrasonographer, cooperative interchange between the ultrasonographer and the nurse facilitates the procedure. In addition, the transducer gel should be warmed to the same temperature as the infant's incubator to minimize heat loss. A diaper or other pad placed under the imaged area and quick removal of the gel and drying the skin after the scan also decrease heat loss caused by wet blankets or skin.

It is important to monitor the infant's tolerance of the procedure and provide information that may be of diagnostic importance to the ultrasonographer. In addition, the nurse's presence at the bedside allows for immediate visual feedback and interpretation of the extent of the pathology that may be present. This knowledge allows better support of the infant's parents during further diagnostic testing and treatment decisions after their discussions with the medical staff. Interaction with the ultrasonographer at the bedside may also help the nurse to anticipate future health care needs of both an immediate and long-term nature.

REFERENCES

Alpen, E. L. (1990). *Radiation biophysics*. Englewood Cliffs, NJ: Prentice Hall.

Bushong, S. C. (1992). *Radiologic science for technologists: Physics, biology & protection* (5th ed.). St. Louis: C. V. Mosby.

Fanaroff, A. A., & Martin, R. J. (Eds.). (1992). *Neonatal-perinatal medicine* (5th ed.). St. Louis: C. V. Mosby.

Gofman, J. W. (1983). *Radiation and human health*. New York: Pantheon Books.

Gyll, C. (1985). *A handbook of pediatric radiography* (2nd ed.). Oxford: Blackwell Scientific Publications.

Gyll, C., & Blake, N. (1986). *Pediatric diagnostic imaging*. London: William Heinemann Medical Books.

Haller, J. O., & Slovis, T. L. (1984). *Introduction to radiology in clinical pediatrics*. Chicago: Year Book Medical Publishers.

Hilton, S. von W., & Edwards, D. K. (1994). *Practical pediatric radiology* (2nd ed.). Philadelphia: W. B. Saunders.

Horowitz, A. L. (1995). *Magnetic resonance imaging: Physics for radiologists* (3rd ed.). New York: Springer-Verlag.

Juhl, J. H., & Crummy, A. B. (Eds.). (1993). *Paul and Juhl's essentials of radiologic imaging* (6th ed.). Philadelphia: J. B. Lippincott.

Kelsey, C. A. (1985). *Essentials of radiology physics*. St. Louis: Warren H. Green.

Kirks, D. R. (1984). *Practical pediatric imaging*. Boston: Little, Brown.

Martin, D. J. (1985). Neonatal disorders diagnosed with ultrasound. *Clinics in Perinatology, 12*, 219–242.

Moss, A. A., Ring, E. G., & Higgins, C. B. (Eds.). (1984). *NMR, CT and interventional radiology*. San Francisco: University of California Printing Department.

Noz, M. E., & Maguire, G. Q. (1985). *Radiation protection in the radiologic and health sciences* (2nd ed.). Philadelphia: Lea & Febiger.

Poznanski, A. K. (1976). *Practical approaches to pediatric radiology*. Chicago: Year Book Medical Publishers.

Poznanski, A. K., Kanellitsas, C., Roloff, D. W., & Borer, R. C. (1974). Radiation exposure to personnel in a neonatal nursery. *Pediatrics, 54*, 139–141.

Shapiro, J. (1990). *Radiation protection* (3rd ed.). Cambridge, MA: Harvard University Press.

Siddiqui, A. R. (1985). *Nuclear imaging in pediatrics*. Chicago: Year Book Medical Publishers.

Squire, L. F., & Novelline, R. A. (1988). *Fundamentals of radiology* (4th ed.). Cambridge: Harvard University Press.

Swischuk, L. E. (1989). *Imaging of the newborn, infant, and young child* (3rd ed.). Baltimore: Williams & Wilkins.

Swischuk, L. E. (1995). *Differential diagnosis in pediatric radiology* (2nd ed.). Baltimore: Williams & Wilkins.

Treves, S. T. (Ed.). (1990). *Pediatric nuclear medicine*. (2nd ed.). New York: Springer-Verlag.

Vogler, J. B., Helms, C. A., & Collen, P. W. (1986). *Normal variants and pitfalls in imaging*. Philadelphia: W. B. Saunders.

Walker, J. M., & Margouleff, D. (Eds.). (1984). *A clinical manual of nuclear medicine*. Norwalk, CT: Appleton-Century-Crofts.

Wesenberg, R. L. (1973). *The newborn chest*. Hagerstown, MD: Harper & Row.

Whaler, J. P., & Balter, S. (1984). *Radiation risks in medical imaging*. Chicago: Year Book Medical Publishers.

CHAPTER 25

Diagnostic Tests and Laboratory Values

LABORATORY VALUES

A wide variety of laboratory tests are available for use in both diagnosis and care of the neonate. Although a general range of normal values is established, many hospitals have compiled their own list of acceptable values; specific laboratories should be contacted when evaluating laboratory results. (See tables in Appendix A.)

CARDIOLOGY PROCEDURES

Cardiac Catheterization

Use of radiopaque dye allows for clarification of congenital heart defects. A radiopaque catheter is inserted into an arm or leg vessel by percutaneous puncture or cutdown. Under fluoroscopy, the catheter is visualized and passed into the heart. Selected chambers and vessels of the heart can then be evaluated for size and function. Intracardiac pressures and oxygen saturations can also be measured during this procedure.

Immobilization of the neonate and constant monitoring are required during cardiac catheterization. The infant must be restrained to maintain supine positioning. Electrocardiographic electrodes must also be placed to provide constant vital sign monitoring. To maintain proper positioning during the procedure, sedation may be a consideration.

After the desired information is obtained, the catheter used to obtain this information is carefully removed. If a cutdown was performed, the vessel is ligated and the skin is sutured. Pressure should be applied over a percutaneous puncture site to enhance clot formation. For continued bleeding problems, pressure dressings may be applied to the insertion site; these must be checked frequently for active bleeding.

After cardiac catheterization, vital signs should be measured frequently, comparing them with precatheterization baseline vital signs. Evaluation for localized bleeding or signs of hypotension resulting in changes in heart rate and blood pressure is essential. Assessment of the insertion site and affected extremity for bleeding, color, peripheral pulses, temperature, and capillary refill should continue for at least 24 hours after the procedure.

Complications of catheterization may include hypovolemia (as a result of bleeding or fluid loss during the procedure), infection, thrombosis, or tissue necrosis. Peripheral intravenous fluids may be required to compensate for fluid losses. Localized infection of the catheterization site may be demonstrated by redness, swelling, warmth, or drainage. Management usually involves use of antibiotic ointment on the site followed by protection with a dry sterile dressing. Assessments of skin color and temperature, as well as quality and characteristics of bilateral peripheral pulses, are essential after cardiac catheterization.

Echocardiography

Echocardiography is a noninvasive diagnostic procedure. Single-dimension echocardiography allows for evaluation of anatomic structures, including valves, chambers, and vessels. Two-dimensional echocardiography provides more in-depth information about relationships between the heart and the great vessels (Flanagan & Fyler, 1994).

Echocardiographic examination also allows for evaluation of structural function within the heart. This information can be important not only in preoperative assessment of cardiac defects but also in postoperative evaluation of procedures.

Doppler echocardiography is used in various forms to evaluate characteristics of blood flow through the heart, valves, and great vessels. It can measure not only cardiac output but also flow velocity changes, as demonstrated in stenotic lesions. Regurgitation through insufficiently functioning valves can also be identified through Doppler studies. Directional Doppler echocardiography can also be used to identify shunting through a patent ductus arteriosus (Hohn & Stanton, 1995).

Electrocardiography

Electrocardiography is used in conjunction with other diagnostic measures to evaluate cardiac function—specifically, circulatory demands placed on individual heart chambers. Dysrhythmias may also be diagnosed by the use of electrocardiography (Flanagan & Fyler, 1994).

GENETIC PROCEDURES

Chromosome Analysis

Analysis of chromosome composition can assist in identification of various genetic disorders. A blood specimen is obtained from the infant and used to harvest an actual set of chromosomes. During active cell division, usually during metaphase, the chromosomes are photographed and then arranged in pairs by number. This karyotype is then evaluated for the appropriate number of pairs, chromosome size, and structure.

Sweat Chloride Testing

The sweat chloride test is an evaluation of sodium and chloride content in sweat and is used to diagnose cystic fibrosis. Sweat, produced by an electrical current, is collected onto a gauze pad or filter paper. The sweat content is then evaluated; a sweat chloride value of greater than 60 mEq/L is consistent with cystic fibrosis (Vanderhoof, Zach, & Adrian, 1994).

GASTROINTESTINAL PROCEDURES

Barium Enema

A barium enema is used to evaluate the structure and function of the large intestine. The diagnosis of disorders such as Hirschsprung's disease and meconium plug syndrome can easily be supported by the use of this procedure.

In the enema procedure, a contrast medium such as barium sulfate is instilled and a series of films are taken under fluoroscopy. The infant must be well restrained. The procedure is started with the infant supine. As the contrast medium is instilled, its flow through the bowel is observed as the infant's position is changed. A series of abdominal radiographs should be taken once the bowel has been filled with contrast medium. Follow-up films may also be necessary to document evacuation of the contrast medium from the bowel. Evaluation of the bowel is essential after this procedure to prevent constipation or obstruction. Assessment of bowel elimination is important after barium enema.

Upper Gastrointestinal Series With Small Bowel Follow-Through

As in a barium enema, barium sulfate or other water-soluble contrast media are used in this procedure. However, the contrast medium is swallowed to examine the upper gastrointestinal tract. Three main areas are examined (Kenner, Harjo, & Brueggemeyer, 1988): (1) the esophagus, for size, patency, reflux, and presence of a fistula or swallowing abnormality; (2) the stomach, for anatomic abnormalities, patency, and motility; and (3) the small intestine, for structures, patency, and function.

Follow-up radiographs may be needed to evaluate the emptying ability of the stomach and intestinal motility as the contrast medium moves through the small bowel. Again, care includes assessment of temperature and cardiac and respiratory status throughout the procedure. The nurse should be alert for reflux or vomiting, which can be accompanied by aspiration. Evacuation of contrast medium from the bowel remains a concern after an upper gastrointestinal series with small bowel follow-through and should be monitored by the nurse. It is also possible for fluid to be pulled out of the vascular compartment and into the bowel. The side effects are thus fluid loss and hypotension.

Rectal Suction Biopsy

Rectal biopsy is a procedure commonly used to evaluate the presence or absence of ganglion cells in the bowel (the latter being seen in Hirschsprung's disease). Before a rectal biopsy, it is essential to obtain bleeding times, prothrombin times, partial thromboplastin times, and platelet counts as well as a spun hematocrit to ensure that the infant is not in danger of excessive bleeding. The procedure is as follows:

- The infant is positioned supine with legs held toward the abdomen.
- With a suction blade apparatus inserted into the bowel through the

anus, small specimens of rectal tissue from the mucosa and submucosa levels are excised.

- Specimens are evaluated by the pathology department for the composition of ganglion cells.

After this procedure, care should focus on assessments for bleeding or intestinal perforation. Included are evaluation of vital signs for increased heart rate or decreased blood pressure, fever, persistent guaiac-positive stools, or frank rectal bleeding (Kenner, Harjo, & Brueggemeyer, 1988).

Liver Biopsy

Open liver biopsy is a surgical procedure that requires general anesthesia, whereas a closed liver biopsy may be done using local anesthetic. Coagulation studies including bleeding time, platelet count, and spun hematocrit are essential. Preoperative care may include sedation of the infant, requiring frequent monitoring of vital signs. Throughout the procedure, assessment of vital signs remains essential in identifying changes in hemodynamics or respiratory states. After the procedure, assessment of vital signs for signs and symptoms of hemorrhage is essential. Indications of hemorrhage also include decreases in the hemoglobin and hematocrit, thus making laboratory monitoring an important element of postbiopsy care. The biopsy site must be evaluated for signs of active bleeding, ecchymosis, swelling, or infection.

GENITOURINARY PROCEDURES

Cystoscopy

Cystoscopy provides direct visualization of the urinary structures, including the bladder, urethra, and urethral orifices. It enables the diagnosis of abnormalities in the structure of the bladder and urinary tract.

A cystoscopy is performed with the infant under general anesthesia. The urethral opening is prepared with an antiseptic solution followed by sterile draping. The lubricated cystoscope is inserted through the urethra, and visualization of the urinary structures is performed.

As with any postanesthesia patient, postprocedural care includes vital sign assessment. However, particular attention should be paid toward assessing for adequate urinary output and the presence of hematuria (Spitzer, Bernstein, Boichis, & Edelmann, 1995).

Radioisotope Renal Scan

This procedure includes the intravenous injection of a radioisotope, after which radioactive counters monitor the movement of the radioisotope through the urinary system. Comparison of the kidneys is made possible by this procedure in terms of blood flow, renal tubule function, and excretion. After injection of the radioisotope, films are taken approximately every 5 minutes for at least 30 minutes. Follow-up films may be desirable if compromised kidney function is suspected.

It must be remembered that the infant's urine is radioactive for 24 hours after injection of the radioisotope. Consequently, gloves should be worn when changing diapers or handling soiled diapers. Also, provisions must be made for linens or trash that is contaminated with radioactive urine.

Voiding Cystourethrogram

The purpose of this procedure is to visualize the lower urinary tract after instillation of contrast medium through urethral catheterization. The infant's bladder is emptied after catheterization and then filled with the contrast medium. Serial films under fluoroscopy in a variety of positions are taken during voiding. After voiding, additional films are obtained. Pathologic results of a voiding cystourethrogram demonstrate residual urine in the bladder, as with a neurogenic bladder, posterior valve obstructions, or vesicoureteral reflux.

As with the cystoscopy procedure, the infant should be evaluated for hematuria. In addition, symptoms of infection as a result of contaminated catheterization should be evaluated (fever, cloudy or sedimented urine, foul-smelling urine).

NEUROLOGIC PROCEDURES

Electroencephalography

Electroencephalographic examination records the electrical activity of the brain. Numerous electrodes are placed at precise locations on the infant's head to record electrical impulses from various parts of the brain. This procedure can be important in diagnosing lesions or tumors, identifying nonfunctional areas of the brain, or pinpointing the focus of seizure activity.

The infant may require sedation during this procedure to prevent crying or movement. As much equipment as is safely possible should be removed to decrease electrical interference. Also, calming procedures such as decreasing light stimulation or warming the environment may assist in quieting the infant during electroencephalography. The infant should be closely observed throughout the procedure for any signs of seizure activity.

Radioisotope Brain Scan

Intravenous injection of radioisotope solution and monitoring of uptake in the brain constitute a diagnostic procedure used in neonates. At specified intervals, various views of the brain are taken, showing the presence of the radioisotope in abnormal brain tissue. Tumors or abscesses as well as areas of hematoma or infarct can be identified with this procedure.

RESPIRATORY PROCEDURES

Laryngoscopy and Bronchoscopy

These procedures are commonly done in tandem with the infant under general anesthesia. Examination of structures by direct visualization provides the opportunity to identify congenital anomalies, obstructions, masses, or mucus plugs and to evaluate stridor or respiratory dysfunction.

Possible complications related to these procedures include bronchospasm, laryngeal spasms, laryngeal edema, and pneumothorax or bradycardia resulting in hypoxia. Close respiratory observation in the immediate postoperative period is essential to maintain a patent airway and promote optimal gas exchange. In addition, bleeding may occur after possible tissue biopsy, but frank bleeding is abnormal and should be investigated (Nickerson, Barnhart, & Czervinske, 1995).

REFERENCES

Flanagan, M. F., & Fyler, D. C. (1994). Cardiac disease. In G. B. Avery, M. A. Fletcher, & M. G. MacDonald. (Eds.). *Neonatology: Pathophysiology and management of the neonate* (4th ed., pp. 516–559). Philadelphia: J. B. Lippincott.

Hohn, A. R., & Stanton, R. E. (1995). The cardiovascular system. In A. A. Fanaroff, & R. J. Martin (Eds.), *Neonatal-perinatal medicine: Diseases of the fetus and infant* (5th ed., pp. 883–940). St. Louis: C. V. Mosby.

Kenner, C. A., Harjo, J., & Brueggemeyer, A. (1988). *Neonatal surgery: A nursing perspective.* Orlando, FL: Grune & Stratton.

Nickerson, B. G., Barnhart, S. L., & Czervinske, M. P. (1995). Bronchoscopy. In S. L. Barnhart, & M. P. Czervinske (Eds.), *Perinatal and pediatric respiratory care* (pp. 103–113). Philadelphia: W. B. Saunders.

Spitzer, A., Bernstein, J., Boichis, H., & Edelmann, C. M., Jr. (1995). Kidney and urinary tract. In A. A. Fanaroff, & R. J. Martin (Eds.), *Neonatal-perinatal medicine: Diseases of the fetus and infant* (5th ed., pp. 1293–1327). St. Louis: C. V. Mosby.

Vanderhoof, J. A., Zach, T. L, & Adrian, T. E. (1994). Gastrointestinal disease. In G. B. Avery, M. A. Fletcher, & M. G. MacDonald (Eds.), *Neonatology: Pathophysiology and management of the neonate* (4th ed., pp. 605–629). Philadelphia: J. B. Lippincott.

Special Clinical Concerns

• •

CHAPTER 26

Surgical Neonate

PREOPERATIVE PERIOD

Stabilization of the neonate in the preoperative period will determine the infant's ability to survive the trauma of surgical intervention. The major factors to be considered in effective stabilization include oxygenation, acid–base balance, thermoregulation, fluid and electrolyte balance, and pharmacologic support.

Oxygenation

Adequate tissue oxygenation is mandatory in the prevention of irreversible organ damage as a result of hypoxia. Establishment of effective ventilation is a primary concern in providing optimal air exchange and oxygenation.

Ventilatory insufficiency can occur with various surgical problems. For example, airway obstruction occurs with choanal atresia, whereas an ineffective airway clearance mechanism is experienced with a tracheoesophageal fistula with esophageal atresia.

Hypoventilation is encountered with a diaphragmatic hernia as well as with those defects causing increased abdominal pressure on the diaphragm and lungs. Defects that manifest this type of problem include omphalocele or gastroschisis, necrotizing enterocolitis, and bowel obstructions.

A surgical neonate is not immune to problems such as prematurity, respiratory distress syndrome, persistent pulmonary hypertension, atelectasis, aspiration pneumonia, or bronchopulmonary dysplasia. Neonates are obligate nose breathers. With choanal atresia, an oral airway will be required to establish adequate ventilation. Intubation, if required, will need to be performed through the orotracheal route.

Any intra-abdominal pressure changes can lead to respiratory compromise. To minimize this problem the infant should be positioned to avoid abdominal pressure from an abdominal wall defect. The side-lying or semi-side-lying position may relieve diaphragmatic pressure from the defects and enhance ventilator assistance and pulmonary function.

Omphalocele or gastroschisis, necrotizing enterocolitis, and bowel obstructions all cause increased abdominal distention.

Gastric decompression is necessary to decrease this source of pressure on the diaphragm and the increasing difficulty in lung expansion. This decompression is achieved by use of an orogastric or nasogastric tube to gravity drain or suction and the maintenance of tube patency.

Continued abdominal distention may further compromise respiratory effort. Increased oxygenation or ventilation needs may reflect unresolved abdominal distention and worsening of the disease process. In addition, the ascites encountered in renal defects such as ureteropelvic junction obstructions can cause respiratory difficulty. Mechanical ventilation may be required until surgical intervention relieves the abdominal pressure.

A neonate with a diaphragmatic hernia has special respiratory needs.

- Mask ventilation *must be avoided* at all costs. It is contraindicated because air is forced into the gastrointestinal tract, causing the volume to be increased in the chest and thus increasing the respiratory compromise in an infant with already limited lung function.
- Use of the minimal pressures is necessary to provide adequate oxygenation but avoid damage to the functional lung.
- Persistent pulmonary hypertension must be prevented.
  - Adequate ventilation is provided—to avoid hypoxia, hypercarbia, and acidosis, which are known influencing factors in pulmonary hypertension.

Considerations in management of an infant with tracheoesophageal fistula/esophageal atresia include the following:

- Mask ventilation is contraindicated when a tracheoesophageal fistula with esophageal atresia is present because of rupture of the esophageal pouch and overdistention of the stomach.
- Reflux of stomach contents can occur through the fistula into the trachea, causing pneumonia.
  - Proper endotracheal tube positioning should be maintained.
  - Minimal ventilator pressure is used to minimize these complications.
- Aspiration pneumonia should be prevented.
  - If the blind esophageal pouch fills with saliva, overflow occurs into the lungs, causing pneumonia.
  - The patency of a double-lumen suction tube should be maintained to drain the esophageal pouch. If diagnostic testing is necessary to evaluate the esophageal pouch, one should try to keep the contrast medium from spilling out of the pouch. A plain anteroposterior chest and abdominal radiograph is taken with a radiopaque tube placed in the esophageal pouch. The esophageal pouch will be clearly outlined, and air in the stomach will confirm the presence of a tracheoesophageal fistula. Positioning the infant with the head of the bed elevated and/or prone minimizes possible reflux of gastric secretions.

Maintenance of a patent airway can be of concern with various defects. In some circumstances, intubations may be avoided if proper positioning is employed. Extension of the neck may be necessary in cases in which a large, obstructing cystic hygroma is present. Hydrocephalus of severe proportions may also require slight extension of the neck and turning of the head to either side.

Regardless of the type of defect present, nursing priorities in regard to oxygenation status include the following:

- Respiratory assessment for the quantity and quality of respiratory effort
- Investigation of wide changes in respiratory rate
- Adequate ventilation
  - Ease of respirations
  - Absence of retractions or nasal flaring
  - Pink color of lips, mucous membranes, or nail beds

Acid–Base Balance

Alterations in acid–base balance can be caused by a variety of factors in the surgical neonate. Major areas that can result in acidosis include inadequate respiratory support and fluid or electrolyte imbalances. The effects of sepsis and tissue necrosis are also significant causes of acidosis. Acidosis in the surgical neonate can be respiratory, metabolic, or mixed.

Respiratory acidosis could occur with decreased ventilation, resulting in increased PCO_2 levels and decreased pH. An overproduction of acids may occur with any condition that causes decreased oxygenation or decreased perfusion.

- Impaired kidney function: acute renal failure or renal tubular necrosis decreases elimination of hydrogen ions, contributing to the development of metabolic acidosis.
- Bicarbonate losses: severe diarrhea, intestinal fistulas, vomiting and gastric drainage result in metabolic acidosis.

The neonate with a diaphragmatic hernia is at great risk for development of respiratory or metabolic acidosis or both. Aggressive ventilation and administration of a buffering agent (e.g., sodium bicarbonate, tromethamine) to prevent acidosis, which could contribute to the development of primary pulmonary hypertension will be necessary.

Poor tissue perfusion causes acidosis, as occurs in infants with multiple gastrointestinal anomalies that are accompanied by large fluid losses, such as the following:

- Tracheoesophageal fistula with esophageal atresia
- Ruptured omphalocele/gastroschisis
- Bowel obstructions
- Necrotizing enterocolitis

Adequately replenishing fluid or blood volume usually corrects this metabolic acidosis. However, in cases in which necrosis or perforation occurs, the acidosis may not be correctable until the necrotic bowel is removed and any resulting sepsis is treated.

Thermoregulation

The large body surface area in association with the lack of insulating subcutaneous fat enhances heat loss. Oxygen consumption increases as the metabolic rate increases to maintain body temperature. This increased metabolic work results in acidosis and tissue hypoxia.

Prevention of hypothermia is imperative to the surgical neonate in the preoperative period. Maintenance of a neutral thermal environment is a constant challenge. Any prolonged deviations from the neutral thermal environment will further stress the neonate.

Heat loss occurs through evaporation, conduction, convection, and radiation. Evaporative heat loss occurs with situations such as exposure of the intestinal contents of a ruptured omphalocele/gastroschisis, an unprotected spinal cord (encephalocele or a myelomeningocele), or an exposed bladder mucosa (exstrophy of the bladder). Prevention of this heat loss can be accomplished by applying warm dressings to the defects followed by the covering of these areas with plastic.

Conductive heat loss occurs from direct skin contact on a cold surface, such as from cold or wet linens, a weight scale, an examining table, x-ray plates, and unwarmed bed. Avoidance of this type of heat loss can be done by the following:

- Prewarm linens.
- Prewarm bed or incubator.
- Warm examining or x-ray tables with heat lamps before and during procedure.
- Replace wet linens.
- Cover x-ray plates and scales with warmed linens.

Convection occurs with air blowing over the infant. To decrease this type of heat loss, the following should be done:

- Use warmed oxygen in head hoods and ventilators.
- Do not open incubator door for prolonged periods.
- Perform insertion of nasogastric tubes, placement of intravenous lines, x-rays, physical examination, and phlebotomy procedures through the incubator portholes.
- Place an additional heat source over the incubator when the door must be open.

Heat loss by radiation is the most difficult to control. This type of heat loss occurs during transportation through cold hallways, in cold examining rooms, and in a cold operating room. Preventing this cold stress is done by covering the infant with warmed linens during transport and prewarming examining and operating rooms to well above the comfortable temperature. Nursing care should focus on the following:

- Maintenance of a constant temperature, whether inside an incubator or in a radiant warmer bed
- Using warmed solutions for suctioning and dressing changes
- Frequent temperature monitoring
- Consistency in measuring temperature
- Appropriate documentation of temperature

Prevention of cold stress will decrease the chance of surgical complications. This is one of the reasons more neonatal surgical procedures such as patent ductus arteriosus ligations are being performed within the neonatal intensive care unit.

Fluid and Electrolyte Balance

FLUID LOSSES

Adequate fluid volume is required to ensure adequate perfusion of all organ systems. An inadequate vascular volume interferes with the oxygen supply to peripheral tissues, resulting in cellular damage and accompanying acidosis.

All fluid losses must be accurately measured to allow for adequate replacement. Estimation of insensible fluid losses is essential, including those caused by humidification through ventilation, radiant heating, and phototherapy. Unexpected fluid losses and inadequate fluid replacement will delay the neonate's preoperative stabilization.

With an esophageal atresia, there are continuous losses of saliva suctioned from the esophageal pouch. These must be measured and this loss corrected. In the case of a ruptured omphalocele or gastroschisis, correction of these losses may involve up to twice the normal maintenance fluids. If an omphalocele is protected by a membranous sac, less fluid requirement is needed. In gastrointestinal obstructions, losses can occur from vomiting and from suctioning required for gastric decompression. Peritonitis, as occurs with perforations demonstrated in necrotizing enterocolitis, midgut volvulus, or ruptured meconium ileus, causes third spacing of fluid or fluid shifts into the bowel. Additionally, cerebrospinal fluid can be lost from a leaking myelomeningocele.

Third spacing of fluids, or capillary leak syndrome, is the result of trauma to the gastrointestinal system. The capillary membrane's permeability is changed. This phenomenon may be due to the body's natural fibronectin, a glycoprotein secreted by epithelial cells in the pulmonary and gastrointestinal trees. It is secreted in response to stimulation of the immune system in an attempt to heal a wound. Unfortunately, it alters the capillary permeability and shifts fluid, resulting in a leaky capillary and the third spacing of fluid. The body's compensatory response to any gastrointestinal trauma then can result in a movement of fluid across this "leaky" membrane. Fluid moves out of the vascular compartment and into the tissues. The infant becomes swollen with generalized edema. Abdominal swelling creates pressure on the thoracic cavity, increasing the work of breathing. Gas exchange and ventilation are compromised as a result of the following:

- Pressure
- Decreased circulation
- Increased cardiac workload
- Loss of the buffer system through decreased kidney perfusion and gastric losses

The immediate reaction by inexperienced health care professionals is to restrict fluids in this edematous infant without realizing that the vascular compartment is severely depleted of fluids. The infant is hypotensive, increasing the risk of cardiopulmonary compromise. Thus, liberalization of fluids is necessary if total vascular collapse is to be avoided.

The performance of diagnostic enemas with hyperosmolar solutions can have catastrophic results in a neonate who is not properly hydrated. Adequate intravenous access and good hydration are essential. Vascular collapse and even shock can occur rapidly if the fluid is shifted from the vascular bed into the bowel and the fluid is extracted with the enema and not appropriately replaced.

GLUCOSE

Fluctuation in the glucose level is a major indication of stress as well as infection. Preoperative hyperglycemia can result from sepsis or excessive intravenous administration of glucose. Hypoglycemia may result from the following:

- Reduced glycogen stores in prematurity and intrauterine growth retardation
- Excessive insulin production in the infant of a diabetic mother
- With sudden or prolonged cessation of glucose infusions: difficult or delayed intravenous line insertions
- Abnormalities in glucose metabolism: sepsis, shock, and asphyxia, as well as with various central nervous system abnormalities

Careful titration of glucose infusions is necessary to provide adequate hydration while slowly restoring the serum glucose value to an acceptable level, avoiding extremes.

ELECTROLYTE IMBALANCES

Fluid losses as well as inadequate intake result in hypokalemia and/or hyponatremia. Hyperkalemia occurs with acidosis, excessive potassium intake, and renal failure. Renal failure may be evidenced in genitourinary obstructions or as a result of sepsis and poor perfusion, as seen in necrotizing enterocolitis with perforation and/or peritonitis. Hypernatremia results from excessive intake of sodium, which results from the following:

- Administration of hypertonic solutions
- Intravenous flushes with normal saline and/or heparinized normal saline
- Administration of sodium bicarbonate
- Use of antibiotics such as ampicillin

Return to proper fluid and electrolyte balance is needed to improve the neonate's ability to tolerate any necessary operative procedure and to reduce potential complications.

Pharmacologic Support

Calculations of medication doses must be carefully individualized. The neonate's weight is only one factor to be considered in these calculations. An immature renal and hepatic system may result in a decreased ability to metabolize as well as excrete drugs that are administered. To prevent toxicity, serum levels of medications should be closely monitored.

Preoperative antibiotic therapy may be required for the treatment of sepsis. Untreated sepsis may progress, causing deterioration of the respiratory and cardiovascular systems. Respiratory distress requires increased ventilation. Inotropic drugs may be needed to support the cardiovascular system. In many neonatal intensive care units, gentamicin is used in combination with aminoglycoside therapy as treatment for sepsis. This antibiotic increases the sodium intake and must be considered in monitoring electrolyte balance. Clindamycin is an effective agent used in the treatment of anaerobic organisms, which are generally found in the gastrointestinal infections.

With suspected gastrointestinal obstructions, antibiotics may be needed to treat peritonitis or enterocolitis. The progression of necrotizing enterocolitis may be slowed with vigorous antibiotic therapy. Treatment of omphalocele/gastroschisis should include antibiotics to protect the exposed gastrointestinal contents and to help prevent ischemic injury to the abdominal contents. If pneumonia accompanies an esophageal atresia with tracheoesophageal fistula, aggressive antibiotic treatment should be instituted to clear the pneumonia and promote an optimal surgical repair of the defect. A myelomeningocele will require antibiotic treatment to prevent meningitis from an exposed spinal cord.

Inotropic agents may be necessary to improve cardiac function and thus improve organ perfusion that has been impaired as a result of sepsis and stress. Dobutamine achieves organ perfusion by increasing cardiac output. Dopamine, used in low to moderate doses, causes vasodilation with resultant improvement in cardiac, renal, gastrointestinal, and cerebral blood flow. However, use of dopamine at high doses causes vasoconstriction of renal as well as gastrointestinal vessels. This vasoconstriction could worsen a renal system affected by obstruction or poor flow status, as well as the gastrointestinal system already compromised in necrotizing enterocolitis, omphalocele/gastroschisis, or obstructions. Thus, dobutamine and dopamine doses must be carefully calculated and continually titrated to achieve the desired effect. They are incompatible with many other drugs. For example, alkaline solutions such as sodium bicarbonate, ampicillin, gentamicin, and furosemide can inactivate dobutamine and dopamine. These inotropic agents are also irritating to vessels, so close monitoring of intravenous sites for infiltration is essential.

A buffering agent may be required to treat the acidosis that may accompany a diaphragmatic hernia, necrotizing enterocolitis, omphalocele/gastroschisis, or obstruction with resulting ischemic injury. It is imperative that adequate ventilation and tissue perfusion be established and maintained before medication is used to treat acidotic conditions.

OPERATIVE PERIOD

Timing of the Operation

The proper timing of a surgical procedure is an important factor in minimizing the stress. A surgical neonate may suffer from a multitude of medical as well as surgical problems. A complete evaluation is needed. A metabolically stable, growing infant is a much better surgical risk than an unstable, acidotic, premature infant. Also, the emergent nature of any surgical problem takes precedence over minor defects.

Perforation of the stomach or intestines is one of the few reasons an emergency surgical repair is performed. If this perforation is not treated, hypovolemia, acidosis, and shock will occur. Delay in treating necrotizing enterocolitis with perforation or midgut volvulus will result in further infarction of an already compromised bowel, leading to shock and death. The physiologic response to perforation will not be correctable until the diseased bowel is resected. Even in these emergent situations, hypovolemia must be aggressively treated to attain an optimal surgical outcome.

Treatment of a congenital diaphragmatic hernia is directed toward aggressive stabilization of respiratory status before the repair of the hernia, including extracorporeal membrane oxygenation. The repair is performed when the infant is stable and still on oxygenation.

An infant with a tracheoesophageal fistula with an esophageal atresia will receive a gastrostomy tube as soon as possible to prevent reflux of gastric contents into the lungs through the fistula. The repair of the atresia and fistula can be delayed until the infant's condition is stable and a complete evaluation is performed for other anomalies. The fistula may be ligated and the esophageal anastomosis delayed to allow for better growth and an optimal surgical outcome. Treatment of any pneumonia that may be present must be done before any surgical procedure is undertaken.

When a neonate is not stable enough for primary closure of an omphalocele/gastroschisis or the defect is too large, a Silastic pouch, or "silo," may be performed. This pouch helps to prevent infection, alleviate the restriction of venous return to the extremities, and reduce renal compromise. This procedure will relieve abdominal pressure, which may cause respiratory compromise by suspending the defect above the abdomen. Slow, daily reduction of this silo over 7 to 10 days allows closure of the defect with minimal complications.

A myelomeningocele can be protected with sterile normal saline–soaked dressings to allow for full evaluation of the infant's neurologic status before repairing the defect. An ultrasound evaluation of the head helps determine if placement of a ventriculoperitoneal shunt is needed. Evaluation by an orthopedist for determination of potential intervention for the lower extremities can be delayed until the back repair has been done and is healing.

If the infant with an encephalocele is stable, a full evaluation should be performed to reveal the type of tissue and vascular access involved in the defect. Removal of an encephalocele can be assisted by this information and allows for preparation of the family for the infant's postoperative prognosis.

The timing factor is important when a sacrococcygeal teratoma is present. Evaluation of the defect preoperatively is essential to determine the surgical technique and the postoperative outcome. For instance, is the spinal cord involved? Is the defect extremely vascular? What will be the result if the defect is excised? A great loss of blood can occur and will need to be anticipated. Preoperative stabilization of the infant's hematologic status is imperative to optimize surgical outcome.

An infant with an imperforate anus requires radiologic evaluation to identify the location of the rectum. This evaluation will determine the surgical procedure, that is, whether an anoplasty or a colostomy is required.

The effects of anesthesia during the surgical procedure present additional problems. Vascular access must be established to rapidly give drugs, fluids, and blood products. Arterial lines may be needed to monitor blood gases and arterial pressures. Critical assessments of vital signs and exact fluid management will directly affect the positive or negative outcome of surgical intervention.

Oxygenation

A number of factors can limit gas exchange during anesthesia in the neonate. The gestational age and birth weight of the infant dictate the size of the endotracheal tube used for intubation. Smaller-gauge tubes create increased airway resistance and, thus, increased difficulty in ventilation. Specific defects such as diaphragmatic hernia and omphalocele/gastroschisis cause additional considerations. When the abdominal contents of the defects are replaced in the abdominal cavity, pressure on the diaphragm is increased and ventilation must be adjusted to compensate for this change. Stress and fatigue in the infant also decrease respiratory effort and necessitate prolonged manual or mechanical ventilation.

Anesthetic agents can cause respiratory depression, as can narcotic and sedative medications. The capacity of the neonate to tolerate anesthesia for a prolonged period is limited. The residual effect of anesthesia can delay the recovery of the infant from the surgical procedure, as evidenced by decreased respiratory effort or apnea. Oxygenation of the neonate should be directed toward maintenance of a Po_2 in the range of 60 to 80 mm Hg or an oxygen saturation range of 90 to 95 percent.

Acid–Base Balance

The effects of sepsis and tissue necrosis as well as poor tissue perfusion add to the potential for an acidotic state. Acid–base balance may also continue to be altered as a result of impaired renal function or prolonged fluid imbalances. Monitoring of blood gas levels and the administration of buffering agents are important aspects of patient care.

Thermoregulation

Concerns related to temperature regulation continue during the intraoperative period. Although it is always helpful for a normal core temperature to be achieved before surgery, this is not always possible. Nursing measures regarding thermoregulation are as follows:

- Monitor temperature (skin or rectal probe) throughout the procedure.
- Use a radiant warmer during line placement, preparation, draping, and induction of anesthesia.
- Use a warming blanket.
- Increase room temperature.
- Humidify and warm anesthetic gases.

- Warm blood products, irrigation fluids, and intravenous fluids.
- Replace surgical drapes, if possible, when they become wet.
- Cover infant with warmed linen during transport.
- During the operative procedure, keep the bed warm to allow for some warmth during transport postoperatively.

Fluid and Electrolyte Balance

Maintenance of the fluid and electrolyte balance requires the following:

- Constant monitoring of fluid balance
- Early treatment of hypovolemia
- Monitoring of intravenous fluid administration to prevent fluid boluses, which could compromise fluid and electrolyte balance
- Monitoring and correcting fluid loss from the surgical defect and blood loss during the operative procedure
- Knowing that metabolic response to surgery may also alter fluid and electrolyte balance
  - Hyperglycemia may be a response to surgical stress.
  - Cold stress adds to metabolic response.

Glucose stability is an additional consideration during surgery. Glucose metabolism is not stable in the neonate, and prematurity magnifies this problem. The glucose level should be monitored frequently. Infusions of intravenous fluids should be monitored closely to prevent inaccurate rates of administration, resulting in hypoglycemia or hyperglycemia.

Pharmacologic Support

Irregular patterns of metabolism, immature or compromised renal function, and variations in hepatic blood flow can influence the action and effectiveness of medications. Bradycardia can result from narcotics such as fentanyl and morphine, inhalation anesthetics, and muscle relaxants. The resultant hypoxia must be considered a major problem and must be resolved quickly.

When considering the use of muscle relaxants, it must be remembered that neonates are particularly sensitive to succinylcholine. Bradycardia can be associated with this drug, and a predose of atropine may be given to avoid this complication. Intermediate and long-acting muscle relaxants such as pancuronium are commonly preferred for their ability to achieve or maintain a hemostatic state by increasing the heart rate and blood pressure.

Inhalation anesthetics and intravenous anesthetics have been known to depress the ventilatory response to hypoxemia and hypercarbia. An increased pulmonary uptake of some agents causes high tissue levels and eventual cardiac compromise. However, the successful use of inhalation anesthetics in combination with narcotics has been achieved in the neonatal population (Reyes & Vidyasagar, 1989). Careful monitoring of fluid status and cardiovascular and renal function is essential.

POSTOPERATIVE PERIOD

The initial postoperative period is a critical time in the recovery of the surgical neonate. The skillful assessment and management of the neonate is required to achieve a positive surgical outcome. This requires experience and collaborative care before, during, and after surgery.

Close monitoring includes frequent assessment of the following:

- Core temperature
- Surface temperature
- Heart and respiratory rate
- Blood pressure
- Perfusion
- Oxygen saturation

Ventilatory assistance is evaluated for rate, pressure, and oxygen administration. The rate of intravenous infusions is assessed to ensure adequate urine output of at least 1 to 2 ml/kg/hr (Ingelfinger, 1985). Serum glucose levels should be monitored and adjusted.

Oxygenation

The respiratory tract can be traumatized by intubation, anesthetic gases, and the stress of the procedure. Depression of respiratory drive can also be seen as a residual effect of anesthesia. Airway clearance may also be difficult to maintain. These alterations in respiratory mechanics may lead to respiratory insufficiency and the need for prolonged mechanical support (Leape, 1987). Although specific respiratory needs may vary depending on the surgical procedure, a conservative approach to respiratory care is essential to maintain optimum oxygenation. An aggressive plan of weaning may cause recurring acidosis, hypoxia, or damage to the surgical repair.

In the postoperative neonate with diaphragmatic hernia, care should be geared toward prevention of persistent pulmonary hypertension, caused by pulmonary vasoconstriction, and prevention of damage to the "good lung," resulting from excessive ventilator pressures. Paralysis with pancuronium can be beneficial in the postoperative period to assist in adequate ventilation and oxygenation. This infant should be weaned from respiratory support very cautiously.

Respiratory support for the postoperative infant with tracheoesophageal fistula may range from humidified mist to endotracheal intubation, depending on the type of repair and the complications encountered in surgery (Kenner, Harjo, & Brueggemeyer, 1988). Frequent suctioning is necessary to minimize both endotracheal and oropharyngeal secretions. A measured catheter should be used to avoid damage to the surgical sites. A thoracotomy may also be done to prevent atelectasis or pneumothorax and promote expansion of the lung.

Respiratory compromise is a common complication after primary closure of an omphalocele/gastroschisis. Excessive pressure on the diaphragm and poor peripheral perfusion related to pressure on the inferior vena cava may require ventilatory support to improve lung expansion and oxygenation status. Paralysis with pancuronium may be helpful with ventilation as well as preventing rupture of incisions.

Postoperative care of the neonate with necrotizing enterocolitis includes aggressive ventilation. Many of these infants are small, premature, and of low birth weight with already compromised lung function. The stresses of severe infection, the surgical procedure itself, and premature lungs may require a prolonged ventilation with a slow weaning process.

Acid–Base Balance

As in the preoperative and intraoperative periods, acid–base balance continues to present a challenge to the neonate postoperatively. Although the neonate's initial reaction to the stress of surgery will influence this balance, the concern over acidosis will continue for a significant period of time. Blood gases should be monitored, attention paid to fluid balance, and appropriate respiratory support delivered. As sepsis is resolved, fluid status is stabilized, and urine output is optimized, acid–base balance will also stabilize.

Thermoregulation

Use of radiant warmers is a method of choice in maintaining both core and surface temperatures. The premature, small infant may require enclosure in an incubator to maintain consistent temperature control.

The principles of thermoregulation used in the preoperative and intraoperative periods are again useful in the postoperative plan of care for the surgical neonate.

Fluid and Electrolyte Balance

The goal is to provide fluid and electrolyte balance without overhydration. Hypovolemia is a major cause of hypotension and must be resolved quickly to ensure adequate perfusion to all organ systems and to combat acidosis. However, extreme care must be taken in administering fluids because premature infants are susceptible to third spacing of fluids and edema. Neonates are also very easily overloaded with excessive fluids. Nursing management includes the following:

- Frequently monitor vital signs: initially every 15 to 30 minutes.
  - Drastic changes in heart rate and/or blood pressure could indicate shock or undetected fluid loss for which the body is trying to compensate.
  - Assessment of temperature continues to be an important factor and must be considered when evaluating fluid needs.
- Evaluate serum electrolyte and glucose levels: immediately postoperatively and then every 4 to 6 hours until stable.
  - Sodium losses may continue through wound drainage or gastric decompression.
  - Maintain and correct losses with intravenous fluids.
- Know that glucose metabolism may be altered as a response to surgery.
  - Monitor serum glucose levels every 1 to 2 hours after surgery (Kenner, Harjo, & Brueggemeyer, 1988).
  - Overzealous attempts to correct glucose or electrolyte problems can result in a rebound effect.

The neonate moves from a catabolic to an anabolic state fairly rapidly compared with an older child or adult. These phases may occur over a few days or weeks in the infant instead of months as in the adult. Additional nursing considerations are as follows:

- Obtain baseline serum electrolyte and glucose levels. Repeat every 1 to 4 hours, depending on how extreme the levels are.
- When any intervention is needed, increase or decrease levels slowly and in small increments. Follow by repeated determination of serum levels, and closely monitor the infant.
- Third spacing of fluids causing edema in the first few postoperative days is an additional consideration. Evaluate: weight, renal function, and nutritional needs.
- Maintain skin integrity.

Nutritional Needs

Concern during the convalescent period for some surgical neonates goes beyond fluid and electrolyte balance. The nutritional needs of infants with altered function of the gastrointestinal tract present unique problems. A small stomach size with altered emptying ability, as sometimes seen with diaphragmatic hernia, gastroschisis/omphalocele, and bowel resections, may present paramount problems in providing proper nutrition when feedings are started. The use of continuous feedings may help with these problems.

Gastroesophageal reflux may present challenges to feeding. Assessments of vomiting and large gastric aspirates must be made. Treatment of reflux may include positioning the infant prone and/or in an upright position after feedings and thickening of feedings. Continued reflux without appropriate weight gain is cause for evaluation for surgical intervention such as pyloroplasty or pyloromyotomy.

The neonate with bowel resection after perforation, as occurs in necrotizing enterocolitis, can present a significant challenge. Concerns should center around the following:

- Vomiting
- Diarrhea
- Distention
- Presence of glucose or blood in the stool

Tolerance of standard formulas may not be achievable, and an alternate formula such as Pregestimil may be required.

Pharmacologic Support

During the postoperative period, antibiotic therapy remains aggressive. Ampicillin and gentamicin remain the most commonly used combination of drugs. However, penicillin G, clindamycin, cefotaxime, and ceftriaxone are also frequently used.

Inotropic agents, dopamine and dobutamine, may be needed postoperatively to maintain organ perfusion and renal function. As fluid balance is achieved and cardiac compromise resolves, monitoring and titration of these drugs remains essential as noted previously.

Management of pain in the surgical neonate is an ongoing challenge in the postoperative period. Narcotic analgesics possess both advantages and disadvantages. Although they are potent and achieve effective analgesia in all age groups, their most adverse effect is the respiratory depression and apnea produced. The sedative effect of narcotics can be advantageous in the immediate postoperative period. However, when unstable vital signs are present, potential bradycardia and hypotension, which can be side effects of a variety of narcotic preparations, must be considered.

Use of acetaminophen is common when concerns about respiratory depression exist. Combined with low-dose narcotics, acetaminophen may achieve satisfactory analgesia with minimal complications. Also, acetaminophen has no significant effect on platelet aggregation, thus causing no risk for increased bleeding (Reyes & Vidyasagar, 1989).

REFERENCES

Ingelfinger, J. R. (1985). Renal conditions in the newborn period. In J. P. Cloherty & A. R. Stark (Eds.), *Manual of neonatal care* (2nd ed., pp. 377–394). Boston: Little, Brown.

Kenner, C., Harjo, J., & Brueggemeyer, A. (1988). *Neonatal surgery: A nursing perspective*. Orlando, FL: Grune & Stratton.

Leape, L. L. (1987). *Patient care in pediatric surgery*. Boston: Little, Brown.

Reyes, H., & Vidyasagar, D. (1989). Neonatal surgery: Preface. *Clinics in Perinatology, 16*(1), xi–xii.

CHAPTER 27

Identification, Management, and Prevention of Pain in the Neonate

Before the middle 1970s, neonates were thought incapable of experiencing pain owing to their immature nervous system and incomplete myelinization. However, it was not until the discovery that up to 80 percent of fibers that transmit pain information remain unmyelinated in the adult (Price & Dubner, 1977) that the potential for infants with immature (largely unmyelinated) nervous systems to perceive pain was recognized and fully appreciated.

Concurrent to the developments in pain science, three factors led to the emergence of an imperative for the treatment of infant pain: (1) the advent of neonatal intensive care; (2) realization of the influence of environment on the developing central nervous system (CNS); and (3) the emergence of an ethical mandate for pain management.

THE EFFECTS OF PAIN

Immediate Effects

Pain causes adverse physiologic effects in all major organ systems that can be life-threatening in the acutely ill patient. These effects include the following:

- Reduced tidal volume and vital capacity in the lungs
- Increased demands of the cardiovascular system
- Hypermetabolism resulting in neuroendocrine imbalances (Kehlet, 1986) and increased oxygen consumption, hypoxemia, and myocardial ischemia
- Mobilization of endocrine and metabolic resources resulting in changes in blood pressure (which can be either increased or decreased), changes in skin color, and temperature
- Lack of autoregulation of cerebrovascular bed, predisposing to intraventricular hemorrhage (Brazy, 1988)
- Endorphin release, which may also affect blood pressure and respiration
- Prolonged catabolic reactions and circulatory and metabolic complications after surgery when anesthetic agents were not administered or were inadequate (Anand & Aynsley-Green, 1988a, 1988b; Anand, Sippell & Aynsley-Green, 1987)

589

Effects of Anesthesia

In the neonate, anesthesia effectively does the following (Anand & Carr, 1989; Anand & Hickey, 1992):

- Reduces the magnitude of the hormonal-metabolic stress response
- Decreases the stress response

Increased Sensitivity of Premature Neonates

There are a number of reasons for increased sensitivity of premature neonates:

- Excessive light and noise in the neonatal intensive care unit (NICU) elicit dramatic physiologic and behavioral stress responses.
- Handling and caregiving procedures cause significant physiologic distress, including blood pressure, heart rate instability, and hypoxia.
- Cardiorespiratory effects of handling may result from increased circulating catecholamines, particularly norepinephrine, and cortisol (Gunnar, Connors, & Isensee, 1989; Lagercrantz, Nilsson, Redham, & Hjemdahl, 1986)
- For the premature neonate, social interaction (e.g., the human voice and face) can cause physiologic and behavioral distress similar to caregiving procedures (Table 27–1).

Potential Long-Term Effects

The developing human brain is most vulnerable to environmental influences during periods of rapid growth that occur between 10 to 18 weeks' gestation

---

TABLE 27–1. Minimal Handling Protocol (Children's Hospital, Oakland)

Protect from Light
Shade infant's eyes with blanket over isolette or table or use cut-out box over infant's head.

Protect from Noise
Do not talk over infant.
Set speakers as low as possible.
Do not have phones ring in room.
Close isolette doors softly.
Do not set bottles or other objects on top of isolettes.
Remove all sources of loud, jarring noise (e.g., trash receptacles with lids that bang shut).

Protect from Overstimulation
Cluster nursing care activities.
Allow 2 to 3 hours of undisturbed rest.
Do not routinely suction or perform postural drainage (PRN only).
Contain limbs (swaddle) during suctioning or other procedures.

Provide Boundaries
Position prone or sidelying.
Cover/wrap/swaddle.

and again between 30 weeks' gestation and 3 months' postnatal age (Dobbing & Smart, 1974). Although the infant brain undergoes a tremendous period of growth, the process of neuronal competition for synaptic connections (particularly during the third trimester) results in a large amount of cell death and remodeling of the neuronal structure (Volpe, 1987). It is on this process that environmental influences can have the most profound effects. Patterned neuronal activity serves to select those cell populations that will proliferate from those that will degenerate (Janowsky & Finlay, 1986). The amount and frequency of painful stimuli inflicted on the infant receiving intensive care could possibly result in a reallocation of cortical resources and in permanent alterations in cerebral neuroanatomy.

The arousal resulting from a painful event may be overwhelming for the infant, who will attempt to shut out all stimuli, altering interactions with caregivers and sleep patterns (Emde et al., 1971; Marshall et al., 1982). It has been suggested that a mismatch between the environmental demands of the NICU and the infant's neurobehavioral maturity can result in aberrant patterns of social interaction that may persist beyond infancy (Als, 1983).

Modulation of the negative effects with modifications of the NICU environment can improve developmental outcome (Als et al., 1986; Barnard & Bee, 1983). Premature infants who spend the neonatal period in the NICU are at risk for developmental delays, permanent CNS handicap, and emotional disorders (Sell, 1986). The neonatal CNS must be considered as an organ system at risk, as important as the cardiovascular or pulmonary systems, and protected from adverse environmental events, including pain.

MEASUREMENT OF INFANT PAIN RESPONSES

Neonatal pain assessment is gathered from three categories of responses: behavioral, physiologic/autonomic, and neuroendocrine.

Behavioral Responses

Behavioral responses are strongly influenced by neuromuscular maturation and severity of illness (Coll, 1990; Tronick, Scanlon, & Scanlon, 1990) and may not be a reliable indicator of the presence or absence of pain. Premature neonates demonstrate decreased behavioral responsiveness to painful stressors (Stevens & Johnston, 1994). Some neonatal behavioral responses to pain are described below:

- Infant pain cries have been shown to be spectrographically distinct in terms of frequency and pitch from cries due to other stimuli (Fuller, 1991; Levine & Gordon, 1982).
- "Cry face," or facial expression in response to painful stimuli, includes brow bulge, eye squeeze, and deepening of the nasolabial folds.
- Premature neonates have less robust facial expressions that can be accurately and reliably detected and correlated with physiologic signs of pain.
- Healthy infants display vigorous gross motor movements and attempt to withdraw from the painful stimulus (Franck, 1986).
- Critically ill or premature infants may exhibit diffuse, disorganized

behavior but quickly become limp and flaccid in response to noxious stimuli.

- Flexor reflex is evoked by a cutaneous mechanical stimulus to the heel producing a clear, distinct withdrawal of the leg.
- Repeated heelsticks lower the flexor reflex threshold. Hypersensitivity of the injured heel was reversed with application a topical local anesthetic.

If an overt response is absent, it does not necessarily indicate lack of pain perception. The response to pain stimuli may also be delayed or cumulative. Also, an immature CNS has a limited ability to withstand stress. The absence of response may only indicate the depletion of response capability.

Agitation in the ill neonate can be disruptive to physiologic processes. Distinguishing irritable, restless behavior due to pain from that due to agitation or other causes is one of the most challenging tasks of infant pain management.

Physiologic/Autonomic Responses

Measurement of neonatal physiologic responses to painful stimuli include the following:

- Changes in heart rate, respiratory rate, blood pressure, transcutaneous oxygen and carbon dioxide levels, oxygen saturation, intracranial pressure, cardiac vagal tone, and palmar sweat
- Heart rate variability. Examining the amplitude of beat-to-beat changes in heart rate to estimate the parasympathetic and/or sympathetic influences due to pain may be helpful.

Neuroendocrine Responses

Neuroendocrine responses are difficult to measure but occur from the following:

- Release of catecholamines, cortisol, endorphins, and other chemicals with neuroendocrine effects in response to pain
- Changes in plasma, urinary, and salivary cortisol levels observed in response to painful stressors. The degree of cortisol responsiveness correlates closely with the intensity of the stressor (Gunnar, 1992)

Variability in Neonatal Responses to Pain

Expression of neonatal stress responses is further modulated by the following:

- Increased sensitivity of premature neonates to sensory stimuli
- Initial behavioral state of the neonate
- The neonate's ability to habituate

CLINICAL ASSESSMENT OF INFANT PAIN

The following is a summary of existing pain scales:

- Neonatal Infant Pain Scale (NIPS): this has been shown to be a valid and reliable measure of infant responses (including facial expression, cry, breathing pattern, arm and leg movement, and behavioral state) to needle puncture (arterial, venous, or capillary) (Lawrence et al., 1993).

- CRIES: this scoring tool combines both physiologic and behavioral indices (Krechel & Bildner, 1995)
- The Premature Infant Pain Profile (PIPP): this profile rates changes in heart rate, oxygen saturation, facial action (degree of brow bulge, eye squeeze, and nasolabial furrow) on a three-point scale. Gestational age and behavioral state are also factored into the pain score (Stevens, Johnston, Petryshen & Taddio, 1994).

Incorporating a standardized pain assessment protocol (no matter how imperfect the tool) emphasizes the importance of pain management for infants. Once consciousness has been raised, then interventions can be tailored to alter care to increase comfort level to promote rest and recovery.

MANAGEMENT OF NEONATAL PAIN

The goals of pain management in infants are to minimize the intensity, duration, and physiologic cost of the pain experience and to maximize the infant's ability to cope with and recover from the painful experience (Tables 27–2 and 27–3).

Nonpharmacologic Management

Nonpharmacologic management of pain includes the following:

- Gentle handling
- Quick, efficient, and skilled execution of invasive procedures
- Rest periods between procedures
- Proper support during the procedure
- Swaddling, assisting the infant with hand-to-mouth contact, or nonnutritive sucking (Campos, 1989; Field & Goldson, 1984)
- Reduction of environmental stimuli by dimming lights, talking softly at the bedside, and quietly closing portholes on the isolette
- Offering pacifiers to mechanically ventilated neonates to reduce behavioral and physiologic distress during painful procedures (Miller & Andrews, 1993)
- Contralateral tactile stimulation, which has been shown to result in a significant decreased sensitivity to pain

Pharmacologic Management

Pharmacologic agents are often required to alleviate the pain caused by invasive procedures.

OPIOIDS

Opioids can cause respiratory depression. Neonates may require higher concentrations of opioids than older patients to provide adequate analgesia.

TABLE 27–2. Question Guide to Determining Infant Pain Treatment

---

Assessment

What behavior is the infant displaying that is actually or potentially harmful? Is there interference with adequate ventilation, circulation, nutrition, sleep-wake, or social development?

Is the infant compromised physiologically?

Can any precipitating factors be identified?

Is ventilation/oxygenation optimized?

    Is the oxygen delivery system functioning adequately?

    Does the infant need to be suctioned?

    Is the infant breathing in synchrony with the ventilator?

Have painful procedures been recently performed?

Will painful procedures be performed frequently?

Does the infant have a painful condition?

Nonpharmacologic Support

Have nonpharmacologic comfort measures been attempted?

    Is the infant's temperature stable?

    Has wet diaper or bedding been removed?

    Has abdominal distention been relieved?

    Has the infant been repositioned, swaddled?

    Has the infant been offered nonnutritive sucking?

Has a minimal handling protocol been implemented?

Selecting Appropriate Analgesics

What routes are available for delivery of medication?

Is a brief period of analgesia needed for an invasive procedure?

Is prolonged analgesia required for a painful condition?

What is the drug half-life?

What are the side effects?

Will blood levels be helpful in assessing efficacy or toxicity?

How many doses will need to be given before the drug reaches steady state?

Evaluation of Drug Treatment

Did the drug achieve the desired effect?

Was the drug given at an appropriate interval for an appropriate period of time (to achieve steady state)?

Were there any side effects?

How will weaning from pharmacologic support be achieved?

TABLE 27–3. Strategies to Prevent or Minimize Pain in the Critically Ill/ Premature Infant

---

Group blood drawing periods to minimize the number of venipunctures per day.

Use noninvasive monitoring devices when possible.

Establish central vessel access to minimize vein and artery punctures.

Have only expert staff attempt intravenous access on the most unstable patients.

Use minimal amount of tape and remove tape gently.

Ensure proper premedication before invasive procedures.

Increased clearance and decreased half-life of opioids are exhibited as gestational age increases (Bhat, Chari, & Iver, 1994). Rapid maturation of opioid metabolic mechanisms occurs during postnatal life, with clearance levels approaching the clearance levels of adults by 6 months of age (Lynn & Slattery, 1987).

Morphine

The effects of morphine are as follows:

- Mean elimination half-life after a single dose ranges from 2.6 to 14 hours (Bhat et al., 1990; Bhat, Chari, & Iver, 1994).
- Neonates younger than 40 weeks' gestation have longer elimination half lives and delayed clearance than older neonates (Lynn & Slattery, 1987) after bolus administration.
- Eighty percent of morphine is unbound by plasma proteins, accounting for increased CNS concentrations of morphine (Kupferberg & Way, 1963).

Morphine has few effects on the neonatal cardiovascular system in the well-hydrated neonate. However, hypotension commonly occurs in dehydrated patients. Decreased intestinal motility and abdominal distension may also occur.

Meperidine

During the first two days of life, more meperidine than normeperidine is excreted. By 3 days of age the reverse is true. Because normeperidine is an active metabolite, delayed respiratory depression and reduction in seizure threshold can occur with meperidine administration.

Fentanyl

The characteristics of fentanyl are listed below:

- Used to provide anesthesia
- Short acting
- Must be administered as a continuous infusion or as an intravenous bolus every 1 to 2 hours.
- Has mean elimination half-life after a single dose of 6 to 32 hours (Collins et al., 1985; Gauntlett et al., 1988; Koehntop et al., 1986)
- Has lower serum concentrations in neonates than in older infants and children
- More than 90 percent metabolized by the liver (Gauntlett et al., 1988)
- Has elimination half-life that can be tripled by increased intra-abdominal pressure, probably because of reduced hepatic artery blood flow (Koehntop et al., 1986)
- Rarely can significantly reduce chest wall compliance (stiff chest syndrome). This naloxone-reversible side effect can be prevented by slow infusion (as opposed to rapid bolus administration), administration of doses less than 3 μg/kg, or concomitant use of muscle relaxants.
- Blunts increases in pulmonary vascular resistance and pressure in stressed (but normoxic) neonates

A major problem with long-term fentanyl administration is the development of tolerance and physical dependence (Franck & Vilardi, 1995). A morphine infusion can provide similar pain relief, better sedative effects, and less tolerance and physical dependence when long-term use of an opioid is required (Franck & Vilardi, 1995).

Sufentanil and Alfentanil

Sufentanil is ten times more potent than fentanyl and is used to provide anesthesia for neonates undergoing cardiac surgery. The volume of distribution of sufentanil is about half as large in infants as it is in older patients. The shorter elimination half-life and smaller volume of distribution shorten the duration of anesthesia. Sufentanil has a mild negative inotropic effect and reduces serum catecholamine concentrations in infants. This drug has been used to premedicate children for surgery. However, the dose required often causes decreased lung compliance, which is a significant risk for the spontaneously breathing infant. More recently, sufentanil was administered to premature neonates in a continuous infusion and was well tolerated with no decrease in heart rate or blood pressure.

Alfentanil is also very short acting and is used in older children for brief procedures in which rapid return to consciousness is desired. The elimination half-life is approximately 30 percent shorter in neonates than in adults. Decreased lung compliance may occur in neonates, and clinicians should be prepared to intervene.

Methadone

Methadone is more commonly known for its use in the opioid-dependent pregnant woman. However, its long-acting properties and good oral bioavailability make it an attractive option to treat postoperative pain and prevent neonatal abstinence syndrome.

Epidural Administration of Opioids

Improvements in catheter design and insertion technique have made the epidural route an effective mode of analgesia administration for neonates. Morphine or fentanyl administered alone or in combination with local anesthetics can provide good intraoperative anesthesia and postoperative analgesia after abdominal or lower extremity surgery. Use of epidural analgesia may potentially expedite extubation (Murrell, Gibson, & Cohen, 1993; Valley & Bailey, 1991). Because the opioids act directly on the neurons in the spinal cord, lower doses are used for epidural or intrathecal administration and fewer opioid side effects are generally seen. Opioid side effects can still occur and require careful monitoring of the patient for side effects such as respiratory depression, hypotension, or urinary retention. Catheter-related side effects include systemic overdose related to catheter migration or infection. Epidural analgesia should not be used in the septic patient.

Cardiovascular and Respiratory Side-Effects of Opioids

Although opioids may depress respiratory efforts, this effect seems less significant than previously thought. Cardiovascular effects of opioids vary depending on the specific opioid administered as well as on the route and rate of administration. Hydration status is also a key factor in the maintenance of cardiovascular stability, with opioid-induced hypotension more likely to occur in the hypovolemic neonate than in the normovolemic neonate (Gregory, 1994a, 1994b; Yaster & Deshpande, 1988).

LOCAL ANESTHETICS

Local infiltration of anesthetics (e.g., 0.25 to 0.5 ml/kg of 25 percent bupivacaine or 0.5 to 1.0 percent lidocaine) can be used for procedures such as lumbar puncture or intravenous catheter insertion.

Topical Application of Local Anesthetics

Use of topical anesthetics for procedures such as venipuncture has significantly improved the management of pain in pediatrics (Yaster, Tobin, Fisher, & Maxwell, 1994). The effectiveness of topical local anesthesia for reducing pain in neonates has not been as clearly demonstrated. While use of EMLA (eutectic mixture of local anesthetics; Astra Pharmaceuticals) decreased behavioral and physiologic responses to circumcision (Benini, Johnston, Faucher, & Aranda, 1993), it was not effective for heelstick procedures (Barker & Rutter, 1995a, 1995b).

Nerve Blocks

Peripheral nerve and caudal epidural blocks using local anesthesia (or a combination of local anesthetic and an opioid) can be used to provide intraoperative regional or general anesthesia and postoperative pain relief for neonates (Yaster, et al., 1994). Careful monitoring of the patient during the postoperative period is required to assess for potential complications, including bleeding, compartment syndrome, excessive sensorimotor blockade, or systemic local anesthetic toxicity (Yaster & Maxwell, 1989). In addition to pain assessment, nurses caring for infants receiving local anesthetics by epidural infusion will need to assess the patient sensorimotor blockade by eliciting withdrawal reflex of the legs every few hours.

NONOPIOID ANALGESICS

Acetaminophen is useful for treating mild to moderate pain in children. The use of acetaminophen in neonates is limited because it can only be administered orally or rectally.

USE OF ADJUNCTIVE DRUGS

Sedatives should only be used when pain has been ruled out (Hartley, Franck, & Lundergan, 1989).

Benzodiazepines

Some guidelines for the use of specific benzodiazepines are provided here.

Diazepam

- Do not administer on a fixed schedule because of its long half-life (approximately 31 hours).
- Administer only as clinical signs indicate.

Midazolam

- Short-acting, rapid onset provides sedation for mechanically ventilated neonates.
- Ninety percent is protein bound so if administered to a neonate with low serum protein, increased midazolam enters the CNS with increased sedation and respiratory depression.
- Metabolism occurs in the liver by microsomal oxidation.
- In normoxic neonates, it is not associated with hypotension.
- Elimination $T_{1/2}$ is estimated at 6.5 hours in the critically ill neonate.
- Intravenous bolus can cause hypotension and decreased cerebral blood flow in ill neonates (van Straaten, Rademaker, & de Vries, 1992).

Lorazepam

- Indications are for sedation and for the prevention of seizures.
- Heart rate is not affected, and it does not cause apnea.
- With renal failure, repeated doses can cause hypotension, apnea, or delayed weaning from mechanical ventilation.
- Dose of benzyl alcohol preservative in lorazepam is below the dose known to cause fatal toxicity in premature neonates (100 to 400 mg/kg/day); however, with frequent dosing, benzyl alcohol toxicity is a potential risk.
- Oral administration is a useful alternative to chloral hydrate for the nonventilated infant with chronic lung disease who requires ongoing or intermittent sedation to prevent respiratory distress associated with activity or agitation.

Chloral Hydrate

- Effective sedation of neonates is provided during pulmonary function, radiographic, and other diagnostic testing where the patient must lie still.
- Alternative sedatives (e.g., benzodiazepines) should be used whenever possible because chloral hydrate has other gastrointestinal side effects and may be associated with direct hyperbilirubinemia.
- It has a long half-life (greater than 72 hours); this increases the risk of toxicity with repeated administration, which may be manifest as increased agitation.

Phenobarbital, Pentobarbital, Secobarbital

Phenobarbital is commonly given to control seizures in neonates and does have a sedative effect that is short lived. Secobarbital has also been used to provide sedation to mechanically ventilated neonates but has been reported to cause prolonged sedation 24 to 96 hours after the last dose (Nahata, Starling & Edwards, 1991).

Care must be taken to assess analgesia as opposed to simply sedation; prolonged use may potentially impair development due to amnesiac effects.

Pharmacologic Pain Management for Specific Procedures

CIRCUMCISION

Circumcision is performed on healthy, spontaneously breathing newborns, and provision of analgesia is perceived by some clinicians as overly risky. In fact, dorsal penile nerve block is a safe and effective method of providing local anesthesia to infants during circumcision. Numerous studies have demonstrated safety and efficacy, with a reduction in physiologic and behavioral distress with the use of dorsal penile nerve block (Dixon, Snider, Holve, & Bromberger, 1984; Stang et al., 1988). However, many physicians remain reluctant to use the technique. Infants who received comfort measures such as music, intrauterine sounds, and/or pacifier exhibited the same degree of behavioral distress as did control infants who received no intervention during circumcision. Acetaminophen has also been shown to have no effect in reducing distress during and after circumcision. Provision of a sucrose-dipped pacifier or topical local anesthesia decreased distress as compared with no treatment at all (Benini et al., 1993).

PREPROCEDURE ANESTHESIA/ANALGESIA

Local anesthesia is used to prevent pain for other procedures performed in the NICU such as chest tube insertion (Franck, 1987) and lumbar puncture. Use of topically applied local anesthesia for heelstick has also been reported (Fitzgerald, Millard, & McIntosh, 1989).

Local anesthesia may not be sufficient for procedures that affect deeper tissue, such as chest tube insertion of surgical cutdown of vessels. Central analgesia is then required to prevent pain.

For the nonventilated patient, when there is concern for the respiratory depressant effects of opioids, one half the standard dose may be administered. For the infant who is receiving opioid analgesics on a regular basis, a higher dose may be required to provide adequate analgesia during an invasive procedure.

ANESTHESIA FOR SURGICAL PROCEDURES

Anesthesia is required for prolonged surgical procedures involving deep tissue. Nurses should assist physicians and parents in weighing the risks and benefits and understanding the need for anesthesia in infants undergoing surgery.

Opioids are efficacious in attenuating hemodynamic, hormonal, and metabolic effects of surgical stress. Some clinicians now advocate use of 50 to 100 μg/kg of fentanyl anesthesia and continuation of a 10- to 15-μg/kg fentanyl infusion during the early postoperative period to prevent neuroendocrine stress responses and hemodynamic instability in infants undergoing cardiac surgery (Wessel, 1993).

POSTOPERATIVE ANALGESIA

Adequate analgesia is important during the immediate postoperative period for the optimal recovery of the patient. Unrelieved pain can interfere with ventilation and delay weaning. Use of low-dose continuous infusion of narcotic analgesics is proven effective in the care of the postoperative adult patient and can provide more constant, effective neonatal pain relief with less drug (Truog & Anand, 1989).

MECHANICAL VENTILATION

Opioids are frequently used to sedate, promote respiratory synchrony, improve ventilation, and relieve pain or discomfort in neonates (Bell & Ellis, 1987; Koren & Maurice, 1989).

EXTRACORPOREAL MEMBRANE OXYGENATION

Most patients on ECMO are given an anesthetic dose of an opioid (usually fentanyl) for cannulation and then kept sedated with a continuous fentanyl drip. Often benzodiazepines (lorazepam or midazolam) are also used, and additional injections of morphine are given. Rapid tolerance to fentanyl has been reported as well as severe withdrawal after decannulation and weaning of drug (Arnold & Truog, 1990). Continuous morphine infusion may provide better sedation than fentanyl and reduce the incidence of post-ECMO opioid withdrawal symptoms (Franck & Vilardi, 1995).

PREVENTION OF WITHDRAWAL SYMPTOMS

Infants, like adults, will develop physical dependence to psychoactive drugs, including opioids and benzodiazepines given over time (as little as several hours with some agents). Opioid analgesics, sedatives, or antianxiety agents given around the clock should never be discontinued abruptly (Maguire & Maloney, 1988). To prevent withdrawal symptoms, the infant should be weaned from opioid and sedative drugs. Abstinence scoring methods commonly used in the care of the infant with prenatal drug exposure must be used in assessing the infant during the opioid weaning (Franck & Vilardi, 1995).

NURSING MANAGEMENT

Providing comfort and relieving pain are two central goals of nursing care. Fear of addiction and disproportionate concern for side effects have resulted in severe underutilization of narcotic analgesics for acute postoperative pain (Schechter, 1989). Patients often suffer needlessly because of the nurse or physician's unfounded fears of addiction or misinformation about analgesics.

Nurses must be prepared to respond to questions from parents and encourage parent participation in providing nonpharmacologic comfort measures to their infant. The nurse is also obligated to find effective methods to communicate her assessments and recommendations to maximize the collaboration between members of the health care team in providing effective pain management.

REFERENCES

Als, H. (1983). Infant individuality: Assessing patterns of very early development. In J. Calls, E. Galenson, & R. Tuson (Eds.), *Frontiers of infant psychiatry* (pp. 363–378). New York: Basic Books.

Als, H., Lawhon, G., Brown, E., et al. (1986). Individualized behavioral and environmental care for very low birth weight preterm infants at high risk for bronchopulmonary dysplasia: Neonatal intensive care unit and developmental outcome. *Pediatrics, 78,* 1123–1132.

Anand, K. J., & Aynsley-Green, A. (1988a). Does the newborn infant require potent anesthesia during surgery? Answers from a randomized trial of halothane anesthesia. In R. Dubner, G. F. Gebhart, & M. R. Bond (Eds.), *Proceedings of the 5th World Congress on Pain* (pp. 329–335). New York: Elsevier.

Anand, K. J., & Aynsley-Green, A. (1988b). Measuring the severity of surgical stress in newborn infants. *Journal of Pediatric Surgery, 23,* 297–305.

Anand, K. J. & Carr, D. B. (1989). The neuroanatomy, neurophysiology, and neurochemistry of pain, stress, and analgesia in newborns and children. [Review]. *Pediatric Clinics of North American, 36,* 795–822.

Anand, K. J., & Hickey, P. R. (1992). Halothane-morphine compared with high dose sufentanil for anesthesia and post-operative analgesia in neonatal cardiac surgery. *New England Journal of Medicine, 326,* 1–9.

Anand, K. J. S., Sippell, W. G., & Aynsley-Green, A. (1987). Randomized trial of fentanyl anaesthesia in preterm babies undergoing surgery: Effects on the stress response. *Lancet, 1,* 234.

Arnold, J. H., & Truog, R. D. (1990). For infants undergoing extracorporeal membrane oxygenation. [Abstract]. Presented at ECMO Conference.

Barker, D. P., & Rutter, N. (1995a). Exposure to invasive procedures in neonatal intensive care unit admissions. *Archives of Disease in Childhood, 72*(1), F47–F48.

Barker, D. P., & Rutter, N. (1995b). Lignucaine ointment and local anaesthesia in preterm infants. *Archives of Disease in Childhood, 72*(3), F203–F204.

Barnard, K. E., & Bee, H. L. (1983). The impact of temporally patterned stimulation on the development of preterm infants. *Child Development, 54,* 1156–1167.

Bell, S. G., & Ellis, L. J. (1987). Use of fentanyl for sedation of mechanically ventilated neonates. *Neonatal Network, 6,* 27–31.

Benini, F., Johnston, C. C., Faucher, D., & Aranda, J. V. (1993). Topical anesthesia during circumcision in newborn infants. *JAMA, 270*(7), 850–853.

Bhat, R., Chari, G., Gulati, A., et al. (1990). Pharmacokinetics of a single dose of morphine in preterm infants during the first week of life. *Journal of Pediatrics, 117,* 477–481.

Bhat, R., Chari, G., & Iver, R. (1994). Postconceptual age influences pharmacokinetics and metabolism of morphine in sick neonates. *Pediatric Research, 35*(4, pt. 2), 81A.

Brazy, J. E. (1988). Effects of crying on cerebral blood flow and cytochrome aa3. *Journal of Pediatrics, 112,* 457–461.

Campos, R. G. (1989). Soothing pain-elicited distress in infants with swaddling and pacifiers. *Child Development, 60,* 781–792.

Coll, C. G. (1990). Behavioral responsivity in preterm infants. *Clinics in Perinatology, 17,* 113–123.

Collins, C., Koren, G., Crean, P., et al. (1985). Fentanyl pharmacokinetics and hemodynamic effects in preterm infants during ligation of patent ductus arteriosus. *Anesthesia and Analgesia, 64,* 1078–1080.

Dixon, S., Snyder, J., Holve, R., & Bromberger, P. (1984). Behavioral effects of circumcision with and without anesthesia. *Development and Behavioral Pediatrics, 5,* 246–250.

Dobbing, J., & Smart, J. L. (1974). Vulnerability of developing brain and behaviour. *British Medical Bulletin, 30,* 164–168.

Emde, R. N., Harmon, R. J., Metcalf, D., et al. (1971). Stress and neonatal sleep. *Psychosomatic Medicine, 33,* 491–497.

Field, T., & Goldson, E. (1984). Pacifying effects of nonnutritive sucking on term and preterm neonates during heelstick procedures. *Pediatrics, 74,* 1012–1015.

Fitzgerald, M., Millard, C., & McIntosh, N. (1989). Cutaneous hypersensitivity following peripheral tissue damage in newborn infants and its reversal with topical anaesthesia. *Pain, 39,* 31–36.

Franck, L. S. (1986). A new method to quantitatively describe pain behavior in infants. *Nursing Research, 35,* 28–31.

Franck, L. S. (1987). A national survey of the assessment of pain and agitation in the national intensive care unit. *Journal of Obstetric, Gynecologic, and Neonatal Nursing, 16,* 387–393.

Franck, L., & Vilardi, J. (1995). Assessment and management of opioid withdrawal in ill neonates. *Neonatal Network, 14*(2), 39–48.

Fuller, B. F. (1991). Acoustic discrimination of three types of infant cries. *Nursing Research, 40*(3), 156–160.

Gauntlett, I. S., Fisher, D. M., Hertzka, R. E., et al. (1988). Pharmacokinetics of fentanyl in neonatal humans and lambs. *Anesthesiology, 69,* 683–687.

Gregory, G. A. (1994a). Pharmacology. In G. A. Gregory (Ed.), *Pediatric anesthesia* (3rd. ed., pp. 13–45). New York: Churchill Livingstone.

Gregory, G. A. (1994b). Anesthesia for premature infants. In G. A. Gregory (Ed.). *Pediatric anesthesia* (3rd. ed., pp. 351–373). New York: Churchill Livingstone.

Gunnar, M. R. (1992). Reactivity of hypothalamic-pituitary-adrenocortical system to stressors in normal infants and children. *Pediatrics, 90,* 491–497.

Gunnar, M. R., Connors, J., & Isensee, J. (1989). Lack of stability in neonatal adrenocortical reactivity because of rapid habituation of the adrenocortical response. *Developmental Psychobiology, 22,* 221–233.

Hartley, S., Franck, L. S., & Lundergan, F. (1989). Maintenance sedation of agitated infants in the NICU with chloral hydrate: New concerns. *Journal of Perinatology, 9*(2), 162–164.

Janowsky, J. S. & Finlay, B. L. (1986). The outcome of perinatal damage: The role of normal neuron loss and axon retraction. [Review]. *Developmental Medicine and Child Neurology, 28,* 375–389.

Kehlet, H. (1986). Pain relief and modification of the stress response. In M. F. Cousins & G. D. Phillips (Eds.), *Acute pain management* (pp. 49–76). New York: Churchill-Livingstone.

Koehntop, D. E., Rodman, J. H., Brundage, D. M., et al. (1986). Pharmacokinetics of fentanyl in neonates. *Anesthesia & Analgesia, 65,* 227–232.

Koren, G., & Maurice, L. (1989). Pediatric uses of opioids. *Pediatric Clinics of North America, 36,* 1141–1156.

Krechel, S. W., & Bildner, J. (1995). Cries: A new neonatal postoperative pain measurement score: Initial testing of validity and reliability. *Pediatric Anaesthesia, 5,* 53–61.

Kupferberg, H. J., & Way, E. L. (1963). Pharmacologic basis for the increased sensitivity of the newborn rat to morphine. *Journal of Pharmacology and Experimental Therapy, 141,* 105–112.

Lagercrantz, H., Nilsson, E., Redham, I., & Hjemdahl, P. (1986). Plasma catecholamines following nursing procedures in a neonatal ward. *Early Human Development, 14,* 61–65.

Lawrence, J., Alcock, D., McGrath, P., et al. (1993). The development of a tool to assess neonatal pain. *Neonatal Network, 12*(6), 59–66.

Levine, J. D., & Gordon, N. C. (1982). Pain in prelingual children and its evaluation by pain-induced vocalization. *Pain, 14,* 85–93.

Lynn, A. M., & Slattery, J. T. (1987). Morphine pharmacokinetics in early infancy. *Anesthesiology, 66,* 136–139.

Maguire, D. P., & Maloney, P. (1988). A comparison of fentanyl and morphine use in neonates. *Neonatal Network, 7*(1), 27–32.

Marshall, R. E., Porter, F. L., Rogers, A. G., et al. (1982). Circumcision: II. Effects upon mother-infant interaction. *Early Human Development, 7,* 367–374.

Miller, H. D., & Anderson, G. C. (1993). Nonnutritive sucking: Effects on crying and heart rate in intubated infants requiring assisted mechanical ventilation. *Nursing Research, 42,* 305–307.

Murrell, D., Gibson, P. R., & Cohen, R. C. (1993). Continuous epidural analgesia in newborn infants undergoing major surgery. *Journal of Pediatric Surgery, 28,* 548–553.

Nahata, M. C., Starling, S., & Edwards, R. C. (1991). Prolonged sedation associated with secobarbital in newborn infants receiving ventilatory support. *American Journal of Perinatology, 8*(1), 35–36.

Price, D. D., & Dubner, R. (1977). Neurons that subserve the sensory-discriminative aspects of pain. [Review]. *Pain, 3,* 307–338.

Schechter, N. L. (1989). The undertreatment of pain in children: An overview. [Review]. *Pediatric Clinics of North America, 36,* 781–794.

Sell, E. J. (1986). Outcome of very very low birth weight infants. *Clinics in Perinatology, 13,* 451–459.

Stang, H. J., Gunnar, M. R., Snellman, L., et al. (1988). Local anesthesia for neonatal circumcision: Effects on distress and cortisol response. *Journal of the American Medical Association, 259,* 1507–1511.

Stevens, B. J., & Johnston, C. C. (1994). Physiological responses of premature infants to a painful stimulus. *Nursing Research, 43,* 226–231.

Stevens, B., Johnson, C. C., Petryshen, P., Taddio, A. (1994). The development and validation of a measure to assess pain in premature infants. Paper presented at the 3rd International Symposium on Pediatric Pain, Philadelphia, PA, June 6–9.

Tronick, E. Z., Scanlon, K. B., & Scanlon, J. W. (1990). Protective apathy, a hypothesis about the behavioral organization and its regulation to clinical and physiological status of the preterm infant during the newborn period. *Clinics in Perinatology, 17,* 125–154.

Truog, R., & Anand, K. J. S. (1989). Management of pain in the postoperative neonate. [Review]. *Clinics in Perinatology, 16,* 61–78.

Valley, R. D., & Bailey, A. G. (1991). Caudal morphine for postoperative analgesia in infants and children: A report of 138 cases. *Anesthesia and Analgesia, 72,* 120–124.

van Straaten, H. L., Rademaker, C. M., & de Vries, L. S. (1992). Comparison of the effect of midazolam or vercuronium on blood pressure and cerebral blood flow velocity in the premature newborn. *Developmental Pharmacology Therapeutics, 19,* 191–195.

Volpe, J. J. (1987). Neuronal proliferation, migration, organization and myelination. In *Neurology of the newborn* (2nd ed.). Philadelphia: W. B. Saunders.

Wessel, D. L. (1993). Hemodynamic responses to perioperative pain and stress in infants. *Critical Care Medicine, 21*(9 Suppl.), S361–S362.

Yaster, M., & Deshpande, J. K. (1988). Management of pediatric pain with opioid analgesics. *Journal of Pediatrics, 113,* 421–429.

Yaster, M. & Maxwell, L. G. (1989). Pediatric regional anesthesia. *Anesthesiology, 70,* 324–338.

Yaster, M., Tobin, J. R., Fisher, Q. A., & Maxwell, L. G. (1994). Local anesthetics in the management of acute pain in children. *Journal of Pediatrics, 124,* 165–176.

Principles of Neonatal Drug Therapy

The principles that govern the use of medications in the neonatal population are no different from those in other age groups. However, the neonate is significantly different physiologically from other populations, and this physiology affects the way that the neonate responds to medication therapy.

GENERAL PRINCIPLES

One of the most important considerations when one prescribes or administers medications to any patient is the understanding of what is expected from the administration of the drug. It is important to design a monitoring plan that establishes the limits of toxicity that will be tolerated as well as the expected therapeutic benefit of the drug regimen. The manner in which a patient responds to therapy is influenced by the following patient characteristics:

- Age
- Size
- Development
- Concomitant administration of other medications
- Concurrent disease states
- Organ function

The prevention of drug-related morbidity and mortality is the responsibility of all patient care providers. Drug-related problems can be divided into eight categories (Helper & Strand, 1989):

1. The patient has a medical problem that requires drug therapy but is not receiving a drug for that indication.
2. The patient has a drug indication but is taking the wrong drug.
3. The patient has a medical problem that is being treated with a subtherapeutic dose of the right drug.
4. The patient has a medical problem that is the result of the patient not receiving the drug (e.g., formulation or drug-delivery problems).
5. The patient has a medical problem that is the result of an adverse drug reaction or side effect.
6. The patient has a medical problem that is being treated with too much of the right drug.
7. The patient has a medical problem that is the result of a drug–drug, drug–food, or drug–laboratory interaction.
8. The patient has received a medication for no medically valid indication.

Health care providers should evaluate medication regimens and ensure that a drug-related problem does not exist. Tools such as laboratory tests and other diagnostic aids should be incorporated into the overall plan for the patient's medication regimen.

ADVERSE DRUG REACTIONS

Adverse drug reactions (ADRs) are defined as any effect or response from a drug that is noxious and unintended when the drug is given in appropriate dosages (Fincham, 1992). An adverse reaction may be caused by either the active drug or an inert component of the drug, such as a filler or preservative. ADRs may be considered to be either bothersome events that allow the drug to be continued or toxic events that require discontinuation of therapy. An adverse reaction is designated into one of these categories, based on several factors:

- Temporal relationship to administration of drug and occurrence of adverse event
- Improvement of patient symptoms with discontinuation of medication (dechallenge)
- Reappearance of adverse reactions when the medication is restarted (rechallenge)
- Absence of concomitant medications or disease states that could possibly be responsible for an adverse event

ADRs are a common reason for hospitalization of patients and also a major reason for delay in discharge of hospitalized patients (Manasse, 1989). Each hospital has its own system for monitoring and evaluating ADRs. The U.S. Food and Drug Administration (FDA) has also established a MedWatch program for reporting of ADRs nationally (Department of Health and Human Services, FDA Drug Bulletin, 1993).

DRUG INTERACTIONS

Understanding drug interactions, not only with other medications but also with food and other laboratory tests, is important. Whenever a patient's response to a prescribed regimen is different from expected, or laboratory values are inconsistent with clinical findings, it is important to consider a drug interaction. The potential for a drug interaction should be evaluated in any patient receiving multiple drugs.

Drug interactions may be of many types (Hansten & Horn, 1993). It is important to consider the expected time course of the drug interaction when one evaluates a potential interaction. Not all interactions occur immediately when two drugs are administered to the same patient. Each interaction has a time course of maximal risk.

Drug–drug interactions may be grouped into several categories. Certain drugs may interfere with the absorption of other medications from the gastrointestinal tract. This interference can result from altered motility, altered gastrointestinal pH, alterations in gastrointestinal flora, and actual drug binding within the gut lumen. Antacids not only alter the gastric pH but also may bind to medications within the gastrointestinal tract, resulting in inactivation of medications. Prokinetic agents, cisapride and metoclopramide, may decrease gastrointestinal transit time and therefore reduce the time available for drug absorption of other medications.

Drug–drug interactions can also occur because of altered plasma or tissue protein binding. One drug may interfere with the metabolism or excretion of another medication, thereby increasing effectiveness, creating toxicity, or producing subtherapeutic levels. Rifampin and phenobarbital are classic examples of medications that induce liver enzymes (Hansten & Horn, 1993). Medications such as cimetidine reduce enzyme activity and result in a decreased clearance of certain medications.

Drugs may also be interfered with by concurrent disease states. Congestive heart failure results in blood flow alterations to the liver, thereby decreasing the metabolism of medications that require hepatic biotransformation (Rowland & Tozer, 1989). Interferences such as these are referred to as drug–disease state interactions.

MEDICATION ADMINISTRATION

Oral Formulations

Many of the medications that are used orally are available only as tablets or capsules. Therefore, oral medications administered for the neonatal population are often extemporaneously prepared in the pharmacy. These preparations are usually formulated from available literature on in vitro stability. However, little is usually known about the bioavailability of the product, that is, the extent to which the active ingredient is absorbed and the time at which a maximal serum concentration in achieved. Some ingredients necessary for the preparation of these medications may not be readily available and therefore make acquisition difficult after discharge from the hospital.

Of the medications that are commercially available as suspensions and oral solutions, often the volume of medication is not appropriate for the neonate. The product may be concentrated such that accurate measuring for a neonatal dose is difficult. These preparations may also contain "silent" or inert ingredients such as preservatives that are harmless in adults but when administered frequently to neonates may result in toxicity.

Osmolality must also be considered when providing neonatal enteral medications. Substances with high osmolality that are administered to the neonate have been associated with many adverse effects, including the development of necrotizing enterocolitis and decreased transit time (Ernst, Glick, Williams, & Lemons, 1983). Many enteral medications add a significant osmolar load to the formula or breast milk (White & Harkavy, 1982). It is important to *stagger* neonatal enteral medication administration to avoid simultaneous administration of highly osmolar medications.

Intravenous Administration

Accurate neonatal medication delivery is critical to the interpretation of the efficacy or toxicity of a prescribed regimen.

Factors that may affect the rate and completeness of drug administration include the following:

- Site of injection
- Rate of intravenous fluid administration
- Medication dosage

- Fluid volume
- Administration of multiple medications
- Properties of the drug solution such as specific gravity, osmolality, and pH (Gould & Roberts, 1979)
- Incomplete medication administration, secondary to the low flow of intravenous fluids

Neonatal fluid administration may be by several methods:

- *Antegrade system.* Medications are administered at a port (Y-site, flashball) and are assumed to flow to the patient from that site (Roberts, 1981). In this system the time to peak effect and the total drug delivery are dependent on the volume of medication administered, the rate of administration of the intravenous fluid, and the site of injection. It is often difficult to predict when the time to peak effect will be with this method.
- *Retrograde system* (Benzing & Loggie, 1973). Two three-way stopcocks are used, separated by an extension tubing that becomes part of the maintenance infusion line. The medication is infused at the most proximal port, and the dose is injected away from the patient and displaces fluid in the tubing up into a syringe on the distal stopcock. Then both stopcocks are opened to the patient and the intravenous line, resulting in delivery of medication to the patient. This method is more reliable than the anterograde method but is still influenced by drug dosage volumes, the intravenous fluid rate, and the tubing diameter.

Syringe pumps provide a rate of medication delivery that is independent of the rate of the intravenous fluid and dosage volume. Complicated medication regimens in which there is a lot of tubing between the syringe pump and the patient will still be influenced by factors such as drug volume and intravenous fluid rate.

Many of the available intravenous medications are provided in concentrations that prohibit accurate measurement and administration of neonatal doses. This can affect the interpretation of the infant's response to the therapy. Another important consideration is the concentration of fluid that the infant is receiving through an intravenous line; many medications may be hyperosmolar and cause irritation at the site of infusion. Administration of intermittent medications into a line that is dedicated to a continuous infusion of a medication may result in an inadvertent bolus of that medication that potentially could be harmful to the patient. This is particularly troublesome with vasoactive medications, sedatives, and narcotics. Sudden changes in drug delivery may also occur when medication lines are changed.

Extravasation and *infiltration* are terms used interchangeably in the literature; both terms reflect a misdirection of intravenous fluid or medication into the tissue surrounding the intravenous site (MacCara, 1983). The extent of damage that follows such an event depends on the extravasated substance and the volume of the fluid that has leaked into the interstitium. The best prevention is close attention to the intravenous site where the medication is infusing. Extravasation of medications with alpha-adrenergic activity (e.g., epinephrine, dopamine) may be treated with the alpha-adrenergic blocking agent phentolamine. Hyaluronidase, an enzyme that destroys tissue cement, may be useful for the treatment of other extravasations.

Aerosolized Medications Administration

The delivery of medications to the lung would appear to be optimal because this is the desired site of action of many therapies prescribed in the neonatal population. The particle size produced by various inhalers and nebulized solutions may be much larger than the airway diameter itself. This discrepancy may preclude the premature infant from receiving the most benefit from a medication administered by inhalation because the larger particles of the drug may deposit in the airway before reaching the intended site of activity.

PHARMACOKINETICS

Pharmacokinetics is the study of the movement of a substance through the various body compartments (Levy, 1992). It reflects a time-dependent relationship between a drug dosage and the measurable concentration of medication that results, usually in the serum or plasma. Measurement of blood levels is usually much simpler than measurement of tissue levels. Pharmacodynamics is the study of how that substance affects the body and the clinical effect that is desired when a medication is administered (Lalonde, 1992).

Volume of distribution refers to an imaginary space into which a medication distributes once it reaches the blood stream and assumes an equal distribution of drug throughout all body compartments (Rowland & Tozer, 1989). It is the mathematical relationship between the dose administered and the serum concentration of the medication. A volume of distribution for a medication depends on the chemical properties of the drug itself and the physiologic state of the patient. Factors such as extent of plasma and tissue binding, lipid solubility, an increased volume of distribution for medications that distribute into body water, increases in a patient's intravascular and extravascular fluid, changes in protein concentration and binding capacity, and fat content can alter a volume of distribution.

Half-life describes the time it takes for the serum concentration of a medication to decrease by one half of its original concentration (Winter, 1988). Half-life may be influenced by other medications, tissue perfusion, and organ function.

Steady state refers to the point in time at which for each dosing interval the patient is receiving the same amount of drug that is being excreted by the body: the rate of drug administration equals the rate of drug elimination. In clinical practice, steady state is considered to be achieved after about four to five half-lives of the drug have passed (Shargel & Yu, 1985).

Clearance refers to the amount of drug cleared from the blood stream per unit of time (Rowland & Tozer, 1989). Clearance of a medication depends on many factors, including the volume of distribution, the half-life, the physiologic status of the patient, blood flow to the organs, organ function, and the properties of the medication itself.

In clinical practice, clearance is generally referred to as linear (*first order*) or nonlinear (*zero order*). For a drug whose clearance follows linear pharmacokinetics, an increase in the dose will proportionately and predictably increase the serum proportional to the concentration of drug achieved at steady state. The majority of medications used in neonates (aminoglycosides, vancomycin, phenobarbital, caffeine, and catecholamines) follow this type of elimination. Theophylline is also eliminated on a linear basis when concentrations are in the normally accepted therapeutic range. However, when concentrations above the therapeutic range are exceeded, theophylline deviates from linear elimination.

A drug that follows nonlinear pharmacokinetics may have a rapid rise in serum concentration in response to a small increase in dose. This unpredictable dose response is a result of enzyme saturation in the liver. Elimination now becomes dose dependent. All medications cleared hepatically follow nonlinear pharmacokinetics; however, elimination may appear linear over the therapeutic range and change to nonlinear elimination when levels exceed the therapeutic range. An increase in dose yields a predictable increase in serum concentration unless the serum concentration exceeds what is normally considered therapeutic. At these elevated serum concentrations, the nonlinear pharmacokinetic parameters are observed. Phenytoin is a classic example of a medication with nonlinear kinetics; once the enzymes responsible for the elimination of phenytoin are saturated, elimination can no longer occur at the rate of drug administration. A proportional increase in clearance is not seen with a dosage increase; rather, serum concentrations become excessively elevated with small dosage increases. Elimination of medication through this saturable enzyme process is often referred to as Michaelis-Menton kinetics (Rowland & Tozer, 1989).

Loading Doses

Medications will gradually accumulate in the body over time. When there is an immediate need to achieve a desired therapeutic concentration to elicit an effect and accumulation of drug is expected, a loading dose of medication may be necessary. This is true of medications including antiarrhythmic agents, phenobarbital, caffeine, gentamicin, and theophylline. If a loading dose is not given, it may take hours to days to achieve the desired therapeutic concentration (Table 28–1).

Therapeutic Drug Monitoring

A *therapeutic range* is a definable range of drug concentrations in which the drug is expected to exert the desired effect with little or low toxicity.

TABLE 28–1. Common Pharmacokinetic Equations

$$\text{Volume of distribution (Vd)} = \frac{\text{dose (mg/kg)}}{\text{peak conc (mg/L)}}$$

$$\text{Half-life } (t_{1/2}) = \frac{0.693}{k_e}$$

$$\text{Clearance (Cl)} = \frac{0.693 \times \text{Vd}}{t_{1/2}}$$

$$\text{Elimination rate constant } (k_e) = \frac{\ln \text{conc}_a - \ln \text{conc}_b}{\Delta t}$$

Therapeutic drug monitoring requires an assay be available to measure serum concentrations and is part of the day-to-day monitoring of drug therapy. For some medications (e.g., aminoglycosides) it is important to evaluate both peak and trough serum concentrations.

- Generally, if trough concentrations are elevated, this reflects an inability of the body to eliminate a medication and the dosing interval should be extended.
- Conversely, if the trough concentration is below a desired level, shortening the dosage interval is needed.
- Subtherapeutic or elevated peak levels require actual dosage adjustment instead of interval changes. For other medications, it is most important to be able to determine that the serum drug concentration remains within the therapeutic range throughout the dosing interval (e.g., antiepileptics, cardiac medications, theophylline, caffeine). In such cases, an evaluation of a trough concentration will provide the most benefit. For these medications, peak concentrations are obtained only if the patient exhibits signs of toxicity.

Obtaining levels once a patient achieves steady-state concentrations will usually provide the health care provider with the most accurate information concerning how the patient may handle the medication on a long-term basis. Because obtaining serum concentrations may require significant volumes of blood in a neonate, assessing the patient's clinical status may provide more useful information than obtaining serial serum concentrations of drugs.

Certain medications are highly protein bound. For these medications, two types of assays may be available: total and free serum concentrations. Free levels indicate the amount of free, unbound drug that is available to exert its effects on target tissues. Phenytoin, for example, should be monitored by evaluating free levels in the neonate because it is highly bound to plasma proteins and its pharmacokinetic parameters are significantly altered in this age group. If free phenytoin serum assays are not available, caution must be used in the interpretation of total serum concentrations. Levels may be falsely interpreted as low when the actual amount of active drug is adequate or toxic.

FACTORS UNIQUE TO THE NEONATE

Absorption

No absorption phase is required for intravenous or intra-arterial administration of medications. Other routes of administration, such as intramuscular, oral, topical, rectal, and subcutaneous, require absorption of the medication from the site of administration for the drug to be recovered from the blood stream.

Absorption of a medication from an intramuscular injection is influenced by muscle tone, muscle mass, and regional blood flow to the area (Stewart & Hampton, 1987). Neonates, especially premature infants, may have significantly decreased muscle mass and decreased tone. Blood flow to the muscle tissue itself can be complicated by hypoxemia, sepsis, shock, and congestive heart failure. Intramuscular injections of some medications may result in a delay in therapy because of poor or erratic absorption. A longer duration of action and a delay in the time to peak serum concentration may occur with intramuscular administration of medications to neonates, thus the intramuscular route should be avoided unless absolutely necessary for the patient to receive the drug therapy.

Absorption from the gastrointestinal tract depends on many variables, including gastrointestinal pH, gastric emptying time, microbial colonization of the gastrointestinal tract, intestinal transit time, pancreatic enzyme activity, biliary function, and the clinical status of the infant (Morselli, Franco-Morselli, & Bossi, 1980). Neonates have a gastric pH that differs significantly from that of adults. The gastric pH at birth is 6 to 8. Gastric acid production is initiated soon after birth and then decreases over the first 30 days of life. Those medications that are weak acids (e.g., phenobarbital, phenytoin, acetaminophen) will be more poorly absorbed. Medications that are weak bases, such as penicillin, will be absorbed to a much greater extent. This difference in absorption may result in either a lack of drug absorption or in excess absorption as compared to intravenously administered medications, but usually results in a longer duration of action. The differences in gastrointestinal absorption may or may not be clinically significant.

Absorption and time for peak serum concentration are influenced by the contact time of the medication with the absorptive surface. Gastric emptying time is delayed in the neonate, especially in the premature infant (Morselli, Franco-Morselli, & Bossi, 1980). The slow intestinal transit time may influence the timing and peak effect of medications absorbed in the small intestine.

The presence of diarrhea will increase the gastrointestinal motility, resulting in less absorption of drug. Patients receiving narcotics usually develop a prolonged transit time that may result in increased absorption of other medications the patient is receiving.

Neonates have a relative state of pancreatic insufficiency. Pancreatic enzymes are required for the intraluminal hydrolysis of some medications (e.g., chloramphenicol, clindamycin).

Biliary function and the bile acid pool increase over the first month of life (Watkins et al., 1973). The relative state of bile acid depletion affects medications administered with food. Bile acids are required for absorption of fat-soluble vitamins; patients with poor biliary function may have difficulty absorbing these nutrients.

The microbial gut colonization facilitates the breakdown of some medications and is involved in the enterohepatic recirculation of some medications. Changes in the gut flora may influence the metabolism of some drugs and influence some drug–drug interactions.

The absorption of medications through the skin depends on the skin integrity, blood flow to the skin, and the amount of subcutaneous fat (Stewart & Hampton, 1987). Premature infants have a skin to body surface area ratio that is three times that of an adult. Along with decreased amounts of subcutaneous fat and an overall decreased skin barrier, agents topically applied can be absorbed to a significant degree. This enhanced absorption can lead to toxicity, but it can also be exploited therapeutically.

Rectal administration of medications may be a valuable means of providing certain medications (e.g., aspirin, acetaminophen, diazepam, and Kayexalate) when other routes of administration are not available. Rectal absorption depends on blood flow, retention of the drug in the rectum, and chemical properties of the drug and its formation.

Distribution

Once the medication has reached the blood stream, the next step is its distribution to other body compartments. This distribution phase is affected by the following:

- Binding to tissue or plasma proteins
- Nature and size of available body compartments
- Chemical properties of drugs

Most medications that are protein bound bind to serum albumin. Serum albumin and serum total protein levels are decreased during infancy and rise slowly over the first year of life to adult values (Brodersen & Honore, 1989). Newborns also have a higher serum concentration of substances (i.e., maternal estrogens and bilirubin) that compete with medications for binding sites on albumin. Only the amount of medication that is biologically active is the free or unbound fraction. Decreased available sites for protein binding and increased displacement may influence therapeutic efficacy and toxicity at lower measured serum concentrations than would be evident in an adult. Patients with hepatic dysfunction or renal failure have alterations in protein binding and also have increased amounts of free or unbound drug (Besunder, Reed, & Blumer, 1988). Trimethoprim-sulfamethoxazole and phenytoin are examples of highly protein bound medications that may result in the availability of increased free drug depending on the age of the patient and organ function.

Total body water and the distribution of it in the intracellular and extracellular spaces varies with the gestational age of the infant (Stewart & Hampton, 1987). As the fetus matures, total body water decreases to a total of 75 percent at term, with only about half of that as extracellular fluid.

The central nervous system of neonates is immature (Levin, 1988). The formation of the blood-brain barrier is also incomplete, resulting in an increased accessibility of drugs to the central nervous system. Increased sensitivity to many drugs, especially those with sedative and central nervous system effects, may occur in the neonatal period.

Medications that are hydrophilic have a much higher volume of distribution as compared with adult data. Therefore, neonatal dosing will be higher on a per kilogram basis. Likewise, medications that are lipophilic have a much smaller distribution volume in a neonate as compared with an adult, because less of a neonate's body mass is composed of adipose tissue. Neonatal dosing of medications that are lipophilic will probably be smaller on a per kilogram basis as compared with the adult dosing.

Metabolism

Many drugs undergo metabolism before elimination from the body. The process of biotransformation occurs mainly in the liver, although other tissues may also be involved (Reed & Besunder, 1989). There are many pathways available for the metabolism of drugs, and each pathway matures at a different rate.

Consideration must also be given to medications that the mother might have taken during her pregnancy. During intrauterine life, the fetus depends on both the mother's liver as well as its own liver to detoxify compounds. There is some evidence that prenatal exposure to drugs that have the capacity to induce hepatic enzymes may affect neonatal metabolism (Rudd & Brazy, 1988).

Excretion

The primary route of elimination of medications from the body is through the kidney. Glomerular filtration rate is lower in infants than adults and significantly lower in premature infants than those born at term. The first increase in glomerular filtration rate is seen at 34 weeks of postconceptual age. Tubular reabsorption and secretion are also decreased in the neonate. Therefore, drugs excreted primarily by the renal route must have extended dosing intervals as compared with the adult dosing. Dosing intervals may need to be extended. For example, gentamicin is administered only once or sometimes twice a day in most neonates compared with adult dosing of three times a day.

SPECIAL NEONATAL POPULATIONS

Patients on extracorporeal membrane oxygenation (ECMO) are often treated with numerous medications, including antibiotics, sedatives, analgesics, inotropes, diuretics, and antiepileptics. Medications may be administered to patients on ECMO either into the ECMO circuit or directly to the patient.

Medications delivered into the ECMO circuit may be injected directly into the venous reservoir either before the filter or after the filter. The effects of the pump may cause an incomplete admixture of the medication depending on the site of injection. More consistent distribution and delivery of medication occurs when drugs are injected after the filter. Administration into this site places the patient at risk for development of air emboli, and administration of medications here should be done with great caution. Medications injected directly into the reservoir or prefilter usually result in a prolonged time of actual drug delivery to the patient and incomplete drug administration. There is often a delay in peak effect for these patients, resulting in false interpretation of serum peak levels for aminoglycoside antibiotics.

In addition to the pharmacokinetic influences of ECMO, drugs such as heparin and fentanyl bind to the ECMO circuit, resulting in a reduced amount of bioavailable drug for the patient (Hynynen, 1987). Once the circuit becomes saturated with these medications, bioavailability ceases to be an issue. Therefore, increased doses may be required initially when these medications are used or when the circuit is changed during ECMO therapy.

Patients placed on ECMO often have underlying hepatic and renal dysfunction secondary to hypoxic insults. The physiology of ECMO further compounds this dysfunction. Frequently, renal function continues to deteriorate during ECMO. Dosing adjustments for any medications cleared renally need to be made (Southgate, DiPiro, & Robertson, 1989).

FETAL AND INFANT EXPOSURE TO MATERNAL MEDICATIONS

Fetal Exposure

Virtually any medication or substance given to the mother either intentionally or inadvertently can cross the placental membrane. The fetal effects seen depend on the agent, amount of substance, and the stage of gestation when the fetal exposure occurs.

The amount of drug that passes into the fetal circulation is dependent on several factors:

- Molecular weight of the substance
- Protein binding
- Lipid solubility
- Ionization of drug
- Maternal serum concentrations
- Integrity of the placental barrier

Lactation Exposure

Drugs may reach the breast milk after binding to fat or protein or by the passage of lipid-soluble drugs into the milk. Protein binding, degree of ionization, and concentration of drug in the maternal circulation also contribute to the amount of drug that reaches the milk supply. Considerations concerning the amount of medication the infant will receive also include the following:

- Time the medication is taken in relation to the period of nursing
- Amount or dose of medication
- Length of nursing
- Amount of milk ingested

The American Academy of Pediatrics Committee on Drugs publishes guidelines regarding the transfer of drugs and chemicals into human milk (Committee on Drugs, 1994). These guidelines include a list of medications and chemicals for which data are available evaluating the transfer of a substance into the mother's milk and the subsequent effects to expect in the nursing infant. If a breast-fed infant develops any adverse effects from a medication prescribed to the mother, this information should be documented.

REFERENCES

Benzing, G., III, & Loggie, J. (1973). A new retrograde method for administering drugs intravenously. *Pediatrics, 52,* 420–425.

Besunder, J. B., Reed, M. D., & Blumer, J. C. (1988). Principles of drug biodisposition in the neonate: Part I. [Review]. *Clinical Pharmacokinetics, 14,* 261–286.

Brodersen, R., & Honore, B. (1989). Drug binding properties of neonatal albumin. *Acta Paediatrica Scandinavica, 78,* 342–346.

Committee on Drugs. (1994). The transfer of drugs and other chemicals into human milk. *Pediatrics, 93,* 137–150.

Department of Health and Human Services. (1993). Med Watch Reporting Program. *FDA Medical Bulletin, 23*(2), insert.

Ernst, J., Williams, J., Glick, M., & Lemons, J. (1983). Osmolality of substances used in the intensive care nursery. *Pediatrics, 72,* 347–352.

Fincham, J. (1992). Monitoring and managing adverse drug reactions. *American Pharmacy, 32*(2), 74–81.

Gould, T., & Roberts, R. (1979). Therapeutic problems arising from the use of the intravenous route for drug administration. *Journal of Pediatrics, 95,* 456–471.

Hansten, P., & Horn, J. (1993). *Drug interactions & updates quarterly* (pp. 1–25, 95–99, 119–1240). Spokane, WA: Applied Therapeutics.

Helper, C., & Strand, L. (1989). Opportunities and responsibilities in pharmaceutical care. *American Journal of Pharmaceutical Education,* Winter Suppl., p. 7s.

Hynynen, M. (1987). Binding of fentanyl and alfentanyl to the extracorporeal circuit. *Acta Anaesthesiologica Scandinavica, 31,* 706–710.

LaLonde, R. (1992). Pharmacodynamics. In W. E. Evans, J. J. Schentag, & W.J. Jusko. (Eds.), *Applied pharmacokinetics principles of therapeutic drug monitoring* (pp. 1–31). Spokane, WA: Applied Therapeutics.

Levin, R. (1988). Pediatric and Neonatal Therapy. In E. T. Herfindal, D. R. Gourley, & L. L. Hart (Eds.), *Clinical pharmacy and therapeutics* (pp. 1011–1029). Baltimore: Williams & Wilkins.

Levy, G. (1992). Applied pharmacokinetics—a prospectus. In W. E. Evans, J. J., Schentag, & W. J. Jusko (Eds.). *Applied pharmacokinetics principles of therapeutic drug monitoring* (pp. 1–8). Spokane, WA: Applied Therapeutics.

MacCara, M. (1983). Extravasation: A hazard of intravenous therapy. *Drug Intelligence and Clinical Pharmacy, 17,* 713–717.

Manasse, H., Jr. (1989). Medication use in an imperfect world: Drug misadventuring as an issue of public policy: I. *American Journal of Hospital Pharmacy, 46,* 929–944.

Morselli, P., Franco-Morselli, R., & Bossi, L. (1980). Clinical pharmacokinetics in newborns and infants: Age-related differences and therapeutic implication. [Review]. *Clinical Pharmacokinetics, 5,* 485–527.

Reed, M., & Besunder, J. (1989). Developmental pharmacology: Ontogenic basis of drug disposition. *Pediatric Clinics of North America, 36,* 1053–1074.

Roberts, R. (1981). Intravenous administration of medication in pediatric patients: Problems and solutions. *Pediatric Clinics of North America, 28,* 23–34.

Rowland, M., & Tozer, T. N. (1989). *Clinical pharmacokinetics concepts and applications* (2nd. ed., pp. 17–31, 156–158, 182–187). Philadelphia: Lea & Febiger.

Rudd, C., & Brazy, J. (1988). Drugs in the perinatal period: Implications for the preterm infant. *Comprehensive Therapy, 14,* 30–37.

Shargel, L., & Yu, A. (1985). *Applied biopharmaceutics and pharmacokinetics* (2nd ed.). Norwalk, CT: Appleton-Century-Crofts.

Southgate, W. M., DiPiro, J. T., & Robertson, A. F. (1989). Pharmacokinetics of gentamicin in neonates on extracorporeal membrane oxygenation. *Antimicrobial Agents and Chemotherapy, 33,* 817–819.

Stewart, C. F., & Hampton, E. M. (1987). Effect of maturation on drug disposition in pediatric patients. [Review]. *Clinical Pharmacy, 6,* 548–564.

Watkins, J. B., Ingall, D., Szczepanek, P., et al. (1973). Bile salt metabolism in the newborn: Measurement of pool size and synthesis by stable isotope technic. *The New England Journal of Medicine, 288,* 431–434.

White, K., & Harkavy, K. (1982). Hypertonie formula resulting from added oral medications. *American Journal of Diseases of Children, 136,* 931–933.

Winter, M. (1988). *Basic clinical pharmacokinetics* (2nd. ed., pp. 7–63). Spokane, WA: Applied Therapeutics.

CHAPTER 29

The Drug-Exposed Neonate

The effects of prenatal exposure to tobacco, cocaine, heroin, and alcohol are considered separately in this chapter, but multiple substances are often simultaneously abused, making it difficult to ascertain which effect is caused by which substance.

TOBACCO

Risk Factors Associated With Maternal Smoking

MATERNAL HAZARDS

The risks to the mother of smoking during pregnancy are listed as follows:

- Reduced fertility (Lincoln, 1986; McGarry, 1983) by altered tubal motility and antiestrogen effects
- Increased incidence of spontaneous abortion
- Unexplained vaginal bleeding
- Abruptio placentae
- Placenta previa
- Risk 2.3 times greater than nonsmokers of having an anomalous child

FETAL HAZARDS

The fetus may have any of the following:

- Reduced birth weight
- Increased incidence of prematurity
- Morbidity associated with prematurity
- Reduced fetal heart rate variability
- Fetal movement is reduced
- The placenta's aging process is hastened, which makes the uterine environment less favorable for fetal habitation.
- Nitrosamines are known carcinogens (Enkin, 1984).
- Carbon monoxide competes with oxygen for the binding sites on the hemoglobin, forming carboxyhemoglobin and thus lowering the fetal oxygen partial pressure and impairing tissue oxygenation (Longo, 1976).
- Polycythemia is a compensatory mechanism that increases available oxygen binding sites, which further reduces blood flow and increases the hypoxia. This leads to the development of venous thrombi and hyperbilirubinemia.
- Chronic intrauterine hypoxia stimulates the fetal stress response. This causes secretion of glucocorticoids, which facilitates surfactant production.

- Nicotine has the same vasoconstrictive properties as carbon monoxide. This vasoconstriction reduces the uteroplacental blood flow and consequently reduces fetal-placental exchange.
- Cyanide is present in a small amount and readily crosses the placenta. It inhibits cellular respiration and, in sufficient doses, can readily induce death.

INFANT HAZARDS

The following may occur in infants as a result of maternal smoking:

- Neonatal thyroid enlargement
- Strabismus
- Sudden infant death syndrome (SIDS)
- More frequent episodes of upper respiratory tract infections and otitis media than their nonsmoking counterparts (Rantakallio, 1983)

COCAINE

Mechanism of Action

Cocaine is a central nervous system (CNS) stimulant that was first synthesized from the *Erythroxylon coca* leaves in 1858 (Stimmel, 1979). In 1884, cocaine was first used as a topical anesthetic (Cregler & Mark, 1985). Its vasoconstrictive properties provide a relatively bloodless field. These same vasoconstrictive properties are the basis for many of the complications of systemic cocaine use, such as hypertensive episodes and tachycardia.

Metabolism

Cocaine is metabolized by the esterase enzymes, which are produced within the liver and are present in the plasma. According to Chasnoff, Burns, and Burns (1987), if a woman has ingested cocaine 2 to 3 days before delivery, her urine will contain metabolites for 24 hours and the neonate's urine will continue to test positive for 4 to 7 days. However, the more immature the fetal liver, the longer the cocaine metabolites may linger in the fetal system (Udell, 1989).

Hazards of Cocaine Addiction

Potential complications specific to pregnancy are listed below:

- Spontaneous abortion
- Increased rate of placental abruption, which is associated with stillbirths
- Preterm labor and delivery of infants with low birth weight and who are small for gestational age
- Abnormalities noted in fetal monitoring
- Fetal meconium staining (Chasnoff, Burns, & Burns, 1987; MacGregor et al., 1987)

FETAL EFFECTS

Fetal/neonatal effects include the following:

- Symmetrical growth retardation
- Intrauterine hypoxic episodes, fetal "stroke" in utero
- Fetal heart rate arrhythmias
- Necrotizing enterocolitis
- Visceral anomalies, including gastroschisis
- Hyperreflexia
- Irritability
- Difficulty in consoling
- Difficulty in holding secondary to neonate's hyperextension, posturing, and being easily overloaded by sensory stimulation
- Abnormal electroencephalograms during the first 12 months of life

HEROIN

Mechanism of Action

Heroin is a derivative of the opium poppy. It is a CNS depressant that is six times as potent as morphine and is highly addictive (Malseed & Harrigan, 1989).

General Risk Factors Associated With Heroin Abuse

Typical attributes of women addicted to heroin are as follows:

- Substandard living conditions
- Transient, homeless lifestyle
- Poor nutrition
- Lack of adequate prenatal care
- Poor personal hygiene
- High incidence of prostitution to finance their addiction
- Exposure to sexually transmitted diseases (herpes, syphilis, gonorrhea), hepatitis, and the acquired immunodeficiency syndrome
- Anovulation and associated amenorrhea

Generally, the pregnant addict is placed on methadone maintenance and given prenatal care, nutritional assistance, and counseling. Once the child is delivered, detoxification may be attempted (Connaughton, Reeser, Schut, & Finnegan, 1977).

Fetal/Neonatal Effects

The risks to the fetus and neonate include the following:

- Low birth weight
- Fetal distress
- Meconium staining/aspiration pneumonia
- Increased incidence of breech presentation among heroin-exposed infants, which is believed to be from heightened fetal activity during episodes of hypoxia (Connaughton, Finnegan, Schut, & Emich, 1975).

Neonatal Abstinence Syndrome

The majority of infants born to women addicted to heroin undergo withdrawal (Naeye, Blanc, LeBlanc, & Khatamee, 1973; Reddy, Harper, & Stern, 1971; Zelson, Rubio, & Wasserman, 1971), with an onset of withdrawal symptoms up to day 6 of life (Reddy, Harper, & Stern, 1971). Symptoms may persist for 8 to 16 weeks (Philips, 1986). The term *neonatal abstinence syndrome* (NAS) was coined because of the consistent pattern of symptoms. Heroin-exposed infants are small for gestational age and have CNS and gastrointestinal symptoms.

Being small for gestational age results from maternal factors (e.g., poor nutrition, no prenatal care) and from the intermittent hypoxia associated with erratic heroin supply.

CNS symptomatology is the first to appear and includes such behaviors as hyperactivity, irritability, tremors (Reddy, Harper, & Stern, 1971), high-pitched cry, hypertonicity, and convulsions (Zelson, Rubio, & Wasserman, 1971).

Symptoms related to the gastrointestinal tract appear on day 4 to 6 of life and include regurgitation, poor feeding, vomiting, and diarrhea. Incessant crying associated with withdrawal often makes the caregiver think that the infant is hungry. This may lead to overfeeding or caregiver frustration when the infant continues crying instead of sucking from the bottle.

Less frequent symptoms are hyperpyrexia, nasal congestion, tachypnea (Reddy, Harper, & Stern, 1971), yawning, and sweating (Zelson, Rubio, & Wasserman, 1971).

Physiologic jaundice is less frequent among infants of addicted women than among nonaddicted infants.

Increased lung maturity with a lowered rate of respiratory distress syndrome is believed to be a result of repeated stimulation of the fetal stress response or a direct action that heroin may exert on the fetal lung to enhance pulmonary surfactant production (Glass & Evans, 1977).

Signs and symptoms of withdrawal can be categorized and scored (Table 29–1 and Fig. 29–1). NAS has been reported to last longer in infants born to mothers maintained on methadone. It may be treated with medications such as methadone, oral morphine, phenobarbital, paregoric, opium, chlorpromazine, or diazepam, depending on the maternal substance or substances used (D'Apolito & McRorie, 1996).

TABLE 29–1. Neonatal Abstinence Syndrome: Clinical Manifestations

Gastrointestinal	Central Nervous System	Other
Regurgitation	First to appear	Small for gestational age
Poor feeding	Hyperactivity	Hyperpyrexia
Vomiting	Irritability	Nasal congestion
Diarrhea	Tremors	Tachypnea
	High-pitched cry	Yawning
	Hypertonicity	Sweating
	Convulsions	
	Incessant crying	

NEONATAL ABSTINENCE SCORING SYSTEM

SYSTEM	SIGNS AND SYMPTOMS	SCORE	A^M	P^M	COMMENTS
CENTRAL NERVOUS SYSTEM DISTURBANCES	Excessive High Pitched (Or other) Cry Continuous High Pitched (Or other) Cry	2 3			Daily Weight:
	Sleeps < 1 Hour After Feeding Sleeps < 2 Hours After Feeding Sleeps < 3 Hours After Feeding	3 2 1			
	Hyperactive Moro Reflex Markedly Hyperactive Moro Reflex	2 3			
	Mild Tremors Disturbed Moderate-Severe Tremors Disturbed	1 2			
	Mild Tremors Undisturbed Moderate-Severe Tremors Undisturbed	3 4			
	Increased Muscle Tone	2			
	Excoriation (Specific Area)	1			
	Myoclonic Jerks	3			
	Generalized Convulsions	5			

		1													
METABOLIC/VASOMOTOR/RESPIRATORY DISTURBANCES	Sweating	1													
	Fever<101 (99-100.8 F./37.2-38.2C.)	1													
	Fever>101 (38.4C. and Higher)	2													
	Frequent Yawning (> 3-4 Times/Interval)	1													
	Mottling	1													
	Nasal Stuffiness	1													
	Sneezing (> 3-4 Times/Interval)	1													
	Nasal Flaring	2													
	Respiratory Rate > 60/min	1													
	Respiratory Rate > 60/min with Retractions	2													
GASTRO-INTESTINAL DISTURBANCES	Excessive Sucking	1													
	Poor Feeding	2													
	Regurgitation	2													
	Projectile Vomiting	3													
	Loose Stools	2													
	Watery Stools	3													
	TOTAL SCORE														
	INITIALS OF SCORER														

FIGURE 29–1. Neonatal abstinence scoring system. (From Finnegan, L. P. [1986]. Neonatal abstinence syndrome: Assessment and pharmacotherapy. In F. F. Rubaltelli & B. Granati [Eds.], *Neonatal therapy: An update.* New York: Excerpta Medica. Reprinted with permission.)

PROFILE OF THE DRUG-ADDICTED WOMAN

Common attributes of the drug-addicted woman are listed below:

- May have an underlying personality disorder that requires in-depth psychotherapy (Atkins, 1988)
- Was raised in a dysfunctional family, being victim of abuse and rape
- Lacks "healthy" parental role model
- Is socially isolated as a consequence of her addiction
- Has low self-esteem
- Is often poorly equipped to earn a living
- Has unrealistic expectations of her infant

ALCOHOL

Alcohol-induced aberrations fall on a continuum ranging from mild to severe, with some children manifesting all or more characteristics and others exhibiting few or none. In fact, two classifications of alcohol-related effects exist. *Fetal alcohol syndrome* is on the severe end of the continuum, and the term *fetal alcohol effects* refers to mild symptomatology.

Diagnosis of FAS

Fetal alcohol syndrome is often undiagnosed during the neonatal period unless the mother is admitted in labor while intoxicated and/or if the amniotic fluid smells of alcohol (Little, Snell, Rosenfeld, & Gilstrap, 1990). No definitive test for fetal alcohol syndrome exists, so the diagnosis is based on a positive drinking history during pregnancy and on the findings of dysmorphic characteristics, CNS dysfunction, and growth deficiency.

Common manifestations include failure to thrive, persistent behavioral problems, and/or academic failure.

Biological parents who are caring for their children will need to cope with the guilt from the realization of how they harmed their child through prenatal drinking. They should receive treatment to achieve/maintain sobriety, cope with emotional issues underpinning their addiction, and learn consistent parenting strategies.

Risk Factors Associated With Alchohol Abuse

Women who drink heavily often smoke and are poorly nourished (Little, 1977; Wright, 1986). Heavy drinkers are at risk for a poor state of health related to inadequate diet and direct effects of alcohol (e.g., cirrhosis, alcoholic cardiac myopathy). Pregnancy-associated risks include increased incidence of spontaneous abortion and an infant with low birth weight.

FETAL ALCOHOL SYNDROME

Fetal alcohol syndrome is diagnosed by reported maternal alcohol consumption during pregnancy as well as characteristic neonatal features. These findings revolve around three areas: (1) prenatal and postnatal growth deficiency; (2) dysmorphic characteristics; and (3) CNS dysfunction (Lipson, 1988; Jones & Smith, 1973; Jones, Smith, Ulleland, & Streissguth, 1973; Streissguth, Clarren, & Jones, 1985, Streissguth & LaDue, 1985).

Growth Deficiency
- Small at birth
- Failure to demonstrate catch-up growth
- Failure to thrive in spite of adequate calorie intake (Jones et al., 1973; Streissguth, Clarren, & Jones, 1985)
- Weight for height and head circumference below the tenth percentile

Dysmorphic Characteristics
- Facial anomalies:
  - Microcephaly
  - Short palpebral fissures
  - Flat midface
  - Indistinct philtrum
  - Thin upper lip
  - Epicanthal folds
  - Low nasal bridge
  - Minor ear anomalies
  - Short nose
  - Micrognathia (Streissguth, Clarren, & Jones, 1985)
- Abnormal palmar creases
- Congenital heart disease, mainly septal defects

Central Nervous System Dysfunction
- Irritability and tremulousness
- Poor suck with subsequent feeding problems
- Disturbed by sensory stimulation (Clarren, Bowden, & Astley, 1985; Warren & Bast, 1988)
- Hyperactivity

ASSESSMENT

Part of the admission protocol for all women should include a systematic routine assessment for substance use/abuse.

NURSING INTERVENTIONS FOR INFANTS BORN TO SUBSTANCE-ABUSING MOTHERS

Care Related to Central Nervous System Manifestations

Neonatal intervention is largely supportive and dependent on the type of symptoms experienced by the infant. If irritability is a problem, the following can be done:
- Regulate environment.

- Reduce the quantity and variety of sensory input (e.g., dimming nursery lights or covering the incubator with a blanket, reducing noise by not talking loudly at the bedside, keeping radios and intercom volumes low, silencing alarms after responding, and quietly closing incubator doors).
- Minimize handling.
  - Provide group care to the level of infant tolerance.
  - Use electronic monitoring capabilities for routine vital signs.
  - Avoid routine laboratory work.
  - Use infant behavioral cues as a basis for directing the amount of stimulation to be given.

The infant's tolerance of each sensory modality (visual, tactile, auditory, kinesthetic, gustatory) should be evaluated.

Care Related to Gastrointestinal Manifestations

Substance-exposed infants are often of low birth weight and have a poorly coordinated suck-swallow reflex. Heroin-exposed infants may experience abdominal cramping with diarrhea. Intense crying is often misinterpreted as hunger, with overfeeding creating abdominal distention, vomiting, and diarrhea. Nursing care for gastrointestinal disorders includes the following:

- Small frequent feedings
- Accurate measurement of intake and output
- Use of indwelling, small-diameter (e.g., 5 French) nasogastric feeding tube to gavage portion of milk that infant is unable to nipple or to provide nutrition if infant is sleeping so rest can be maintained
- Meeting sucking needs with use of pacifier or hand sucking during gavage feedings
- Calming measures such as swaddling, holding the infant in a flexed position, with the infant's hands past midline, hand holding, vertical rocking, and use of a pacifier (Griffith, 1988)
- Daily weight and head circumference measurements to track growth

Drug screens should be done on breast milk specimens, because cocaine, heroin, and alcohol cross into human milk. Mothers should be informed of this crossover, and, unless abstinence has been achieved, bottle feeding should be encouraged.

Pharmacologic Intervention

Infants who are withdrawing from opiates or who are manifesting neonatal abstinence syndrome constitute the population who may need pharmacologic intervention during withdrawal. Signs and symptoms of withdrawal include the following (Chasnoff, 1988):

- Fever
- Vomiting and diarrhea
- High-pitched cry
- Sweating
- Sneezing

• Agitation, tremors, seizures

Pharmacologic intervention is indicated if there has been any of the following (Chasnoff, 1988):

- Weight loss from gastrointestinal symptoms or hyperactivity associated with withdrawal or both
- Inability of the infant to rest
- Fever unrelated to infection
- Seizures

THERAPEUTIC DRUGS

Paregoric

- Improves sucking ability and is correlated with weight gain
- Provides direct relief by its cross-dependence with heroin
- Has direct effect on the gastrointestinal system to reduce diarrhea

Diazepam

- Depresses sucking, heart rate, and respirations
- Is contraindicated in an infant who is jaundiced
- Late-onset seizures after diazepam discontinuance (Chasnoff, 1988)

Phenobarbital

- Reduces symptoms associated with NAS (van Baar, Soepatmi, Gunning, & Akkerhuis, 1994).

Care Related to Risk for Infection

Care should be taken to maintain universal isolation precautions, because there is an increased incidence of hepatitis and acquired immunodeficiency syndrome among these women and their infants. Common signs and symptoms suggestive of sepsis are as follows:

- Temperature instability
- Hypotonicity
- Color changes (pale or mottled)
- Feeding intolerance
- Episodes of apnea
- Bradycardia

Care Related to Facilitating Maternal-Child Attachment

Appropriate nursing intervention includes the following:

- Parents need to be educated about the expected behavioral manifestations in the infant.
- Withdrawal, if it is occurring, should be discussed.

- Parents can be shown when the infant appears receptive to interaction.
- Significant others need to be involved.
- Discharge should be interdisciplinary and include follow-up care.
- Referrals should be made to a drug rehabilitation program and other appropriate community resources (e.g., the Women, Infants, and Children [WIC] program).

REFERENCES

Atkins, W. (1988). Cocaine: The drug of choice. In I. Chasnoff (Ed.), *Drugs, alcohol, pregnancy and parenting* (pp. 91–96). Hingham, MA: Kluwer Academic Publishers.

Chasnoff, I. J. (1988). Newborn infants with drug withdrawal symptoms. [Review]. *Pediatrics in Review, 9,* 273–277.

Chasnoff, I. J., Burns, K. A., & Burns, W. J. (1987). Cocaine use in pregnancy: Perinatal morbidity and mortality. *Neurotoxicology and Teratology, 9,* 291–293.

Clarren, S., Bowden, D., & Astley, S. (1985, Fall). The brain in the fetal alcohol syndrome: Observation in human and nonhuman primates. *Alcohol Health and Research World, 10,* 20–25.

Connaughton, J. F. Jr., Finnegan, L., Schut, J., & Emich, J. P. (1975). Current concepts in the management of the pregnant opiate addict. *Addictive Diseases: An International Journal, 2*(1–2), 21–35.

Connaughton, J. F., Reeser, D., Schut, J., & Finnegan, L. P. (1977). Perinatal addiction: Outcome and management. *American Journal of Obstetrics and Gynecology, 129,* 679–686.

Cregler, L. L., & Mark, H. (1985). Relation of acute myocardial infarction to cocaine abuse. *American Journal of Cardiology, 56,* 794.

D'Apolito, K. C. & McRorie, T. I. Pharmacologic management of neonatal abstinence syndrome. *The Journal of Perinatal & Neonatal Nursing, 9*(4), 70–80.

Enkin, M. W. (1984). Smoking and pregnancy—A new look. *Birth, 11,* 225–229.

Glass L., & Evans, H. (1977). Physiological effects of intrauterine exposure to narcotics. In J. L. Rementeria (Ed.), *Drug abuse in pregnancy and neonatal effects* (pp. 108–115). St. Louis: C. V. Mosby.

Griffith, D. (1988). The effects of perinatal cocaine exposure on infant neurobehavior and early mother-infant interactions. In I. Chasnoff (Ed.), *Drugs, alcohol, pregnancy, and parenting* (pp. 105–113). Hingham, MA: Kluwer Academic Publishers.

Jones, K. L., & Smith, D. W. (1973). Recognition of the fetal alcohol syndrome in early infancy. *Lancet, 2,* 999–1001.

Jones, K. L., Smith, D. W., Ulleland, C. N., & Streissguth, P. (1973). Pattern of malformation in offspring of chronic alcoholic mothers. *Lancet, 1,* 1267–1271.

Lincoln, R. (1986). Smoking and reproduction. [Review]. *Family Planning Perspectives, 18,* 79–84.

Lipson, T. (1988). Fetal alcohol syndrome. [Review]. *Australian Family Physician, 17,* 385–386.

Little, R. (1977). Moderate alcohol use during pregnancy and decreased infant birth weight. *American Journal of Public Health, 67,* 1154–1156.

Little, B. B., Snell, L. M., Rosenfeld, C. R., & Gilstrap, L. C. III (1990). Failure to recognize fetal alcohol syndrome in newborn infants. *American Journal of Diseases in Children, 144,* 1142–1146.

Longo, L. D. (1976). Carbon monoxide: Effects on oxygenation of the fetus in utero. *Science, 194,* 523–525.

MacGregor, S. N., Keith, L. G., Chasnoff, I. J., et al. (1987). Cocaine use during pregnancy: Adverse perinatal outcome. *American Journal of Obstetrics and Gynecology, 157,* 686–690.

Malseed, R., & Harrigan, G. (1989). *Textbook of pharmacology & nursing care: Using the nursing process.* Philadelphia: J. B. Lippincott.

McGarry, J. (1983, February). Smoking in pregnancy—A 25-year survey. *Midwives Chronicle and Nursing Notes, 96,* 51–55.

Naeye, R. L., Blanc, W., LeBlanc, W., & Khatamee, M. A. (1973). Fetal complications of maternal heroin addiction: Abnormal growth, infections, and episodes of stress. *Journal of Pediatrics, 83,* 1055–1061.

Philips, K. (1986). Neonatal drug addicts. *Nursing Times, 82*(12), 36–38.

Rantakallio, P. (1983). A follow-up study up to the age 14 of children whose mothers smoked during pregnancy. *Acta Paediatrica Scandinavica, 72,* 747–753.

Reddy, A. M., Harper, R. G., & Stern, G. (1971). Observations on heroin and methadone withdrawal in the newborn. *Pediatrics, 48,* 353–358.

Stimmel, B. (1979). *Cardiovascular effects of mood altering drugs.* New York: Raven Press.

Streissguth, A. P., Clarren, S. K., & Jones, K. L. (1985). Natural history of the fetal alcohol syndrome: A 10-year follow-up of 11 patients. *Lancet 2,* 85–91.

Streissguth, A., & LaDue, R. (1985, Fall). Psychological and behavioral effects in children prenatally exposed to alcohol. *Alcohol Health and Research World, 10,* 6–12.

Udell, B. (1989). Crack cocaine. In *Special currents: Cocaine babies* (pp. 5–8). Columbus, OH: Ross Laboratories.

van Baar, A. L., Soepatmi, S., Gunning, W. B., & Akkerhuis, G. W. (1994). Development after prenatal exposure to cocaine, heroin and methadone. *Acta Paediatrics Supplement, 404,* 40–46.

Warren, K. R., & Bast, R. J. (1988). Alcohol-related birth defects: An update. [Review]. *Public Health Reports, 103,* 638–642.

Wright, J. (1986). Fetal alcohol syndrome. *Nursing Times, 82,* 34–35.

Zelson, C., Rubio, E., & Wasserman, E. (1971). Neonatal narcotic addiction: 10 year observation. *Pediatrics, 48,* 178–189.

CHAPTER 30

Procedures

Many types of procedures are required in neonatal care, usually as a result of operative procedures to correct surgical defects. Although hospital policies may vary, many procedures are similar in their purpose and function. Some adaptations may be required in light of resources and expenses.

CENTRAL LINE CARE

Central lines provide optimal nutrition when intravenous (IV) access has become compromised. When enteral nutrition is inadequate for growth, as in short gut syndrome (short bowel syndrome), or prolonged parenteral nutrition is required, central lines are invaluable.

The following procedures are performed to decrease the risk of infection that may accompany the use of indwelling central venous catheters.

INTRAVENOUS (IV) TUBING CHANGE

Changing central line (CL) tubing only once during a 24-hour period using sterile technique assists in preventing infection of the line and septicemia.

Equipment Needed

- IV fluids
- Appropriate IV tubing, including an air elimination filter and pump tubing
- Pourable povidone-iodine
- Pourable 10 percent rubbing alcohol
- Mask
- Sterile gloves
- Two sterile towels or barriers
- Sterile 3 × 3-inch gauze pads (four packages)

Procedure (Kenner, Harjo, & Brueggemeyer, 1988)

1. Wash hands.
2. Prime fluids to be infused through tubing, keeping the end of the tubing protected to avoid contamination.
3. Clean work area with alcohol.
4. Prepare sterile field with mask on:
   a. Open sterile barrier, holding by the corners only, and place on work area.
   b. Open and place each package of sterile gauze pads on the sterile field, without touching gauze pads.

    c. Saturate one set of gauze pads with povidone-iodine and the other with alcohol.

5. Prepare the patient by restraining extremities to avoid contamination during the procedure.
6. Prepare line for tubing change:
   a. Place new, primed tubing close to patient.
   b. Untape junction of catheter and IV tubing.
   c. Open the second sterile barrier, touching only the corners, and place under the CL catheter.
7. Scrub junction of CL catheter and IV tubing.
   a. Put on sterile gloves.
   b. Hold CL catheter with dry gauze pad in nondominant hand during entire procedure.
   c. Scrub junction with povidone-iodine–soaked gauze pad in dominant hand for 1 minute.
   d. Allow junction to air dry for 1 minute.
   e. Scrub junction with alcohol-soaked gauze pad in dominant hand for 1 minute.
8. Change tubing:
   a. Pinch-clamp CL catheter with dry gauze pad in dominant hand.
   b. Remove old IV fluid lines and discard.
   c. Pick up new tubing with nondominant hand.
   d. Drip new fluids into the hub of the CL catheter to fill the hub, preventing air flow into the line.
   e. Attach new tubing to the CL catheter and unclamp the CL clamp.
9. Set infusion pumps according to ordered rates and amounts. Check pressure limit and alarm.
10. Tape any connections that are without Luer-Lok.

DRESSING CHANGE

To monitor the condition of the CL site, dressings should be changed at least once a week (hospital policies may vary). An indication for more frequent changes is a nonocclusive dressing; note leakage at the site, bleeding, or signs of infection. Collect a specimen from the insertion site for culturing if infection is suggested. Daily dressing changes are necessary if a local site infection occurs, until it is cleared.

Equipment Needed

- Sterile dressing tray containing:
  - Applicators or swabs with hydrogen peroxide
  - Applicators or swabs with povidone-iodine
  - Povidone-iodine ointment
  - Sterile gauze pads
  - 3 × 3-inch gauze pads
  - Nonadherent gauze pad
  - Scissors, tape, mask, sterile gloves
  - Tape
- Gloves and mask
- Transparent dressing such as Op-Site or Tegaderm

Procedure (Kenner, Harjo, & Brueggemeyer, 1988) (Fig. 30–1)

1. Wash hands.
2. Restrain patient to prevent contamination during procedure.
3. Remove any clothing around site.
4. Open dressing-kit tray.
5. Put on mask and remove package of gloves.
6. Open transparent dressing and place on tray field, maintaining sterility.
7. Remove old dressing and tape.
8. Inspect CL site for redness, or drainage or puffiness, and note if catheter cuff is exposed.
   a. Collect culture of site if infection is suggested.
   b. Catheter may need to be replaced if cuff is exposed.
9. Cleanse insertion site:
   a. Put on mask and sterile gloves.
   b. Cut tape: one slit piece, one chevron piece, one wide protecting piece.
   c. Cleanse skin with hydrogen peroxide; use a circular motion starting at the line site and work away from the site cleaning the area covered by the dressing. Pat the skin dry with a sterile gauze pad, covering the area under the catheter.
   d. Cleanse skin with povidone-iodine using the same technique just described. Pat dry with sterile gauze pad leaving it in place while cutting tape.
10. Apply dressing:
    a. Cut tape: one slit piece, one chevron piece, one wide protecting piece (see Fig. 30–1). Place small drop of povidone-iodine ointment at insertion exit site.

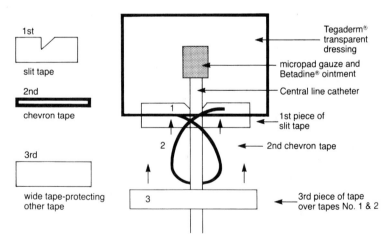

FIGURE 30–1. Central line dressing. (From Kenner, C., Harjo, J., & Brueggemeyer, A. [1988]. *Neonatal surgery: A nursing perspective* [p. 354]. Orlando, FL: Grune & Stratton. Reprinted with permission.)

   b. Place small square of nonadherent gauze dressing over insertion exit site

   c. Place transparent dressing over CL site; secure dressing to allow CL catheter to be positioned safely, that is, away from colostomy, gastrostomy, or incision line.

11. Gloves may be removed.

12. Tape bottom edge of dressing to ensure occlusiveness.

   a. Slit piece should measure as long as the lower edge of the dressing.

   b. Cut and place the slit tape in the center of this piece of tape and fit tape around the catheter line at the edge of the transparent dressing.

   c. Chevron piece should be narrow; tape around the catheter to secure in place.

   d. Secure the chevron piece with the third wide strip.

   e. Place the date and time of the dressing change on this final piece along with initials.

CAPPING AND HEPARINIZATION

When an infant has reached the goal of full enteral nutrition, the CL catheter can be capped. This capping allows for future use if necessary. Although hospital policies may vary, the Centers for Disease Control and Prevention recommends changing the cap every 72 hours to prevent bacterial growth. CL catheters are usually heparinized daily, although some multilumen catheters may require flushing as often as every 8 to 12 hours (Vaill, 1990).

CHANGING CAPPING

Gather equipment and clean work area with alcohol.

Equipment Needed

- Mask
- Sterile gloves
- Two sterile barriers
- Sterile gauze pads (3 × 3 inch), four packages
- Pourable povidone-iodine
- Pourable 10 percent rubbing alcohol
- 3.5- or 3-ml syringe without separate needle
- Separate needle or needleless cannula
- One vial heparinized normal saline (2 units/ml)
- One injection cap

Procedure (Kenner, Harjo, & Brueggemeyer, 1988)

1. Wash hands.
2. Clean work area with alcohol.
3. Restrain infant to prevent contamination during procedure.
4. Prepare sterile field (see procedure for IV fluid tubing change).
5. Add syringe and injection cap to sterile field.
6. Place needle or syringe cannula on the edge of sterile field.

7. Swab the top of the heparinized normal saline vial with alcohol sponge.
8. Untape CL.
9. Place sterile barrier under CL.
10. Swab the top of the vial with alcohol.
11. Draw up heparinized normal saline:
    a. Glove dominant hand to hold syringe.
    b. Place needle or cannula on the syringe with ungloved hand and remove covering needle cap without touching syringe or needle.
    c. Hold heparinized normal saline vial with ungloved hand.
    d. Fill syringe with gloved hand; draw up 2 ml and place syringe with needle or cannula on sterile field of heparinized normal saline.
    e. Place glove on nondominant hand.
12. Fill injection cap with heparinized normal saline, leaving syringe with needle or cannula syringe attached.
13. Carefully remove all air bubbles in cap.
14. Scrub the junction of the CL catheter and injection cap (see procedure for IV fluid tubing change).
15. Change the cap:
    a. Pinch-clamp CL catheter.
    b. Holding one sterile gauze pad, remove old cap using a sterile gauze pad; remove old injection cap.
    c. Pick up new cap with syringe and drip several drops of heparinized normal saline into the hub of the CL catheter to prevent air bubbles.
16. Apply new injection cap:
    a. Attach new cap to the catheter and release pinch-clamp in line.
    b. Inject heparinized normal saline into the catheter.
    c. As the last 0.25 ml of solution is injected, slowly withdraw the syringe needle from the injection cap. You may clamp the line before removing the syringe from the cap. Both methods are used to prevent aspirating blood into the catheter and possibly causing clotting.
17. Tape connection and secure to patient.

HEPARINIZATION

Equipment Needed

- One vial heparinized normal saline solution (2 units/ml)
- Two sterile alcohol swab sticks
- One sterile povidone-iodine swab stick
- 2- or 3-ml syringe with needle or needleless cannula

Procedure (Kenner, Harjo, & Brueggemeyer, 1988)

1. Wash hands.
2. Untape CL catheter.
3. Restrain patient to prevent contamination during procedure.
4. Swab top of heparinized normal saline vial with alcohol sponge.

5. Draw up 2 ml heparinized normal saline for injection.
6. Scrub top of injection cap port for 1 minute; scrub port with povidone-iodine swab stick for 1 minute.
7. Allow to air dry for 1 minute.
8. Scrub top of injection cap for 1 minute; scrub port with alcohol swab stick for 1 minute.
9. Inject heparinized normal saline into CL through injection cap.
10. As the last 0.25 ml is injected, slowly withdraw the syringe, withdraw the needle from the injection cap, or clamp catheter before withdrawing syringe. These steps will prevent aspiration of blood into the catheter and possible clotting.
11. Tape connection.
12. Secure CL catheter to patient.

●●●●●●●●●●●●●●●●●●●●●
Aspirating a Clotted Line

This procedure may be necessary to safely aspirate a clot and restore patency to the CL. This procedure is not frequently used, and the nurse should be very cautious when attempting to aspirate a clot. Central venous catheter resource nurses and members of the nutritional support team experienced in this procedure may need to assist when a clot aspiration is necessary.

Equipment Needed

- Mask
- Sterile gloves
- Two sterile barriers for field
- Sterile gauze pads (3 × 3 inch), four packages
- Pourable povidone-iodine
- Pourable 10 percent rubbing alcohol
- One tuberculin syringe without needle
- Two 3-ml syringes without needle
- Two separate needles or needleless cannulas
- One vial of heparinized normal saline solution (2 units/ml); use 2 ml

Procedure (Kenner, Harjo, & Brueggemeyer, 1988)

1. Wash hands.
2. Clean work area with alcohol.
3. Restrain patient to prevent contamination during procedure.
4. Set up sterile field (see procedure for IV tubing change).
5. Add syringes to sterile field.
6. Place needles or cannulas at the edge of sterile field.
7. Swab top of heparinized normal saline vial with alcohol sponge.
8. Draw up heparinized normal saline solution (see IV Tubing Change, Capping CL Catheter).
9. Scrub junction of catheter and tubing (see IV Tubing Change).
10. Pinch-clamp CL catheter.
11. Using one sterile gauze pad, disconnect tubing and place needle or cannula over tubing to maintain sterility.

12. Attach tuberculin syringe to the catheter.
13. Unclamp catheter.
14. Slowly attempt to aspirate clot.
15. Pinch-clamp catheter.
16. Remove clot-filled syringe.
17. Drip several drops of heparinized normal saline into the hub of the catheter and connect syringe to catheter.
18. Attach syringe containing heparinized normal saline to the catheter.
19. Unclamp catheter and flush with heparinized normal saline.
20. Pinch-clamp catheter.
21. Drip several drops of IV fluids into catheter hub; attach tubing.
22. Unclamp catheter and resume IV infusion.

If Unable To Aspirate Clot:

1. Pinch-clamp catheter.
2. Remove tuberculin syringe.
3. Drip several drops of heparinized normal saline solution into the catheter hub of the catheter and attempt to flush catheter GENTLY!!!

If, after several attempts to aspirate and flush or if flush resistance is met, clamp the catheter and leave syringe attached to catheter. Central venous catheter resource nurses or physicians need to be contacted. Notify the nutritional support team (if not already involved) or the physician for further assistance. Instillation of urokinase or other agents to dissolve clots should be done according to hospital policy.

COLOSTOMY CARE

· · · · · · · · · · · · · · · · · · · ·
OSTOMY DRESSINGS

Dressings should be used in the immediate postoperative period to monitor the integrity of the stoma. When the condition of the stoma is no longer dark or bleeding and stool has been passed, ostomy pouches may be used. Dressings may also be needed any time that skin excoriation occurs.

Equipment Needed
- Absorbent square gauze pads
- Soap and water; towel, and washcloth
- Petrolatum (Vaseline) gauze
- Protective cream
- Surgical mask (tie type) with metal wire removed (to avoid discomfort or injury to the infant); any securing device may be used to avoid using tape (e.g., Montgomery straps, twill tape ties, or surgical mask; avoid tape because this may result in skin breakdown).

Procedure (Kenner, Harjo, & Brueggemeyer, 1988)

1. Change dressing at least every 4 hours to monitor the condition of the stoma and the surrounding skin.

2. Carefully remove old dressings; moisten as needed to prevent irritation to the stoma and skin.
3. Clean area around stoma carefully to remove any drainage to avoid irritation:
    a. Wash with mild soap and water and dry thoroughly; liberally apply protective cream around stoma.
    b. Monitor stoma for bleeding and/or discoloration.
    c. Wrap petrolatum gauze around stoma to keep moist.
    d. Observe surrounding skin for further excoriation.
    e. Liberally apply protective cream to surrounding skin.
    f. Place absorbent gauze pads around and over stoma; secure dressings.

POUCHES (BAGS)

The pouch is a clear plastic device that fits around the stoma, allowing modification for individual patients, to collect stool. The bottom is open to allow emptying without removing the bag. It can be closed with a rubber band or other closure devices. There are several types of pouch-wafer systems available. Some pouches are permanently attached to the protective wafer. These one-piece appliances are easier to apply. A two-piece system requires the application of a protective wafer to the pouch. Pouches are used as soon as the infant is stooling consistently and for home care.

Equipment Needed

- Byram premie pouch or other small ostomy appliance that allows modification for individual patients
- Protective wafer for two-piece systems
- Sharp scissors
- Pattern for stoma size
- Soap and water; towel, and washcloth
- Skin preparation/sealant: spray, liquid, gel, or wipes
- Skin barrier: Stomahesive or karaya paste

Procedure (Kenner, Harjo, & Brueggemeyer, 1988)

1. Change pouch when loose or leaking. Any stool that is allowed to remain on the surrounding skin will cause excoriation.
2. Prepare one-piece pouch:
    a. Measure stoma.
    b. Cut appropriate-sized opening in pouch, ensuring the fit is not too tight for stoma but not leaving surrounding skin unprotected.
3. Prepare two-piece pouch.
    a. Cut protective wafer to the size of pouch.
    b. Measure stoma.
    c. Cut appropriate sized openings in pouch, as noted with one-piece pouch.
4. Carefully remove old pouch by gently pulling from skin.
5. Clean around stoma and dry well. Monitor for any skin breakdown. Observe stoma for prolapse or retraction.
6. Cut Stomahesive square to fit adherent base of pouch.

7. Measure stoma; cut appropriate-sized opening in Stomahesive and pouch.
8. Apply skin preparation/sealant to skin and allow to dry.
9. If skin breakdown is present, apply protective barrier.
10. Remove paper from adhesive part of pouch and attach nonadherent side of protective wafer to pouch.
11. Apply prepared pouch to skin, fitting opening securely around stoma.
12. Position the pouch on the abdomen so that it lies to the patient's side and away from CL site, gastrostomy tube, or incisions.
13. Fold bottom of pouch several times and clamp with available closure system.

Empty the pouch several times a day, when half full with stool or if air is accumulating. Unfold the ends of the pouch and drain stool; cleaning the ends of the pouch before refolding. It may be beneficial, especially in terms of home care, to have a number of pouches precut for ease of changing when the bag becomes loose or leaks.

GASTROSTOMY CARE

A gastrostomy tube (GT) may be placed as an aid to gastric decompression after any bowel resection, such as occurs with necrotizing enterocolitis or the various intestinal atresias, and after the closure of an omphalocele or gastroschisis. To prevent reflux of gastric contents through a tracheoesophageal fistula, a GT may be inserted.

GTs are inserted for infants who are not able to suck and/or swallow enough for adequate nutrition. These infants may have problems with their mouth (e.g., a cleft palate); esophagus (e.g., esophageal atresia); stomach (e.g., gastroesophageal reflux); intestines (e.g., necrotizing enterocolitis, omphalocele/gastroschisis, bowel obstructions); heart surgery; prolonged ventilator dependency; or neurologic deficits. Feedings can be given as a bolus or continuously.

Various types of GTs can be used. Malecot catheters are soft and have a mushroom end that allows the tube to stay in place. Foley catheters and MIC (Medical Innovations Corporation, 1990) catheters have a balloon that is inflated to hold it in place.

Routine gastrostomy care focuses on the prevention of infection and avoidance of displacement. Care is usually performed only once per day. If excessive drainage is noted or skin breakdown is present, the care should be increased to two to three times per day, which may also assist with difficulties encountered with feeding. Gastric decompression may be accomplished with a GT after any bowel resection, such as occurs with necrotizing enterocolitis or the various intestinal atresias. The closure of an omphalocele or gastroschisis requires gastric decompression, which can be facilitated with a GT.

The prevention of reflux of gastric contents through a tracheoesophageal fistula requires the insertion of a GT. As a feeding aid, the GT may be used to deliver continuous gastric feedings for those infants unable to tolerate the load of a bolus feeding. This intolerance occurs after resection of bowel, as occurs in necrotizing enterocolitis or intestinal atresias, as well as after repair of an omphalocele or gastroschisis. For the infant with short bowel syndrome, the GT with continuous gastric feedings is a necessity.

The GT can be used to assist in bolus feedings when the infant is unable to consume total bottle feedings. This may occur with the repair of a tracheoesophageal fistula or diaphragmatic hernia.

The routine care of a GT focuses on the prevention of infection and the avoidance of displacement.

ROUTINE GASTROSTOMY CARE

Routine gastrostomy care is usually done only once a day. If excessive drainage or skin breakdown is present, the care should be increased to two or three times a day until the condition improves.

Equipment Needed

- Two strips of ½-inch adhesive tape, 3 to 4 inches long
- Two strips of 1-inch paper/micropore tape, 5 to 6 inches long
- Hydrogen peroxide
- Cotton-tipped applicators
- Clean towel or gauze sponge
- Baby-bottle nipple or other securing device
- One package 2 × 2-inch gauze dressing, if needed

Procedure (Kenner, Harjo, Brueggemeyer, 1988) (Fig. 30–2)

1. Wash hands.
2. Gather supplies.
3. Cut tapes to desired lengths.
4. Pour a small amount of hydrogen peroxide into a clean container. (If skin appears irritated, use one-half strength by mixing equal amounts of water with hydrogen peroxide.)
5. Prepare nipple: cut tip off and cut small holes at each notch of the nipple.
6. Nipple should be changed every week or if soiled. Slide new nipple onto tube while infant is quiet. Restrain infant as needed.
7. Remove old tape and nipple; keeping one hand on the base of the tube to prevent dislodgment.
8. Dry skin around tube.
9. Slide new nipple onto tube.
10. Apply adhesive tape (see Fig. 30–2):
    a. Fold down each end of tape to make tabs for easy removal.
    b. Place one piece on each side of tube.
    c. Do not twist tape around tube, just press tape down the side. This will prevent dislodgment of tube with care.
    d. Change position of tape every day to minimize skin irritation.
    e. Clean tube and the surrounding skin with applicators soaked with hydrogen peroxide until all drainage is removed.
11. Apply strips of adhesive tape, one on each side of tube; fold down top edge of tape to make tab.

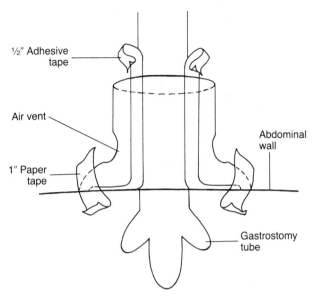

FIGURE 30–2. Gastrostomy tube.

    a. Do not twist tape around tube, just press down the side of the
       tube onto the skin (for ease of removal with next dressing change).
    b. Change position of these tapes daily to minimize skin irritation.
12. If needed, place 2 × 2-inch gauze dressing around base of tube next
    to skin.
13. After removing old nipple, slide clean nipple down to skin.
14. Apply strips of paper/micropore tapes:
    a. Fold down ends of tape to form tabs.
    b. Tape one piece on each side of nipple to hold in place. Two pieces
       may not be sufficient for an active infant, one on each side. Tape
       over edges of the nipple to secure.
15. Change position of these tapes daily to minimize skin irritation.

ROUTINE CARE FOR MIC (MEDICAL INNOVATION CORPORATION) TUBES

Equipment Needed (See Care of Malecot and Foley
Catheters)

- No tape is required.
- Use 2 × 2-inch gauze dressings only if necessary.
- No nipple is needed.

Procedure

Daily care should be performed as noted for Malecot and Foley catheters. The area under the Secur-Lok ring next to the skin should also be carefully cleansed. This ring needs to be rotated with each cleaning. Remember to always dry the skin thoroughly after care. These tubes do not require any taping.

DISLODGMENT OF THE GASTROSTOMY TUBE

1. Don't panic!
2. Cover the stoma with a gauze dressing, cloth diaper, or washcloth to absorb gastric contents.
3. Take the infant to the pediatrician's office, if appropriate (some pediatricians are skilled in GT reinsertion), or the emergency department to have the tube reinserted.
4. Bring the old tube with you so that the correct size can be reinserted.
5. Replacement of the GT should be done within 4 hours, before the tract becomes narrowed or closes, to allow for ease of insertion.
6. Occasionally, parents may be taught to reinsert the GT. This should be discussed with the physician before discharge.
7. Hospital replacement should be performed by a surgeon or someone experienced in GT placements.
8. After discharge the infant may need to come to the emergency department for placement of tube. Pediatricians, if properly trained, may insert tubes in their office. Parents are taught by some surgeons to reinsert tubes themselves.
9. Always keep an extra tube of the appropriate size available or have the old tube available to identify appropriate size.
10. A GT introducer will be needed to reinsert the tube.
11. Clean site and secure tube appropriately after reinsertion.
12. Radiographic confirmation of proper placement may be done.

CONTINUOUS GASTROSTOMY FEEDING

Infants who do not tolerate bolus feedings due to malabsorption or other intestinal dysfunction will benefit from continuous feedings. These feedings can be given over 24 hours or for shorter periods with windows for oral feedings if tolerated. Pump feedings may be needed for intermittent feedings for those infants who are sensitive to rapid rates of feedings. As previously mentioned, continuous gastrostomy feedings may be used in infants who, because of bowel dysfunction, do not tolerate bolus feedings without malabsorptive consequences.

Equipment Needed

- Kangaroo or feeding bag
- Farrell or reflux bag
- Kangaroo or feeding pump

Procedure

1. Wash hands.
2. Measure appropriate amount of feeding, plus enough to prime tubing. Feedings are usually hung for 8 hours.
3. Connect reflux system to feeding bag and tubing.
4. Prime feeding through tubing displacing all air.
5. Place feeding tubing into the pump. Set infusion, using appropriate rate and volume limit to complete the 8-hour infusion.
6. Set appropriate infusion rate and volume limit.
7. Check gastric aspirates every 4 hours, if needed, to ensure that the infant is tolerant of feedings.

As the infant grows and tolerance of feedings improves, the continuous feedings may be weaned and oral/bolus feedings will be used, supplemented by bolus feedings in anticipation of discharge.

BOLUS GASTROSTOMY FEEDINGS

Equipment Needed

- Large catheter-tipped syringe (35 or 60 ml)
- Measured amount of formula, warmed to room temperature
- Water for flushing tube

Procedure (Kenner, Harjo, & Brueggemeyer, 1988)

1. Wash hands.
2. Position infant on side with head slightly elevated.
3. Connect syringe to GT while clamped.
4. Unclamp GT; pull back on plunger of syringe to check gastric measure stomach aspirates.
5. Reinsert aspirate slowly and reclamp gastrostomy.
6. Hold feeding and notify physician if large amounts of aspirates are above accepted level.
7. If aspirate levels are acceptable, remove plunger from syringe. Place syringe barrel into the gastrostomy tube and unclamp.
8. Pour formula into syringe. Allow formula to slowly flow into tube by gravity over 20 to 30 minutes. Raise or lower the tube to control the flow of feeding.
9. Assess infant throughout feeding for gagging, coughing, or vomiting. If this occurs, slow or stop feeding until infant recovers.
10. Rinse tube with 5 to 10 ml of water after feeding.
11. Reclamp GT and remove syringe. If infant has problems with reflux, is vomiting, and/or has discomfort with feedings, the tube may be vented for 30 to 60 minutes after feeding.
12. Offer a pacifier during the feeding and hold it if tolerated to encourage sucking.
13. Burp infant after feeding is completed.
14. Clean equipment with hot soapy water; rinse thoroughly.
15. Syringes may be reused until rubber tip of plunger becomes stiff, making aspiration difficult, or until the measurements on the syringe are illegible.

DILATIONS

. . . .
ESOPHAGEAL DILATIONS

Dilating the esophagus may be necessary after a repair for esophageal atresia. This dilation is necessary when stenosis occurs at the site of the anastomosis. Stenosis may occur at any time from weeks to months after the repair. Occasionally, dilations are necessary for 1 to 2 years.

Equipment Needed

- Graduated sizes of tapered metal or rubber dilators
- Esophageal string/black suture material
- Lubricating gel

Procedure

Dilations are usually performed under general anesthesia but may be done at the bedside with sedation. Dilators are lubricated and then guided down the esophagus through the nose or the mouth. These dilators are passed out through the gastrostomy site. The size of the dilator is increased after each dilation attempt.

An esophageal string, made with black suture material, may be passed along the dilation path and secured in place to the infant's cheek and gastrostomy site. This allows for ease with future dilations without general anesthesia.

The infant's feeding schedule may be resumed after this procedure after awake from the anesthesia. The esophageal string, if left in place, will not disrupt oral feedings (Kenner, Harjo, & Brueggemeyer, 1988).

. . . .
RECTAL DILATIONS

Dilation of the rectum may be required to establish or maintain the patency of the anus. This may be used when the rectum is completely formed but the anal opening is covered by a membrane. Infants with a rectal fistula or rectal stenosis will also benefit from dilations.

Equipment Needed

- Size 8 to 18 French red rubber catheters.
- Lubricating gel
- Gloves

Procedure (Kenner, Harjo, & Brueggemeyer, 1988)

1. Wash hands.
2. Position infant on abdomen or on side.
3. Individual catheters are lubricated and inserted into the anus to dilate.
4. The size of the dilating catheters may be increased until the desired effect is achieved.
5. Monitor the infant for bleeding after the procedure.
6. Passage of stool must be observed to evaluate the effectiveness of the dilations.

7. Feedings can be resumed after the dilation.
8. If required, parents will be taught this procedure before discharge.

NURSING MANAGEMENT

Use of these procedures varies in scope and magnitude at many institutions. Nursing management must, however, center on procedural policy, daily care, and family teaching.

Policies must be followed carefully to the letter. If nurses find that a particular procedure is lacking or that a particular method is not meeting the patient's/family's needs, policies should be revised or modified.

Staff education needs to be a priority for those who are unfamiliar with this care. Parents are eager to learn and understand their infant's care. Structured teaching sessions along with consistent reinforcement and follow-up and reinforcement are essential. In addition to teaching parents, it can also be beneficial to educate another caregiver (e.g., a grandparent or other relative). Families should be encouraged to take responsibility for their infant's daily care as soon as teaching sessions have been completed so that troubleshooting and problem-solving can take place well in advance of discharge.

REFERENCES

Kenner, C., Harjo, J., & Brueggemeyer, A. (1988). *Neonatal surgery: A nursing perspective*. Orlando, FL: Grune & Stratton.

Medical Innovation Corporation. (1990). *Gastrostomy care for the MIC Gastrostomy Tube*. Milpitas, CA.

Vaill, C. D. (1990). Your complete guide to central venous catheters. *Nursing '90, 20*(2), 34–42.

Long-Term Development of the Neonate

. . . .

Systematic Assessment and Home Follow-Up: A Basis for Monitoring the Neonate's Integration Into the Family Unit

NEED FOR HOME FOLLOW-UP OF PRETERM INFANTS

It has long been known that there is a prevalence of disabling neurodevelopmental conditions among infants of low birth weight (Bennett, 1984; Field & Sostek, 1983). Preterm infants are especially vulnerable because of both their biologic status (i.e., being preterm) and environmental factors that interact to put them at high risk for later problems. Within the home environment, the parent–infant interaction was found to be the best predictive factor for later positive development in preterm infants (Barnard, et al. 1989; Barrera, Rosenbaum, & Cunningham, 1986; Bendersky & Lewis, 1986; Crnic & Greenberg, 1987; Field, 1987; Greenberg & Crnic, 1988; Ramey, Farram, & Campbell, 1979; Schraeder, Rappaport, & Courtwright, 1987).

PRETERM INFANT CHARACTERISTICS AND THEIR EFFECT ON CAREGIVER INTERACTION

Studies comparing term and preterm infants found preterm infants to be different from their full-term counterparts in several ways—ways that have a tremendous influence on the parent–infant interaction. First, preterm infants as a group were found to be less neurologically mature than full-term infants. This lack of maturity produces infants who are less regulatory (organized) in their behavior, making it harder to understand and predict how they will behave. This lack of neurologic maturity is directly related to how premature they are—the younger the preterm infant gestationally, the less mature and the more disorganized the infant. Second, preterm infants as a group exhibited a lower level of behavioral social responsiveness, were less persistent and adaptable, and tended to respond in more negative ways than full-term infants (Anders & Keener, 1985; Barnard, 1980; Barnard & Bee, 1981; Bennett, 1984; Schwartz, Horowitz, & Mitchell, 1984; Tekolste & Bennett, 1987; Telzrow et al., 1982).

These characteristics result in infants who give hard-to-read cues, making it difficult for their parents to know when to feed, when to soothe, when to leave them alone, and when to play with them. Preterm infants, sensitive to stimuli and limited in energy reserves, respond to their parents' attempt to interact by turning away, dropping off to sleep, or crying inconsolably, behavior that parents see as negative and difficult to cope with and under-stand. If we think of parent–infant interaction as a sort of "dance" in which each participant (here parent and infant) must give clear and readable cues that can be read by the partner, be motorically and neurologically alert to respond quickly and positively to the partner's cues, and retain enough energy to keep the dance going in a smooth and rhythmical way, we can see why interacting (dancing) with a preterm infant may not be the positive experience most parents expect it to be. Because parents often expect their preterm infant to behave like a full-term infant, they become confused when this does not occur. In essence, a parent is dancing with a partner who does not hold up his or her side of the dance duo, resulting in dyssynchrony and discord. Even the most positive of parents can lose confidence in their ability to parent.

These characteristics of giving unclear cues and being more negative and less socially responsive may also account for the report by parents of preterm infants that they are harder to care for and have a more difficult tempera-ment than full-term infants. Several researchers have studied the tempera-ment of preterm infants. In general, their findings suggest that older (34 to 37 weeks), heavier (>1200 g), and healthier preterm infants show no differ-ences in temperament from term infants by parent report, whereas the younger (<34 weeks), lighter (<1200 g), and sicker preterm infants are described by parents as being more difficult in temperament than those in reports by parents of full-term infants.

These characteristics seem to affect strongly the adaptation between these infants and their caregivers. However, parents who are aware, understand, and adapt to the behavioral and temperament characteristics of their preterm infant report that their preterm infants are easier to care for and more enjoyable to be around. Unfortunately, not all parents are able to adapt.

PARENTAL RESPONSE TO THEIR PRETERM INFANT'S BEHAVIOR

Parental burnout, superparent syndrome, vulnerable child syndrome, and higher potential for child abuse are four phenomena described in the literature as maladaptive responses by parents possibly related to the behaviors of preterm infants. Beckwith and Cohen (1980) first described parental burnout in their follow-up study of preterm infants. They found that the level of maternal responsiveness changes over time and is related to the infant's behavior. Generally, in normal full-term infants, the more responsive the infant, the more responsive the mother. However, they found that preterm infants who had more health problems and who were more premature tended to have mothers who became less socially responsive over the first year of life. They concluded that there was a need for some reinforcement from the infant to keep the mother responding to her infant's behavior in a positive way. If this reinforcement did not occur, then over time the mother responded less and less. Furthermore, they found that there is a limit to how long parents will respond without any reinforcement. If no reinforcement is forthcoming, parents become exhausted trying and eventually "burn out" (Beckwith & Cohen, 1980).

Maygary (1987), in discussing Beckwith and Cohen's "burnout," describes how some parents when confronted with this low social responsiveness in their infant become "hyperactive" in their interactions. That is, in compensating for the lower level of social responsiveness of the preterm infant, the parent tries harder and harder to get the infant to respond. As the parent heightens his or her response, the infant withdraws further, becoming less and less responsive in an attempt to deal with the increased stimulation. This "superparent syndrome," as Maygary describes it, leads to the parental burnout described by Beckwith and Cohen, in which the parent eventually gives up when the responsiveness needed by the infant does not occur (Maygary, 1987). When maladaptation between the infant and the caregiver occurs, as in the case of parental burnout and the superparent syndrome, then the positive integration of the infant into the family unit suffers.

Vulnerable child syndrome, a term first coined by Green and Solnit in 1964, has been associated with preterm infants (Culley, Perrin, & Chaberski, 1989; Macey, Harmon, & Easterbrooks, 1987; McCormick, Shapiro, & Starfield, 1982; Perrin, West, & Culley, 1989). In this phenomenon, parents continue to see their infant as vulnerable (susceptibility to a negative outcome) despite evidence to the contrary—that the infant is physically and developmentally normal. This results in maladaptive behavior both on the part of the parent (usually the mother) and the infant. Reported parental behaviors include overprotectiveness (i.e., less willingness to leave infant alone, discouragement of infant exploration), skewed perception of the infant's capabilities, and frequent visits to the hospital or clinic. Behaviors reported in infants and children include less exploration, infantilization, separation anxiety, and psychosocial problems such as somatic complaints and problems in school (Bidder, Crowe, & Gray, 1974; Forsyth & Canny, 1985; Jeffcoate, Humphrey, & Lloyd; 1979; Levy, 1984; Macey, Harmon, & Easterbrooks, 1987; McCormick, Shapiro, & Starfield, 1982).

Another phenomenon reported to be associated with preterm infants is child abuse. As with the other three phenomena discussed, reasons for the increased risk of abuse seem to be the combination of infant behavioral characteristics (irritability, lack of clear cues, and low social responsiveness) and certain parental experiences and characteristics (lack of social support, history of violence as a child or with a spouse, insensitivity to their child, annoyance or anger when the infant cries). However, rather than reacting with a lack of responsiveness to the infant (parental burnout), an increase in infant stimulation (superparent syndrome), or overprotectiveness (vulnerable child syndrome), the parent instead abuses the child (Beckwith, 1990; Clark, 1989; Elmer & Gregg, 1967; Klein & Stern, 1979; Ricciuti, 1983; Schmitt & Kempe, 1975).

SYSTEMATIC ASSESSMENTS

An important component of any follow-up is the use of systematic assessment. Systematic assessment is the use of validated measures to organize the collection of information that can be used to promote strengths, identify concerns, and suggest areas for further evaluation or referral (Barnard, Eyres, Lobo, & Snyder, 1983). Bailey and Simeonsson (1988) identified the home environment and parent–infant interaction as important areas to include in any family assessment related to early intervention.

Tekolste and Bennett (1987) identified areas in which nurses could make a difference in home follow-up. Areas included (1) monitoring and providing support, instructions, and problem solving in the areas of feeding, weight gain and growth, sleeping, and developmental and behavioral concerns, and (2) as a complementary liaison with the primary care physician (Tekolste & Bennett, 1987). Based on these findings, it seems logical then to use measures that assess those areas needed and not being universally monitored, such as sleep–wake organization, parent–infant interaction, and conditions of the home environment.

Nursing Child Assessment Satellite Training Scales

An important aspect of any assessment measure is that it be married to the realities of the health care system, that is, the measure should be easy to use, complement current practice, provide information (for both professional and client), and assess factors found through research to be predictive of a child's later development. In addition, measures should address areas of parent concern to ensure the interest and motivation of the parent in incorporating whatever recommendations are warranted from the assessment (Delerian, 1988). The Nursing Child Assessment Satellite Training (NCAST) scales are examples of assessment measures that fit these criteria. Developed under the direction of Dr. Kathryn Barnard, a nurse, they are a result of her research examining characteristics present in families early on that predicted later child outcomes. In addition to assessing the areas of sleep–wake organization, feeding, parent–infant interaction, and the home environment, these scales are useful as a clinical tool to (1) provide information and support to the parent; (2) document the infant and parent current behavior; and (3) provide information about predictability of behavior over time, support for positive behavior, and improvement in problem areas when repeated measurements of the same assessment are used (Barnard, et al., 1989; Bee et al., 1982; Censullo, 1986; Johnson-Crowley & Sumner, 1987a; Ruff, 1987).

Another advantage is that assessments completed over time generate a picture of the child's changing behavior in a realistic way. This cuts down on exaggeration or understatement of the infant's problems and helps produce a more realistic perception of the infant for the parents.

Professionals find these assessments clinically useful because they help organize the home visit and give them a baseline from which to identify the following:

- The developing sleep–wake patterns
- The appropriateness of the amount and type of infant feedings
- Areas of strength to build the parents' confidence in the care of their infant
- Problem areas and areas of concern to be relayed to the parent
- When and where further assessments need to be performed
- Documented evidence of the behavior of the parent and the child (Johnson-Crowley & Sumner, 1987a, 1987b)

Studies using these scales have found correlations with later cognitive performance and behavioral outcomes (Barnard & Eyres, 1977, 1979; Barnard, Booth, Mitchell, & Telzrow, 1983a, 1983b; Eyres, Barnard, & Gray, 1979; Gottfried, 1984; Hammond, Bee, Barnard, & Eyres, 1983; Slater, Naqvi, Andrew, & Haynes, 1987). The four NCAST assessments are described in the following sections.

Nursing Child Assessment Sleep–Activity Record

The Nursing Child Assessment Sleep–Activity (NCASA) record is a 24-hour record that requires the parent (or caregiver) to keep an hour-by-hour record of the infant's sleep and activity for 1 week (Barnard, 1987). The record is set up in graph form with each square representing 60 minutes. Caregivers record sleep–wake times; when the child is content and when the child is fussy or crying, feeding, or playing; and any other activity for which the parent or nurse identifies a need. An advantage of this record is that symbols are used to represent the activities recorded (Fig. 31–1). The use of symbols has made it useful for those parents and caregivers who have little education, difficulty reading, or are non–English speaking (Johnson-Crowley, 1988).

Because the NCASA record is completed over 24 hours and can be filled out week after week, it generates a picture of the child's "increasing temporal integration of activities" (Barnard, 1989). This change means that over time one can see the neuromaturational behavior of the infant—a relative de-

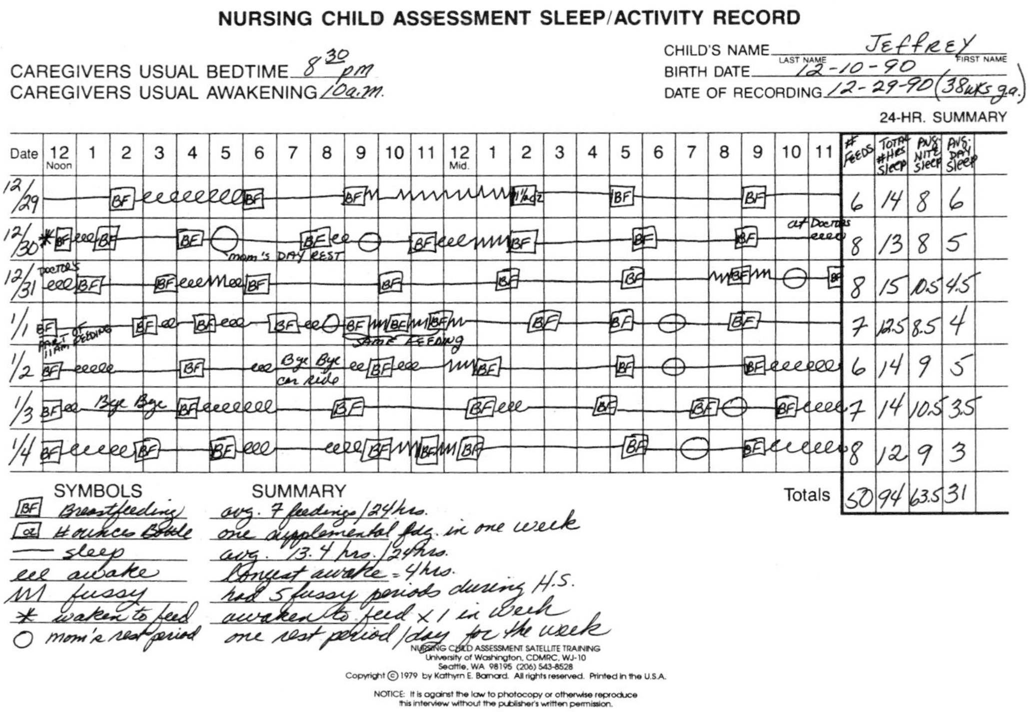

FIGURE 31-1. NCASA record completed by mother of a preterm infant, 38 weeks' gestational age. (Courtesy of Kathryn E. Barnard.)

crease in the amount of feedings and night awakenings in infants as they grow and mature. With this decrease comes an increase in the amount of time spent awake and more time for play and parent–infant interaction. Parents have found the NCASA record useful in organizing their activities and providing an ongoing view of their infant's changing behavior, which is an important process for parents of preterm infants, in whom developmental strides may be slow and seemingly nonexistent at times (Johnson-Crowley, 1986).

Nursing Child Assessment Feeding Scale

Whereas the NCASA scale gives a picture of the amount and frequency of feedings the infant is getting, the Nursing Child Assessment Feeding Scale (NCAFS) assesses certain tasks that the parent and the child have for ensuring a positive interactional relationship during feeding, so that the feeding is set in as positive an atmosphere as possible for both parent and child (Barnard, 1987; Barnard & Kelly, 1990). For preterm infants and their families, who may experience feeding as a long, arduous, and often negative process, this scale can provide a very important way to change conditions so that the feeding is a more positive experience. If one realizes that during the early months of life the feeding episode may provide the only times the preterm infant is awake and one of the few times the parent and infant are together and interacting for any length of time, it becomes additionally important that this be as pleasant a time as possible (especially for the parent), because it may set the stage for later interactions (Johnson-Crowley & Sumner, 1987a).

Areas of assessment include the infant's ability to provide clear cues to the parent and respond appropriately and positively to the parent's attempt to interact. For the parents, their abilities during the feeding to be sensitive to the infant's cues, respond sympathetically to any distress the infant might experience, provide social and emotional activities that are affectionate and social, and present activities that enhance the infant's cognitive development are assessed as well.

The NCAFS works well as a follow-up to the use of the NCASA record should any feeding difficulties be identified. For instance, should a review of the NCASA record reveal that a breastfeeding preterm infant is getting fewer than the recommended number of feedings per day and discussions with the parent reveal difficulties in getting the infant to eat, then use of the NCAFS may reveal areas in the parent–infant interaction that may be affecting this, such as the parent's inability to read the infant cues (Johnson-Crowley & Sumner, 1987a, 1987b). Use of the NCAFS after discussion of the NCASA record is an example of how assessment measures can complement and build on one another, providing information related to a similar topic (in this case feeding) but in different areas. In this way a more comprehensive view of the parent, infant, and the situation is obtained by using multiple assessment measures, making assessment, intervention, and evaluation easier and more complete.

Nursing Child Assessment Teaching Scale

The Nursing Child Assessment Teaching Scale (NCATS) assesses the interaction between parent and child while the parent is teaching the child a simple task (Barnard, 1987; Barnard & Kelly, 1990). Although the tasks are chosen by the observer, the parent chooses how he or she wishes to present and teach the task. The areas assessed are similar to those in the NCAFS scale just described, but around a different topic, teaching instead of feeding. Both the NCAFS and NCATS have been shown to be reliable and valid measurements of the parent–infant interaction. Although both assessments measure parent–infant interaction, analysis of the assessments has shown that they offer different and important glimpses of the parent–infant interaction (Barnard et al., 1989).

There are other differences as well. First, the NCAFS (feeding) assessment takes as long as a feeding lasts, possibly 15 minutes to more than an hour; the NCATS (teaching) assessment is brief, usually lasting between 1 and 5 minutes. The NCAFS is validated for use up to 12 months of an infant's life, whereas the NCATS can be performed up to age 36 months (Barnard et al., 1989). The investigators point out that the feeding situation, because it occurs six times a day, 7 days a week, may be a more familiar, well-rehearsed situation that places few demands on the parent–infant pair. The teaching situation, in contrast, set up by the observer, is more novel in approach and places some stress on the parent–infant interaction, possibly resulting in more restrictive behavior on the part of the parent (Barnard & Kelly, 1990; Barnard et al., 1989). Barnard and colleagues (1989) state, "Added together, the two scales give us a richer look at the interactive patterns than either taken separately, but each can be used independently when the situation calls for or allows only one" (p. 47). In addition, the NCAFS (feeding) is useful for measuring parent–infant interaction only as long as the infant and parent are involved in the feeding situation. When the infant is older (older than 1 year), most parents allow infants to feed themselves while parents are engaged in other activities. At this time, the NCATS may be more useful to get a more accurate picture of the parent–infant interaction.

Home Observation for Measurement of the Environment

This instrument, designed by Caldwell, Bradley, and their colleagues, measures "the quality and quantity of support for cognitive, social and emotional development available to the child in the home environment" (Bradley & Caldwell, 1988, p. 97). This assessment is administered using a combination of interview and observation. Both the animate (i.e., people) and the inanimate (e.g., toys) aspects of the home environment are assessed (Caldwell & Snyder, 1978). A review of several studies using the Home Observation for Measurement of the Environment (HOME) assessment measure has demonstrated that the HOME is a powerful predictor of later cognitive skills both in term and preterm infants (Gottfried, 1984). Its ease of use, broad perspective, and extensive use in research make it a popular assessment measure in clinical practice.

Used together in any home follow-up program, the NCASA, NCAFS, NCATS, and HOME assessments offer a way for the health care professional to monitor the ongoing integration of the preterm infant into the family unit by identifying strengths that increase a parent's confidence and competence, assessing systematically those areas found problematic for this population, providing organization to clinical practice, planning individual intervention, measuring outcomes, and, most important, providing a way to give support and direction to the parents related to caregiving for their child.

HOME-BASED PROTOCOLS: PRETERM INFANTS AND FAMILIES

Home follow-up of preterm infants and their families needs to attach the assessment component to a plan of prevention and intervention. This plan should entail a predesigned set of protocols outlining strategies of care. Protocols set up plans of care that are based on the population being served but allow flexibility to take into account individual differences. For instance, in the case of the preterm infant, these protocols of care would involve instructions for monitoring weight and growth parameters. Feeding issues and sleep–wake organization would also be included. Although these protocols would be based on the needs of preterm infants and their families, they should include components important to the growth and development of any infant. Protocols have been found to be extremely useful in organizing nursing practice and creating satisfaction in providing care and increasing optimal parenting (Barnard, 1985). In a report on five nurse entrepreneurs, four of the five described the use of nursing protocols as an aid to their practice (Hartman, 1988).

There is much evidence in support of providing prevention and intervention-type programs for families with preterm infants. Patteson and Barnard (1990), in a comprehensive review of intervention programs, found 16 of the 19 studies identified had positive outcomes. Elements believed to be effective in producing these positive results included the use of both hospital and home contacts or home contacts alone and the enlistment and involvement of the parent in the intervention and in interaction with the child. Urging further research in the area of infant intervention, Patteson and Barnard (1990) stated that continued focus should be on "testing ways to help parents cope with the emotional crises of having a low birth weight infant, enhancing positive interactions with their infant, and increasing their knowledge of infant developmental and care needs" (p. 53).

Nursing Systems Toward Effective Parenting—Preterm

Nursing Systems Toward Effective Parenting—Preterm (NSTEP-P) is an example of one type of parent-focused home follow-up intervention program designed specifically to address the problems of parenting a preterm infant. A component of this program is specific protocols of care that help the nurse get organized, allowing him or her to meet the needs of the family in a way that is comfortable, thorough, supportive, and efficient, thereby increasing nurse satisfaction. The original NSTEP-P program was developed in 1984, through a Continuing Education Grant from Maternal-Child Health Service (Grant #MCJ-009035-01-0), the University of Washington, Department of Parent and Child Nursing, under the direction of Dr. Kathryn Barnard, to test the efficacy of providing nursing services to preterm infants and their families. The nursing protocol that was an integral part of the program was based on research of preterm infants, parenting, and "ecology" of infants and families previously discussed in this chapter (Barnard, 1985).

This home follow-up program was tested in six sites across the nation and involved 23 public health nurses making eight home visits at specific times. Evaluation data were collected and analyzed on 76 mothers and their preterm infants. The results from this research indicated that the program was successful. Nurses reported that it was helpful to their practice. In addition, measures used to assess parent–infant interaction (NCAFS and NCATS) demonstrated that the techniques used to modulate the infant's sleep–wake state had significantly improved the parent–infant interaction. Additional measures of family function, perceived support, and child growth and development were all positive. Follow-up of a subset of these children revealed higher scores on the NCATS, NCAFS, and HOME measurements at 24 months of chronologic age than there were at 5 months of corrected age. Denver Developmental Screening Test (DDST) scores revealed that 95 percent of the children tested normal at 24 months of chronologic age in the area of fine motor, gross motor, and personal-social development. In the area of language, all of the children were normal (Johnson-Crowley, 1987).

A revised version is being tested with a population of low socioeconomic parents and their preterm infants. Although the final results are still pending, components of the original program included in the present program continue to show positive results (Barnard, 1989).

OVERVIEW

The overall framework for the NSTEP-P program is the therapeutic relationship in which the nurse structures the interaction to be sensitive to the parents' need while at the same time providing information that will help them learn parenting techniques for the preterm infant who has difficulty feeding, tends to have a less well-organized state regulation, and tends not to be responsive to the caregiver (Johnson-Crowley & Sumner, 1987b).

The protocols designed as part of the NSTEP-P program are intended to complement a health agency's current strategy of care. Nurses are encouraged to use their agency's routines as well as to incorporate any existing preterm follow-up programs in the community. Although comprehensive in scope, the NSTEP-P program is not designed to take the place of physician/ nurse visits. In fact, an important part of this program is to monitor families to make sure that they continue to see their physicians for well-child check-ups or for specific health concerns (Johnson-Crowley, 1988).

CONTENT

The program is built on the established characteristics and problems of the preterm infant reported in research and is centered around two main areas: content for the family and content for the health professional.

Content for the Family

As might be expected, issues involving health and state modulation (especially in relation to feeding) take priority early in the program, with less time spent discussing the other content areas. Later, as the problems and concerns in health and state modulation resolve, the content areas of parent–infant interaction and the infant's environment become more paramount. Parental coping and support continues to be a focus throughout the entire home visit program.

Health-Related Concerns. These issues have to do with feeding and nutrition, safety and temperature, illness and infection control, and growth and development. Special health problems more common to the preterm infant are also included, such as anemia, hernias, and vision and hearing problems.

State Modulation. This involves infant state organization, alertness, maintaining state arousal, and stimulation related to the state of the infant.

Parent–Infant Interaction. This area covers behavioral cues, behavioral differences, parent–infant interaction, importance in developing social competence in children, and the preterm infant's effect on his or her caregiver.

Infant's Environment. This content includes stimulation as provided by the animate and inanimate environment, elements of parent involvement, the important role of fathers and siblings, stimulation of the preterm infant, and the importance of playing with and enjoying the infant.

Parental Coping and Support. This content involves parental support (family and professional networks), problem-solving, stress appraisal, parental coping, and the challenges of parenting a preterm infant.

Content for the Health Care Professional

Systematic assessments are given special emphasis because they are critical to the delivery and evaluation of the NSTEP-P program. During delivery of the program, assessments (infant health, parent–infant interaction, parental support, and the home environment) identify potential problems before they develop and delineate when intervention would be most effective. During evaluation, systematic assessments document accomplishment of program goals and promote professional accountability. Assessments found important to the success of the NSTEP-P program are anthropometric measures, including height, weight, and head circumference, as well as measures of developmental assessment; the NCAST assessment measures, including the NCASA, NCAFS, NCATS, and HOME; and the network survey, a measurement of the family's support network, including a section assessing support from family, friends, and coworkers and a section assessing support from health agencies and health care professionals.

Therapeutic Process. This content involves contract setting, therapeutic relationships, and closure (termination) with families.

Intervention Strategies. These strategies involve the use of systematic assessments, prescriptions of care, and integrated handouts.

Structured Protocols. These protocols involve the organization of practice, step-by-step home visiting instructions, and detailed record keeping.

STRUCTURE

The NSTEP-P program involves a series of home visits starting from hospital discharge to 5 months of corrected age. One visit is designed to be made before the infant's discharge from the hospital to aid transition to home, and a "check-in" visit is scheduled between 9 and 12 months of corrected age to monitor the progress of the family. More visits are made in the beginning, when the parents are most anxious and desirous of contact. As the infant matures and parental confidence increases, the visits are spaced farther apart. More visits may occur during the home visit program and after the program has concluded, depending on the needs of the family and at the discretion of the home visitor. This allows for flexibility and takes into account the individual differences and needs of each family.

FORMAT

Presentation of the content information is formulated around a structured format that is consistent from visit to visit. This format, which includes a brief introduction, review of previous content, presentation of new content, summary of the visit, anticipatory guidance, nursing prescriptions, and termination, provides structure for the NSTEP-P families during a period of family disorganization and disequilibrium. This structure and consistency allow nurses and parents to know what to expect with each visit, which reduces the possibility of ambiguity, confusion, and miscommunication. Having clearly defined role expectations helps lessen the parent's need to mobilize additional energy for the nurse's visits.

PARENT HANDOUTS

Handouts are an important source of information for parents. When designed well (a key point), handouts present much of the information—some of it complex—in a format that is easy to read and geared to the interest and education level of the parent. Whenever possible, pictures are used rather than words to convey the information. Use of pictures is critical, because parents who might be exhausted and overburdened do not need pages of material to read when important information can be presented simply, visually, and attractively.

Designed for parents with an eighth grade education, these handouts would be a problem for parents who cannot read at an eighth grade level or for those who do not read English. However, because the protocol requires that the content of the handouts be explained fully, most professionals have found them applicable for those with less than an eighth grade education. Parents who do not read English often have found another family member to translate the information if they see the value in that information.

Most handouts present information related to the content, but handouts can be used in additional ways, such as the following:

- An avenue for assessment of the infant by the nurse or parent
- A means for the nurse to model appropriate behavior for the parent
- A way to transmit information to other members of the family or support network

• A record for the parent and nurse of the home visit

In the NSTEP-P program all of these functions—providing information, assessing the infant, modeling behavior, relaying information to other family members, and recording the visit—are promoted through handouts (Johnson-Crowley, 1988b).

The *Symptoms of Illness* handout is an example of a handout designed as a means for the nurse to model appropriate behavior for the parent and for assessing certain behaviors in the infant. This checklist-type handout is designed with a list of symptoms that might be seen should the child become ill or have some other health problem. It is used by the nurse during a home visit if the parent states the child might be ill. The nurse systematically reviews the list of symptoms in an attempt to identify exactly what behavior the infant is exhibiting that makes the parent believe the child is ill. The nurse then discusses the list with the parent and provides feedback as to whether the child's symptoms bear monitoring, are serious enough to warrant seeing the physician, or are not worrisome. Modeling by the nurse gives a chance for the parent to observe how the form is to be used and is an effective mechanism for the nurse to gather important data about the child, as well as to point out what information is important to communicate to the physician. Blank copies of the form are left with the parents to fill out, so that when they call the physician or make a clinic visit they have an accurate list of the infant's symptoms that required physician attention. When the form is used in this way, the physician gets accurate information and parental confidence is increased.

Another parent handout, the *Parent Activities Sheet*, is an example of a handout that can be used as a record of the home visit. On this sheet, important information about the infant is recorded, such as the infant's current age, weight, height, and head circumference, as well as when the next visit to the physician or clinic is scheduled. Activities and content discussed throughout the visit are listed, as well as suggestions made for problems or concerns the parent and the nurse addressed. Nursing prescriptions written down outline information to read and areas for the parent to follow up until the nurse's next visit. Finally, referrals are listed along with the scheduled date, day, and time of the next visit. Spaces for the nurse's name, agency, and telephone number are also filled in. These forms are produced so that a carbon copy is made. The nurse keeps one copy, and another copy is given to the parent.

The copy for the nurse becomes a record of the nurse's visits and in some agencies is placed in the child's chart, giving clear documentation of what was accomplished (or not accomplished) during the visit. Nurses who use the handout as documentation of the visit report that the *Parent Activities Sheet* has cut down on the amount of information they need to write in the chart. They simply place a copy of the sheet into the chart and refer to it in the nursing notes, thereby cutting down the need for transcribing the entire visit. This also presents a more accurate picture of nursing care, because many nurses do not list all activities carried out during visits with families.

The copy left with the parents allows them a chance to review what was discussed, is a reminder of what to do or whom to call between visits, and is a way to convey information to other family members about the care of the infant. It also cuts down on the discrepancies about what was discussed. When the nurse returns for the following visit, the *Parent Activities Sheet* can be reviewed to clarify any misunderstandings and help to ensure smooth and positive communication between the parent and the nurse.

These handouts are three of the many ways information (and any other activities deemed important) can be conveyed to parents in a positive and supportive way. They are an important part of the NSTEP-P protocols of care.

Summary

The NSTEP-P program is an example of what should be included in any quality parent-focused follow-up program for preterm infants and their families. Important components to keep in mind for any follow-up program of this population include the following:

- Home visiting to monitor and provide support
- Measures for systematically assessing the infant and family for identification of problem areas, providing intervention, and evaluating outcomes
- Protocols of care that are structured, flexible, and consistent from visit to visit
- Parent involvement in all aspects of care, including assessment, intervention, and evaluation
- Content encompassing important areas for normal growth and development, yet specific to the needs and problems of preterm infants
- Methods that are research based and supported

Those programs that include these important components will be on their way to ensuring not only that graduates of neonatal intensive care units survive but also that they develop optimally and as normally as possible—one of the most important considerations for all health care professionals, parents, and families.

For information about the NCAST Assessments and the NSTEP-P program, contact NCAST, WJ-10, University of Washington, Seattle, WA 98195, (206) 543–8528, fax 206-685–3284.

REFERENCES

Anders, T. F., & Keener, F. (1985). Developmental course of nighttime sleep-wake patterns in full-term and premature infants during the first year of life. *Sleep, 8,* 173–192.

Bailey, D. B., & Simeonsson, R. J. (1988). *Family assessment in early intervention.* Columbus, OH: Merrill Publishing Company.

Barnard, K. E. (1980). Sleep organization and motor development in prematures. In E. J. Sell (Ed.), *Follow-up of the high-risk newborn: A practical approach.* Springfield, IL: Charles C Thomas.

Barnard, K. E. (1985). *Nursing systems toward effective parenting-preterm.* Final report supported by Maternal and Child Health Training. Grant #MCH-009035, Bureau of HCDA, HRSA, PHS, DHHS.

Barnard, K. E. (1987). *Nursing child assessment learner manual.* Seattle, WA: NCAST Publications.

Barnard, K. E. (1989). *State modulation*. Presented at the NCAST Nursing Systems Toward Effective Parenting-Preterm Training Workshop, Seattle, May 1989.

Barnard, K. E., & Bee, H. L. (1981). Premature infant refocus project, School of Nursing and the Child Development and Mental Retardation Center, University of Washington, Seattle, Washington.

Barnard, K. E., Booth, C. L., Mitchell, A., & Telzrow, R. (1983). Final report: Newborn nursing models, Grant #RO1 NU-00719-03. Seattle, WA: NCAST Publications.

Barnard, K. E., & Eyres, S. J. (1977). Nursing child assessment project final report: The first 12 months of life. Final report to the Division of Nursing, BHRD, PHS, HRA, DHEW.

Barnard, K. E., & Eyres, S. J. (Eds.). (1979). *Child health assessment, part 2: The first year of life*. DHEW Publication No. (HRA) 79–25. Seattle, WA: NCAST Publications.

Barnard, K. E., Eyres, S. J., Lobo, M., & Snyder, D. (1983). An ecological paradigm for assessment and intervention. In T. B. Brazelton & B. M. Lester (Eds.), *New approach to developmental screening of infants*. New York: Academic Press.

Barnard, K. E., Hammond, M., Booth, C. L., et al. (1989). Measurement and meaning of parent–child interaction. In F. Morrison, C. Lord, & D. Keating (Eds.), *Applied developmental psychology* (vol. III, pp. 39–80). New York: Academic Press.

Barnard, K. E., & Kelly, J. F. (1990). Assessment of parent–infant interaction. In S. J. Meisels & J. P. Shonkoff (Eds.), *Handbook of early childhood intervention*. Cambridge, England: Cambridge University Press.

Barrera, M. E., Rosenbaum, P. L., & Cunningham, C. E. (1986). Early home intervention with low birth weight infants and their parents. *Child Development, 57,* 20–33.

Beckwith, L. (1990). Adaptive and maladaptive parenting: Implications for intervention. In S. J. Meisels & J. P. Shonkoff (Eds.), *Handbook of early childhood intervention*. Cambridge, England: Cambridge University Press.

Beckwith, L., & Cohen, S. E. (1980). Interactions of preterm infants with their caregivers and test performance at age 2. In T. M. Field, S. Goldberg, D. Stern, & A. Sostek (Eds.), *High-risk infants and children: Adult and peer interactions*. New York: Academic Press.

Bee, H. L., Barnard, K. E., Eyres, S. J., et al. (1982). Prediction of IQ and language skill from perinatal status, child performance, family characteristics, and mother–infant interaction. *Child Development, 53,* 1134–1156.

Bendersky, M., & Lewis, M. (1986). The impact of birth order on mother-infant interactions in preterm and sick infants. *Developmental and Behavioral Pediatrics, 7,* 242–246.

Bennett, F. C. (1984). Neurodevelopmental outcome of low birth weight infants. In V. C. Kelby (Ed.), *Practice of pediatrics* (vol. 2). New York: Harper & Row.

Bidder, R. T., Crowe, E. A., & Gray, O. P. (1974). Mothers' attitudes to preterm infants. *Archives of Diseases in Childhood, 49,* 776–777.

Bradley, R. H., & Caldwell, B. M. (1988). Using the HOME inventory to assess the family environment. *Pediatric Nursing, 14*(2), 97–102.

Caldwell, B. M., & Snyder, C. (1978). *HOME—Home observation for measurement of the environment*. Seattle, WA: NCAST Publications.

Censullo, M. (1986). Home care of the high-risk newborn. *Journal of Obstetric, Gynecologic, and Neonatal Nursing, 15,* 146–153.

Clark, M. C. (1989). In what ways, if any, are child abusers different from other parents? *Health Visit, 62,* 268–270.

Crnic, D. A., Greenberg, M. T., & Slough, M. M. (1986). Early stress and social support influences on mothers' and high risk infants' functioning in late infancy. *Infant Mental Health Journal, 7,* 19–48.

Culley, B. S., Perrin, E. C., & Chaberski, M. J. (1989). Parental perception of vulnerability of formerly premature infants. *Journal of Pediatric Health Care, 3,* 237–245.

658   *Unit VII: Long-Term Development of the Neonate*

Delerian, D. (1988). Focus on patient education. Seminar presented by The Continuing Education Project, Seattle, WA.

Elmer, E., & Gregg, G. (1967). Developmental characteristics of abused children. *Pediatrics, 40,* 596–602.

Eyres, S. J., Barnard, K. E., & Gray, C. A. (1979). Child health assessment, part 3: 2–4 years. Final report, Grant #RO2-NU-00559. Seattle, WA: NCAST Publications.

Field, T. M. (1987). Interaction and attachment in normal and atypical infants. *Journal of Consulting and Clinical Psychology, 55,* 853–859.

Field, T. M., & Sostek, A. (Eds.). (1983). *Infants born at risk: Physiological, perceptual and cognitive processes.* New York: Grune & Stratton.

Forsyth, B. W., & Canny, P. (1985). Long-term implications of problems of feeding and crying behavior in early infancy: A 3½ year follow-up. Presented at the annual meeting of the Ambulatory Pediatric Association, Washington, DC, May 1985.

Gottfried, A. (1984). *Home environment and early cognitive development.* New York: Academic Press.

Green, M., & Solnit, A. J. (1964). Reactions to the threatened loss of a child: A vulnerable child syndrome. *Pediatrics, 34,* 58–66.

Greenberg, M. T., & Crnic, K. A. (1988). Longitudinal predictors of developmental status and social interaction in premature and full-term infants at age two. *Child Development, 59,* 554–570.

Hammond, M. A., Bee, H. L., Barnard, K. E., & Eyres, S. J. (1983). Child health assessment, part 4: Follow-up of second grade. Final report of project supported by Grant #RO1 NU 00816. Seattle, WA: NCAST Publications.

Hartman, K. (Ed.). (1988). Nurses offer home health-care alternatives—Part II. *NAACOG Newsletter, 15*(5), 4–8.

Jeffcoate, J., Humphrey, M., & Lloyd, J. (1979). Disturbance in parent–child relationship following preterm delivery. *Developmental Medicine and Child Neurology, 21,* 344–352.

Johnson-Crowley, N. (1986). Guidelines for nursing intervention NCASA record with prematures. *NCAST National News, II*(2), 2–4.

Johnson-Crowley, N. (1987). NSTEP-P: A home visit program for preterm infants and their families. A poster session presented at the Fifth Biennial National Training Institute for National Center for Clinical Infant Programs, Washington, DC.

Johnson-Crowley, N. (1988). NSTEP-P: A Home visit program for preterm infants and their families. Presentation at the Annual Pediatric Nursing Conference, Chicago, Illinois.

Johnson-Crowley, N., & Sumner, G. A. (1987a). *Concept manual: Nursing systems toward effective parenting—preterm.* Seattle, WA: NCAST Publications.

Johnson-Crowley, N., & Sumner, G. A. (1987b). *Protocol manual: Nursing systems toward effective parenting—preterm.* Seattle, WA: NCAST Publications.

Klein, M., & Stern, L. (1979). Low birthweight and the battered child syndrome. *American Journal of Diseases of Children, 122,* 15–18.

Levy, J. C. (1984). Vulnerable children: Parents' perceptions and the use of medical care. *Pediatrics, 65,* 956–963.

Macey, T. J., Harmon, R. J., & Easterbrooks, M. A. (1987). Impact of premature birth on the development of the infant in the family. *Journal of Consulting and Clinical Psychology, 55,* 846–852.

Maygary, D. (1987). Parent–infant interaction. In N. Johnson-Crowley & G. A. Sumner (Eds.), *Nursing systems toward effective parenting—preterm.* Seattle, WA: NCAST Publications.

McCormick, M. C., Shapiro, S., & Starfield, B. (1982). Factors associated with maternal opinion of infant development—Clues to the vulnerable child? *Pediatrics, 69,* 537–543.

Patteson, D. M., & Barnard, K. E. (Spring, 1990). Parenting of low-birthweight infants: A review of issues and interventions. *Infant Mental Health Journal,* 37–56.

Perrin, E. C., West, P. S., & Culley, B. S. (1989). Is my child normal yet? Correlates of vulnerability. *Pediatrics, 83*, 355–363.

Ramey, C. T., Farram, D. C., & Campbell, F. A. (1979). Predicting IQ from mother-infant interactions. *Child Development, 50*, 804–814.

Ricciuti, H. N. (1983). Interaction of multiple factors contributing to high-risk parenting. In V. J. Sasserath (Ed.), *Minimizing high-risk parenting—Pediatric round table: 7*. Skillman, NJ: Johnson & Johnson Baby Products.

Ruff, C. C. (1987). How well do adolescents mother? *Journal of Maternal-Child Nursing (MCN), 12*, 249–253.

Schmitt, B., & Kempe, H. (1975). Neglect and abuse of children. In V. Vaughan & R. McKay (Eds.), *Nelson textbook of pediatrics* (pp. 108–111). Philadelphia: W. B. Saunders.

Schraeder, B. D., Rappaport, J., & Courtwright, L. (1987). Preschool development of very low birthweight infants. *IMAGE: Journal of Nursing Scholarship, 19*(4), 174–177.

Schwartz, S. F., Howowitz, F. D., & Mitchell, D. W. (1984). A comparison of the behaviors of preterm and full term infants: Implications for mother-infant interaction. In abstracts of papers presented at the Fourth International Conference on Infant Studies. *Infant Behavior and Development*, p. 7.

Slater, M. A., Naqvi, M., Andrew, L., & Haynes, K. (1987). Neurodevelopment of monitored versus non-monitored very low birth weight infants: The importance of family influences. *Developmental and Behavioral Pediatrics, 8*, 278–285.

Tekolste, K. A., & Bennett, F. C. (1987). State of the art, the high risk infant: Transitions in health, development, and family during the first years of life. *Journal of Perinatology, 7*, 368–377.

Telzrow, R. W., Kang, R., Mitchell, S. K., et al. (1982). An assessment of the behavior of the premature infant of 40 weeks conceptional age. In L. P. Lipsitt & T. M. Field (Eds.), *Perinatal risk and newborn behavior*. Norwood, NJ: Ablex.

CHAPTER 32

Neonatal Development

FETAL AND NEONATAL CENTRAL NERVOUS SYSTEM DEVELOPMENT

The development of the central nervous system (CNS) can be divided into six overlapping stages. The first three stages of CNS development (dorsal induction, ventral induction, and neurogenesis) are completed before the fourth month of gestation. However, the last three stages (neuron migration, synaptogenesis and arborization, and myelinization) continue during the time many infants are in the neonatal intensive care unit (NICU) (Volpe, 1995).

Areas of development during the last part of gestation that are particularly critical in considering neurobehavioral vulnerabilities of ill or immature infants include the following:

- Autonomic homeostatic control
- Alterations in the germinal matrix
- Pattern of dendritic connections
- Growth of the cerebellum

From 28 to 32 weeks of gestation, preterm infants begin to achieve some degree of physiologic homeostasis, with increasing control of the sympathetic system over their autonomic functioning, at least at the subcortical level. With increasing autonomic control, the infant develops greater autonomic stability.

The pattern of dendritic connections between neurons is a critical growth process that begins during the sixth month of gestation and may be particularly vulnerable to insults from the effects of the NICU environment. The interconnections between individual neurons constitute the "wiring" of the brain. Dendritic connections, or arborization, are critical for processing of impulses and for cell-to-cell communication. Lack of connections can result in hypersensitivity, poorly modulated behaviors, and all-or-nothing responses, which can often be observed in preterm infants in the NICU.

The cerebellum is primarily concerned with control of muscles and coordination of movements; it undergoes a critical growth spurt at 30 to 32 weeks of gestation. Insults may lead to the altered sequences of motor development seen in some preterm infants (Nelson, 1987).

NEONATAL NEUROBEHAVIORAL DEVELOPMENT

The synactive theory of development (Als, 1982) provides a model through which one can specify the degree of differentiation of behavior and the ability of infants to organize and control their behavior. This model is based on the assumption that the infant's primary route of communicating both functional stability and the limits for stress is through behavior (Als, 1986).

660

Infants are seen as being in continual interaction with their environment through five subsystems:

- Autonomic/physiologic
- Motor
- State/organizational
- Attentional/interactive
- Self-regulatory

These subsystems mature sequentially, and within each subsystem a developmental sequence can be observed. Thus, at each stage of development, new tasks and organizations are learned against the backdrop of previous development. The subsystems are interdependent and interrelated.

Instability in the autonomic system can be seen in the pattern of respiration (pauses, tachypnea), color changes (red, pale, dusky, mottled), and various visceral signs (regurgitation, twitching, stooling). Organization of the motor system is assessed by observing the infant's tone and posture (flexed, extended, hyperflexed, flaccid); specific movement patterns of the extremities, head, trunk, and face; and level of activity. The development of motor responses is closely linked to state organization (Als, 1986). The organization of neuromotor responses moves from minimal capacity for response, to a phase of obligatory, autonomic (all-or-nothing) response, to development of smoother, more organized responses with more individual variation (Sammons & Lewis, 1985).

The state system is understood by noting the available range of states of consciousness (sleep to arousal, awake to alert, crying), how well defined each state is (in terms of behavioral and physiologic parameters), transitions between states, and the quality of organization of these states.

Sleep–Wake States

Sleeping and waking states are clusters of behaviors that tend to occur together and represent the level of the arousal of the individual, the individual's responsivity to external stimulation, and the underlying activation of the central nervous system (Ashton, 1973). Three states have been identified in adults: wakefulness, non-REM (rapid eye movement) sleep, and REM sleep. In infants, it is also possible to identify states within waking and states that are transitional between waking and sleeping because infants are less able to make rapid changes between states than are adults. Infants also have more difficulty sustaining alertness when awake. Because the electrophysiologic patterns associated with sleeping and waking states in infants are somewhat different than those in adults (Anders, Emde, & Parmelee, 1971), the sleep states are usually designated active and quiet sleep, rather than REM and non-REM sleep.

Autonomic, Motor, and State Systems

Initially, preterm infants tend to be unstable and fragile, with sudden changes in their autonomic, motor, and state systems. These infants often have all-or-nothing responses, that is, they may have minimal response to handling or other sensory input until a threshold is reached, then quickly develop a cascade of responses, ending in several color changes, flaccidity, bradycardia, and apnea. As the infant matures, the responses are more variable and the infant is less likely to totally decompensate (Als, 1986, 1996).

The attentional/interactive system involves the infant's ability to orient and focus on sensory stimuli, such as faces, sounds, or objects—the external environment. This system also includes the range of abilities in states of consciousness: how well-defined periods of alertness are and transitions into and out of alertness. At first, this alertness may be very brief, with a dull look or glassy-eyed stare. As this system matures, the infant is able to interact with greater ease and for longer periods. Social responsiveness requires that the infant has enough state control to sustain some awake and alert states (Als, 1986; Sammons & Lewis, 1985).

The self-regulatory system includes behaviors the infant uses to maintain the integrity and balance of the other subsystems, to integrate the other systems, and to move smoothly between states.

Assessment of Neonatal Neurobehavioral Development

Historically, two types of neonatal assessments have evolved, the neurologic examination and the behavioral examination. The neurologic examination assesses the function of the CNS and typically includes assessment of motor tone and reflex behaviors within the context of infant state. The behavioral examination complements and elaborates on the neurologic assessment (Gorski, Lewkowicz, & Huntington, 1987). An assumption underlying the behavioral examination is that the observable behavior of an infant is a reflection of her or his underlying neurologic status. The behavioral examination seeks to describe the quality of behavioral performance. More recently, these two forms of assessment have been combined into the neurodevelopmental or neurobehavioral assessment.

The neurodevelopmental examination is important because it yields a large pool of early observable behavior, including information about the infant's neurologic status and abilities to cope and interact with the environment.

NEUROBEHAVIORAL ASSESSMENT IN THE NICU

Neurobehavioral assessment can be performed at several different levels and is an essential part of comprehensive care of the high-risk infant in the NICU. Individuals such as Brazelton, Als, and their colleagues have sought to assess preterm and term newborn behavior and adaptations. Their work is based on an understanding of newborns as competent individuals with emerging developmental processes who are engaged in dynamic interactions and negotiations with their environment. As a result, several tools have been developed to describe and quantify neurobehavioral organization of both preterm and term newborns.

Brazelton Neonatal Behavioral Assessment Scale

The NBAS combines evaluation of basic reflex responses with the integration of motor capacity, state regulation, and interactive abilities (Brazelton,

1984). Infants are followed through the various states of sleep, arousal, and wakefulness and assessed on their ability to self-regulate in the face of increasingly vigorous activity. The results are an assessment of the infant's ability to do the following:

- Organize states
- Habituate to external stimulation
- Regulate motoric activity in the face of increasing sensory input
- Respond to reflex testing
- Alert and orient to visual and auditory stimuli
- Interact with a caregiver
- Self-console

Assessment of Preterm Infant Behavior

The APIB is based on the synactive theory of development. It is particularly useful for the preterm and term high-risk infant from birth to 44 weeks' postconceptional age. The purpose is to determine how infants cope with the intense environment of the NICU and organization of the CNS. The focus is not on assessment of skill performance or specific responses to various stimuli only but on the unique way each individual infant deals and interacts with his or her world.

Thoman State Scoring System

Another state scoring system is the Thoman (Thoman, 1985, 1990). This system consists of 10 sleeping and waking states: alert, nonalert waking activity, fuss, cry, daze, drowse, sleep–wake transition, active sleep, active-quiet transitional sleep, and quiet sleep. This is a little more difficult to learn than the NBAS because it calls for subtle distinctions between behaviors.

Anderson Behavioral State Scale

Anderson developed a 12-state scoring system, the ABSS, to be used with preterm infants. The ABSS divides the sleep–wake states into very quiet sleep, quiet sleep with irregular drowsy, alert inactivity, quiet awake, restless awake, very restless awake, fussing, crying, and hard crying (Gill et al., 1988). This scale assumes a linear relationship between the states and heart rates and energy consumption (Ludington, 1990; McNeely, 1987). It, too, is difficult to learn owing to the need to make subtle distinctions in the assessment.

Neonatal Individualized Development Care and Assessment Program

The NIDCAP incorporates several levels of developmental training in assessment techniques and intervention planning for high-risk preterm and full-term infants. Included in this program is an observation tool (level 1 NIDCAP—naturalistic behavioral observation), which is extremely useful for the NICU nurse. This assessment involves an observation of the infant before, during, and after a routine caregiving episode. It provides the NICU nurse with information on the infant's individual cues for both stress and stable, organized function. The nurse can then structure the infant's experiences, including caregiving interventions and the physical and social environment, to support the infant at the current level of tolerance.

Assessment Beyond Neonatal Development in the NICU

As the infant matures, moves out of the neonatal period, and becomes a "long termer" in the NICU with chronic respiratory or other problems, neurodevelopmental assessments continue to provide important information. For the infant who requires prolonged hospitalization, a developmental assessment at the bedside can provide information on how the infant interacts with objects and people, organizes behavior, and copes with the environment, as well as on the infant's neurologic status. No formal developmental assessments have been standardized for these NICU populations. Most developmental psychologists or specialists adapt items from other examinations such as the Bayley scales of infant development (Bayley, 1969).

Owing to the nature and severity of their illness, these infants may not be able to tolerate a complete examination at one session. Important areas of assessment include the following:

- Availability of alerting
- Ability to use interventions for consoling or developmental activities
- Self-soothing capacity
- Motor activities and strengths
- Tolerance for handling (how long? with whom?)
- Degree of fragility
- Degree of distractibility
- Hand use
- Parts of body available for use
- Respiratory capacity and tolerance

NEONATAL INTENSIVE CARE UNIT ENVIRONMENT

White-Traut and others (1994) have noted that although the last two sensory systems to become functional are the visual and auditory systems, these two systems commonly receive the most, and often random, stimulation in the NICU environment. Thus, the NICU environment is inconsistent with the preterm infant's level of development and quite different from the intrauterine one.

Intrauterine Environment

The intrauterine environment provides a variety of stimuli to the fetus while modifying the intensity and nature of the sensory input. Characteristics of the intrauterine milieu include (1) auditory input, such as the maternal heartbeat, bowel sounds, and muffled sounds from the extrauterine environment; (2) vestibular, tactile, and kinesthetic stimuli from maternal and fetal movements; and (3) rhythmic and cyclic recurrent stimuli, such as the maternal heartbeat, maternal sleep and activity patterns, and neurohormonal cycles (Blackburn & Barnard, 1985).

NICU Environment

SOUND

Sound and noise levels in the NICU are of concern for two reasons: (1) potential damage to the cochlea with hearing loss; and (2) arousal (Douek et al., 1976; Thomas, 1989). Arousal is a particular concern with immature infants, who are unable to inhibit responses. Noise interferes with sleep and causes fatigue in adults and older infants. It increases heart rate and blood pressure, leads to vasoconstriction, and alters respiratory patterns and endocrine function (Peabody & Lewis, 1985; Raymond, 1991). Vasoconstriction of blood vessels in the ear may lead to ischemia and hearing loss (Ciesielski, Kopka, & Kidawa, 1980). Sudden loud noises are associated with agitation, crying, irritability, increased intracranial pressure, and decreased oxygenation (Long, Lucey, & Phillips, 1980; Peabody & Lewis, 1985). Desaturation episodes correlated with peak noise bursts (Satish & Doll-Speck, 1993). Concerns have also been raised about the possible additive effects of drugs and environmental noise.

Loudness of sound is measured in decibels. Ambient sound levels in the NICU have been documented at 50 to 90 dB, which is higher than in the average office or home (Thomas, 1989). Normal adult speech in conversation is usually recorded at a loudness of 45 to 50 dB. Sound levels inside infant incubators have been reported to range from 50 to 80 dB (Agnagnostakis, Petmezakis, Messaritakis, & Matsaniotis, 1980; Bess, Finlayson-Peek, & Chapman, 1979). In adults, levels above 80 to 85 dB have been associated with hearing loss in some individuals. Decibel levels are even higher inside incubators of infants with ventilatory support equipment. However, the incubator does muffle external sounds, an advantage that is not experienced by infants in open radiant warmers.

Transported infants are exposed to both high noise levels and vibration. Rotary wing aircraft have the most vibration and noise, often exceeding 90 dB, followed by fixed wing air and ground transport (Campbell et al., 1984). Infants on high-frequency ventilation are also exposed to vibration and noise. Specific effects on an infant of these conditions are not known, but noise and vibration may have a synergistic effect on hearing loss (Hamernik, Ahroon, Davis, & Axelsson, 1989).

Sound levels in NICUs have two characteristic patterns. There is the relatively loud and continuous pattern of background noise (50–90 dB), which has little diurnal rhythm. Interposed with this constant background noise are peak noises, which can significantly increase the decibel level (Bess, Finlayson-Peek, & Chapman, 1979; Thomas, 1989).

LIGHT

If the light intensity is seldom changed, as is the case in many NICUs, the infant never experiences diurnal rhythmic patterns necessary for development. Another concern is that intense stimuli, whether light or noise, have a potentially arousing effect on the CNS. This effect may be especially problematic for neonates, who cannot regulate incoming stimuli, leading to wasted energy and sensory overload.

Environmental lighting has been suggested as a factor increasing risks of retinopathy of prematurity (ROP) in infants of very low birth weight, although current studies are inconclusive with many methodologic problems (Ackerman, Sherwonit, & Williams, 1989; Glass et al., 1985; Seiberth, Linderkamp, Knorz, & Liesinhoff, 1994).

Preterm infants are more vulnerable to retinal light damage. Factors influencing the amount of light reaching the retina include lens translucency (increased in preterm infants), amount of time the eye is open (increased in VLBW infant), pupil reactivity (decreased <30 weeks), density of optic media (less dense in preterms), macular pigment (immature retinal structures and vascularity), as well as infant position (e.g., facing artificial light sources or windows) and bed position in relation to windows (Glotzbach et al., 1993; Robinson & Fielder, 1990, 1992; Robinson, Bayliss, & Fielder, 1991; Robinson, Moseley, Thompson, & Fielder, 1989).

Common measurements used in describing light environments are irradiance (what kind of light) or the amount of radiant energy (W/cm^2) emitted over specific wavelength bands and illuminance (how much light) in lux (lumens/m^2) or foot-candles (ft-c). Lux divided by 10 is roughly equivalent to foot-candles. Light intensity in the NICU ranges from 192 to 1488 lux (19 to 148 ft-c), with greater intensity during day than night hours (Glotzbach, et al. 1993; Landry, Scheidt, & Hammond, 1985; MacLeod & Stern, 1972). Treatment lights and warming lamps used in the NICU average 200 to 350 ft-c (or higher), and lights used to treat bilirubinemia may be as high as 10,000 ft-c (Glass, 1990; Glass et al., 1985)

For many years, NICU lighting was bright and continuous throughout the 24-hour day. This lack of diurnal rhythmicity may interfere with the development of natural rhythms. Many nurseries have instituted some dimming of lights at night. Reports have shown that infants experiencing reduced light levels for a portion of the 24-hour period had reduced heart rate, decreased activity, enhanced biological rhythms, increased sleep, and improved feeding and weight gain (Blackburn & Patteson, 1991; Lotus, 1992; Mann et al., 1986; Miller et al., 1995; Shiroiwa et al., 1986; Tenreiro et al., 1991). Thus, reducing light levels may facilitate rest and subsequent energy conservation and promote organization and growth.

ANIMATE ENVIRONMENT

An important component of the infant's animate environment is the opportunity for contingent caregiving, that is, care in which the experiences and caregiver responses are dependent on the infant's behavior. In this way, infants begin to learn that their behavior influences their environment and vice versa (Blackburn, 1983; Blackburn & Barnard, 1985). Contingent interaction between the infant and caregiver depends on three characteristics (Sammons & Lewis, 1985):

- Readability or clarity of behaviors and cues
- Predictability of the other in anticipating behavior from immediately preceding behaviors
- Responsiveness or reactions of the other with appropriate behaviors within a short latency period

Developmental Intervention Approach

The developmental intervention approach is based on the synactive theory (Als, 1982) and focuses on fostering neurobehavioral and physiologic organization. Intervention strategies are individualized for each infant and based on ongoing assessment of that infant. An assumption underlying this approach is that the high-risk infant is vulnerable to sensory overload and overstimulation and demonstrates this by a variety of physiologic, state, motoric, and attentional cues. Therefore, the goal is not to focus on achievement of developmental milestones or to offer stimulation to foster specific skills but rather to help the infant stabilize at each stage of maturation and to support the infant's emerging behaviors and organization while reducing stress.

Sensory input is an important and critical parameter in fostering CNS development. However, sensory input is provided only when appropriate to the infant's physiologic and neurobehavioral status.

CUE-BASED CARE

Caregiving is based on infant cues that provide communications about an infant's needs and status at any given time. These cues include infant state and behavioral capabilities and signs of stress, overstimulation, and stability. Caregiving based on infant cues involves attention to messages from the infant that may indicate timing for interventions, such as when to provide care, or opportunities for sensory input and interaction. These cues also indicate how the infant handles stimuli, signals sensory overload, and tolerates stimulation.

GUIDELINES FOR PROVIDING DEVELOPMENTAL SUPPORT

Goals of developmental interventions are as follows:

- Promote an understanding with the parents of their infant's behavior, including manifestations of stress and stability
- Facilitate neurobehavioral organization based on individualized assessment of the infant's capacity
- Enhance infant recovery
- Promote CNS organization
- Facilitate self-regulatory capabilities
- Preserve energy and promote growth
- Reduce stress and prevent agitation
- Normalize the environment to the extent that medical care permits (VandenBerg 1985, 1995)

Once the infant's current level of organization has been documented, a plan of care can be developed that delineates the degree and kind of environmental support necessary to promote organization and development. This plan should be based on the following guidelines (VandenBerg, 1985):

1. Interventions must seek to normalize or modify the NICU environment to the extent that medical care permits.
2. Interventions must be consistent with the infant's level of maturity and gestational age.

3. Interventions must be appropriately timed in terms of the infant's state, physiologic status, and behavioral responses.
4. Interventions must be individualized to a given infant and be altered with changes in the infant's health status and neurobehavioral maturation.
5. Interventions must be sensitive to the infant's cues.
6. Interventions must take into account how much stimuli each infant can tolerate.

An individualized behaviorally based developmental and family-focused care approach stabilizes the infant, reduces stress during NICU hospitalization, and improves neurodevelopmental and medical outcome after premature birth.

INTERVENTION STRATEGIES

Environmental Manipulations

Auditory Environment: Reducing Noise Levels

Sound levels vary in different NICUs and over time within a unit. These levels should be monitored regularly so that problem areas can be identified and modified. Sound levels can be reduced by attending to events that increase both background and peak noise. Increased noise levels result from closing portholes with a snap. Removing water bubbling in oxygen and ventilator tubing decreases background noise, as will eliminating radios. Peak noises can also be reduced if staff avoid tapping or banging tops of incubators.

Location of the infant's bed in relation to equipment (including monitors) and to surrounding traffic and activity also needs to be evaluated. By determining from which point on the equipment sounds and alarms emanate, the infant can be repositioned to modify this component of the auditory environment. Noise from equipment belonging to both the infant being cared for and surrounding infants must be considered.

Other sources of noise that should be considered are the volume of music boxes, tape recorders, and musical toys. The volume can be kept low or muffled with a blanket as needed. These should not be used with infants who are easily disorganized. Audible telephone ringers can be replaced with light signals on telephones. Staff should quietly close garbage cans, linen hampers, and equipment carts. Felt stripping can be placed on this equipment and drawers to reduce sound levels. Placing thick, soundproof blankets or other materials around incubators, warmers, and cribs reduces both sound and light. In addition, bottles and other equipment can be placed on blankets or pads rather than directly on the incubator hood.

Sound levels can also be reduced by eliminating the use of radios, by talking and walking softly, and by avoiding shouting. Some units have instituted the concept of a daily quiet hour.

Visual Environment: Reducing Light Levels

Individually controlled lights at each bedside allow the nurse to control lighting for each infant. Indirect full-spectrum light, which does not have the side effects of cool white light, can be used at the bedside (Peabody &

Lewis, 1985). Covering incubators, radiant warmers, and cribs reduces infant exposure to bright overhead lights or daylight. Complete covering can be used for sleep periods, with partial covering during awake times. Dimmer switches, window shades, and curtains increase staff control over the light environment. Dimming lights at night may promote development of diurnal cycles. Adjusting lighting levels during other periods fosters state transition and periods of alertness or sleep. Infants who are having brief, predictable alert periods need semi-dim light until they are ready to maintain longer periods of alertness.

Visual Environment: Reducing Visual Clutter

The entire visual environment of the infant needs to be evaluated regularly and simplified. Infants in the NICU can accumulate an amazing clutter of toys, pictures, and other equipment, and this is easily modified.

Congestion and Traffic Patterns

Disorganization increases arousal and stress in older children and adults. Infants need to be assessed and monitored to identify environmental events, such as reports when changing shifts and nursing or medical rounds, that are disruptive. Infants for whom these events are a problem can be moved out of unit traffic patterns, and reports and rounds can be moved away from the bedside.

Altering Patterns of Care

Most NICU infants are being monitored for a variety of physiologic parameters with sophisticated equipment. The data from this equipment can be used to decrease disruption of the infants by routine activities such as monitoring of vital signs. Nonemergency interventions, including monitoring of vital signs, feeding, bathing, diapering, and administration of routine medications, can be done in states other than quiet sleep (infants do not stay in quiet sleep periods for long; often less than 5 to 10 minutes). Because infants spend very little time in the quiet alert state, aversive procedures should be avoided during this state. Duxbury and coworkers (1984) found that infants who received care (except for emergency procedures) only after beginning to awaken spontaneously had improved growth and physiologic function and a significantly decreased length of hospital stay.

Caregiving interventions can also be grouped or clustered to provide longer uninterrupted rest periods. Caregiving involves a significant amount of sensory input and energy utilization. Although some infants do well with clustering of care, others become exhausted and overloaded. Some infants tolerate having aversive interventions (e.g., blood drawing, injections, suctioning) clustered; others do not. Some infants tolerate clustering of these procedures with infant care interventions (e.g., feedings, diapering); others do not. The amount of time between clusters must be monitored to provide adequate time for recovery and rest (Evans, 1994). Time of interventions within a cluster is also an important consideration, not only in terms of potential side effects but also in terms of avoiding exhausting an infant before feeding him or her (Gorski, 1985; VandenBerg, 1990).

Interventions With Overstimulated or Stressed Infants

For the immature or fragile infant, any handling may be stressful, even handling that staff or parents perceive as positive, such as holding, stroking, or talking to the infant. When an infant becomes "overloaded," interventions can be implemented to help the infant recover and reorganize.

Interventions with overstimulated infants include time out with no or minimal handling or sensory input, containment or swaddling the infant with one's hands or a blanket, holding the infant quietly and providing no other sensory input (e.g., do not talk to, stroke, or jiggle the infant), placing blanket rolls at the infant's back and feet, or placing one's hands on the soles of the infant's feet.

Positioning

Positioning of the sick or immature infant includes consideration of the effects of gravity along with neuromuscular characteristics, such as variable weak muscle tone and decreased flexion in the limbs, trunk, and pelvis. These infants are at risk for positioning disorders such as widely abducted hips (frog-leg position), retracted and abducted shoulders, ankle and foot eversion, increased neck extension with a right-sided head preference, and increased trunk extension with arching of the neck and back. These positioning disorders affect later development because of their impact on the ability of the child to bear weight, bring the shoulders forward and hands to midline, and rotate the head (Updike et al., 1986). Therefore, in addition to improved physiologic status, developmental goals of positioning include enhancement of flexion in the limbs and trunk, extensor balance, and facilitation of midline skills.

These goals are superseded, however, by the importance of stress reduction and enhancement of organized motor system function. This means prevention of ongoing frantic activity (flailing) and frequent recurrent extensions of the extremities and neck. These responses are very costly to the infant in terms of energy expenditure, respiratory function, and oxygenation.

Thus, the immature or sick neonate requires support from caregivers to facilitate and maintain postures that enhance motor control and physiologic functioning and reduce stress. Most infants can be routinely placed in side-lying and prone positions and rotated every 2 to 3 hours. Supine positions are generally avoided. Infants who must be placed supine should be positioned to promote flexion and proper alignment.

Covering, swaddling, and placing blanket rolls around the infant help him or her maintain the desired posture and prevent loss of control of the flexed position. The use of these rolls provides containment and boundaries for the infant, promoting feelings of security, quiescence, and energy conservation. Nesting is often an effective way of reducing agitation (Lawhon, 1986). Placing rolls at the infant's feet also provides the infant with something to brace against during stressful interventions (Als, 1986; Lawhon, 1986; Lawhon & Melzar, 1988).

When infants need to be moved and/or repositioned, they should be unwrapped and repositioned slowly with containment of the limbs and support of the head and neck. When repositioning the infant, it is important to ensure that the infant is covered or swaddled if possible; if covering is not possible for medical reasons, partial wrapping is encouraged. Swaddling with blankets or containment with the caregiver's hands also reduces stress during procedures.

Sheepskin or lambskin promotes flexion, provides tactile input, and reduces skin abrasion. Waterbeds and slings also promote flexion. In addition, waterbeds provide contingent stimuli (movement in response to the infant's movement) and kinesthetic input.

Handling

The *individualization* of caregiving for each infant includes flexibility and willingness on the part of the caregiver to adapt handling to specific infant needs to reduce stress and prevent agitation. The caregiver must also recognize that infant's needs change.

Appropriate *timing* of handling is also essential to avoid overtiring or overstimulating infants or increasing stress. Infants can improve their abilities to regulate their own movements, states, and autonomic function when caregiving activities are offered in sequence and with sensitivity to their degree of tolerance.

Infants in an NICU, no matter how sick or how small, are experiencing and reacting to every aspect of care and the surrounding environment. A goal of neonatal care is to avoid costly stress in these infants. Slow, sensitive handling for medical procedures and routine caregiving is required to accomplish this goal. Before gently touching an infant, the caregiver should talk softly. This reduces startling, tremors, or other stress responses from the infant's suddenly being moved by "hands out of nowhere." Minimal handling protocols are necessary for immature, fragile infants (Lawhon, 1986; Vanden-Berg & Franck, 1990). These protocols involve reduction of environmental stimuli, positioning techniques, and pacing caregiving routines to allow for up to 3 hours of undisturbed rest.

State Modulation

Initially, state modulation efforts are directed toward protecting the infant from environmental stressors and aversive sensory input by reducing arousal through implementing time-out maneuvers. These early interventions are directed toward protecting the infant from disorganization and decompensation.

Infants are most responsive to the environment when in the waking states and, in particular, when alert. When alert, the infants eyes are open and scanning. Motor activity is typically low, particularly in full-term newborns, but premature infants may be motorically active. Alertness is the state in which the infant exhibits focused attention on sources of stimulation (Brazelton, 1984). This state is optimal for feeding. In this state, infants are most receptive to interactions with caregivers, but this is limited in the premature infant.

Crying, another waking state, serves a communication function. However, the meaning of cries differs in different situations and may depend on their intensity (Hopkins & Palthe, 1987; Thoman, Acebo, & Becker, 1983). Although crying that occurs when the infant is alone may elicit parental attention, crying that occurs during social exchanges may actually disrupt the parent–infant relationship. An infant who spends time crying will burn more calories and use more oxygen.

The final waking state, nonalert waking activity, is characterized by periods when the infant shows motor activity but is not alert or crying. Usually the infant's eyes are open.

There are two major sleep states—active sleep and quiet sleep—although some state systems define a transitional state between them. In active sleep, the infant's respiration is uneven and primarily costal. Sporadic motor movements occur, but muscle tone is low between these movements. The most distinct characteristic of this state is rapid eye movements that occur intermittently. Active sleep is the most common state from birth throughout infancy.

Quiet sleep is characterized by a lack of body movements and the presence of regular respiration. A tonic level of motor tone is maintained. The major purpose of quiet sleep seems to be rest and growth. The amount of quiet sleep depends on environmental factors. Thus, this, as well as the other states, must be considered in developmentally supportive interventions.

INTERVENTIONS

Interventions to organize state include helping these infants to organize their sleep, alerting, and crying. To promote sleep, the caregiver can modify the environment to reduce light, noise, and traffic around the infant's bed. Use of boundaries, prone positioning, minimal handling, and support of flexion, along with predictable routines, will also facilitate sleep organization. Interventions to prevent irritability and crying include predictable routines, reducing environmental stress, timing procedures or other caregiving according to infant cues, and soothing infants when they become stressed. Periods of irritability can be minimized if signs of stress and sensory overload are recognized early and appropriate interventions initiated. Soothing interventions for the immature or ill infant include containment and swaddling, providing time out for recovery, reducing stimulation, holding the infant's hands or feet, prone positioning, and providing sucking opportunities (Als, 1986; Lawhon, 1986; VandenBerg, 1990, 1995).

Immature infants will initially spend very little time in alert states. When they do achieve an alert state, these states are transient and easily disrupted. Caregivers need to approach infants who have reached a quiet alert state carefully. It is often an exciting event when an infant finally opens her or his eyes and reaches a quiet alert state. Unfortunately, caregivers often try to capitalize on this time by providing input and reinforcement that is "too much, too soon." A more appropriate response to interacting with these infants is to allow the infant to initiate and control the interaction.

Alerting activities with healthy term or more mature, stable preterm infants include talking to the infant, varying the pitch and intensity of one's voice; unwrapping the infant, even if only the upper extremities; providing a drowsy infant with visual or auditory stimuli; putting the infant in an upright position, such as up on one's shoulder; and eliciting the rooting or sucking reflexes. Activities to soothe include talking in a slow, steady monotone; swaddling the infant with hands or blanket; providing a pacifier or helping the infant get her or his fingers or hand into the mouth; and placing one's hands against the soles of the infant's feet (Blackburn & Kang, 1991). As with the more fragile infants, these infants should also be observed for their stress and stability cues in response to each intervention.

Provision of Sensory Input

Specific considerations for providing sensory input to high-risk infants include the following:

- Vulnerability to sensory overload
- Benefit from positive experiences
- Recovery optimal with minimized sensory input
- Longer time needed to inhibit responses
- Withstanding of only a small amount of stimuli at a time and at a slower rate
- Handling of only unimodal rather than multimodal stimuli

Feeding

Feeding is a very demanding task, often exceeding what has been asked of an infant up to that point. If the infant is preterm, he or she has an immature CNS with weak movement patterns, disorganized states, and oral structures that do not function as those of a term neonate. Tongue and jaw movements are affected by immature development, leading to poorer control of suck, swallow, and breathing patterns (Morris & Klein, 1987). Behavioral patterns include weak, poorly sustained sucking and inadequate state control during feeding. This interferes with coordination of suck and swallow with breathing. Nippling even small amounts can lead to exhaustion and flaccidity with disruption of respiratory control. Compounding the problem is staff and parental anxiety over weight gain and growth.

Usually, these infants can suck and swallow a small amount adequately. They then lose control, developing poor coordination of sucking and swallowing with breathing, an inability to sustain sucking, poor suck and swallow rhythm, respiratory irregularities, or exhaustion. This pattern of behavior has been called the "disorganized feeder," as opposed to the "dysfunctional feeder" (VandenBerg, 1990). Abnormal oral muscle tone and reflexes are frequently present in this group of infants; professional intervention is required for improvement.

The goal for the disorganized feeder is to learn self-regulation of autonomic, motoric, and state systems to eventually nipple adequately. To do this, the infant must be able to *simultaneously* (1) coordinate suck and swallow with respirations while maintaining heart rate and color; (2) coordinate movement patterns, posture, and tone; and (3) remain in a calm, organized state.

Environmental modifications include a quiet setting with indirect lighting and minimal congestion and traffic. Positioning to facilitate feeding includes promoting generalized body flexion to reduce hypertonia and to assist with swallowing, maintaining the head in midline with hands close to face, providing hip flexion, and swaddling.

Nonnutritive Sucking

Infants demonstrate two modes of sucking—nutritive and nonnutritive—each with a specific pattern of organization (Medoff-Cooper, 1991). Nonnutritive sucking has a pattern of short, alternating bursts of sucking and rest in contrast to the longer, continuous, rhythmic patterns characteristic of nutritive sucking (Medoff-Cooper, Weininger, & Zukowsky, 1989). Nonnutritive sucking is present in the fetus as early as 4½ months of gestation (Dubignon & Campbell, 1968).

Nonnutritive sucking is induced by placing a nipple in the infant's mouth without presentation of food. Nonnutritive sucking and rhythmic mouthing (seen in quiet sleep) have similar temporal organization, with regularity of the sucking–pause pattern. Nonnutritive sucking is a state modulation and organizing activity that is used during gavage feeding and interfeeding intervals. It has been associated with improved oxygenation; decreased, more stable intracranial pressure; increased quiet sleep; decreased activity and crying; increased alertness; increased readiness for nipple feeding; better weight gain; and shorter hospital stays (Anderson, Burroughs, & Measel, 1983; Burroughs, Asonye, Anderson-Shanklin, & Vidyasagar, 1978; Field & Goldson, 1984; Field et al., 1982).

Strategies to facilitate development of nonnutritive sucking in intubated infants are as follows:

- Using nasal rather than oral intubation
- Minimizing touch and stress to the oral musculature (and, when necessary, using gentle, slow touch)
- Placing in side-lying position with hands together
- Positioning with hands tucked under chin or so that hands touch parts of face
- Providing pacifiers. After extubation, infants can be positioned with their hands together at the mouth or hands touching their face. In addition, pacifiers can be provided during nasogastric feedings and between feedings.

Kangaroo Care

The kangaroo method of care involves placing a stable term or preterm newborn, who requires no assistance with breathing, skin-to-skin in a vertical position between the mother's breasts. The warmth of the skin-to-skin contact and other sensations foster close contact between mother and infant. The infant usually wears only a diaper. The mother wears a loose blouse, dress, or gown that opens in the front and that can be easily wrapped around the infant once placed on the mother's chest. The infant is kept warm by the heat generated by the mother's body and is covered by her clothing, so heat loss is avoided. In fact, most nurses report that close monitoring of the infant's temperature is important during kangaroo care so as to avoid overheating rather than underheating. Infants weighing as little as 1000 g and who are stable have been placed with their mothers kangaroo style.

Interventions With Parents

Interventions with parents include the following (Blackburn, 1983; Blackburn & Kang, 1991):

- Discussing discrepancies between the parents' expectations of their infant's appearance and behavior and reality
- Encouraging approaches appropriate to the infant's status and maturity
- Placing parents in situations in which they will succeed in interacting positively with their infants
- Avoiding remarks that unfavorably compare infant responses to parents with infant responses to other caregivers
- Involving parents in identifying effective techniques for interacting with their infants
- Identifying infant behavioral responses, including subtle signs of attention and response to the parent's touch or voice (e.g., decreased activity, more regular respirations, or increased oxygenation)
- Teaching parents to recognize and use infant states and stress and stability cues in interacting with their infants and techniques for alerting and consoling their infant that are appropriate to the infant's maturity and health status
- Providing anticipatory guidance as the infant matures

Goals in Nursing Management

The goals in nursing management in addressing the neurobehavioral needs of high-risk infants are listed below:
- Provide an environment that enhances and supports the infant's developing capabilities.
- Protect the infant from sensory overload and minimize stressors.
- Assist parents in understanding their infant's unique abilities.
- Help parents interact with their infant in ways appropriate to the infant's health status, state, and level of maturity.
- Use the infant's needs and capabilities to foster more positive parent–infant interaction.

REFERENCES

Ackerman, B., Sherwonit, E., & Williams, J. (1989). Reduced incidental light exposure: Effect on the development of retinopathy of prematurity in low birthweight infants. *Pediatrics, 83,* 956–962.

Agnagnostakis, D., Petmezakis, J., Messaritakis, J., & Matsaniotis, N. (1980). Noise pollution in neonatal units: A potential health hazard. *Acta Paediatrica Scandinavica, 69,* 771–773.

Als, H. (1982). Toward a synactive theory of development: Promise for the assessment and support of infant individuality. *Infant Mental Health Journal, 3,* 229–243.

Als, H. (1986). A synactive model of neonatal behavioral organization: Framework for the assessment of neurobehavioral development in the premature infant and for the support of infants and parents in the neonatal intensive care environment. *Physical and Occupational Therapy in Pediatrics, 6*(3–4), 3–53.

Als, H. (1996). The Very Immature Infant—Environmental and Care Issues. Paper presented at The Physical and Developmental Environment of the High Risk Neonate. Clearwater Beach, FL: University of South Florida College of Medicine.

Anders, T., Emde, R., & Parmelee, A. (Eds.). (1971). *A manual of standardized terminology, techniques and criteria for scoring of states of sleep and wakefulness in newborn infants.* Los Angeles: UCLA Brain Information Service/BRI Publications Office.

Anderson, G. C., Burroughs, A. K., & Measel, C. P. (1983). Nonnutritive sucking opportunities: A safe and effective treatment for preterm neonates. In T. M. Field, A. K. Sostek (Eds.), *Infants born at risk: Physiological, perceptual and cognitive processes* (pp. 129–146). New York: Grune & Stratton.

Ashton, R. (1973). The state variable in neonatal research: A review. *Merrill Palmer Quarterly, 19,* 3–20.

Bayley, N. (1969). *Bayley scales of infant development.* New York: The Psychological Corporation.

Bess, F. H., Finlayson-Peek, B., & Chapman, J. J. (1979). Further observations of noise levels in infant incubators. *Pediatrics, 63,* 100–106.

Blackburn, S. (1983). Fostering behavioral development of high risk neonates. *Journal of Obstetric, Gynecologic, and Neonatal Nursing, 12*(3 Suppl.), 76s–86s.

Blackburn, S., & Barnard, K. E. (1985). Analysis of caregiving events in preterm infants in the special care unit. In A. Gottfried & J. Gaiter (Eds.), *Infants under stress: Environmental neonatology* (pp. 113–129). Baltimore: University Park Press.

Blackburn, S., & Kang, R. E. (1991). *Early parent–infant relationships* (2nd ed.). White Plains, NY: March of Dimes Birth Defects Foundation.

Blackburn, S., & Patteson, D. (1991). Effects of cycled lighting on activity state and cardiorespiratory function in preterm infants. *Journal of Perinatal and Neonatal Nursing, 4*(4), 47–54.

Brazelton, T.B. (1984). *Neonatal behavioral assessment scale* (2nd ed.). Philadelphia: J. B. Lippincott.

Burroughs, A. K., Asonye, U. O., Anderson-Shanklin, G. C., & Vidyasagar, D. (1978). The effect of nonnutritive sucking on transcutaneous oxygen tension in noncrying preterm neonates. *Research in Nursing and Health, 1*(2), 69–75.

Campbell, A. N., Lightstone, A. D., Smith, J. M., et al. (1984). Mechanical vibration and sound levels experienced in neonatal transport. *American Journal of Diseases of Children, 138,* 967–970.

Ciesielski, S., Kopka, J. & Kidawa, B. (1980). Incubator noise and vibration—possible iatrogenic influence on the neonate. *International Journal of Pediatric Otohinolaryngology, 1,* 309–316.

Douek, E., Dodson, H. C., Bannister, L. H., et al. (1976). Effects of incubator noise on the cochlea of the newborn. *Lancet, 2,* 1110–1113.

Dubignon, J., & Campbell, D. (1968). The relationship between laboratory measures of sucking, food intake, and perinatal factors during the newborn period. *Child Development, 40,* 1107–1120.

Duxbury, M. L., Henly, S. J., Broz, L. J., et al. (1984). Caregiver disruptions and sleep of high risk infants. *Heart and Lung, 13,* 141–147.

Evans, J. C. (1994). Comparison of two NICU patterns of caregiving over 24 hours for preterm infants. *Neonatal Network, 13*(5), 87.

Field, T., & Goldson, E. (1984). Pacifying effects of nonnutritive sucking on term and preterm neonates during heelstick procedures. *Pediatrics, 74,* 1012–1015.

Field, T. M., Ignatoff, E., Stringer, S., et al. (1982). Nonnutritive sucking during tube feedings: Effects on preterm neonates in an intensive care unit. *Pediatrics, 70,* 381–384.

Gill, N. E., Behnke, M., Conlon, M., et al. (1988). Effect of nonnutritive sucking on behavioral state in preterm infants before feeding. *Nursing Research, 37,* 347–350.

Glass, P. (1990). *Environmental manipulations in the NICU: Innovations in practice.* Paper presented at Conference on Developmental Interventions in Neonatal Care, Contemporary Forums, Washington, DC.

Glass, P., Avery, G. B., Subramanian, K. N., et al. (1985). Effect of bright light in the hospital nursery on the incidence of retinopathy of prematurity. *New England Journal of Medicine, 313,* 401–404.

Glotzbach, S. F., Rowlett, E. A., Edgar, D. M., et al. (1993). Light variability in the modern neonatal nursery: Chronobiological issues. *Medical Hypotheses 41,* 217–224.

Gorski, P. A. (1985). Behavioral and environmental care: New frontiers in neonatal nursing. *Neonatal Network, 10*(4), 8–11.

Gorski, P. A., Lewkowicz, D. J., & Huntington, L. (1987). Advances in neonatal and infant behavioral assessment: Toward a comprehensive evaluation of early patterns of development. [Review]. *Journal of Developmental and Behavioral Pediatrics, 8*(1), 39–50.

Hamernik, R. P., Ahroon, W. A., Davis, R. I., & Axelsson, A. (1989). Noise and vibration interactions: Effects on hearing. *Journal of Acoustic Society of America, 86,* 2129–2137.

Hopkins, B. & Palthe, T. V. W. (1987). The development of the crying state during early infancy. *Developmental Psychobiology, 20,* 165–175.

Landry, R. J., Scheidt, P. C., & Hammond, R. W. (1985). Ambient light and phototherapy conditions of eight neonatal care units: A summary report. *Pediatrics 75*(2 pt. 2), 434–436.

Lawhon, G. (1986). Management of stress in premature infants. In D. J. Angelini, C. M. Knapp, & R. M. Gibes (Eds.), *Perinatal/neonatal nursing: A clinical handbook* (pp. 319–328). Boston: Blackwell Scientific Publications.

Lawhon, G., & Melzar, A. (1988). Developmental care of the very low birth weight infant. *Journal of Perinatal and Neonatal Nursing, 2*(1), 56–65.

Long, J. G., Lucey, J. F., & Philips, A. G. (1980). Noise and hypoxemia in the intensive care nursery. *Pediatrics, 65,* 143–145.

Lotus, M. J. (1992). Effects of light and sound in the neonatal intensive care unit environment on the low-birth-weight infants. *NAACOG's Clinical Issues in Perinatal and Women's Health Nursing 3*(1), 34–44.

Ludington, S. M. (1990). Energy conservation during skin-to-skin contact between premature infants and their mothers. *Heart and Lung, 19*(5 pt. 1), 445–451.

MacLeod, P., & Stern, L. (1972). Natural variations in environmental illumination in a newborn nursery. *Pediatrics 50,* 131–133.

Mann, N. P., Haddow, R., Stokes, L., et al. (1986). Effect of night and day on preterm infants in a newborn nursery: Randomized trial. *British Medical Journal Clinical Research Edition, 293,* 1265–1267.

McNeely, J. B. (1987). *Preterm heart rate in twelve behavioral states.* Unpublished master's thesis, University of Florida, Gainesville.

Medoff-Cooper, B. (1991). Changes in nutritive sucking patterns with increasing gestational age. *Nursing Research, 40,* 245–247.

Medoff-Cooper, B., Weininger, S., & Zukowsky, K. (1989). Neonatal sucking as a clinical assessment tool: Preliminary findings. *Nursing Research, 38,* 162–165..

Miller, C. L., White, R., Whitman, T. L., et al. (1995). The effects of cycled and noncycled lighting on growth and development in preterm infants. *Infant Behavior and Development 18*(1), 87–95.

Morris, S. E., & Klein, D. K. (1987). *Prefeeding skills.* Tucson: Therapy Skills Builders.

Nelson, M. (1987). *Development of the newborn.* Presented at the Conference on Developmental Interventions in Neonatal Care, Chicago.

Peabody, J. L., & Lewis, K. (1985). Consequences of neonatal intensive care. In A. Gottfried & J. Gaiter (Eds.), *Infants under stress: Environmental neonatology* (pp. 199–226). Baltimore: University Park Press.

Raymond, L. W. (1991). Neuroendocrine, immunologic, and gastrointestinal effects of noise. In T. H. Fay (Ed.). *Noise and health.* New York: New York Academy of Medicine, 27–40.

Robinson, J., Bayliss, S. C. & Fielder, A. R. (1991). Transmission of light across the adult and neonatal eyelid in vivo. *Vision Research 31,* 1837–1840.

Robinson, J., & Fielder, A. R. (1990). Pupillary diameter and reaction to light in preterm neonates. *Archives of Diseases in Childhood 65*(1 Spec. No.), 35–38.

Robinson, J., & Fielder, A. R. (1992). Light and the immature visual system. [Review]. *Eye 6*(pt. 2), 166–172.

Robinson, J., Moseley, M. J., & Fielder, A. R. (1990). Illuminance of neonatal units. *Archives of Diseases of Childhood 65*(7 Spec. No.), 679–682.

Robinson, J., Moseley, M. J., Thompson, J. R., & Fielder, A. R, (1989). Eyelid opening in preterm neonates. *Archives of Diseases in Childhood 64*(7 Spec. No.), 943–948.

Sammons, W. A. H., & Lewis, J. M. (1985). *Premature babies: A different beginning.* St. Louis: C. V. Mosby.

Satish, M., & Doll-Speck, L. (1993). Elevated sound levels increase desaturation episodes in sick preterm infants. Paper presented at the Annual Meeting, American Academy of Pediatrics, Washington, DC.

Seiberth, V., Linderkamp, O., Knorz, M. C., & Liesinhoff, H. (1994). A controlled trial of light and retinopathy of prematurity. *American Journal of Ophthalmology 118,* 492–495.

Shiroiwa, Y., Kamiya, V., Uchibori, S., et al. (1986). Activity, cardiac and respiratory responses of blindfold preterm infants in a neonatal intensive care unit. *Early Human Development 14,* 259–265

Tenreiro, S., Dowse, H. B., D'Souza, S., et al. (1991). The development of ultradian and circadian rhythms in premature babies maintained in constant conditions. *Early Human Development 27,* 33–152.

Thoman, E. B. (1985). *Sleep and waking states of the neonate* (rev. ed.). (Unpublished manuscript available from E. B. Thoman, Box U-154, Graduate Program in Biobehavioral Sciences, 3107 Horsebarn Hill Road, University of Connecticut, Storrs, Connecticut 06268 USA.)

Thoman, E. B. (1990). Sleeping and waking states in infancy: A functional perspective. *Neuroscience and Biobehavioral Reviews, 14,* 93–107.

Thoman, E. B., Acebo, C., & Becker, P. T. (1983). Infant crying and stability in the mother–infant relationship: A systems analysis. *Child Development, 54,* 653–659.

Thomas, K. A. (1989). How the NICU environment sounds to a preterm infant. *American Journal of Maternal Child Nursing (MCN), 14,* 249–251.

Updike, C., Schmidt, R. E., Macke, C., et al. (1986). Positional support for premature infants. *American Journal of Occupational Therapy, 40,* 712–715.

VandenBerg, K. A. (1985). Revising the traditional model: An individualized approach to developmental interventions in the intensive care nursery. *Neonatal Network, 3*(5), 32–38.

VandenBerg, K. A.(1990). The management of oral nippling in the sick neonate: The disorganized feeder. *Neonatal Network, 9*(1), 9–16.

VandenBerg, K. A. (1995). Behaviorally supportive care for the extremely premature infant. In L. P. Gunderson & C. Kenner (Eds.), *Care of the 24–25 week gestational age infant (small baby protocol)* (2nd ed., pp. 145–170). Petaluma, CA: NICU Ink.

VandenBerg, K. A., & Franck, L. (1990). Behavioral issues for infants with BPD. In C. Lund (Ed.), *BPD: Strategies for total patient care.* Petaluma, CA: Neonatal Network.

Volpe, J. J. (1995). *Neurology of the newborn.* Philadelphia: W. B. Saunders.

White-Traut, R. C., Nelson, M. N., Burns, K., & Cunningham, N. (1994). Environmental influences on the developing premature infants: Theoretical issues and applications to practice. [Review]. *Journal of Obstetric, Gynecologic and Neonatal Nursing, 23,* 393–401.

Assessment and Management of the Transition to Home and Home Care

PARENTAL TRANSITION

Transition involves change—leaving behind the familiar and trying something new. Taking on a new role requires energy, commitment, and, most of all, a change in the pattern of functioning—thus, a transition. A new role requires an adjustment, a setting of new priorities, and an examination of new expectations. The role of becoming a parent is a good example of the transition process.

Transition as a Crisis

Baird (1986) describes a crisis as a state of upset and disequilibrium. It is also a time when an individual or family has the opportunity to grow, mature, and become better able to handle future life problems (Baird, 1986; Mercer, Nichols, & Doyle, 1989). When the usual coping methods do not return the person to a state of equilibrium, a crisis will evolve.

A crisis situation usually lasts 4 to 6 weeks and is characterized by the following (Baird, 1986):

- The event itself
- The meaning of the event to the family
- The family's resources in dealing with the event

Factors that may precipitate a crisis surrounding an infant's discharge from an NICU are listed below:

- Less thought is given to the support available to or needed by a family during discharge than when the infant is in the NICU (Noga, 1982).
- Parents worry about the infant's chances of survival.
- High parental anxiety interferes with "hearing" and integrating information (Kersten, 1984).
- Parents have been totally dependent on other people to care for their infant, so they are unfamiliar with parenting roles, especially parenting roles associated with premature or sick infants (Simone, 1986).
- Families have often deferred many of their early responses to the preterm or problematic birth because the NICU demanded their attention, and, once home, these feelings and responses reemerge (Simone, 1986).
- Friends and family believe that the crisis is over once the infant is

679

discharged and are less available to the parents for support (Simone, 1986).

- Parents often become overwhelmed by the demands and dependence of their infant (Simone, 1986).
- The infant often continues to have fluctuations in progress and may even regress, thus affecting the parents' ability to cope (Simone, 1986).
- The premature infant's behavior (e.g. sleeping much of the time, not being socially engaging) leaves the parent, especially the mother, feeling like a failure.

Characteristics of crisis intervention are as follows:

- Intervention is most effective when applied as close to the time of the crisis as possible.
- Intervention is aimed at helping the person to deal with the present problem, relying on past history only as it pertains to the present situation.
- Resolution of the crisis is related to the mother's stress level, the social support that is received, and the mother's understanding of the infant's behavior pattern (Zimpelmann, 1990).

Nursing interventions for parents in crisis may include the following:

- Anticipatory planning for future crisis situations (Baird, 1986) through reviewing with the family their coping strategies and preparing parents for what to expect so that they feel prepared to handle the situation
- Recognizing the stressors associated with infant discharge and teaching parents how to recognize anxiety, how to use relaxation techniques, and how these tools could be used (Cobiella, Mabe, & Forehand, 1990)
- Providing parents with transition programs, such as one case management–home care program in Utah called Welcome Home (Scholtes et al., 1994). This program was specifically designed to allow parents of medically fragile infants in the NICU to learn how to take care of their child before discharge.

Parental Concerns

Kenner (1988) and Bagwell and associates (1990) found that parents from level II and III units had similar concerns. Their concerns fell into five categories: (1) informational needs; (2) grief; (3) parent–child development; (4) stress and coping; and (5) social support.

INFORMATIONAL NEEDS

Common information needs of parents are listed below:

- How to provide routine newborn care
- How to recognize normal newborn characteristics, both physical and behavioral
- How to keep the infant healthy after discharge
- Parents' responsibilities about how to provide care
- Understanding equipment used on their infant while in the NICU

- Explanation of the medical diagnosis and the expected prognosis (McKim, 1993)

GRIEF EXPERIENCED BY PARENTS

Examples of grief by parents include the following:

- Parents express the loss of their idealized child.
- Parents worry that their infant might die or be chronically ill.
- Grief is exacerbated by comparing their NICU infant to other well siblings.
- Sense of loss over their expected parenting role is superimposed upon the feeling of loss of their prepregnancy life that is an exaggeration of the loss of previous roles experienced by parents of well infants.

PARENT–CHILD DEVELOPMENT

This category refers to the parental and child role expectations. New parents of healthy infants make adjustments in how they carry out the tasks of daily living once their newborn is at home. Each time a new member is introduced into the family, adjustments are made. When there is a problem with the infant that requires special care, parents may have to set aside their ideal expectations of what their role will be like. The hospitalization may reinforce their role or may hinder it. Women especially have need to have some control over their role and their interactions with health care professionals (Rothman, 1996). Nurses can help them achieve this by anticipating this need.

STRESS AND COPING

For many families, there is no warning that a problem is pending with the infant's birth or that the infant will be sick. Therefore, there is a lack of preparation and a suddenness that come with the reality of a sick neonate. The expected feelings of joy and the months of anticipation are replaced by sharply contrasting feelings of fear, shock, and overwhelming sadness.

Adaptation coping is necessary to reach a stage of conditional acceptance. This form of coping comes about through the identification of the family's stresses from their own perspective. It also requires a determination of the resources that are available to the family. These resources might be parent support groups, parent hotlines, extended family members, friends, financial resources, or home care. Adaptation also requires a change of attitude. Information and acknowledgment of feelings before and after discharge both help to ease the transition process to home and into the role of parent. By acknowledging that other parents have been scared about assuming responsibility for their infant's care and by introducing them to successful parents, the stress is decreased and coping increased.

SOCIAL SUPPORT

Parents expressed the feeling that social support has both positive and negative facets. They meant that they saw the NICU nurses as having a lot of power and the potential to explain their infant's progress. They also believed that nurses had the potential to explain why medical treatment plans changed when there were house staff changes in teaching institutions. Yet, parents did not feel that, for the most part, nurses fulfilled their role as advocate. The NICU nurses did not anticipate that the parents might be confused, and the parents readily admitted that they were too confused or intimidated by the health care professionals to ask questions.

For most parents, the physician was the gatekeeper regarding what they were allowed to know about their infant. Physicians even regulated communication to parents through the nursing staff. Even after discharge, parents believed that the physician's permission was necessary to make even the smallest change in the infant's routine that had been established in the hospital.

The positive side of support was also expressed—the caring attitude by some professionals, the friendly hug, the taking time to talk with the parents, even if it was about something other than their infant's problem. Acknowledgment of the mother's own physical discomfort conveyed a caring and supportive attitude. The availability of a phone number and the potential for a home visit were viewed as positive. Home visits provided encouragement and support of their parenting skills, a time to answer questions, and an objective person to vent their frustrations related to their infant's hospitalization and course of recovery.

Parents also believed that many times family and friends withdrew their support. For others, family and friends were afraid to approach the parents for fear of doing the wrong thing. Other times, parents believed that their family and friends wanted to tell them what they were doing wrong and how they should parent their infant. The positive side of this involvement was when family and friends would tell the parents what a good job they were doing with their infant, how well they were coping, or how their feelings of inadequacy were normal for any parent. Social support differs, however, depending on whether it is professional or personal.

INTERVENTION STRATEGIES PLANNING FOR THE TRANSITION HOME

Nursing strategies to plan for the transition home may include the following:

- Spend more time and effort preparing parents to care for their child at home by themselves. Actively listening to the parents' concerns is a first step toward effective discharge planning (Barnard, Snyder, & Spietz, 1984).
- Coordinate a collaborative, interdisciplinary plan of care, including discharge and follow-up, that includes parents demonstrating competence and comfort with routine newborn care.
- Provide for continuity of care.
- Know that parents need to be able to express their concerns openly.
- Know that parents also need to be informed and reminded that even though their infant is 6 months old by chronological age, he or she may be only 3 months old by conceptual age.
- Provide tips on helping the infant adapt to home, such as leaving

radios and lights on to help the infant adapt to the new environment (Simone, 1986).
- Establish care-by-parent units where parents assume responsibility for their infant's care before discharge while nurses are available.
- Evaluate the need for home care and provide the appropriate planning if extended home care is needed.

INTERVENTION STRATEGIES FOR HOME CARE

Short-Term Care

Characteristics of short-term care include the following:

- Short-term care is usually less than 6 months in duration.
- It includes such procedures as phototherapy, administration of supplemental oxygen, home monitoring for apnea, medication administration, and gavage feedings.
- Treatments are attended to by the parents/primary caregivers in the home after education and training by nurses.
- Nurses provide close supervision and are available.
- The condition is usually self-limiting, and the home therapy can be discontinued at a predetermined endpoint.

Long-Term Care

Characteristics of long-term care include the following:

- Duration of the condition and the need for care will exceed 6 months.
- It includes conditions such as bronchopulmonary dysplasia, short bowel or short gut syndrome, congenital heart disease, physical and cosmetic defects, neurologic and metabolic disorders, and numerous other prolonged pathologic conditions.
- On discharge, health care workers provide direct care and over time gradually integrate families into the health care routine.
- Family responsibility changes as the infant's condition evolves.
- The primary care physician must be closely involved and should be able to rely comfortably on the caregiver's judgment for making assessments and alterations in the home care plan.
- Long-term home care requires open communication between the family, community physicians, tertiary resources, community health care providers, home medical equipment providers, and financial providers.

Hospice Care

Hospice care is a philosophy of caring when cure is no longer a reasonable expectation. This care is not strictly a kind of terminal care but rather an effort to maximize present quality of life without giving up all interest in a cure (Corr & Corr, 1985). Hospice provides comfort measures and focuses on alleviation of symptoms.

Essential to the success of these types of programs, however, is the family's desire and the parents' confidence in their ability to care for the child at home. In addition, they must be assured of regularly scheduled home visits and the availability of program personnel to respond when needed (Lauer & Camitta, 1980). Most facilities require a physician's certification that the child will die within 6 months. The remaining time a child has left is very often difficult to predict. Another serious barrier is the lack of financial reimbursement for care or the inadequacy of the reimbursement to cover the cost of hospice care (Rhymes, 1990).

Respite Care

The daily routine for parents may be time consuming and exhausting. Practical problems arise that were not issues during hospitalization. Family and friends outside of the household cannot appreciate the constant strain that is experienced by the immediate family. Social activities become restricted and ungratifying. Even routine outings such as grocery shopping become cumbersome. The child is often too fragile to take to the store, and appropriate child care is often scarce. The resulting fatigue and frustration can threaten the quality of care provided for the child and other family members.

Parents need to maintain time for themselves. Privacy and recreation for parents are essential if they are to meet the challenge of caring for a sick infant at home successfully. Various community services are making available relief care for overburdened families. Families should be encouraged to seek and take advantage of any available family or community source of respite care.

Day Care

Models of special day care centers are emerging across the country. These facilities offer a protected environment, medical technology, and professional nursing care in a day care setting.

Day care for medically fragile, technology-dependent infants is a concept with great potential for future growth. This new alternative offers a much needed care delivery system to special-needs infants and their families. This avenue of care also presents to nursing a challenge and an opportunity to expand professional knowledge and nursing expertise.

Foster Care

Parents and families of infants with complex medical conditions and complex health care needs may find themselves unable to assume the responsibility of caring for their child. The child's health status requires monitoring, compliance with medical and developmental protocols, and timely interventions. These demands are often beyond the capabilities of birth families.

The number of low birth weight infants and infants with developmental delays born to teenagers, substance-using mothers, and homeless women continues to grow rapidly (Lima & Seliger, 1990). Because of the circumstances surrounding the birth and the dysfunctional dynamics of these families, many infants are assumed to be at high risk for abuse, neglect, and abandonment. For these infants and children, medical foster care is an option.

Long-Term Implications for the Family Unit

The following is a list of the advantages of home care for medically fragile children:

- Parents are free to interact with their infants in their own home in a spontaneous fashion.
- Trips to the hospital are eliminated so the family can reestablish daily routines.
- Parents believe they can assume the parent role as primary caregiver in their home, which facilitates attachment/bonding.
- Home care reduces the long-term complications associated with institutionalization, such as delayed growth and development, abandonment, nosocomial infections, and financial expense.
- Home care provides an alternative to care when insurance coverage is depleted. Parents need to be advised of the maximum lifetime insurance available because prolonged hospitalization in the NICU can consume the entire family's lifetime health insurance coverage.

The following is a list of adverse effects of long-term care of a medically fragile child:

- Breakdown of family communication with disintegration of marriages and altered relationships with friends and family secondary to the incessant demands of caring for the medically fragile child
- Negative sibling reactions, including sibling behaviors of anxiety, jealousy, decreased attention span, enuresis, encopresis, and speech regression. Some siblings express feelings of isolation, rejection, and anger.
- Worsening of preexisting problems. The family's plans and goals may need to be altered. Issues such as family planning often need to be reevaluated. Career plans are frequently interrupted. The financial responsibility for a sick child can be devastating to an already burdened family.
- Increased risk for child abuse, neglect, nonorganic failure to thrive, and developmental and behavioral problems (Brown et al., 1989; Klein, 1990; Tobey & Schraeder, 1990)
- Caregiver stress and burnout or infant neglect
- Compensatory parenting, in which the mother feels guilty for having a neonate in the NICU and attempts to make up for this by providing extra experiences to foster development and shields the infant from other life situations to protect him or her from further hurt (Miles & Holditch-Davis, 1995)
- Fatigue, irritation, and frustration of parents owing to unanticipated demands and limitations of the new child. In spite of comprehensive discharge teaching, many caregivers doubt their ability to maintain the level of care they have observed in the security of the NICU.
- Loss of privacy owing to the presence of a nurse and technical equipment, which is also a constant reminder of additional medical expenses

- Unresolved feelings of chronic sorrow and grieving that incapacitate them. They cannot attach, or they withdraw from attaching to the sick infant. When some parents are confronted with the actual care of their child, they become overwhelmed and resistant to learning the necessary care techniques.
- Financial impact of home care on the family. This must be evaluated before the child is discharged. Although it has been shown that home care can result in significantly lower costs over hospitalized care, the family does not necessarily directly benefit from the cost saving. Families incur incremental costs as a result of undertaking home care of the chronically ill and handicapped infant. Often, the actual costs to the family are hidden or overlooked. Direct and indirect costs can become an enormous burden. Direct costs include such items as physician care, equipment, durable supplies and goods, home renovations, transportation, and home health services. Indirect costs include the time spent transporting and in caregiving activities, time from work, forgone leisure time, and forgone income of the caregiver. The provision of room and board is a usual hidden cost (Jacobs & McDermott, 1989).

Occasionally, families believe that there are no other alternatives to home care. For the technology-dependent child, some options include hospital transitional wards, rehabilitation or chronic care hospitals, pediatric skilled nursing facilities, specialized community group care, or foster care. In reality, some families have no other options.

Parents who take medically fragile children home and assume their care need support. They need support from family, friends, health care professionals, and, most importantly, the community.

CRITERIA FOR HOME CARE

The decision to facilitate early discharge from hospital care to home care must be based on standards that are safe and that provide effective ongoing therapy. Criteria for discharge to home care must be met by the infant, the family, and the follow-up health care system.

Infant Criteria

The infant's home health care needs must be assessed as to technical feasibility and medical requirement. The following is a list of factors that need to be evaluated:

- Nutritional support: feeding technique, frequency, and special formulas
- Pharmacologic support: types of medication, route of administration, desired effects and side effects
- Respiratory support: supplemental oxygen, respiratory therapy treatments, or chest physical therapy

Level of care required must be matched to the ability and skills of the home care providers.

Family Criteria

The assessment of the family's commitment to home care is perhaps the most critical factor determining the success or failure of home health care. After extensive discharge teaching, skills development, and repetitive occasions of caregiving, the parents must want the child at home and under their care. They must be willing and able to devote the time and energy required to meet the physical and emotional needs of the child. These factors are essential to the well-being of the family unit.

Home Equipment Criteria

The most common equipment needed for neonates includes that for cardio-pulmonary monitoring, oxygen provision, suctioning, and feeding. Once the equipment company has been selected, the following factors need to be addressed:

- Instructions for parents on neonatal cardiopulmonary resuscitation (CPR), including written instructions to take home and a checklist for the CPR procedure that can be clearly posted
- Instructions on operation of cardiopulmonary monitoring, including troubleshooting common monitor problems
- Instructions on operating suctioning equipment for patients who have had a tracheostomy. This equipment requires electricity and running water. There must be a portable and battery powered unit for trips to and from the clinic and other excursions out of the home. Both types of units should have a regulator valve to adjust the amount of suction. Parents should be taught both clean and sterile suctioning technique, using clean technique as long as there is no grave danger of cross-contamination with other infectious agents in the home, as may be the case when siblings are ill. Signs that indicate the need for suctioning are the same as used by health care professionals in the NICU and include restlessness, decreased color, coughing, increased respiratory effort, or sounds congested.
- If a portable or stationary oxygen device is needed, it can vary in size and amount of time it will last. They are classified as sizes AA through K, with G, H, and K being large and stationary, whereas the others are portable. It does not require external electricity or battery power sources. These infants will often also need an oxygen concentrator. This concentrator is like the old fashioned mix-box used in the NICU to mix air and oxygen to achieve the desired oxygen concentration. It separates oxygen from nitrogen in room air and collects oxygen (Burstein, 1995). The concentrations that are possible with these home devices are between 45 and 95 percent (Burstein, 1995). They cannot deliver very low flow rates such as 0.5 L/min. They are electrically powered. Portable units are needed outside the home. A backup gas oxygen cylinder is necessary for electrical failures and for outside the home excursions. A list of equipment needed for an infant who has had a tracheostomy is provided in Table 33–1.

Humidification of the airway is necessary for those infants with artificial

TABLE 33–1. Equipment Supply List for a Patient Who Has Had a Tracheostomy

Apnea–bradycardia monitor
Electrodes (2 pairs)
Lead wire (2 pairs)
Belts (2 each)
Tracheostomy tubes (same size) (4 per month)
Tracheostomy tubes (one size smaller) (1 each)
Velcro tracheostomy ties (2 boxes per month)
Twill tape (1 roll)
Free-standing suction machine (1 each)
Portable suction machine
Suction connecting tubing (4 per month)
Suction catheters (4 cases per month)
DeLee traps (6 each)
Portable air compressor—50 psi
Jet nebulizers (4 per month)
Corrugated aerosol tubing (100-ft roll)
Tracheostomy collars (4 per month)
Liquid oxygen with portable reservoir (as needed)
Oxygen connecting tubing (4 each)
Sterile water (2 to 3 cases per month)
Normal saline, 3-ml vials (2 boxes per month)
Heat and moisture exchangers (1 to 2 boxes per month)
Scissors (2 pairs)
Nonsterile gloves (2 boxes per month)
Manual resuscitation bags (2 each)
Sterile cotton-tipped applicators (2 boxes per month)
Hydrogen peroxide (2 bottles per month)
Stethoscope

Adapted with permission from Burstein, L. (1995). Home care. In S. L. Barnhart & M. P. Czervinske (Eds.), *Perinatal and pediatric respiratory care* (pp. 658–679). Philadelphia: W. B. Saunders.

airways to prevent drying and cracking of mucous membranes. It is possible for a tracheostomy stoma to become occluded with dry secretions. Humidification can be provided by volume jet nebulizers with a 50 psi portable air compressor. Humidification levels of 35 to 100 percent can generally be achieved (Burstein, 1995). This compressor should be capable of providing high- or low-pressure aerosol. This capability is important if the infant requires a mist tent at night but during the day is connected to a tracheostomy collar or other airway devices. Some companies will suggest use of a heat and moisture exchanger.

The type of mechanical ventilation needs to be assessed according to the infant's condition and the family's lifestyle. If the parents anticipate movement from home to other areas or other relatives' homes, a portable unit may be best. All portable units must have an internal and external battery. An emergency back-up must be available whether it be housed in the home or at immediate dispatch from the equipment company; it does not matter as long as there is a back-up for those times when there are equipment failures with the portable device. Battery back-up is necessary, too. Usually a 12-volt battery with 74 A/hr potential is suggested. This battery can go 18 to 20 hours without recharge.

These areas of home care monitoring are the most common. Specific instructions on how and what equipment is necessary in each situation should be obtained from a home health care agency who is to provide care, the hospital equipment vendors, and the home health care equipment vendors.

Criteria for home care cannot be complete without accurate assessment of the availability of follow-up after discharge. Environmental conditions and social supports are two of the strongest influences on the ability of the parents to nurture their child in the home (Lang, Behle, & Ballard, 1988). The visiting resource person must be appropriately knowledgeable concerning the physical and emotional needs of the family. To be effective, the home visitor should be sensitive to cultural and ethnic differences and incorporate them into the follow-up plan.

Once the child is in the home, health care becomes a community-oriented case management process, with the primary care pediatrician or nurse practitioner assuming the role of coordinator. The physician implements, evaluates, and subsequently modifies the care plan with the assistance of the family and home care personnel. A home care team usually evolves and consists of the physician, the parents, the community health care providers, the home medical equipment providers, and the sponsors of the funds, if any, to support the home care. The tertiary center then becomes an important resource for support and consultation (Goldberg & Monahan, 1989).

Regularly scheduled home visits by nursing personnel, frequent telephone contacts with the family, and regularly scheduled office visits contribute to the success of the home care program. Parental support can be enhanced by physician–parent and nurse–parent conferences. Consultations with social workers and psychiatric services should be made available periodically for the family members. Referrals to parent support groups and community support services are helpful for the families involved in home care of the sick child.

Complex technology-dependent home care of children continues to be a rapidly expanding field. It has become increasingly important for pediatricians, primary care physicians, and home health nursing personnel to keep abreast of advances in all aspects of post-NICU home care.

REFERENCES

Bagwell, G. A., Kenner, C., Dohme, J., et al. (1990). *Parent transition from a special care nursery to home: A replicative study.* Unpublished master's thesis, University of Cincinnati College of Nursing and Health.

Baird, S. F. (1986). Crisis intervention strategies in nursing assessment and strategies for the family at risk. In S. H. Johnson (Ed.), *High-risk parenting* (2nd ed.). Philadelphia: J. B. Lippincott.

Barnard, K. E., Snyder, C., & Spietz, A. (1984). Supportive measures for high-risk infants and families. In B. S. Raff (Ed.), *Social support and families of vulnerable infants* (pp. 290–329). White Plains, NY: March of Dimes Birth Defects Foundation.

Brown, L. P., Brooten, D., Kumar, S., et al. (1989). A sociodemographic profile of families of low birth weight infants. *Western Journal of Nursing Research, 11*, 520–532.

Burstein, L. (1995). Home Care. In S. L. Barnhart & M. P. Czervinske (Eds.), *Perinatal and pediatric respiratory care* (pp. 658–679). Philadelphia: W. B. Saunders.

Cobiella, C. W., Mabe, P. A., & Forehand, R. L. (1990). A comparison of two stress-reduction treatments for mothers of neonates hospitalized in a neonatal intensive care unit. *Children's Health Care, 19*(2), 93–100.

Corr, C. A., & Corr, D. M. (1985). Pediatric hospice care. *Pediatrics, 76*, 774–780.

Goldberg, A. I. & Monahan, C. A. (1989). Home health care for children assisted by mechanical ventilation: The physician's perspective. *Journal of Pediatrics, 114*, 378–383.

Jacobs, P., & McDermott, S. (1989). Family caregivers' costs of chronically ill and handicapped children: Method and literature review. [Review]. *Public Health Reports, 104*, 158–163.

Kenner, C. A. (1988). *Parent transition from the newborn intensive care unit (NICU) to home.* Unpublished doctoral dissertation, Indiana University, Indianapolis.

Kersten, E. (1984). A premature infant joins the family: The OHN as a health team member. *Occupational Health Nursing, 32*, 530–533.

Klein, M. J. A. (1990). The home health nurse clinician's role in the prevention of nonorganic failure to thrive. *Journal of Pediatric Nursing, 5*, 129–135.

Lang, M. D., Behle, M. B., & Ballard, R. A. (1988). The transition from hospital to home. In R. A. Ballard (Ed.), *Pediatric care of the ICU graduate* (pp. 12–16). Philadelphia: W. B. Saunders.

Lauer, M. E., & Camitta, B. M. (1980). Home care for dying children: A nursing model. *Journal of Pediatrics, 97*, 1032–1035.

Lima, L. & Seliger, J. (1990). Early intervention keeps medically fragile babies at home. *Children Today, 19*(1), 28–32.

McKim, E. (1993). The information and support needs of mothers of premature infants. *Journal of Pediatric Nursing, 8*, 233–244.

Mercer, R. T., Nichols, E. G., & Doyle, G. C. (1989). *Transitions in a woman's life: Major life events in developmental context.* New York: Springer.

Miles, M. S. & Holditch-Davis, D. (1995). Compensatory parenting: How mothers describe parenting their 3-year-old, prematurely born children. *Journal of Pediatric Nursing, 10*, 243–253.

Noga, K. M. (1982). High-risk infants: The need for nursing follow-up. *Journal of Obstetric, Gynecologic, and Neonatal Nursing, 110*, 112–115.

Rhymes, J. (1990). Hospice care in America. *Journal of the American Medical Association, 264*, 369–372.

Rothman, B. K. (1996). Women, providers, and control. *JOGNN, Journal of Obstretric, Gynecologic, and Neonatal Nursing, 25*, 253–256.

Scholtes, P. F., Sherman, J., Griffin, M., et al., (1994). Management of medical fragile infants and children. *Physician Executive, 20*(9), 41–43.

Simone, J. A. (1986). Psychosocial dynamics of high-risk newborn care: The experience of families and the staff's experience. In N. S. Streeter (Ed.), *High-risk neonatal care.* Rockville, MD: Aspen Publishers.

Tobey, G. Y., & Schraeder, B. D. (1990). Impact of caretaker stress on behavioral adjustment of very low birth weight preschool children. *Nursing Research, 39*(2), 84–89.

Zimpelmann, D. G. (1990). *The adaptive process of the preterm infant mother dyad.* Unpublished master's thesis, University of Cincinnati College of Nursing and Health.

Diagnostic Tests and Laboratory Values

TABLE 1. Summary of Common Laboratory Values

Test	Normal Value
Complete Blood Count (CBC)	
Red blood cell count (RBC)	5.1–5.8 (1 million/mm³)
White blood cell count (WBC)	18,000/mm³
Hemoglobin (Hgb)	16.8–18.4 g/dl
Hematocrit (Hct)	52–58% ✘
Platelets	150,000–400,000/mm³
Differential	
Band neutrophils (Bands)	1600/mm³ (9%)
Segmented neutrophils (Segs)	9400/mm³ (52%)
Eosinophils (Eos)	400/mm³ (2.2%)
Basophils (Baso)	100/mm³ (0.6%)
Lymphocytes (Lymphs)	5500/mm³ (31%)
Monocytes (Monos)	1050/mm³ (5.8%)
Serum Electrolytes	
Sodium (Na)	135–145 mEq/L
Potassium (K)	4.5–6.8 mEq/L
Chloride (Cl)	95–110 mEq/L
Carbon dioxide (CO_2)	20–25 mmol/L
Serum Chemistries	
Blood urea nitrogen (BUN)	6.0–30.0 mg/dl
Calcium (Ca)	7–10 mg/dl
Creatinine (Cr)	0.2–0.9 mg/dl
Glucose (G)	40–97 mg/dl
Magnesium (Mg)	1.5–2.5 mg/dl
Phosphorus (P)	5.4–10.9 mg/dl

Data from Fanaroff, A., & Martin, R. (1987). *Neonata–perinatal medicine: Diseases of the fetus and infant* (4th ed.). St. Louis: C.V. Mosby; Cohen, S., Kenner, C., & Hollingsworth, A. (1991). *Maternal, neonatal and women's health nursing.* Springhouse, PA: Springhouse; Kenner, C., Harjo, J., & Brueggemeyer, A. (1988). *Neonatal surgery: A nursing perspective.* Orlando, FL: Grune & Stratton; and Streeter, N.S. (1986). *High risk neonatal care.* Rockville, MD: Aspen Publishers.

TABLE 2. Summary of Normal Urine Laboratory Values

Test	Age	Normal Value
Ammonia	2 to 12 months	4–20 μEq/min/m^2
Calcium	1 week	<2 mg/dl
Chloride	Infant	1.7–8.5 mEq/24 hours
Creatinine	Newborn	7–10 mg/kg/day
Glucose	Preterm	60–130 mg/dl
	Full-term	12–32 mg/dl
Glucose (renal threshold)	Preterm	2.21–2.84 mg/ml
	Full-term	2.20–3.68 mg/ml
Magnesium		180 ± 10 mg/1.73 m^2/dl
Osmolality	Infant	50–600 mOsm/kg
Potassium		26–123 mEq/L
Protein		<100 mg/m^2/dl
Sodium		0.3 to 3.5 mEq/dl (6–10 mEq/m^2)
Specific gravity	Newborn	1.006–1.008

From Ichikawa, I. (1990). *Pediatric textbook of fluids and electrolytes.* Baltimore: Williams & Wilkins. Reprinted with permission.

TABLE 3. Electrocardiographic Data in the Neonate

Parameter	Age			
	0–24 Hours	1–7 Days	8–30 Days	1–3 Months
Heart rate (beats/min)	119 (94–145)*	133 (100–175)	163 (115–190)	154 (124–190)
PR interval (sec)	0.1 (0.07–0.12)	0.09 (0.07–0.12)	0.09 (0.07–0.11)	0.1 (0.07–0.13)
P wave amplitude II	1.5 (0.8–2.3)	1.6 (0.8–2.5)	1.6 (0.8–2.4)	1.6 (0.8–2.4)
QRS duration (sec)	0.065 (0.05–0.08)	0.06 (0.04–0.08)	0.06 (0.04–0.07)	0.06 (0.05–0.08)
QRS axis (degrees)	135 (60–180)	125 (80–160)	110 (60–160)	80 (40–120)
R amplitude V_{1R} (mm)	8.6 (4–14.2)	—	6.3 (3.3–8.5)	5.1 (1.1–10.1)
R amplitude V_1 (mm)	11.9 (4.3–21)	—	11.1 (3.3–18.7)	11.2 (4.5–18)
R amplitude V_5 (mm)	10.2 (4–18)	10.7 (3.4–19)	11.9 (3.5–27)	13.6 (7.3–20.7)
R amplitude V_6 (mm)	3.3 (2.3–7)	5.1 (2.2–13.1)	6.7 (1.7–20.5)	8.4 (3.6–12.9)
S amplitude V_{4R} (mm)	3.8 (0.2–13)	—	1.8 (0.8–4.6)	3.4 (0–9.3)
S amplitude V_1 (mm)	9.7 (1.1–19.1)	—	6.1 (0–15)	7.5 (0.5–17.1)
S amplitude V_5 (mm)	11.9 (0.24)	6.8 (3.6–16.2)	4.8 (2.7–12.3)	4.7 (2–12.7)
S amplitude V_6 (mm)	4.5 (1.6–10.3)	3.3 (0.8–9.9)	2.0 (0.6–9)	2.4 (0.8–5.8)

*Mean (5th to 95th percentile).

From Fanaroff, A., & Martin, R. (1987). *Neonatal-perinatal medicine: Diseases of the fetus and infant* (4th ed., p 1256). St. Louis: C. V. Mosby. As modified from Liebman, J., & Plonsey, R. (1977). Electrocardiography. In A. J. Moss, F. H. Adams, & G. C. Emmanovillides (Eds.), *Heart disease in infants, children and adolescents* (2nd ed.). Baltimore: Williams & Wilkins. Reprinted with permission.

TABLE 4. Time of First Void in 500 Infants

Hours in Delivery Room	395 Full-Term Infants		80 Preterm Infants		25 Postterm Infants	
	No. of Infants	Cumulative (%)	No. of Infants	Cumulative (%)	No. of Infants	Cumulative (%)
<1	51	12.9	17	21.2	3	12
1–8	151	51.1	50	83.7	4	38
9–16	158	91.1	12	98.7	14	84
17–24	35	100	1	100	4	100
>24	0	—	0	—	0	—

From Clark, D. A. (1977). Times of first void and first stool in 500 newborns. *Pediatrics, 60,* 457–459. Reproduced by permission of *Pediatrics.*

TABLE 5. Time of First Stool in 500 Infants

Hours in Delivery Room	395 Full-Term Infants		80 Preterm Infants		25 Postterm Infants	
	No. of Infants	Cumulative (%)	No. of Infants	Cumulative (%)	No. of Infants	Cumulative (%)
<1	66	16.7	4	5	8	32
1–8	169	59.5	22	32.5	9	68
9–16	125	91.1	25	63.8	5	88
17–24	29	98.5	10	76.3	3	100
24–48	6°	100	18†	98.8	0	—
>48	0	—	1‡	100	0	—

°At 25, 26, 27, 28, 33, and 37 hours.

†Five stooled more than 36 hours after birth at 38, 39, 40, 42, and 47 hours.

‡At 59 hours.

From Clark, D. A. (1977). Times of first void and first stool in 500 newborns. *Pediatrics, 60,* 457–459. Reproduced by permission of *Pediatrics.*

TABLE 6. Acid-Base Status

Determination	Sample Source	Birth	1 Hour	3 Hours	24 Hours	2 Days	3 Days
Vigorous Term Infants, Vaginal Delivery							
pH	Umbilical artery	7.26					
	Umbilical vein	7.29					
P_{CO_2} (mm Hg)	Arterial	54.5	38.8	38.3	33.6	34	35
	Venous	42.8					
O_2 saturation	Arterial	19.8	93.8	94.7	93		
	Venous	47.6					
pH	Left atrial		7.30	7.34	7.41	7.39	7.38
						Temporal artery	Temporal artery
CO_2 content (mEq/L)	—	—	20.6	21.9	21.4		
Premature Infants	Capillary (skin puncture)						
pH	<1250 g				7.36	7.35	7.35
P_{CO_2} (mm Hg)					38	44	27
pH	>1250 g				7.39	7.39	7.38
P_{CO_2} (mm Hg)					38	39	38

From Schaffer, A. J. (1971). *Diseases of the newborn* (3rd ed.). Philadelphia: W. B. Saunders. Reprinted with permission.

TABLE 7. Selected Chemistry Values in Full-Term and Preterm Infants

Constituent	Preterm	Term	Reference
Ammonia (μg/dl)	—	90–150	1
Base, excess (mmol/L)	—	−10 to −2	2
Bicarbonate, standard (mmol/L)	18–26	20–26	2
Bilirubin, total (mg/dl)			
Cord	<2.8	<2.8	
24 hours	1–6	2–6	
48 hours	6–8	6–7	
3–5 days	10–12	4–6	
≥1 month	<1.5	<1.5	
Bilirubin, direct	<0.5	<0.5	2
Calcium, total (mg/dl), week 1	6.0–10.0	7.0–12.0	3
Calcium, ionized (mg/dl), 72 hours	2.5–5.0	2.5–5.0	4
Ceruloplasmin (mg/dl)	—	20–40	
Creatinine phosphokinase			
Day 1	—	44–1150	5
(arb U) Day 4	—	14–97	
Creatinine (mg/dl)			
Birth	Mother's level	Mother's level	1, 6
10 days	1.3 ±0.07 (mean ± SD)	0.8–1.4	
1 month	0.6 ±0.05 (mean ± SD)	—	
Gamma-glutamyl transferase (U/L)		14–331	7
Glucose (mg/dl)			
<72 hours	20–125	30–125	8
>72 hours	40–125	40–125	
Lactate dehydrogenase (U/L)	—	357–953	7
Magnesium (mg/dl)	—	1.5–2.8	9
Osmolality (mOsm/L)	—	280–295	2

Table continued on following page

TABLE 7. Selected Chemistry Values in Full-Term and Preterm Infants *Continued*

Constituent	Preterm	Term	Reference
Phosphatase, acid (U/L)	—	7.4–19.4	2
Phosphatase, alkaline (U/L) (mean ± SD)			
26–27 weeks	320 ± 87	164 ± 68	10
28–29	292 ± 87	—	
30–31	281 ± 85	—	
32–33	254 ± 72	—	
34–35	236 ± 62	—	
36	207 ± 60	—	
Phosphorus (mg/dl)			
Birth	5.6–8.0	5.0–7.8	11
Week 1	6.1–11.7	4.9–8.9	
Month 1	6.6–9.4	5.9–9.5	
Aspartate aminotransferase	—	24–81	7
Alanine aminotransferase	—	10–33	7
Urea nitrogen (mg/dl)	—	5–25	2
Uric acid (mg/dl)	—	3.0–7.5	2

....

[1]Meites, S. (1977). *Pediatric clinical chemistry: A survey of normals.* Washington, DC: American Association of Clinical Chemistry.

[2]Wallach, J. B. (1983). *Interpretation of pediatric tests.* Boston: Little, Brown.

[3]Meites, S. (1975). *Critical Reviews in Clinical Laboratory Sciences, 6,* 1.

[4]Brown, D. M., Boen, J., & Bernstein, A. (1972). *Pediatrics, 49,* 841.

[5]Drummond, L. M. (1979). *Archives of Disease in Childhood, 54,* 362.

[6]Stonestreet, B. S., & Oh, W. (1978). *Pediatrics, 61,* 788.

[7]Statlan, B. E., & Freer, D. E. (1978). *Clinical Chemistry, 24,* 1010 [Abstract].

[8]Cornblath, M., & Schwartz, E. (Eds.). (1976). *Disorders of carbohydrate metabolism* (2nd ed.). Philadelphia: W. B. Saunders.

[9]Tsang, R. C. (1972). *American Journal of Diseases of Children, 124,* 282.

[10]Glass, L., et al. (1982). *Archives of Disease in Childhood, 57,* 373.

[11]O'Brien, D. (1974). Interpretation of biochemical values. In C. H. Kempe & H. K. Silver (Eds.), *Current pediatric diagnosis and treatment* (3rd ed.). Los Altos, CA.: Lange Medical Publications.

From Fanaroff, A., & Martin, R. (1987). *Neonatal-perinatal medicine: Diseases of the fetus and infant* (4th ed., p. 1262). St. Louis: C. V. Mosby. Reprinted with permission.

TABLE 8. Serum Total Protein and Electrophoresis Fractions

Fraction	Cord Blood	Age Birth	1 Week	1–3 Months
Total protein	4.78–8.04	4.6–7.0	4.4–7.6	3.64–7.38
Albumin	2.17–4.04	3.2–4.3	2.9–5.5	2.05–4.46
Alpha-1	0.25–0.66	0.1–0.3	0.09–0.25	0.08–0.34
Alpha-2	0.44–0.94	0.2–0.3	0.30–0.46	0.40–1.13
Beta	0.42–1.56	0.3–0.6	0.16–0.60	0.39–1.14
Gamma	0.81–1.61	0.6–1.2	0.35–1.3	0.25–1.05

From Fanaroff, A., & Martin, R. (1987). *Neonatal–perinatal medicine: Diseases of the fetus and infant* (4th ed., p. 1263). St. Louis: C. V. Mosby. Reprinted with permission.

TABLE 9. Heptoglobin Levels in Preterm Infants

Gestation (weeks)	Days After Birth 0	5	10	15	21	28
<32	10 (3)°	—	—	—	—	—
32–34	—	18.5 (2)	51.6 (3)	42.6 (3)	12 (1)	12 (1)
34–36	9.8 (9)	14.9 (11)	11.4 (10)	11.6 (9)	7.1 (7)	16.5 (4)
36–38	13.0 (7)	18.3 (3)	16.6 (5)	16.3 (2)	11 (1)	.7.5 (1)
38+	9.3 (8)	28.3 (6)	20.9 (4)	10.1 (5)	9.2 (3)	7.0 (1)
	10.5 (27)	19.6 (22)	19.5 (22)	16.1 (19)	8.3 (12)	13.2 (7)

° Heptoglobin levels are measured as mg/dl methB binding capacity. Numbers in parentheses indicate number of samples from which mean values were derived.

From Philip, A. G. (1971). Heptoglobins in the newborn: II. Low birth weight babies. *Biology of the Neonate, 19,* 322–328. Reprinted with permission.

TABLE 10. Heptoglobin Levels in Full-Term Infants

	Birth	5 Days
Heptoglobin (mg/dl Hgb binding capacity)	23.9 (10.6–50)	52.3 (14.8–100)

From Fanaroff, A., & Martin, R. (1987). *Neonatal–perinatal medicine: Diseases of the fetus and infant* (4th ed., p. 1263). St. Louis: C. V. Mosby. Reprinted with permission.

TABLE 11. Plasma Immunoglobulin Concentrations in Premature Infants (25–28 Weeks' Gestation)

Age (months)	n	IgG* (mg/dl)	IgM* (mg/dl)	IgA* (mg/dl)
0.25	18	251 (114–552)†	7.6 (1.3–43.3)	1.2 (0.07–20.8)
0.5	14	202 (91–446)	14.1 (3.5–56.1)	3.1 (0.09–10.7)
1	10	158 (57–437)	12.7 (3.0–53.3)	4.5 (0.65–30.9)
1.5	14	134 (59–307)	16.2 (4.4–59.2)	4.3 (0.9–20.9)
2	12	89 (58–136)	16 (5.3–48.9)	4.1 (1.5–11.1)
3	13	60 (23–156)	13.8 (5.3–36.1)	3 (0.6–15.6)
4	10	82 (32–210)	22.2 (11.2–43.9)	6.8 (1–47.8)
6	11	159 (56–455)	41.3 (8.3–205)	9.7 (3–31.2)
8–10	6	273 (94–794)	41.8 (31.1–56.1)	9.5 (0.9–98.6)

°Geometric mean.

†The normal ranges in parentheses were determined by taking the antilog of (mean logarithm ± 2 SD of the logarithms).

From Ballow, M., Cates, K. L., Rowe, J. C., Goetz, C., & Desbonnet, C. (1986). Development of the immune system in very low birth weight (less than 1500 g) premature infants: Concentrations of plasma immunoglobulins and patterns of infections. *Pediatric Research, 20,* 899–904. Reprinted with permission.

TABLE 12. Plasma Immunoglobulin Concentrations in Premature Infants (29–32 Weeks' Gestation)

Age (Months)	n	IgG* (mg.dl)	IgM* (mg/dl)	IgA* (mg/dl)
0.25	42	368 (186–728)†	9.1 (2.1–39.4)	0.6 (0.04–1)
0.5	35	275 (119–637)	13.9 (4.7–41)	0.9 (0.01–7.5)
1	26	209 (94–452)	14.4 (6.3–33)	1.9 (0.3–12)
1.5	22	156 (69–352)	15.4 (5.5–43.2)	2.2 (0.7–6.5)
2	11	123 (64–237)	15.2 (4.9–46.7)	3 (1.1–8.3)
3	14	104 (41–268)	16.3 (7.1–37.2)	3.6 (0.8–15.4)
4	21	128 (39–425)	26.5 (7.7–91.2)	9.8 (2.5–39.3)
6	21	179 (51–634)	29.3 (10.5–81.5)	12.3 (2.7–57.1)
8–10	16	280 (140–561)	34.7 (17–70.8)	20.9 (8.3–53)

°Geometric mean.

†The normal ranges in parentheses were determined by taking the antilog of (mean logarithm ± 2 SD of the logarithms).

From Ballow, M., Cates, K. L., Rowe, J. C., Goetz, C., & Desbonnet, C. (1986). Development of the immune system in very low birth weight (less than 1500 g) premature infants: Concentrations of plasma immunoglobulins and patterns of infections. *Pediatric Research, 20,* 899–904. Reprinted with permission.

TABLE 13. Plasma Amino Acids in Preterm and Full-Term Infants

Amino Acid	Premature, First Day	Newborn, Before First Feeding	16 Days– 4 Months
Taurine	105–255	101–181	
OH-proline	0–80	0	
Aspartic acid	0–20	4–12	17–21
Threonine	155–272	196–238	141–213
Serine	195–345	129–197	104–158
Asp + Glut	655–1155	623–895	
Proline	155–305	155–305	41–245
Glutamic acid	30–100	27–77	
Glycine	185–735	274–412	178–248
Alanine	325–425	274–384	239–345
Valine	80–180	97–175	123–199
Cystine	55–75	49–75	33–51
Methionine	30–40	21–37	15–21
Isoleucine	20–60	31–47	31–47
Leucine	45–95	55–89	56–98
Tyrosine	20–220	53–85	33–75
Phenylalanine	70–110	64–92	45–65
Ornithine	70–110	66–116	37–61
Lysine	130–250	154–246	117–163
Histidine	30–70	61–93	64–92
Arginine	30–70	37–71	53–71
Tryptophan	15–45	15–45	
Citrulline	8.5–23.7	10.8–21.1	
Ethanolamine	13.4–105	23.7–72	
γ-Amino-n-butyric acid	0–29	8.7–20.4	

From Fanaroff, A., & Martin, R. (1987). *Neonatal-perinatal medicine: Diseases of the fetus and infant* (4th ed., p. 1264). St. Louis: C. V. Mosby. Reprinted with permission.

TABLE 14. Urine Amino Acids in Normal Newborns

Amino Acid	μmol/day
Cysteic acid	Tr–3.32
Phosphoethanolamine	Tr–8.86
Taurine	7.59–7.72
OH-proline	0.0–9.81
Aspartic acid	Tr
Threonine	0.176–7.99
Serine	Tr–20.7
Glutamic acid	0–1.78
Proline	0–5.17
Glycine	0.176–65.3
Alanine	Tr–8.03
α-Amino-*n*-butyric acid	0–0.47
Valine	0–7.76
Cystine	0–7.96
Methionine	Tr–0.892
Isoleucine	0–6.11
Tyrosine	0–1.11
Phenylalanine	0–1.66
β-Aminoisobutyric acid	0.264–7.34
Ethanolamine	Tr–79.9
Ornithine	Tr–0.554
Lysine	0.33–9.79
1-Methylhistidine	Tr–8.64
3-Methylhistidine	0.11–3.32
Carnosine	0.044–4.01
Arginine	0.088–0.918
Histidine	Tr–7.04
Leucine	Tr–0.819

Tr, trace.

From Fanaroff, A., & Martin, R. (1987). *Neonatal-perinatal medicine: Diseases of the fetus and infant* (4th ed., p. 1264). St. Louis: C. V. Mosby. Modified from Meites, S. (ed.) (1977). *Pediatric clinical chemistry: A survey of normals, methods and instruments.* Washington, DC: American Association for Clinical Chemistry. Reprinted with permission.

TABLE 15. Cerebrospinal Fluid Values in Healthy Term Newborns

	Age			
	0–24 Hours	*1 Day*	*7 Days*	*>7 Days*
Color	Clear or xanthochromic	Clear or xanthochromic	Clear or xanthochromic	
Red blood cells/mm³	9 (0–1070)°	23 (6–630)	3 (0–48)	
Polymorphonuclear leukocytes/mm³	3 (0–70)	7 (0–26)	2 (0–5)	
Lymphocytes/mm³	2 (0–20)	5 (0–16)	1 (0–4)	
Proteins (mg/dl)	63 (32–240)	73 (40–148)	47 (27–65)	
Glucose (mg/dl)	51 (32–78)	48 (38–64)	55 (48–62)	
Lactate dehydrogenase (IU/L)	22–73	22–73	22–73	0–40

....

°Values are given as mean, with range in parentheses.
    From Fanaroff, A., & Martin, R. (1987). *Neonatal–perinatal medicine: Diseases of the fetus and infant* (4th ed., p. 1265). St. Louis: C. V. Mosby. Reprinted with permission.

TABLE 16. Cerebrospinal Fluid Cytology in 46 Low Birth Weight and Term Neonates

Category	Weight (g)	RBCs/mm³	WBCs/ mm³	Polymorpho- nuclear Leukocytes (%)	Lympho- cytes (%)	Macro- phages (%)
Low birth weight (n = 22)	1437 (652–2438)°	50 (0–431)	7 (0–28)	16 (0–100)	28 (0–100)	56 (0–100)
Normal birth weight (n = 24)	3240 (2665–3997)	131 (0–478)	11 (1–38)	21 (0–100)	20 (0–100)	59 (0–100)

....

°Values are given as mean, with range in parentheses.
    From Pappu, L. D., Purhoit, D. M., Levkoff, A. H., & Kaplan, B. (1982). CSF cytology in the neonate. *American Journal of Diseases of Children, 136,* 297–298. Copyright 1982, American Medical Association. Reprinted with permission.

TABLE 17. Colloid Osmotic Pressure (torr) in Infant's Blood

Term, vaginal delivery	19.5 ± 2.1 (SD)
Term, cesarean section	16.1 ± 2.0
Term, vaginal (sick) (sepsis, asphyxia, heart failure, abdominal surgery)	19.5 ± 3.1
Preterm (700–1980 g) (hyaline membrane disease, asphyxia, necrotizing enterocolitis, etc.)	12.5 ± 2.5

....

From Taeusch, H. W., Ballard, R. A., & Avery, M. E. (Eds.) (1991). *Schaffer and Avery's diseases of the newborn* (6th ed., p. 1078). Philadelphia: W. B. Saunders. Reprinted with permission.

TABLE 18. Thyroid Function in Full-Term and Preterm Infants

| | Serum T₄ Concentration in Premature and Term Infants | | | | | | Serum Free T₄ Index in Premature and Term Infants | | | | |
| | Estimated Gestational Age (wk) | | | | | | Estimated Gestational Age (wk) | | | | |
	30–31	32–33	34–35	36–37	Term		30–31	32–33	34–35	36–37	Term
Cord											
Mean	6.5°	7.5	6.7†	7.5	8.2				5.6	5.6	5.9
SD	1.0	2.1	1.2	2.8	1.8				1.3	2.0	1.1
n	3	8	18	17	37				12	10	14
12–72 hr											
Mean	11.5†	12.3‡	12.4‡	15.5†	19.0		13.1°°	12.9°°	15.5†‡	17.1	19.7
SD	2.1	3.2	3.1	2.6	2.1		2.4	2.7	3.0	3.5	3.5
n	12	18	17	15	6		12	14	14	14	6
3–10 days											
Mean	7.7†	8.5‡	10.0‡	12.7†	15.9		8.3°°	9.0°°	12.0†‡	15.1	16.2
SD	1.8	1.9	2.4	2.5	3.0		1.9	1.8	2.3	0.7	3.2
n	7	8	9	9	29		6	9	5	4	11

11–20 days										
Mean	7.5†	8.3†	10.5	11.2	12.2	8.0§	9.1††	11.8	11.3	12.1
SD	1.8	1.6	1.8	2.9	2.0	1.6	1.9	2.7	1.9	2.0
n	5	11	9	9	8	5	8	8	5	8
21–45 days										
Mean	7.8†	8.0†	9.3†	11.4	12.1	8.4§	9.0††	10.9		11.1
SD	1.5	1.7	1.3	4.2	1.5	1.4	1.6	2.8		1.4
n	11	17	13	5	5	11	17	5		5
			30 to 73 weeks							9.7
48–90 days										1.5
Mean		9.6			10.2	9.4		30 to 35 weeks		10
SD		1.7			1.9	1.4				
n		16			17	13				

° p<.05
† p<.005
‡ p<.001
°° p .001
††p .025
‡‡p .01
§ p .005

For comparison of premature vs. term infants (*t* test).
From Cuestas, R. A. (1982). *Journal of Pediatrics*, 92, 963. Reprinted with permission.

Head Circumference
Measurements

736 need to Report

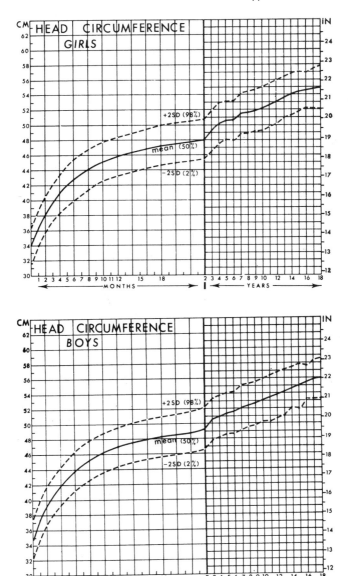

Head circumference records for girls *(top)* and boys *(bottom)*. (From Nelhaus, G. [1968]. Head circumference from birth to eighteen years. Practical composite international and interracial graphs. *Pediatrics, 41,* 106. Copyright American Academy of Pediatrics 1968. Reprinted with permission.)

Index

Note: Page numbers in *italics* refer to illustrations; page numbers followed by t refer to tables.

709

H

R